PROSTAGLANDINS AND RELATED LIPIDS

Peter Ramwell, *Series Editor*

Volume 1: **Prostaglandin Synthetase Inhibitors: New Clinical Applications,** Peter Ramwell, *Editor*

Volume 2: **Prostaglandins and Cancer: First International Conference,** Trevor J. Powles, Richard S. Bockman, Kenneth V. Honn, and Peter Ramwell, *Editors*

Prostaglandins and Cancer: First International Conference

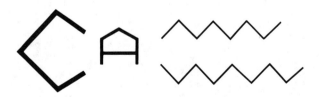

Prostaglandins and Cancer: First International Conference

Proceedings of the First International
Conference on Prostaglandins and Cancer
Washington, D.C., August 30 – September 2, 1981

Editors

Trevor J. Powles
Royal Marsden Hospital
Sutton, Surrey, England

Richard S. Bockman
Memorial Sloan-Kettering Cancer Center
New York, New York

Kenneth V. Honn
Wayne State University
Detroit, Michigan

Peter Ramwell
Georgetown University Medical Center
Washington, D.C.

RC 268.5
I 56
1981

Alan R. Liss, Inc., New York

Library of Congress Cataloging in Publication Data

International Conference on Prostaglandins and
    Cancer (1st: 1981: Washington, D.C.)
    Prostaglandins and cancer.

    (Prostaglandins and related lipids; v. 2)
    Includes index.
    1. Carcinogenesis—Congresses. 2. Prostaglandins
—Physiological effect—Congresses. 3. Cocarcinogenesis—Congresses. I. Powles, Trevor J. II. Title. III. Series. [DNLM: 1. Prostaglandins—Congresses. 2. Medical oncology—Congresses.
3. Neoplasms—Etiology—Congresses. W1 PR771 v. 2/
QZ 202 I568 1981p]
RC268.5.I56 1981   616.99'4071   82-86
ISBN 0-8451-2101-4   AACR2

Contents

Contributors   xv

Preface
Trevor J. Powles   xxxi

GENERAL PRINCIPLES OF PROSTAGLANDIN SYNTHESIS

Prostaglandins, Thromboxanes and Leukotrienes: Biochemical Pathways
Bengt Samuelsson   1

Inhibitors of Arachidonic Acid Metabolism, With Especial Reference to the
Aspirin-Like Drugs
J.R. Vane, R.J. Flower, and J.A. Salmon   21

The Molecular Basis of the Pharmacology of the Arachidonate Metabolites
P.W. Ramwell, J.W. Karanian, and M.L. Foegh   47

Prostaglandin Analogues
J.E. Pike and G. L. Bundy   67

CARCINOGENESIS–INITIATION

The Initiation Stage of Chemical Carcinogenesis: An Introductory Overview
James A. Miller and Elizabeth C. Miller   81

Prostaglandin Synthetase–Dependent Cooxygenation
Lawrence J. Marnett, Michael J. Bienkowski, Marie Leithauser, William
R.Pagels, Augustine Panthananickal, and Gregory A. Reed   97

Oxidation of Chemical Carcinogens by Prostaglandin Synthetase
Thomas Eling, Jeff Boyd, and K. Sivarajah   113

Role of Prostaglandin Endoperoxide Synthetase in Benzidine and 5-Nitro-
furan-Induced Kidney and Bladder Carcinogenesis
T.V. Zenser, S.M. Cohen, M.B. Mattammal, G. Murasaki, and
B.B. Davis   123

Brief Reports

Metabolic Activation of Diethylstilbestrol by Prostaglandin Synthetase as
a Mechanism for its Carcinogenicity
Sharon Bennett, Wayne Marshall, and Peter J. O'Brien   143

The Effects of Vitamin E and/or Selenium Deficiency on Enzymes Involved in the Biosynthesis and Degradation of Prostanoids in Rat Tissues
C.C. Reddy, T.L. Grasso, R.W. Scholz, T. J. Labosh, C. E. Thomas,
and E. J. Massaro   149

Prostaglandin Synthetase Mediated Activation of p-Dimethyl-
Aminoazobenzene (Butter Yellow)
S. Vasdev, Y. Tsuruta, and P.J. O'Brien   155

Prostaglandin Synthetase Catalyzed DNA Strand Breaks by Aromatic
Amines
A. Rahimtula, P. Moldeus, B. Andersson, and M. Nordenskjöld 159

The Involvement of Prostaglandin Intermediates in Covalent Binding to
Nucleic Acids and in Ageing Pigment Formation
Sudesh Vasdev and Peter J. O'Brien 163

Evidence for Lipoxygenase-Peroxidase Activation of N-Hydroxy-2-
Acetylaminofluorene by Rat Mammary Gland Parenchymal Cells
Peter K. Wong, M.J. Hampton, and Robert A. Floyd 167

CARCINOGENESIS–PROMOTION

Overview of Tumor Promotion
R.K. Boutwell 183

Stimulation of Cellular Prostaglandin Production by Phorbolesters and
Growth Factors and Inhibition by Cancer Chemopreventive Agents
Lawrence Levine 189

Prostaglandin Response in Mouse Skin to Tumor Promoters
Edward Bresnick 205

Receptor Binding and Cellular Effects of Tumor Promoters
Ann D. Horowitz and I. Bernard Weinstein 217

On the Role of Prostaglandins in the Induction of Epidermal Proliferation,
Hyperplasia and Tumor Promotion in Mouse Skin
G. Fürstenberger, M. Gross, and F. Marks 239

Modulation of Prostaglandin Synthesis and Tumor Promotion
Susan M. Fischer and Thomas J. Slaga 255

Brief Reports

The Source of Arachidonate for Prostaglandin Synthesis by MDCK Cells
M. Waite, L. Daniel, and G. Beaudry 265

Modulation by Indomethacin, Prostaglandins and Retinylacetate of Rat
Liver Ornithine Decarboxylase Activity Induced by Tumor Promotors in
Vivo
Arnold Bisschop and Lucio A.A. van Rooijen 273

Arachidonic Acid Metabolism and Induction of Plasminogen Activator in
HeLa Cells by Tumor-Promoting Phorbol Ester
David J. Crutchley and James R. Maynard 281

CELL REPLICATION/PROLIFERATION

Platelet Derived Growth Factor Action: A Molelcular Analysis of
BALB/c-3T3 and Transformed BALB/c-3T3 Cells
Charles D. Scher, Ronald L. Dick, Kathryn L. Locatell,
and Charles D. Stiles 291

Endogenous Prostaglandin Production and Cell Replication in Vitro
Sven Hammarström 297

The Regulation of DNA Replication in Animal Cells by Prostaglandin $F_{2\alpha}$
Luis Jimenez de Asua, Angela M. Otto, Marie-Odile Ulrich, Jorge
Martin-Perez, and George Thomas 309

Host Defense: Trilateral Relationships Among Virus Infection, Interferon
Induction and Cellular Prostaglandin Biosynthesis
F.A. Fitzpatrick and D.A. Stringfellow 333

The Possible Roles of Prostaglandin Synthetase and Cytoplasmic Superoxide
Dismutase in Interferon Action in Homologous Cells
K.A. Chandrabose, Raveendran Pottathil, Ernest C. Borden, Rebecca
Fox, and Pedro Cuatrecasas 345

Brief Reports

Structural Activity Requirement for PGA Effects on Tumor Cell Growth
and Differentiation
W.A. Turner, D.R. Bennett, K.C. Thompson, J.D. Taylor, and
K.V. Honn 365

Effects of Prostaglandin "A" Series on Tumor Cells in Vitro
W.A. Turner, J.D. Taylor, and K.V. Honn 369

Thromboxanes and Prostacyclin: Positive and Negative Modulators of
Tumor Cell Proliferation
Kenneth V. Honn, John R. Dunn, and Jay Meyer 375

The Effect of Gamma Radiation on Prostacyclin Production in Cultured
Pulmonary Artery Endothelium
G.L. Hahn, M. Menconi, and P. Polgar 381

Inhibition of Growth of Hamster Pancreatic Ductal Adenocarcinoma
Cells in Vitro by PGE_2 and 16,16-Dimethyl PGE_2 – A Preliminary
Report
David T. Mayschak, Elena Glass, Scott Kacy, William Boerwinkle, Sam
Barranco, M. Wayne Flye, and Courtney M. Townsend, Jr........... 385

Changes in Microtubule-Organization Affect Different Events Regulating
the Initiation of DNA Synthesis Stimulated by Prostaglandin $F_{2\alpha}$ in 3T3
Cells
Angela M. Otto 391

CELL DIFFERENTIATION/MATURATION

Antigenic and Humoral Control of Normal and Leukemic Human
Myelopoiesis
Louis M. Pelus 399

Prostaglandins, T-Lymphocyte Precursors and Cancer
R.S. Bockman 415

Role of Prostaglandins on the Growth and Differentiation of Friend
Erythroleukemia Cells
M.G. Santoro and B.M. Jaffe 425

Role of Prostaglandins in Differentiation of Neuroblastoma Cells in Culture
Kedar N. Prasad 437

Normal and Metaplastic Squamous Differentiation in Diverse Organs
in Vitro
Sam Sorof, Frederick V. Schaefer, and R. Philip Custer 453

Prostaglandins Induce Differentiation and Reduce the Neoplastic Potential
of a Rat Mammary Tumour Stem Cell Line
P.S. Rudland and M.J. Warburton 465

Brief Reports

Evidence for Involvement of the Lipoxygenase Pathway in CSF-Induced
Human and Murine Myeloid Colony Formation
Alan M. Miller, Vincent A. Ziboh, and Adel A. Yunis.................. 481

Relationship of Differentiation and Prostaglandin Production in Human
Promyelocytic Leukemia
David T. Dudley, Ann Louise Olson, and C. Patrick Burns 487

Induction of Glucagon Receptors and Responsiveness in Transformed
Kidney Cells by Prostaglandins
Michael C. Lin, Sue-May Wang, and Suzanne K. Beckner 493

PROSTAGLANDINS, BONE METASTASES, AND HYPERCALCEMIA

Involvement of Prostaglandin Synthesis in Mechanisms of Malignant
Hypercalcemia
Gregory R. Mundy 501

Prostaglandins, Tumor Cells and Bone Metabolism
Armen H. Tashjian, Jr., Edward F. Voelkel, and Lawrence Levine 513

Prostaglandins and Cellular Bone Resorption
T.J. Martin and N.C. Partridge 525

Mechanisms for Development of Bone Metastases and Effects of Anti-
Inflammatory Drugs
T.J. Powles, J. Muindi, and R.C. Coombes 541

Brief Reports

Lymphokine Mediated Bone Resorption Requires Prostaglandin
Synthesis
R.S. Bockman... 555

Morphological Patterns of Bone Destruction by Infiltrating Tumours
R.L. Carter 561

In Vitro Prostaglandin Production by Metastatic Breast Cancer
G.N. Hortobagyi, P. Schultz, R. Cailleau, N. Samaan, and
G. Blumenschein.. 567

Bone Resorptive Activity in Conditioned Medium From Rat Osteosarcoma Cell Line
S.B. Rodan, G.A. Rodan, H.A. Simmons, R.W. Walenga, M.B. Feinstein, and L.G. Raisz 573

HOST TUMOR INTERACTION

Prostaglandins in Relation to Tumour-Host Interactions
Peter Alexander 581

Arachidonate Metabolites and Immunity
Charles W. Parker... 595

The Role of Arachidonic Acid Products in Macrophage Function
W. Dawson 609

Does Prostaglandin Synthesis Effect in Vivo Tumour Growth by Altering Tumour/Host Balance?
Otto J. Plescia 619

Interrelationship of Endogenous Macrophages, Prostaglandin Synthesis and Tumor Cell Clonogenicity in Human Tumor Biopsies
Sydney E. Salmon.. 633

Brief Reports

Differential Effects of Indomethacin and PGE_2 on the Depressed Responses of Cancer Patients
A.B. Tilden, P.A. Dougherty, and C.M. Balch....................... 651

Modulation of Prostaglandins in Hormone Dependent Mammary Carcinoma
M.K. Foecking, R.V. Panganamala, H. Abou-Issa, and J. P. Minton 657

Interferon-Induced Resistance of Human Natural Killer Cells to PGE_2-Mediated Suppression
Kam H. Leung and Hillel S. Koren 663

Leukotrienes Released by Human Monocytes Mediate Tumor Antigen Induced Leukocyte Adherence Inhibition (LAI)
D.M.P. Thomson, Kerry Phelan, and M.K. Bach 667

Inhibition of Tumor Cell Adherence by Prostaglandins
J. Fantone, S. Kunkel, and J. Varani 673

Tumor Antigen Induced Changes in Transmembrane Potential of Leukocytes of Cancer Patients and Modulation by Leukotrienes and Prostaglandins
George Shenouda, D.M.P. Thomson, and M.K. Bach.................. 679

PGE_2-Induced Angiogenesis
David M. Form, Younan A. Sidky, Louis Kubai, and Robert Auerbach 685

Human Lung Cancer and Prostaglandins
I.F. Stamford, A. Bennett, M.A. Carroll, C.N. Hensby, W.F. Whimster, and F. Williams 691

Prostaglandin Production by Squamous Cell Carcinoma of Human
Uterine Cervix in Vitro
Tsuneki Nagasaka, Wendell D. Winters, Olive M. Soriero, and Michael
J.K. Harper 697

Prostaglandins in Tumor-Associated Cells
A. Fulton, A. Rios, S. Loveless, and G. Heppner 701

Prostaglandin Synthesis and Binding by Growing and Regressing
Mammary Carcinoma
Sue C. Liu and Richard A. Knazek 705

Prostaglandin Modulation of ADCC in Human Malignant Melanoma
J. Lee Murray 713

Renal Cell Carcinoma and Urinary Prostaglandin: Case Report
M. Lee Beckman, Francis Deture, and P. W. Ramwell 719

Age Related Immunosuppression: Putative Role of Prostaglandins
Anna Bartocci, Franco M. Maggi, Roy D. Welker, and
Fulvia Veronese 725

PHARMACOLOGICAL MANIPULATION OF PROSTAGLANDIN SYNTHESIS ON TUMOR GROWTH AND METASTASES IN VIVO

Prostacyclin/Thromboxane Ratios in Tumor Growth and Metastasis
Kenneth V. Honn 733

Prostaglandins and Cell Proliferation in Intestinal Tumors in Vivo
P.J.M. Tutton, Frances M. Petry, and D.H. Barkla 753

Effect of Prostaglandin Synthesis Inhibitors on Tumor Growth in Vivo
Alan Bennett 759

Antitumour Activity of Flurbiprofen in Vivo and in Vitro
Kurt Hellman and Barbara A. Pym 767

Effects of Indomethacin on Murine Fibrosarcomas
Neil R. Lynch and J.C. Salomon 775

Brief Reports

Stimulation of PGI$_2$ Biosynthesis by Nafazatrom (Bay g 6575)
T.E. Eling, K.V. Honn, W.D. Busse, F. Seuter, and L.J. Marnett 783

Lipoxygenase Products as Mediators of Tumor Cell Lysosomal Enzyme
Release: Inhibition by Nafazatrom
B.F. Sloane, S. Makim, J.R. Dunn, R. Lacoste, M. Theodorou,
J. Battista, R. Alex, and K.V. Honn 789

Protection Against Misonidazole-Induced Toxicity in Vitro by
Flurbiprofen, a Non-Steroidal Anti-Inflammatory Agent
Barbara C. Millar, Sally Jinks, and Trevor J. Powles 793

Effects of Anti-Inflammatory Agents and Radiotherapy on Esophageal Mucosa and Tumors in Animals
M.G. Northway, A. Bennett, M.A. Carroll, G.L. Eastwood,
M.S. Feldman, H.I. Libshitz, J.J. Mamel, and I.A. Szwarc 799

The Results of Studies of Flurbiprofen in Cancer
G.J. Frank 803

Tumor Cell Induced Platelet Aggregation: Inhibition by Prostacyclin, Thromboxane A₂ and Phosphodiesterase Inhibitors
D. Menter, G. Neagos, J. Dunn, R. Palazzo, T.T. Tchen, J.D. Taylor,
and K.V. Honn 809

Flurbiprofen Does Not Appear to Enhance the Therapeutic Effect of Cyclophosphamide
Susan E. Heckford, Suzanne A. Eccles, T.J. Powles,
and P. Alexander 815

The Effect of Flurbiprofen on Stem Cell Survival Following X Irradiation
R.H. MacDougall, W. Duncan, and Barbara M. Clarke 819

Prostaglandin Administration to Patients With Cancer
T.J. Powles, R.C. Coombes, M. Depledge, J. Muindi, and R. Powles 825

Index 831

Contributors

H. Abou-Issa [657]
Department of Surgery, College of Medicine, The Ohio State University, Columbus, OH 43210

R. Alex [789]
Department of Biological Sciences, Wayne State University, Detroit, MI 48202

Peter Alexander [581, 815]
Division of Tumour Immunology, Institute of Cancer Research, Sutton, Surrey SM2 5PX, England

B. Andersson [159]
Department of Forensic Medicine, Karolinska Institute, Stockholm, Sweden

Robert Auerbach [685]
Department of Zoology, University of Wisconsin, Madison, WI 53706

M.K. Bach [667, 679]
Department of Hypersensitivity Diseases Research, The Upjohn Company, Kalamazoo, MI 49001

C.M. Balch [651]
University of Alabama in Birmingham, University Station, Birmingham, AL 35294

D.H. Barkla [753]
Department of Anatomy, Monash University, Clayton, Victoria 3168, Australia

Sam Barranco [385]
Department of Human Biological Chemistry and Genetics, The University of Texas Medical Branch, Galveston, TX 77550

Anna Bartocci [725]
Laboratory of Chemical Pharmacology, Division of Cancer Treatment, National Cancer Institute, National Institutes of Health, Bethesda, MD 20205

J. Battista [789]
Department of Chemistry, Wayne State University, Detroit, MI 48202

G. Beaudry [265]
Department of Biochemistry, Bowman Gray School of Medicine, Wake Forest University, Winston-Salem, NC 27103

The boldface number in brackets following each contributor's name indicates the opening page number of that author's article.

M. Lee Beckman [719]
Departments of Nephrology and Physiology, Georgetown University School of Medicine, Washington, DC 20007

Suzanne K. Beckner [493]
Laboratory of Nutrition and Endocrinology, NIADDK, National Institutes of Health, Bethesda, MD 20205

Alan Bennett [691, 759, 799]
Department of Surgery, King's College Hospital Medical School, London SE5 8RX, England

D.R. Bennett [365]
Department of Biological Sciences, Wayne State University, Detroit, MI 48202

Sharon Bennett [143]
Department of Biochemistry, Memorial University of Newfoundland, St. John's, Newfoundland A1B 3X9, Canada

Michael J. Bienkowski [97]
Department of Chemistry, Wayne State University, Detroit, MI 48202

Arnold Bisschop [273]
Laboratory for Carcinogenesis and Mutagenesis, National Institute of Public Health, 3720 BA Bilthoven, The Netherlands

G. Blumenschein [567]
The University of Texas System Cancer Center, M.D. Anderson Hospital and Tumor Institute, Houston, TX 77030

R.S. Bockman [415, 555]
Memorial Sloan-Kettering Cancer Center, New York, NY 10021

William Boerwinkle [385]
Department of Human Biological Chemistry and Genetics, The University of Texas Medical Branch, Galveston, TX 77550

Ernest C. Borden [345]
Departments of Human Oncology and Medicine, University of Wisconsin Clinical Cancer Center, Madison, WI 53792

R.K. Boutwell [183]
McArdle Laboratory for Cancer Research, University of Wisconsin, Madison, WI 53706

Jeff Boyd [113]
Laboratory of Pulmonary Function and Toxicology, National Institute of Environmental Health Sciences, Research Triangle Park, NC 27709

Edward Bresnick [205]
Department of Biochemistry, University of Vermont, Burlington, VT 05405

G.L. Bundy [67]
Research Laboratories, The Upjohn Company, Kalamazoo, MI 49001

C. Patrick Burns [487]
Department of Medicine, University of Iowa College of Medicine, Iowa City, IA 52242

W.D. Busse [783]
Bayer AG, Wuppertal, Federal Republic of Germany

R. Cailleau [567]
The University of Texas System Cancer Center, M.D. Anderson Hospital and Tumor Institute, Houston, TX 77030

M.A. Carroll [691, 799]
Department of Surgery, King's College Hospital Medical School, London SE5 8RX, England

R.L. Carter [561]
Haddow Laboratories, Royal Marsden Hospital, Sutton, Surrey SM2 5PX, England

K.A. Chandrabose [345]
Department of Molecular Biology, Wellcome Research Laboratories, Research Triangle Park, NC 27709

Barbara M. Clarke [819]
Department of Clinical Oncology, University of Edinburgh, Western General Hospital, Edinburgh EH4 2XU, Scotland

S.M. Cohen [123]
University of Nebraska, Omaha, NE 68105

R.C. Coombes [541, 825]
Medical Breast Unit, Division of Medicine, Royal Marsden Hospital, Sutton, Surrey SM2 5PX, England

David J. Crutchley [281]
Research Division, Miami Heart Institute, Miami Beach, FL 33140

Pedro Cuatrecasas [345]
Department of Molecular Biology, Wellcome Research Laboratories, Research Triangle Park, NC 27709

R. Phillip Custer [453]
Institute for Cancer Research, Fox Chase Cancer Center, Philadelphia, PA 19111

L. Daniel [265]
Department of Biochemistry, Bowman Gray School of Medicine, Wake Forest University, Winston-Salem, NC 27103

B.B. Davis [123]
VA Medical Center and St. Louis University, St. Louis, MO 63125

W. Dawson [609]
Lilly Research Centre Limited, Earl Wood Manor, Windlesham, Surrey, England

M. Depledge [825]
Department of Medicine, Royal Marsden Hospital, Sutton, Surrey SM2 5PX, England

Francis Deture [719]
Departments of Nephrology and Physiology, Georgetown University School of Medicine, Washington, DC 20007

xviii / Contributors

Ronald L. Dick [291]
Department of Pediatric Oncology, Sidney Farber Cancer Institute, Boston, MA 02115

P.A. Dougherty [651]
University of Alabama in Birmingham, University Station, Birmingham, AL 35294

David T. Dudley [487]
Department of Medicine, University of Iowa College of Medicine, Iowa City, IA 52242

W. Duncan [819]
Department of Clinical Oncology, University of Edinburgh, Western General Hospital, Edinburgh EH4 2XU, Scotland

John R. Dunn [375, 789, 809]
Department of Radiation Oncology, Wayne State University, Detroit, MI 48202

G.L. Eastwood [799]
Department of Gastroenterology, University of Massachusetts Medical School, Worcester, MA 01605

Suzanne A. Eccles [815]
Division of Immunology, Institute of Cancer Research, Sutton, Surrey SM2 5PX, England

Thomas Eling [113, 783]
Laboratory of Pulmonary Function and Toxicology, National Institute of Environmental Health Sciences, Research Triangle Park, NC 27709

J. Fantone [673]
Department of Pathology, University of Michigan School of Medicine, Ann Arbor, MI 48109

M.B. Feinstein [573]
Department of Pharmacology, University of Connecticut School of Medicine, Farmington, CT 06032

M.S. Feldman [799]
Department of Radiotherapy, M.D. Anderson Hospital and Tumor Institute, Houston, TX 77030

Susan M. Fischer [255]
Biology Division, Oak Ridge National Laboratory, Oak Ridge, TN 37830

F.A. Fitzpatrick [333]
Pharmaceutical Research and Development, The Upjohn Company, Kalamazoo, MI 49001

R.J. Flower [21]
Wellcome Research Laboratories, Langley Court, Beckenham, Kent BR3 3BS, England

Robert A. Floyd [167]
Oklahoma Medical Research Foundation, Biomembrane Research Laboratory, Oklahoma City, OK 73104

M. Wayne Flye [385]
Department of Surgery, The University of Texas Medical Branch, Galveston, TX 77550

M.K. Foecking [657]
Department of Physiological Chemistry, The Ohio State University, Columbus, OH 43210

M.L. Foegh [47]
Departments of Physiology and Biophysics and of Medicine, Georgetown University Medical Center, Washington, DC 20007

David M. Form [685]
Department of Zoology, University of Wisconsin, Madison, WI 53706

Rebecca Fox [345]
Departments of Human Oncology and Medicine, University of Wisconsin Clinical Cancer Center, Madison, WI 53792

G.J. Frank [803]
Research Department, The Boots Company Ltd., Nottingham, England

A. Fulton [701]
Department of Immunology, Michigan Cancer Foundation, Detroit, MI 48201

G. Fürstenberger [239]
German Cancer Research Center, Institute of Biochemistry, D-6900 Heidelberg, Federal Republic of Germany

Elena Glass [385]
Department of Surgery, The University of Texas Medical Branch, Galveston, TX 77550

T.L. Grasso [149]
Center for Air Environment Studies, The Pennsylvania State University, University Park, PA 16802

M. Gross [239]
German Cancer Research Center, Institute of Biochemistry, D-6900 Heidelberg, Federal Republic of Germany

G.L. Hahn [381]
Department of Biochemistry, Boston University School of Medicine, Boston, MA 02118

Sven Hammarström [297]
Department of Chemistry, Karolinksa Institute, S-104 01 Stockholm, Sweden

M.J. Hampton [167]
Oklahoma Medical Research Foundation, Biomembrane Research Laboratory, Oklahoma City, OK 73104

Michael J.K. Harper [697]
Department of Obstetrics and Gynecology, The University of Texas Health Science Center at San Antonio, San Antonio, TX 78284

Susan E. Heckford [815]
Division of Immunology, National Cancer Institute, National Institutes of Health, Bethesda, MD 20205

Kurt Hellman [767]
Cancer Chemotherapy Department, Imperial Cancer Research Fund, 44 Lincoln's Inn Fields, London WC2, England

C.N. Hensby [691]
Department of Clinical Pharmacology, Royal Postgraduate Medical School, London W12 DH5, England

G. Heppner [701]
Department of Immunology, Michigan Cancer Foundation, Detroit, MI 48201

Kenneth V. Honn [365, 369, 375, 733, 783, 789, 809]
Departments of Radiation Oncology, Radiology, and Biological Sciences, Wayne State University, Detroit, MI 48202

Ann D. Horowitz [217]
Division of Environmental Science and Cancer Center/Institute of Cancer Research, Columbia University, New York, NY 10032

G.N. Hortobagyi [567]
The University of Texas System Cancer Center, M.D. Anderson Hospital and Tumor Institute, Houston, TX 77030

B.M. Jaffe [425]
Department of Surgery, S.U.N.Y., Downstate Medical Center, Brooklyn, NY 11203

Luis Jimenez de Asua [309]
Department of Cell Biology, Friedrich Miescher-Institut, CH-4002 Basel, Switzerland

Sally Jinks [793]
Radiobiology Unit, Physics Department, Institute of Cancer Research, Sutton, Surrey SM2 5PX, England

Scott Kacy [385]
Department of Surgery, The University of Texas Medical Branch, Galveston, TX 77550

J.W. Karanian [47]
Departments of Physiology and Biophysics and of Medicine, Georgetown University Medical Center, Washington, DC 20007

Richard A. Knazek [705]
Laboratory of Pathophysiology, National Cancer Institute, National Institutes of Health, Bethesda, MD 20205

Hillel S. Koren [663]
Divison of Immunology, Duke Medical Center, Durham, NC 27710

Louis Kubai [685]
Department of Zoology, University of Wisconsin, Madison, WI 53706

S. Kunkel [673]
Department of Pathology, University of Michigan School of Medicine, Ann Arbor, MI 48109

T.J. Labosh [149]
Center for Air Environment Studies and Department of Veterinary Science, The Pennsylvania State University, University Park, PA 16802

R. Lacoste [789]
Department of Biological Sciences, Wayne State University, Detroit, MI 48202

Marie Leithauser [97]
Department of Chemistry, Wayne State University, Detroit, MI 48202

Kam H. Leung [663]
Division of Immunology, Duke Medical Center, Durham, NC 27710

Lawrence Levine [189, 513]
Department of Biochemistry, Brandeis University, Waltham, MA 02254

H.I. Libshitz [799]
Department of Diagnostic Radiology, M.D. Anderson Hospital and Tumor Institute, Houston, TX 77030

Michael C. Lin [493]
Laboratory of Nutrition and Endocrinology, NIADDK, National Institutes of Health, Bethesda, MD 20205

Sue C. Liu [705]
Laboratory of Pathophysiology, National Cancer Institute, National Institutes of Health, Bethesda, MD 20205

Kathryn L. Locatell [291]
Department of Pediatric Oncology, Sidney Farber Cancer Institute, Boston, MA 02115

S. Loveless [701]
Department of Immunology, Michigan Cancer Foundation, Detroit, MI 48201

Neil R. Lynch [775]
Institut de Recherches Scientifiques sur le Cancer, CNRS, Villejuif, France, *presently at* CEPIALET-IND (PAHO-WHO), Aptdo. 4043, Caracas, Venezuela

R.H. MacDougall [819]
Department of Clinical Oncology, University of Edinburgh, Western General Hospital, Edinburgh EH4 2XU, Scotland

Franco M. Maggi [725]
Physiology Department, College of Medicine, Georgetown University, Washington, DC 20007

S. Makim [789]
Department of Biological Sciences, Wayne State University, Detroit, MI 48202

J.J. Mamel [799]
Department of Gastroenterology, University of South Florida, Tampa, FL 33612

F. Marks [239]
German Cancer Research Center, Institute of Biochemistry, D-6900 Heidelberg, Federal Republic of Germany

Lawrence J. Marnett [97, 783]
Department of Chemistry, Wayne State University, Detroit, MI 48202

Wayne Marshall [143]
Department of Biochemistry, Memorial University of Newfoundland, St. John's, Newfoundland A1B 3X9, Canada

T.J. Martin [525]
University of Melbourne, Department of Medicine, Repatriation General Hospital, Victoria 3081, Australia

Jorge Martin-Perez [309]
Department of Cell Biology, Friedrich Miescher-Institut, CH-4002 Basel, Switzerland

E.J. Massaro [149]
Center for Air Environment Studies and Department of Veterinary Science, The Pennsylvania State University, University Park, PA 16802

M.B. Mattammal [123]
VA Medical Center and St. Louis University, St. Louis, MO 63125

James R. Maynard [281]
Research Division, Miami Heart Institute, Miami Beach, FL 33140

David T. Mayschak [385]
Department of Surgery, The University of Texas Medical Branch, Galveston, TX 77550

M. Menconi [381]
Department of Biochemistry, Boston University School of Medicine, Boston, MA 02118

D. Menter [809]
Department of Biological Sciences, Wayne State University, Detroit, MI 48202

Jay Meyer [375]
Department of Radiation Oncology, Wayne State University, Detroit, MI 48202

Barbara C. Millar [793]
Radiobiology Unit, Physics Department, Institute of Cancer Research, Sutton, Surrey, England

Alan M. Miller [481]
Department of Medicine, University of Miami School of Medicine, and the Howard Hughes Medical Institute, Miami, FL 33101

Elizabeth C. Miller [81]
McArdle Laboratory for Cancer Research, The University of Wisconsin Medical School, Madison, WI 53706

James A. Miller [81]
McArdle Laboratory for Cancer Research, The University of Wisconsin Medical School, Madison, WI 53706

J.P. Minton [657]
Department of Surgery, College of Medicine, The Ohio State University, Columbus, OH 43210

P. Moldeus [159]
Department of Forensic Medicine, Karolinksa Institute, Stockholm, Sweden

J. Muindi [541, 825]
Medical Breast Unit, Division of Medicine, Royal Marsden Hospital, Sutton, Surrey SM2 5PX, England

Gregory R. Mundy [501]
Department of Medicine/Endocrinology, University of Texas Health Science Center, San Antonio, TX 78284

G. Murasaki [123]
University of Nebraska, Omaha, NE 68105

J. Lee Murray [713]
Cancer Research Program, Oklahoma Medical Research Foundation, Oklahoma City, OK 73104

Tsuneki Nagasaka [697]
Department of Obstetrics and Gynecology, The University of Texas Health Science Center at San Antonio, San Antonio, TX 78284

G. Neagos [809]
Wayne State University, Detroit, MI 48202

M. Nordenskjöld [159]
Department of Clinical Genetics, Karolinska Institute, Stockholm, Sweden

M.G. Northway [799]
Department of Surgery, King's College Hospital Medical School, London SE5 8RX, England

Peter J. O'Brien [143, 155, 163]
Department of Biochemistry, Memorial University of Newfoundland, St. John's, Newfoundland A1B 3X9, Canada

Ann Louise Olson [487]
Department of Medicine, University of Iowa College of Medicine, Iowa City, IA 52242

Angela M. Otto [309, 391]
Department of Cell Biology, Friedrich Miescher-Institut, CH-4002 Basel, Switzerland

William R. Pagels [97]
Department of Chemistry, Wayne State University, Detroit, MI 48202

R. Palazzo [809]
Wayne State University, Detroit, MI 48202

R.V. Panganamala [657]
Department of Physiological Chemistry, The Ohio State University, Columbus, OH 43210

Augustine Panthananickal [97]
Department of Chemistry, Wayne State University, Detroit, MI 48202

Charles W. Parker [595]
Howard Hughes Medical Institute Laboratory and Department of Internal Medicine, Division of Allergy and Immunology, Washington University School of Medicine, St. Louis, MO 63110

N.C. Partridge [525]
University of Melbourne, Department of Medicine, Repatriation General Hospital, Victoria 3081, Australia

Louis M. Pelus [399]
Department of Developmental Hematopoiesis, Sloan Kettering Institute for Cancer Research, New York, NY 10021

Frances M. Petry [753]
Department of Anatomy, Monash University, Clayton, Victoria 3168, Australia

Kerry Phelan [667]
The Montreal General Hospital Research Institute, Montreal, Quebec H3G 1A4, Canada

J.E. Pike [67]
Research Laboratories, The Upjohn Company, Kalamazoo, MI 49001

Otto J. Plescia [619]
Waksman Institute of Microbiology, Rutgers-The State University of New Jersey, Piscataway, NJ 08854

P. Polgar [381]
Department of Biochemistry, Boston University School of Medicine, Boston, MA 02118

Raveendran Pottathil [345]
Department of Pediatrics, University of Maryland, School of Medicine, Baltimore, MD 21201

R. Powles [825]
Department of Medicine, Royal Marsden Hospital, Sutton, Surrey, England

Trevor J. Powles [xxxi, 541, 793, 815, 825]
Medical Breast Unit, Division of Medicine, Royal Marsden Hospital, Sutton, Surrey SM2 5PX, England

Kedar N. Prasad [437]
University of Colorado Health Sciences Center, School of Medicine, Denver, CO 80262

Barbara A. Pym [767]
Cancer Chemotherapy Department, Imperial Cancer Research Fund, 44 Lincoln's Inn Fields, London WC2, England

A. Rahimtula [159]
Department of Biochemistry, Memorial University of Newfoundland, St. John's, Newfoundland A1B 3X9, Canada

L.G. Raisz [573]
Department of Medicine, University of Connecticut School of Medicine, Farmington, CT 06032

P.W. Ramwell [47, 719]
Departments of Physiology and Biophysics and of Medicine, Georgetown University Medical Center, Washington, DC 20007

C.C. Reddy [149]
Center for Air Environment Studies and Department of Veterinary Science, The Pennsylvania State University, University Park, PA 16802

Gregory A. Reed [97]
Department of Chemistry, Wayne State University, Detroit, MI 48202

A. Rios [701]
Department of Immunology, Michigan Cancer Foundation, Detroit, MI 48201

G.A. Rodan [573]
Department of Oral Biology, University of Connecticut School of Dental Medicine, Farmington, CT 06032

S.B. Rodan [573]
Department of Oral Biology, University of Connecticut School of Dental Medicine, Farmington, CT 06032

P.S. Rudland [465]
Ludwig Institute for Cancer Research (London Branch), Royal Marsden Hospital, Sutton, Surrey SM2 5PX, England

J.A. Salmon [21]
Wellcome Research Laboratories, Langley Court, Beckenham, Kent BR3 3BS, England

Sydney E. Salmon [633]
University of Arizona Cancer Center and Department of Internal Medicine, Hematology/Oncology, Tucson, AZ 85724

J.C. Salomon [775]
Institut de Recherches Scientifiques sur le Cancer, CNRS, Villejuif, France

N. Samaan [567]
The University of Texas System Cancer Center, M.D. Anderson Hospital and Tumor Institute, Houston, TX 77030

Bengt Samuelsson [1]
Department of Physiological Chemistry, Karolinska Institute, S-104 01 Stockholm, Sweden

M.G. Santoro [425]
Centro di Virologia, OORR, San Camillo, Circonvallazione Gianicolense 85, Rome, Italy, *presently at* Department of Surgery, S.U.N.Y., Downstate Medical Center, Brooklyn, NY 11203

Frederick V. Schaefer [453]
Institute for Cancer Research, Fox Chase Cancer Center, Philadelphia, PA 19111

Charles D. Scher [291]
Department of Hematology-Oncology, Sidney Farber Cancer Institute and Children's Hospital Medical Center; and Department of Pediatrics, Harvard Medical School, Boston, MA 02115

R.W. Scholz [149]
Department of Veterinary Science, The Pennsylvania State University, University Park, PA 16802

P. Schultz [567]
The University of Texas System Cancer Center, M.D. Anderson Hospital and Tumor Institute, Houston, TX 77030

F. Seuter [783]
Bayer AG, Wuppertal, Federal Republic of Germany

George Shenouda [679]
The Montreal General Hospital Research Institute, Montreal, Quebec H3G 1A4, Canada

Younan A. Sidky [685]
Department of Zoology, University of Wisconsin, Madison, WI 53706

H.A. Simmons [573]
Department of Medicine, University of Connecticut School of Medicine, Farmington, CT 06032

K. Sivarajah [113]
Laboratory of Pulmonary Function and Toxicology, National Institute of Environmental Health Sciences, Research Triangle Park, NC 27709

Thomas J. Slaga [255]
Biology Division, Oak Ridge National Laboratory, Oak Ridge, TN 37830

B.F. Sloane [789]
Department of Pharmacology, Wayne State University, Detroit, MI 48201

Olive M. Soriero [697]
Department of Obstetrics and Gynecology, The University of Texas Health Science Center at San Antonio, San Antonio, TX 78284

Sam Sorof [453]
Institute for Cancer Research, Fox Chase Cancer Center, Philadelphia, PA 19111

I.F. Stamford [691]
Department of Surgery, King's College Hospital Medical School, London SE5 8RX, England

Charles D. Stiles [291]
Department of Tumor Biology, Sidney Farber Cancer Institute; and Department of Microbiology and Molecular Genetics, Harvard Medical School, Boston, MA 02115

D.A. Stringfellow [333]
Pharmaceutical Research and Development, The Upjohn Company, Kalamazoo, MI 49001

I.A. Szwarc [799]
Department of Diagnostic Radiology, M.D. Anderson Hospital and Tumor Institute, Houston, TX 77030

Armen H. Tashjian, Jr. [513]
Laboratory of Toxicology, Harvard School of Public Health, and Department of Pharmacology, Harvard Medical School, Boston, MA 02115

J.D. Taylor [365, 369, 809]
Department of Biological Sciences, Wayne State University, Detroit, MI 48202

T.T. Tchen [809]
Department of Chemistry, Wayne State University, Detroit, MI 48202

M. Theodorou [789]
Department of Biological Sciences, Wayne State University, Detroit, MI 48202

C.E. Thomas [149]
Center for Air Environment Studies and Department of Veterinary Science, The Pennsylvania State University, University Park, PA 16802

George Thomas [309]
Department of Cell Biology, Friedrich Miescher-Institut, CH-4002 Basel, Switzerland

K.C. Thompson [365]
Department of Biological Sciences, Wayne State University, Detroit, MI 48202

D.M.P. Thomson [667, 679]
The Montreal General Hospital Research Institute, Montreal, Quebec H3G 1A4, Canada

A.B. Tilden [651]
University of Alabama in Birmingham, University Station, Birmingham, AL 35294

Courtney M. Townsend, Jr. [385]
Department of Surgery, The University of Texas Medical Branch, Galveston, TX 77550

Y. Tsuruta [155]
Departments of Biochemistry, Memorial University of Newfoundland, St. John's, Newfoundland A1B 3X9, Canada

W.A. Turner [365, 369]
Department of Biological Sciences, Wayne State University, Detroit, MI 48202

P.J.M. Tutton [753]
Department of Anatomy, Monash University, Clayton, Victoria 3168, Australia

Marie-Odile Ulrich [309]
Friedrich Miescher-Institut, CH-4002 Basel, Switzerland

J.R. Vane [21]
Wellcome Research Laboratories, Langley Court, Beckenham, Kent BR3 3BS, England

Lucio A.A. van Rooijen [273]
Laboratory for Carcinogenesis and Mutagenesis, National Institute of Public Health, 3720 BA Bilthoven, The Netherlands

J. Varani [673]
Department of Pathology, University of Michigan School of Medicine, Ann Arbor, MI 48109

Sudesh Vasdev [155, 163]
Department of Biochemistry, Memorial University of Newfoundland, St. John's, Newfoundland A1B 3X9, Canada

Fulvia Veronese [725]
Laboratory of Viral Carcinogenesis, Frederick Cancer Research Center, National Cancer Institute, National Institutes of Health, Frederick, MD 21701

Edward F. Voelkel [513]
Laboratory of Toxicology, Harvard School of Public Health, Boston, MA 02115

M. Waite [265]
Department of Biochemistry, Bowman Gray School of Medicine, Wake Forest University, Winston-Salem, NC 27103

R.W. Walenga [573]
Department of Pharmacology, University of Connecticut School of Medicine, Farmington, CT 06032

Sue-May Wang [493]
Laboratory of Nutrition and Endocrinology, NIADDK, National Institutes of Health, Bethesda, MD 20205

M.J. Warburton [465]
Ludwig Institute for Cancer Research (London Branch), Royal Marsden Hospital, Sutton, Surrey SM2 5PX, England

I. Bernard Weinstein [217]
Division of Environmental Science and Cancer Center/Institute of Cancer Research, Columbia University, New York, NY 10032

Roy D. Welker [725]
Department of Cell Biology, Litton Bionetics, Inc., Kensington, MD 20795

W.F. Whimster [691]
Department of Morbid Anatomy, King's College Hospital Medical School, London SE5 8RX, England

F. Williams [691]
Department of Clinical Pharmacology, Royal Postgraduate Medical School, London W12 DH5, England

Wendell D. Winters [697]
Department of Microbiology, The University of Texas Health Science Center at San Antonio, San Antonio, TX 78284

Peter K. Wong [167]
Oklahoma Medical Research Foundation, Biomembrane Research Laboratory, Oklahoma City, OK 73104

Adel A. Yunis [481]
Departments of Medicine, Oncology, and Dermatology, University of Miami School of Medicine, and the Howard Hughes Medical Institute, Miami, FL 33101

T.V. Zenser [123]
VA Medical Center and St. Louis University, St. Louis, MO 63125

Vincent A. Ziboh [481]
Department of Dermatology, University of California School of Medicine, Davis, CA 95616

Perhaps one of the most extensive developments in biochemistry and pharmacology which has occurred in the last few years relates to the synthesis in the body of active biological metabolites of arachadonic acid and other similar lipids. These products, particularly the primary prostaglandins, the leucotrienes, thromboxane and prostacyclin, have been the object of intensive research activity relating to most areas of biology.

During the past few years, experimental evidence has accumulated which indicates that some of these active metabolites are involved in mechanisms for initiation and growth of tumours. Furthermore, manipulation of prostaglandin synthesis with analogues and inhibitors will influence development of tumours in animals. Unfortunately the rapid development of biochemical and pharmacological research relating to prostaglandins has made it increasingly difficult for experimental oncology to keep up to date with new developments relevent to cancer research.

The aim of the "Prostaglandin and Cancer Conference 1981" was to bring together scientists involved in prostaglandin research with those involved in cancer research. The main areas of interest included carcinogenesis, cell replication, maturation and differentiation, osteolysis and host/tumour interaction. The meeting commenced with presentations of updated reviews of the chemistry and pharmacology of prostaglandins and related compounds and finished with a session on the overall effects of manipulation of prostaglandin synthesis on tumour growth in animals.

This publication of the papers of the invited speakers and many of the proferred presentations, provides an assessment of the interaction of these two complex areas of research and indications of direction for future research.

Trevor J. Powles,
London, September, 1981.

GENERAL PRINCIPLES OF
PROSTAGLANDIN SYNTHESIS

Prostaglandins and Cancer: First
International Conference, pages 1-19
© 1982 Alan R. Liss, Inc., 150 Fifth Avenue, New York, NY 10011

PROSTAGLANDINS, THROMBOXANES AND LEUKOTRIENES: BIOCHEMICAL

PATHWAYS

BENGT SAMUELSSON

Department of Physiological Chemistry,

Karolinska Institutet, S-10401 Stockholm, Sweden

Evidence for a central role of arachidonic acid as precursor of regulators and mediators of various cell functions
has accumulated during the past few years. The products consist of prostaglandins (including prostacyclin), thromboxanes, and various hydroxylated fatty acids formed in
lipoxygenase catalyzed reactions. Recently, an additional
group of arachidonic acid derived products, the leukotrienes,
was discovered. The present review summarizes some of the
work on the biochemical pathways involved in the formation
of oxygenated derivatives of arachidonic acid and other
polyunsaturated fatty acids.

PROSTAGLANDINS AND THROMBOXANES

The prostaglandins (PGs) are C_{20} unsaturated fatty
acids containing a cyclopentane ring. Each PG is designated
by a letter (PGE, PGF, PGD etc.) indicating the nature of
the cyclopentane substituents and by a subscript (PGE$_1$, PGE$_2$
etc.) which indicates the number of double bonds (Bergström
and Samuelsson, 1965).

The biosynthesis of prostaglandins involves oxygenation
and cyclization of polyunsaturated fatty acids. Dihomo-γ-
linolenic acid (8,11,14-eicosatrienoic acid) and arachidonic
acid, which both belong to the n-6 series of polyunsaturated
fatty acids and thus originate in dietary linoleic acid, are
converted into PG$_1$ and PG$_2$ groups of compounds, respectively
(Fig. 1). Prostaglandins of the "3" series like PGE$_3$ are
formed from eicosapentaenoic acid, which belongs to the n-3
series of unsaturated fatty acids and originates in α-lino-
lenic acid (Samuelsson et al., 1978).

FORMATION OF PG, TX AND LT FROM UNSATURATED FATTY ACIDS

$$\underline{18:1} \quad (\text{N-9})$$

$$\downarrow$$

PG $\longleftarrow\!\!\!|\!\!|$ 20:3 (N-9) $\longrightarrow$ LT$_3$

$$\underline{18:2} \quad (\text{N-6})$$

$$\downarrow$$

PG$_1$ $\longleftarrow$ 20:3 (N-6) $\longrightarrow$ 8,9-LT$_3$

$$\downarrow$$

PG$_2$ $\longleftarrow$ 20:4 (N-6) $\longrightarrow$ LT$_4$

$$\underline{18:3} \quad (\text{N-3})$$

$$\downarrow$$

PG$_3$ $\longleftarrow$ 20:5 (N-3) $\longrightarrow$ LT$_5$

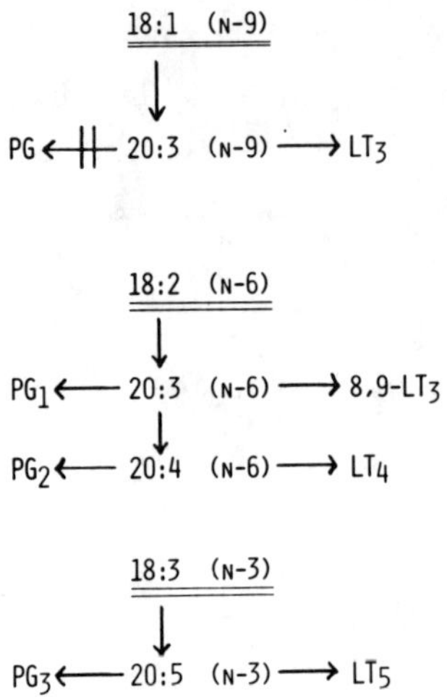

Fig. 1

The precursor fatty acids are normally present in minute amounts in free form and are mainly stored bound in ester form to phospholipids as phosphatidylcholine, phosphatidyl-inositol etc. Upon stimulation of the cells there is activation of phospholipase A$_2$, which catalyzes the hydrolytic release of the precursor acid. In platelets phospholipase C and a diglyceride lipase have been proposed to be involved in the cleavage of the unsaturated fatty acid (Bell et al., 1979). An alternative mechanism consisting of phosphorylation of the diglyceride to phosphatidic acid followed by release of the fatty acid by a phosphatidic acid specific phospholipase A$_2$ has recently been suggested (Billah, Lapetina and Cuatrecasas, 1981). The predominating fatty acid is in most systems arachidonic acid. A detailed mechanism for stimulation of cellular release of polyunsaturated-fatty acids has been suggested (Hirata and Axelrod, 1980).

The prostaglandins are usually not stored in the tissues but released and rapidly metabolized. The transformations includ 15-hydroxy-prostaglandin dehydrogenase and 13,14-reductase cata-lyzed reactions. The resulting products are usually biologically inactive. Further transformation takes place by β-oxidation to C_{18} and C_{16} derivatives and also by ω-oxidation (Samuelsson et al., 1978; Oates et al., 1980).

The formation of prostaglandins from e.g. arachidonic acid has been proposed to be initiated by a lipoxygenase type reaction with introduction of oxygen at C-11 (Fig. 2). Further oxygenation and cyclization yields an unstable endoperoxide intermediate, PGG_2, which is reduced in a peroxidase reaction to give another endoperoxide derivative, PGH_2. The latter compound can be converted to various prostaglandins (Samuelsson et al., 1978).

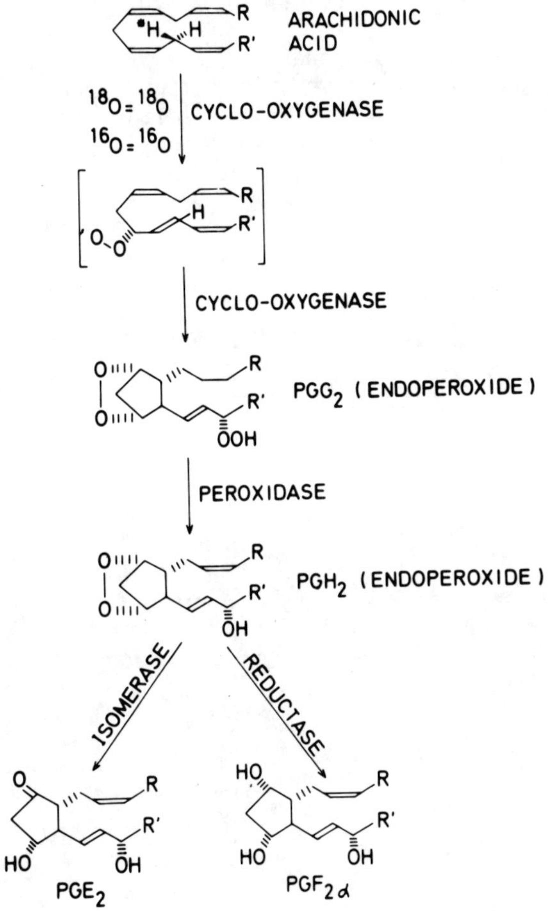

Fig. 2 Mechanism of prostaglandin biosynthesis.

In the course of studies of the biological effects of the endoperoxides, it was recognized that they had effects on platelets (aggregation) which could not be explained by an effect of the endoperoxides per se or of the prostaglandins known at that time. This led to the discovery of the thromboxanes (Hamberg, Svensson and Samuelsson, 1975). Thromboxane A_2 is a highly unstable ($t_{1/2}$ = 30-40 secs.) derivative with potent platelet aggregating and vasoconstrictor effects (Fig. 3). Subsequently it was found that blood vessels could transform the endoperoxide into a compound, PGI_2 or prostacyclin, with opposite effects (Fig. 3) (Moncada and Vane, 1977; Johnson et al., 1976). This pair of arachidonic acid derivatives seem to form a homeostatic mechanism controlling the tonus of blood vessels and the aggregation of platelets.

The peroxidase component of the prostaglandin synthetase mentioned above seems to have the capacity to generate activated forms of oxygen. This reaction was originally discovered with the hydroperoxy-endoperoxide, PGG_2, and also

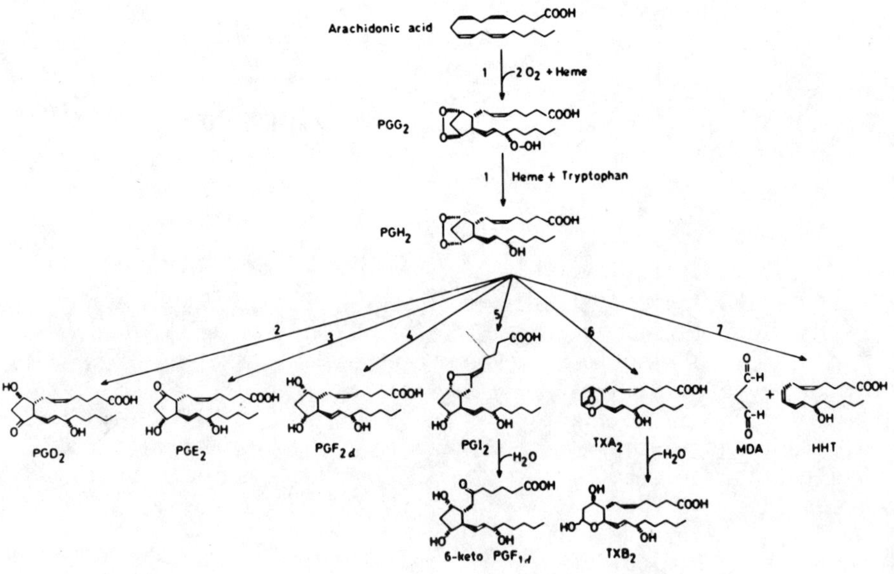

Fig. 3   Transformation of arachidonic acid in human platelets.

with 15-hydroperoxy-eicosatetraenoic acid and the microsomal synthetase (Marnett, Wlodawer and Samuelsson, 1975). The activated oxygen was detected by following chemiluminescence and co-oxygenation of various substrates. This reaction has subsequently been studied in detail both with respect to the enzymes involved and the nature of the activated oxygen (Kuehl et al., 1980). It has been suggested to be of importance in inflammation and also in the transformation and formation of carcinogens and other compounds (Marnett, Wlodawer and Samuelsson, 1975; Kuehl et al., 1980).

LEUKOTRIENES

Non-steroidal antiinflammatory drugs such as aspirin inhibit the enzyme (cyclo-oxygenase) responsible for conversion of arachidonic acid into prostaglandins (Vane, 1971). Antiinflammatory corticosteroids prevent formation of prostaglandins by different mechanism, viz, inhibition of the release of arachidonic acid from the phospholipid stores (Gryglewski et al., 1975; Hong and Levine, 1976). In view of the pronounced differences in the antiinflammatory effects of steroids and aspirin-type drugs it seemed conceivable to us that arachidonic acid might generate additional proinflammatory derivatives the formation of which was not dependent on the cyclo-oxygenase. The production of such products should be inhibited by steroids unless free arachidonic acid was added. To test this hypothesis, the metabolism of arachidonic acid in polymorphonuclear leukocytes was studied.

Using polymorphonuclear leukocytes (PMNL) obtained from the peritoneal cavity of rabbits it was found that 5(S)-hydroxy-6,8,11,14-eicosatetraenoic acid (5-HETE) was the major arachidonic acid derived product (Borgeat, Hamberg and Samuelsson, 1976). Additional work showed that more polar products were also formed. These were identified as 5(S),12(R)-dihydroxy-6,8,10,14-eicosatetraenoic acid (major product) (leukotriene B4, c.f. below), two additional 5(S),12-dihydroxy-6,8,10-trans,14-cis-eicosatetraenoic acids, epimeric at C-12, and two isomeric 5,6-dihydroxy-7,9,11,14-eicosatetraenoic acids (Fig. 4) (Borgeat and Samuelsson, 1979a, 1979b).

Stereochemical analysis, demonstrating formation of two acids with an all trans conjugated triene, epimeric at C-12 and one major isomer (12R) with different configuration of the triene raised the question of the mechanism of formation

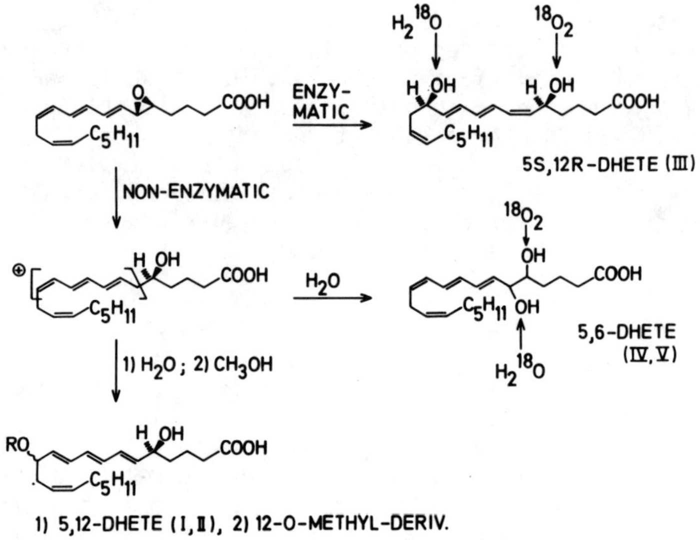

Fig. 4 Formation of dihydroxy derivatives from unstable intermediate. Origin of oxygen and trapping experiments.

(Borgeat and Samuelsson, 1979b). Using isotopic oxygen it could be demonstrated that the oxygen of the alcohol group at C-5 originated in molecular oxygen, whereas the oxygen of the alcohol group at C-12 was derived from water (Fig. 4) (Borgeat and Samuelsson, 1979c). It was therefore postulated that leukocytes generated an unstable intermediate which would undergo nucleophilic attack by water, alcohols, and other nucleophiles.

Based on trapping experiments and other data, the structure 5(S)-oxido-7,9,11,14-eicosatetraenoic acid (Fig. 4) was proposed for the intermediate (Borgeat and Samuelsson, 1979c). The formation of the epoxide from arachidonic acid can be visualized to involve initial formation of 5-hydroperoxy-6,8,11,14-eicosatetraenoic acid (5-HPETE), the precursor of the 5-hydroxy acid (Fig. 5). The epoxide is formed from 5-HPETE by abstraction of a proton at C-10, and elimination of hydroxyl anion from the hydroperoxy group.

The proposed structure (Borgeat and Samuelsson, 1979c), 5,6-oxido-7,9,11,14-eicosatetraenoic acid (leukotriene A_4, c.f. below), of the intermediate has been confirmed by chemi-

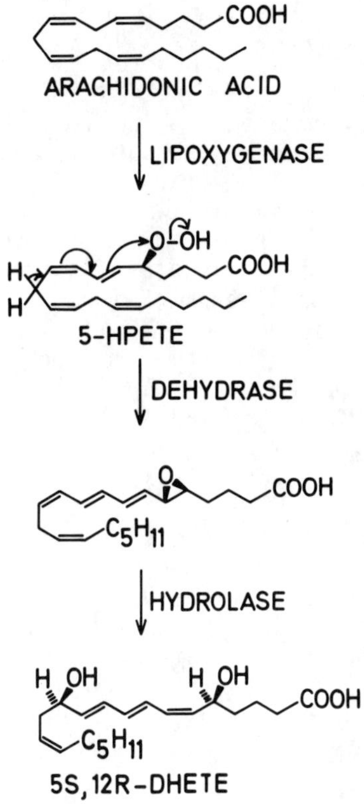
COOH
ARACHIDONIC ACID
LIPOXYGENASE
O-OH
H
COOH
H
5-HPETE
DEHYDRASE
O
COOH
C5H11
HYDROLASE
H OH
H OH
COOH
C5H11
5S,12R-DHETE

Fig. 5 Mechanism of formation of unstable intermediate.

cal synthesis and the stereochemistry has been elucidated (Rådmark et al., 1980a). The configuration of the double bonds of the conjugated triene in leukotriene B_4 was also determined using a synthetic approach (Corey et al., 1980). The allylic epoxide intermediate has recently been isolated from human polymorphonuclear leukocytes (Rådmark et al., 1980b). It can thus exist in free form in cells and tissues.

The concept that the unstable epoxide plays a role in the transformation of arachidonic acid in leukocytes was a prerequisite for the work leading to elucidation of the structure and biogenesis of slow reacting substance of anaphylaxis (SRS-A) (Borgeat and Samuelsson, 1979c). Previous work had indicated that the ionophore A23187 stimulated the release of SRS and that SRS absorbed in the ultraviolet (Conroy, Orange and Lichtenstein, 1976; Morris et al., 1978; Orange et al., 1973). The effects of the ionophore, the UV-absorbance data and other considerations led us to develop the hypothesis that there was a biogenetic link between the unstable allylic epoxide intermediate and SRS-A (Borgeat and Samuelsson, 1979c).

In 1938 Feldberg and Kellaway introduced the term SRS (Slow Reacting Substance) for a smooth muscle containing factor appearing in the perfusate of guinea pig lung following treatment with cobra venom (Feldberg and Kellaway, 1938). Subsequent studies have suggested that SRS is an important mediator in asthma and other types of immediate hypersensitivity reactions (Austen, 1978; Brocklehurst, 1953; Kellaway and Trethewie, 1940; Orange and Austen, 1969). For a review of previous structural work on SRS, see ref. (Murphy, Hammarström and Samuelsson, 1979).

When investigating different methods for production of SRS, we found that murine mastocytoma cells treated with ionophore A23187 and L-cysteine generated SRS. This method proved superior to previously described systems with respect to formation of spasmogenic material antagonized by the SRS antagonist FPL55712 and incorporation of isotopically labeled precursors (see below) (Murphy, Hammarström and Samuelsson, 1979).

The studies on the SRS from mastocytoma cells which have been summarized in detail elsewhere (Murphy, Hammarström and Samuelsson, 1979; Hammarström et al., 1979; Samuelsson et al., 1980a), showed that the structure was 5-hydroxy-6-S-glutationyl-7,9,11,14-eicosatetraenoic acid, leukotriene $(\overline{LT})C_4$ (c.f. below) (Hammarström et al, 1979) (Fig. 6). The structure was confirmed by comparison with synthetic material. The preparation and some properties of corresponding cysteinylglycine derivative (LTD_4) and cysteinyl derivative (LTE_4) were also reported at the same time (Hammarström et al., 1979). These compounds have later been isolated from natural sources (see below). The proposed stereochemistry of LTC_4 was confirmed and unambiguously assigned by total synthesis including preparation of stereoisomers of LTC_4 (Hammarström et al., 1980). The synthetic work was carried out by E.J. Corey et al. LTC_4 is thus 5(S)-hydroxy,6(R)-S-glutathionyl-7,9-trans-11,14-cis-eicosatetraenoic acid. The previously proposed biogenetic relationship between LTA_4 and LTC_4 was recently confirmed by the actual conversion of synthetic LTA_4 into LTC_4 in human polymorphonuclear leukocytes (Fig. 6) (Rådmark, Malmsten and Samuelsson, 1980c).

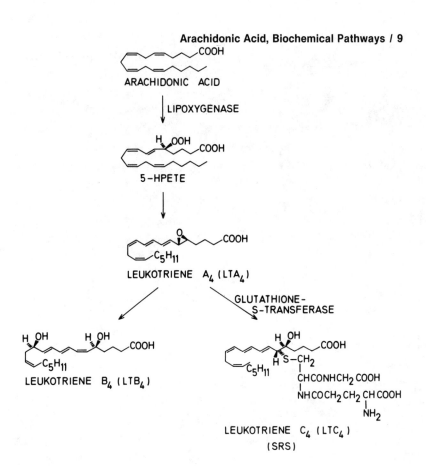

Fig. 6   Formation of leukotrienes.

Additional studies with a different cell type, the RBL-1 cells, demonstrated that the major slow reacting substance was less polar than LTC_4 (Örning, Hammarström and Samuelsson, 1980). Amino acid analyses showed that this product lacked glutamic acid. Edman-degradation indicated that glycine was C-terminal. Incubation of LTC_4 with γ-glutamyl transpeptidase yielded additional proof for the structure. The product 5(S)-hydroxy,6(R)-S-cysteinyl-glycine-7,9-trans-11,14-cis-eicosatetraenoic acid (LTD_4) was identical with the less polar product from RBL-1 cells (Fig. 7).

Following the structure determination of SRS from mastocytoma cells (Hammarström et al., 1979; Murphy, Hammarström and Samuelsson, 1979) and synthetic preparation of LTC_4, LTD_4 and LTE_4 (Hammarström et al., 1979) all of these cysteine con-

SLOW REACTING SUBSTANCE OF ANAPHYLAXIS

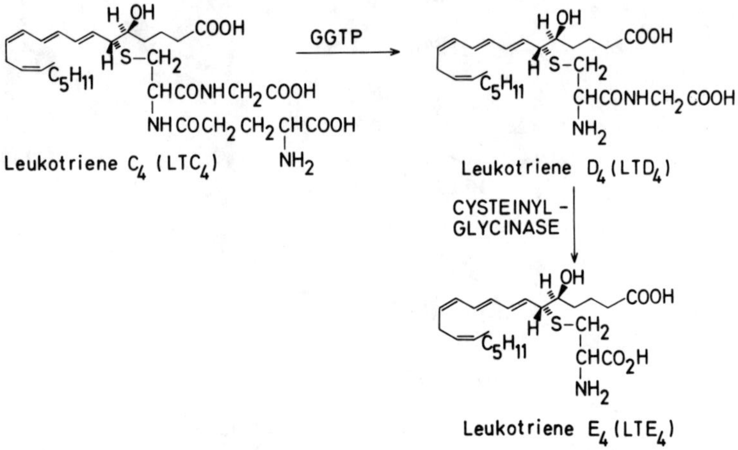

Leukotriene C_4 (LTC_4)

Leukotriene D_4 (LTD_4)

CYSTEINYL - GLYCINASE

Leukotriene E_4 (LTE_4)

Fig. 7 Structures found in preparations of SRS-A.

taining leukotrienes have been found in a variety of biological systems using comparison with synthetic material or partial characterization by chemical or physical methods for
identification. These studies are summarized in Table 1.
SRS-A is thus a mixture of the cysteine containing leukotrienes i.e. the parent compound LTC_4 and the metabolites LTD_4
and LTE_4. The relative proportion of these leukotrienes depends on the procedure used to prepare the SRS-A.

The metabolism of LTC_3 has been investigated using tritium-labeled material of high specific activity and with the
label in the fatty acid part of the molecule (Hammarström,
1981). The results showed that guinea pig lung homogenates
rapidly converted LTC_3 to LTD_3. Liver and kidney homogenates
did not catabolize LTC_3 appreciably. This was apparently due
to high tissue concentrations of glutathione which prevented
LTD_3 formation because LTD_3 was rapidly metabolized by liver
and kidney homogenates through hydrolysis of the peptide bond
to give 5-hydroxy-6-S-cysteinyl-7,9,11-eicotrienoic acid
(LTE_3). In accordance with these finding, labelled LTC_3
administered into the right atrium of male monkey was rapidly transformed into LTD_3 and LTE_3 (Hammarström et al., 1981).

TABLE 1 Identification of leukotrienes from different sources

Source	LTA_4	LTB_4	LTC_4	LTD_4	LTE_4	Reference
Rabbit peritoneal leukocytes	+	+				Borgeat and Samuelsson, 1979a,c
Human peripheral leukocytes	+	+	+			Borgeat and Samuelsson, 1979d; Hansson and Rådmark, 1980; Rådmark et al, 1980b
Mouse mastocytoma cells	+		+	+		Hammarström et al, 1979; Murphy et al, 1979
Rat basophilic leukemia cells				+	+	Morris et al, 1980a; Örning et al, 1980; Parker et al, 1980
Rat peritoneal monocytes			+	+		Bach et al, 1980a,b
Rat peritoneal cells			+	+	+	Lewis et al, 1980a
Rat peripheral leukocytes		+				Ford-Hutchinson, 1981
Rat pleural neutrophils		+				Siegel, 1981
Rat macrophages		+				Doig and Ford-Hutchinson, 1980
Mouse macrophages			+	+		Rouzer et al, 1980
Human lung			+	+		Lewis et al, 1980b
Guinea pig lung				+		Morris et al, 1980b
Cat paws					+	Houglum et al, 1980

The biological significance of the biosynthetic pathways described and the cumbersome systematic names of the compounds involved suggested the introduction of a trivial name for these entities (Samuelsson et al., 1979). The term "leukotriene" was chosen because the compounds were first detected in leukocytes and the common structural feature is a conjugated triene. Various members of the group have been designated alphabetically: leukotrienes A are 5,6-oxido-7,9-trans 11-cis; leukotrienes B, 5(S)12(R)-dihydroxy-6 cis 8,10-trans; leukotrienes C, 5(S)-hydroxy-6(R)-S-γ-glutamyl-cysteinyl-glycyl-7,9-trans-11-cis; leukotrienes D, 5(S)-hydroxy-6(R)-S-cysteinylglycyl-7,9-trans-11-cis; and leukotrienes E, 5(S)-hydroxy-6(R)-S-cysteinyl-7,9-trans-11-cis eicosapolyenoic acids. Since various precursor acids can be converted to leukotrienes containing 3-5 double bonds, a subscript denoting this number is used (Samuelsson and Hammarström, 1980). Leukotriene A_4 is thus the epoxy derivative of arachidonic acid which can be further transformed to leukotrienes B_4, C_4, D_4 and E_4.

It has recently been demonstrated that leukotrienes can also be formed after initial oxygenation at C-15 and C-8. Thus, the unstable 14,15-oxido-5,8,10,12-eicosatetraenoic acid (14,15-LTA_4) is formed via 15-hydroperoxy-eicosatetraenoic acid (15-HPETE) and is transformed into 14,15-dihydroxy-derivatives (14,15-LTB_4) and 8,15-dihydroxy-derivatives (8,15-LTB_4) (Jubiz et al., 1981; Lundberg et al., 1981). Furthermore, bishomo-γ-linolenic acid which is oxygenated to give an 8-hydroperoxy-derivative (Borgeat, Hamberg and Samuelsson, 1976) can be converted to an 8,9-isomer of LTC_3 (Hammarström, 1981).

An isomer of LTB_4, 5S,12S-dihydroxy-6-trans,8-cis,10-trans,14-cis-eicosatetraenoic acid, was recently isolated as a metabolite of arachidonic acid in human leukocytes. This derivative is not formed via the leukotriene pathway and is therefore referred to as 5S,12S-DHETE (Lindgren, Hansson and Samuelsson, 1981).

The suggested importance of SRS-A in asthma and anaphylactic reactions and the finding that SRS-A belonged to the leukotrienes stimulated the interest in studies of the biological effects of these substances.

Recent work using pure leukotrienes has provided more detailed information about the effects on the pulmonary and cardiovascular systems (Hedqvist et al., 1980; Dahlén et al., 1980; Drazen et al., 1980; Smedegård et al., 1981). These studies demonstrate that cysteinyl-containing leukotrienes are bronchoconstrictors of unusual potency. The finding that LTC$_4$ may induce severe bronchoconstriction in a subhuman primate, together with its exquisite potency in isolated human bronchi, suggests that also the human bronchus in situ might be susceptible to these substances. Furthermore, the cysteine containing leukotrienes have specific effects on the micro-circulation (Dahlén et al, 1981) and the dihydroxy-derivative, LTB$_4$, **influences leukocyte migration by causing** leukocyte adhesion to the endothelium in postcapillary venules (Dahlén et al., 1981) and by potent chemotactic effects (Malmsten et al., 1980; Ford-Hutchinson et al., 1980; Goetzl and Pickett, 1980; Palmer et al., 1980). These results indicate that the leukotrienes might be of importance as media-**tors in such host defense mechanisms as immediate hypersensitivity reactions and acute inflammatory reactions.**

The biochemical interrelationship between the cyclo-oxygenase pathway (yielding prostaglandins and thromboxanes) and the leukotriene pathway is illustrated in Fig. 8. Anti-inflammatory steroids prevent the release of the precursor

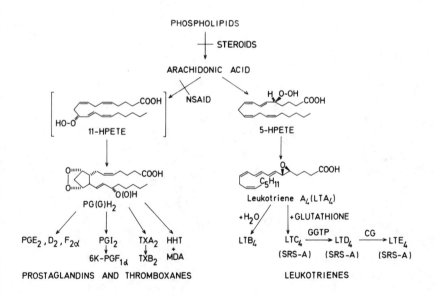

Fig. 8   Formation of prostaglandins, thromboxanes and leukotrienes.

acid, arachidonic acid, whereas cyclo-oxygenase inhibitors
such as aspirin block the transformation of this acid into
prostaglandins and thromboxanes. It has recently been proposed that anti-inflammatory steroids act by stimulating the
synthesis of an inhibitor of phospholipase A_2 (Blackwell et
al., 1980; Hirata et al., 1980). By inhibiting the release
of arachidonic acid steroids prevent formation of not only
prostaglandins and thromboxanes but also leukotrienes and
other oxygenated derivatives. The inhibition of leukotriene
formation might be responsible for some of the therapeutic
effects of steroids which are not shared by aspirin type
drugs.

It is evident that arachidonic acid has a central role
as precursor of biologically active compounds. The increased
knowledge about the biochemistry of the arachidonic acid
derived mediators seems to offer many new possibilities of
exploring the role of this system in physiological and pathophysiological processes.

ACKNOWLEDGEMENT

The work from the author's laboratory was supported by
the Swedish Medical Research Council (project 03X-217).

REFERENCES

Austen KF (1978). Hemostasis of effector systems which can be
    recruited for immunological reactions. J Immunol 121:793.
Bach MK, Brashler JR, Hammarström S, Samuelsson B (1980a).
    Identification of leukotriene C-1 as a major component of
    slow reacting substance from rat mononuclear cells.
    J Immunol 125:115.
Bach MK, Brashler JR, Hammarström S, Samuelsson B (1980b).
    Identification of a component of rat mononuclear cell SRS
    as leukotriene D. Biochem Biophys Res Commun 93:1121.
Bell RL, Kennerly DA, Stanford N, Majerus PW (1979). Diglyce-
    ride lipase: A pathway for arachidonate release from human
    platelets. Proc Natl Acad Sci USA 76:3238.
Bergström S, Samuelsson B (1965). Prostaglandins. Ann Rev
    Biochem 34:101.
Billah MM, Lapetina EG, Cuatrecasas P (1981). Phospholipase
    A_2 activity specific for phosphatidic acid. J Biol Chem
    256:5399.

Blackwell GJ, Carnuccion R, Di R
Persico P (1980). Macrocortin: a polypeptide causing the
anti-phospholipase effect of glucocorticoids. Nature
(London) 287:147.
Borgeat P, Hamberg M, Samuelsson B (1976). Transformation of
arachidonic acid and homo-γ-linolenic acid by rabbit polymorphonuclear leukocytes. J Biol Chem 251:7816.
Borgeat P, Samuelsson B (1979a). Transformation of arachidonic acid by rabbit polymorphonuclear leukocytes. J Biol
Chem 254:2643.
Borgeat P, Samuelsson B (1979b). Metabolism of arachidonic
acid in polymorphonuclar leukocytes. Structural analysis
of novel hydroxylated compounds. J Biol Chem 254:7865.
Borgeat P, Samuelsson B (1979c). Arachidonic acid metabolism
in polymorphonuclear leukocytes: Unstable intermediate in
formation of dihydroxy acids. Proc Natl Acad Sci USA 76:3213.
Borgeat P, Samuelsson B (1979d). Arachidonic acid metabolism
in polymorphonuclear leukocytes: Effects of ionophore
A23187. Proc Natl Acad Sci USA 76:2148.
Brocklehurst WE (1953). J Physiol 120:16P
Conroy MC, Orange RP, Lichtenstein LM (1976). Release of slow-
reacting substance of anaphylaxis (SRS-A) from human leuko-
cytes by the calcium ionophore A23187. J Immunol 116:1677.
Corey EJ, Marfat A, Goto G, Brion F (1980). Leukotriene B.
Total synthesis and assignment of stereochemistry. J Am
Chem Soc 102:7984.
Dahlén SE, Hedqvist P, Hammarström S, Samuelsson B (1980).
Leukotrienes are potent constrictors of human bronchi.
Nature 288:484.
Dahlén SE, Björk J, Hedqvist P, Arfors KE, Hammarström S,
Lindgren JÅ, Samuelsson B (1981). Leukotrienes promote
plasma leakage and leukocyte adhesion in postcapillary
venules: In vivo effects with relevance to the acute in-
flammatory response. Proc Natl Acad Sci USA 78:3887.
Doig MV, Ford-Hutchinson AW (1980). The production and cha-
racterization of products of the lipoxygenase enzyme sys-
tem released by rat peritoneal macrophages. Prostaglandins
20:1007.
Drazen JM, Austen FK, Lewis RA, Clark DA, Goto G, Marfat A,
Corey EJ (1980). Comparative airway and vascular activities of leukotrienes C-1 and D in vivo and in vitro.
Proc Natl Acad Sci USA 77:4354.
Feldberg W, Kellaway CH (1938). Liberation of histamine and
formation of lysolecithin-like substances by cobra venom.
J Physiol 94:187.

Ford-Hutchinson AW, Bray MA, Doig MV, Shipley ME, Smith MJH (1980). Leukotriene B, a potent chemokinetic and aggregating substance released from polymorphonuclear leukocytes. Nature 286:264.

Ford-Hutchinson AW, Bray MA, Cunningham FM, Davidson EM, Smith, MJH (1981). Isomer of leukotriene B_4 possess different biolo gical potencies. Prostaglandins 21:143.

Goetzl EJ, Pickett WC (1980). The human PMN leukocyte chemotactic activity of complex hydroxy-eicosatetraenoic acids (HETEs). J Immunol 125:1789.

Gryglewski R, Panczeko B, Korbut R, Grodzinska L, Ocetkiewicz A (1975). Corticosteroids inhibit prostaglandin release from perfused mesenteric blood vessels of rabbit and from perfused lungs of sensitized guinea pig. Prostaglandins 10:343.

Hamberg M, Svensson J, Samuelsson B (1975). Thromboxanes: A new group of biologically active compounds derived from prostaglandin endoperoxides. Proc Natl Acad Sci USA 72:2994.

Hammarström S, Murphy RC, Samuelsson B, Clark DA, Mioskowski C, Corey EJ (1979). Structure of leukotriene C. Identification of the amino acid part. Biochem Biophys Res Commun 91:1266.

Hammarström S, Samuelsson B, Clark DA, Goto G, Marfat A, Mioskowski C, Corey EJ (1980). Stereochemistry of leukotriene C-1. Biochem Biophys Res Commun 92:946.

Hammarström S (1981). Conversion of dihomo-γ-linolenic acid to an isomer of leukotriene C_3, oxygenated at C-8. J Biol Chem, in press.

Hammarström S, Bernström K, Örning L, Dahlén SE, Hedqvist P, Smedegård G, Revenäs B (1981). Rapid in vivo metabolism of leukotriene C_3 in the monkey. Biochem Biophys Res Commun, in press.

Hansson G, Rådmark O (1980). Leukotriene C_4: Isolation from human polymorphonuclear leukocytes. FEBS Lett 122:87.

Hedqvist P, Dahlén SE, Gustafsson L, Hammarström S, Samuelsson B (1980). Biological profile of leukotrienes C_4 and D_4. Acta Physiol Scand 110:331.

Hirata F, Axelrod J (1980). Phospholipid methylation and biological signal transmission. Science 209:1082.

Hirata F, Schiffmann E, Venkatasubramanian K, Salomon D, Axelrod J (1980). A phospholipase A_2 inhibitory protein in rabbit neturophils induced by glucocorticoids. Proc Natl Acad Sci USA 77:2533.

Hong SCL, Levine L (1976). Inhibition of arachidonic acid release from cells as the biochemical action of anti-inflammatory corticosterodis. Proc Natl Acad Sci USA 73:1730

Houglum J, Pai JK, Atrache V, Sok DE, Sih CJ (1980). Identification of the slow reacting substance from cat paws. Proc Natl Acad Sci USA 77:5688.

Johnson RA, Morton DR, Kinner JH, Gorman RR, McGuire JC, Sun FF, Whittaker N, Bunting S, Salmon J, Moncada S, Vane JR (1976). The chemical structure of prostaglandin X (Prostacyclin). Prostaglandins 12:915.
Jubiz W, Rådmark O, Lindgren JÅ, Malmsten C, Samuelsson B (1981). Novel leukotrienes: Products formed by initial oxygenation of arachidonic acid at C-15. Biochem Biophys Res Commun 99:976.
Kellaway CH, Trethewie ER (1940). The liberation of a slow-reacting smooth muscle-stimulating substance in anaphylaxis. Q J Ex Physiol 30:121.
Kuehl FA Jr, Humes JL, Ham EA, Egan RW, Dougherty HW (1980). Inflammation: The role of peroxidase-derived products. In Samuelsson B, Ramwell PW, Paoletti R (eds): "Adv in Prostaglandin and Thromboxane Research," New York: Raven Press, p 77.
Lewis RA, Drazen JM, Austen KF, Clark DA, Corey EJ (1980a). Identification of the C(6)-S-conjugate of leukotriene A with cysteine as a naturally occurring slow reacting substance of anaphylaxis (SRS-A). Importance of the 11-cis geometry for biological activity. Biochem Biophys Res Commun 96:271.
Lewis RA, Austen KF, Drazen JM, Clark DA, Marfat A, Corey EJ (1980b). Slow reacting substances of anaphylaxis: Identification of leukotrienes C-1 and D from human and rat sources. Prc Natl Acad Sci USA 77:3710.
Lindgren JÅ, Hansson G, Samuelsson B (1981). Formation of novel hydroxylated eicosatetraenoic acids in preparations of human polymorphonuclear leukocytes. FEBS Lett 128:329.
Lundberg U, Rådmark O, Malmsten C, Samuelsson B (1981). Transformation of 15-hydroperoxy-5,9,11,13-eicosatetraenoic acid into novel leukotrienes. FEBS Lett 126:127.
Malmsten CL, Palmblad J, Udén AM, Rådmark O, Engstedt L, Samuelsson B (1980). Leukotriene B_4: A highly potent and stereospecific factor stimulating migration of polymorphonuclear leukocytes. Acta Physiol Scand 110:449.
Marnett L, Wlodawer P, Samuelsson B (1975). Cooxygenation of organic substrates by the prostaglandin synthetase of sheep vesicular gland. J Biol Chem 250:8510.
Moncada S, Vane JR (1977). "The discovery of prostacyclin - a fresh insight into arachidonic acid metabolism, ed 2." New York: Academic Press Inc, p 155.
Morris HR, Taylor GW, Piper PJ, Sirois P, Tippins JR (1978). Slow-reacting substance of anaphylaxis. Purification and characterization. FEBS Lett 87:203.
Morris HR, Taylor GW, Piper PJ, Samhoun MN, Tippins JR (1980a). Slow reacting substances (SRSs): The structure identification of SRSs from rat basophilic leukemia (RBL-1) cells. Prostaglandins 19:185.

Morris HR, Taylor GW, Piper PJ, Tippins JR (1980b). Structure of slow reacting substance of anaphylaxis from guinea pig lung. Nature 285:104.

Murphy R, Hammarström S, Samuelsson B (1979). Leukotriene C: A slow-reacting substance from murine mastocytoma cells. Proc Natl Acad Sci USA 76:4275.

Oates JA, Roberts LJ II, Sweetman, BJ, Maas RL, Gerkens JF, Taber DF (1980). Metabolism of the prostaglandins and thromboxanes. In Samuelsson B, Ramwell PW, Paoletti R (eds): "Adv in Prostaglandin and Thromboxane Research," New York: Raven Press, p 35.

Orange RP, Austen KF (1969). Slow-reacting substance of anaphylaxis. Adv Immunol 10:104.

Orange RP, Murphy RC, Karnovsky ML, Austen KF (1973). The physicochemical characteristics and purification of SRS-A. J Immunol 110:760.

Örning L, Hammarström S, Samuelsson B (1980). Leukotriene D: A slow reacting substance from rat basophilic leukemia cells Proc Natl Acad Sci USA 77:2014.

Palmer RMJ, Stephney RJ, Higgs GA, Eakins KE (1980). Chemokinetic activity of arachidonic acid lipoxygenase products on leukocytes of different species. Prostaglandins 20:411.

Parker CW, Falkenhein SF, Huber MM (1980). Sequential conversion of the glutathionyl side chain of slow reacting substance (SRS) to cysteinyl-glycine and cysteine in rat basophilic leukemia cells stimulated with A-23187. Prostaglandin 20:863.

Rådmark O, Malmsten C, Samuelsson B, Clark DA, Giichi G, Marfat Corey EJ (1980a). Leukotriene A: Stereochemistry and enzymatic conversion to leukotriene B. Biochem Biophys Res Commun 92:954.

Rådmark O, Malmsten C, Samuelsson B, Goto G, Marfat A, Corey EJ (1980b). Leukotriene A: Isolation from human polymorphonuclear leukocytes. J Biol Chem 255:11828.

Rådmark O, Malmsten C, Samuelsson B (1980c). Leukotriene A_4: Enzymatic conversion to leukotriene C_4. Biochem Biophys Res Commun 96:1679.

Rouzer CA, Scott WH, Cohn ZA, Blackburn P, Manning JM (1980). Mouse peritoneal macrophages release leukotriene C in response to a phagocytotic stimulus. Proc Natl Acad Sci USA 77:4928.

Samuelsson B, Goldyne M, Granström E, Hamberg M, Hammarström S, Malmsten C (1978). Prostaglandins and thromboxanes. Ann Rev Biochem 47:997.

Samuelsson B, Borgeat P, Hammarström S, Murphy RC (1979). Introduction of a nomenclature: Leukotrienes. Prostaglandins 17:7

Samuelsson B, Hammarström S (1980). Nomenclature for leukotrienes. Prostaglandins 19:645.
Samuelsson B, Hammarström S, Murphy RC, Borgeat P (1980). Leukotrienes and slow reacting substance of anaphylaxis (SRS-A). Allergy 35:375.
Siegel MI, McConnell RT, Bonser RW, Cuatrecasas P (1981). The production of 5-HETE and leukotriene B in rat neturophils from carrageenan pleural exudates. Prostaglandins 21:123.
Smedegård G, Revenäs B, Hedqvist P, Dahlén SE, Hammarström S, Samuelsson B (1981). Cardiovascular and pulmonary effects of leukotriene C_4 in the monkey (Macaca Iris). Nature, submitted.
Vane JR (1971). Inhibition of prostaglandin synthesis as a mechanism of action for aspirin-like drugs. Nature (New Biol) 231:232.

Prostaglandins and Cancer: First
International Conference, pages 21-45
© 1982 Alan R. Liss, Inc., 150 Fifth Avenue, New York, NY 10011

INHIBITORS OF ARACHIDONIC ACID METABOLISM, WITH ESPECIAL
REFERENCE TO THE ASPIRIN-LIKE DRUGS

J.R. Vane, R.J. Flower and J.A. Salmon

Wellcome Research Laboratories
Langley Court
Beckenham, Kent BR3 3BS, UK

Prostaglandin research has been one of the fastest
growing fields in the biological sciences in the last few
years. Following the detection of prostaglandin activity in
the 1930's (Goldblatt, 1935; Euler, 1936) early landmarks were
the isolation and determination of the structure of the
primary prostaglandins (see Bergstrøm, 1966) and the
realization in 1964 that they are biosynthesized from
essential fatty acids (see Samuelsson, 1972) in almost all
animal cells. A strong impetus was given to the already
burgeoning field by the discovery some ten years ago that the
aspirin-like drugs prevent the biosynthesis of prostaglandins.
This gave both a biochemical basis for the therapeutic
activity of aspirin and a tool for studying further the
physiological and pathological importance of prostaglandins.
It has led (see Robinson and Vane, 1974; Ramwell, 1980) to
considerations of new uses for the aspirin-like drugs, as is
also evidenced by this Symposium.

Prostaglandins are thought to contribute to the
pathogenesis of many conditions including inflammation,
asthma, Bartter's syndrome, dysmenorrhoea, threatened
abortion, premature labour and cancer. Thus, compounds which
inhibit their formation have a wide therapeutic interest.
However, we now know much more about the metabolism of
arachidonic acid than we did in 1971. Many other metabolites
have been characterized as the products of several enzymic
reactions. Each metabolite has a distinct biological profile.
The metabolism of arachidonic acid is the subject of a review
elsewhere in this volume (Samuelsson, 1981) and so it is only
briefly considered here.

Arachidonic acid is metabolized as the free acid and yet it is largely present in the body in esterified form, primarily in the phospholipids of cell membranes. Therefore, the initial and rate limiting step in the biosynthesis of prostaglandins and related compounds is the enzymic liberation of arachidonic acid from the ester pools. The release of arachidonic acid from phospholipids is controlled by either phospholipase A_2 (Lands and Samuelsson, 1968; Vonkeman and Van Dorp, 1968; Kunze and Vogt, 1971; Flower and Blackwell, 1976; Blackwell et al, 1977) or the combined action of phospholipase C and a diglyceride lipase (Bell et al, 1979; Billah, Lapetina and Cuatrecasas, 1979; Lapetina and Cuatrecasas, 1979; Rittenhouse-Simmons, 1979).

Free arachidonic acid can be metabolized by the fatty acid cyclo-oxygenase ("prostaglandin synthetase") present in the microsomal fraction of most animal cells, to the prostaglandin endoperoxides (PGG_2 and PGH_2) which are subsequently converted either enzymically or non-enzymically to prostacyclin (PGI_2), thromboxane A_2 (TXA_2), the stable prostaglandins (PGE_2, $PGF_{2\alpha}$, PGD_2) and a 17-carbon acid, HHT (see Fig. 1). These products have different and frequently opposing pharmacological properties.

Lipoxygenase enzymes also convert free arachidonic acid to hydroperoxy derivatives (hydroperoxy eicosatetraenoic acid; HPETE). These can be reduced to the corresponding hydroxy acids (HETE) either enzymically (glutathione peroxidase) or non-enzymically. One hydroperoxy derivative, 5-HPETE, is of particular interest, for it can be converted to a novel group of compounds now known as leukotrienes . The initial enzymic reaction is the loss of water from 5-HPETE to form an unstable 5,6-epoxide referred to as leukotriene A (LTA_4). LTA_4 is pivotal in the formation of other leukotrienes; it is enzymically hydrolysed to a 5S,12R-dihydroxy acid in which one of three conjugated carbon-carbon double bonds has the <u>cis</u> configuration (LTB_4) or non-enzymically hydrolysed to other isomers of 5,12- and 5,6-dihydroxy acids. Additionally, glutathione can add to LTA_4 to form the 5-hydroxy-6-glutathionyl derivative (LTC_4) which may be further metabolised by gamma glutamyl transpeptidase to LTD_4 (a cysteinyl-glycine derivative). Another product, LTE_4 (containing only cysteine at carbon 6) has also been detected (see Fig. 1). It has not been confirmed whether LTD_4 or LTE_4 can be formed directly from LTA_4. Slow reacting substance in anaphylaxis (SRS-A) consists of a mixture of LTC_4 and LTD_4.

Figure 1

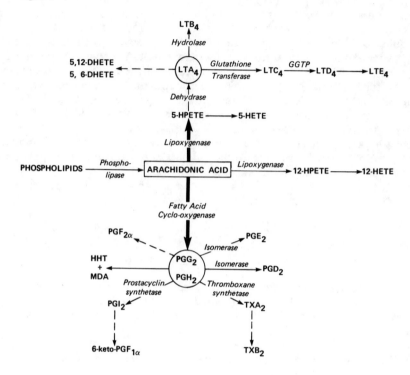

Pathways of arachidonic acid metabolism.

Thus, there are several enzymic reactions controlling arachidonic acid metabolism. In the following section we shall discuss the inhibitors of fatty acid cyclo-oxygenase in some detail. We shall then discuss inhibitors of lipoxygenase, thromboxane synthetase, prostacyclin synthetase and finally, phospholipase.

Inhibition of the Cyclo-oxygenase

An explanation of the therapeutic action of aspirin and its congeners has long been sought in terms of inhibition of a specific enzyme, or group of enzymes. Although these drugs inhibit a wide variety of organic reactions in vitro no convincing relationship could be established with their known anti-inflammatory, antipyretic and analgesic action. In 1971, Vane demonstrated that low concentrations of aspirin and indomethacin inhibited the enzymic production of prostaglandins. At the time of this discovery there was some evidence that prostaglandins participated in the pathogenesis of inflammation and fever, and this reinforced the suggestion that inhibition of prostaglandin biosynthesis could explain the clinical action of these drugs (see Ferreira and Vane, 1974; Ferreira and Vane, 1979; Moncada and Vane, 1979). In the years which have elapsed since the original observations a considerable body of evidence has accumulated which supports this hypothesis. Our knowledge about the inflammatory process has also increased, and the way in which prostaglandins participate in this process has been considerably clarified. The following points should be borne in mind:

a.   All mammalian cell types so far studied (with the possible exception of erythrocytes) have enzymes associated with the microsomal fraction which can synthesize prostaglandins.
b.   Prostaglandins are released when cells are damaged, and have been detected in increased quantities in inflammatory exudates. Cells do not store prostaglandins, so prostaglandin release depends on fresh biosynthesis.
c.   All the aspirin-like drugs (but not other classes) inhibit the biosynthesis and release of prostaglandins in all systems so far tested.

The inhibition of prostaglandin biosynthesis by aspirin and indomethacin was demonstrated simultaneously in three different systems: cell-free homogenates of guinea-pig lungs (Vane, 1971), dog perfused spleen (Ferreira, Moncada and Vane, 1971) and human platelets (Smith and Willis, 1971). In these pioneering experiments prostaglandin synthesis was quantitated biologically, but the basic findings have since been amply confirmed using a wide range of analytical techniques. Furthermore, there are hundreds of different systems in which inhibition of prostaglandin biosynthesis by aspirin, indomethacin or similar compounds has been demonstrated, so this effect is not restricted to any one species or tissue and can be seen in in vitro preparations of subcellular fractions, homogenates, or isolated organs and tissue slices, as well as in vivo. Thus, the effect is a general one depending, in vivo, only on the drug reaching the enzyme (see Flower, 1974). Clearly, the biodistribution and pharmacokinetics will have an important bearing on the activity of the drug (Graf, Glatt and Brune, 1975).

Inhibition of prostaglandin biosynthesis is a property peculiar to drugs of the aspirin type since many otherwise pharmacologically active agents are inactive against this enzyme system. This group of inactive compounds includes centrally acting analgesics (such as opiates), antihistamines, alpha- and beta-adrenoceptor blocking agents and antagonists of acetylcholine and 5-HT. The anti-inflammatory steroids are also inactive against the enzyme although they can also reduce prostaglandin production in other ways (see later).

The aspirin-like drugs inhibit or interfere with a variety of other enzymes and cellular systems; indeed there have been several attempts to explain their clinical effects by these actions. An objection to many of the proposals has been that the concentrations of drug required were unrealistically high. In fact, few of the other enzymes known to be susceptible to aspirin-like drugs are inhibited at concentrations which inhibit the synthetase, although inhibition of other enzymes could contribute to the toxic effects after an overdosage.

Any hypothesis which purports to explain the action of a drug in terms of an anti-enzyme action must satisfy at least two basic criteria. First, the free concentrations achieved in plasma during therapy must be sufficient to inhibit the enzyme in question. Secondly, there must be a reasonable correlation between the anti-enzyme activity and the therapeutic potency.

Certainly, there is good evidence that therapeutic dosage reduces prostaglandin biosynthesis in man. Therapeutic doses of aspirin or indomethacin inhibit prostaglandin production by human platelets and reduce the prostaglandin content of human semen. The most persuasive evidence, however, arises from the work of Hamberg (1972) who monitored the concentrations of the major metabolite of PGE_1 and PGE_2 in the urine of males and females before and after treatment with therapeutic doses of indomethacin, aspirin and salicylate. In females, almost maximal inhibition (63-92 per cent) of prostaglandin turnover was obtained after 1 day's treatment, whereas in males (who generally excreted more metabolite than females) the initial reduction was less, but the output continued to decline throughout the 3 day treatment period. Two days after treatment was discontinued the metabolite excretion had mostly returned to control levels. Indomethacin was the most potent, aspirin and salicylate each being some 15 times less active on a weight basis.

Table 1 also provides evidence to satisfy the criteria. There is a good rank-order correlation between the anti-enzyme activity and the anti-inflammatory activity.

Table 1 (from Flower RJ, Vane JR 1974)

I_{50} Concentrations (in μM) of some common aspirin-like drugs against PG synthetase

Compound	Dog spleen	Source of synthesis BSV	SSV
Melcofenamic acid		0.1	15
Niflumic acid	0.11	125	1.2
Indomethacin	0.17	34	0.5
Mefanamic acid	0.71	NT	2.1
Flufenamic acid	0.64	NT	2.5
Naproxen	NT	425	6.1
Phenylbutazone	7.25	1300	12.6
Ibuprofen	NT	2150	1.5
Aspirin	37.0	9500	83.0

NT = not tested

Other results also point to a close correlation between anti-inflammatory and anti-enzyme activity. Ham and his colleagues (1972) found a good correlation for individual members of a structurally-related group of aspirin-like drugs (except for the fenamates) and a reasonably good overall correlation. More interesting still was that the high degree of stereo specificity exhibited as anti-inflammatory agents in several pairs of enantiomers of alpha methyl aryl-acetic acids, was reflected in their anti-prostaglandin synthetase activity. In each instance the dextro-rotatory isomer was more potent than the levo-rotatory partner. Tomlinson and his colleagues (1972) obtained similar results with enantiomers of naproxen. Naproxen itself was 150 times as potent as aspirin against the synthetase from bovine seminal vesicles, and some 200 times more potent against adjuvant-induced arthritis in rats. The enantiomer of naproxen was much less potent against the synthetase (only twice as potent as aspirin) and had negligible activity in the arthritis test. Indomethacin in the arthritis test was 2000 times more potent than aspirin, and 2140 times more potent against the synthetase. Other workers have also investigated the anti-enzyme activity of several enantiomeric pairs of anti-inflammatory drugs and reported similar findings. The ability of prostaglandin synthetase to distinguish between dextro- and levo-rotatory isomers is a unique one, not shared when anti-inflammatory drugs are tested on other enzymes.

Another example of this type of discrimination is illustrated by the drug sulindac. This is a prodrug, weakly active in itself, but metabolised in vivo to a highly active anti-inflammatory metabolite. Likewise the drug itself has little intrinsic activity against prostaglandin biosynthesis, but the sulfide metabolite is a potent inhibitor.

The degree to which microsomal prostaglandin synthetase preparations from different tissues are inhibited by the aspirin-like drugs also varies considerably, and it is possible that the synthetase system (or at least one component protein) exists in multiple forms within the organism and that each has its own drug specificity. Results with acetaminophen (paracetamol) encourage this idea. Acetaminophen has analgesic and antipyretic effects but little anti-inflammatory activity. It has only weak activity against most cyclo-oxygenase preparations but is considerably more active in diminishing prostaglandin synthesis within the CNS (Flower and Vane, 1972). More recently, Whittle and his colleagues (1980) have shown that damage to the gastric mucosa by certain aspirin-like drugs could be correlated with their ability to inhibit mucosal cyclo-oxygenase. In doses which caused reduction of the prostaglandin content of an inflammatory exudate, aspirin and flurbiprofen seemed even more active on the enzyme in rat gastric mucosa. However, sodium salicylate and BW 755C (Higgs, Flower and Vane, 1979) did not affect mucosal cyclo-oxygenase activity in doses which reduced prostaglandins in inflammatory exudates.

Leukocyte migration into inflamed areas is an important component of inflammation. In doses which block prostaglandin biosynthesis the "classical" aspirin-like drugs - salicylates, pyrazolone derivatives, indomethacin etc. - do not inhibit the formation of products of the 5-lipoxygenase pathway, including the major chemotactic metabolite of arachidonic acid (LTB_4) and may even increase tissue levels. Indeed, treatment with some of these drugs enhances leukocyte infiltration in an experimental model (Higgs et al, 1980).

The mechanism by which the aspirin-like drugs exert their inhibitory effects varies; for example, aspirin acts by acetylating a serine residue at the active site of the cyclo-oxygenase (Roth and Majerus, 1975; Roth, Stanford and Majerus, 1975). Consequently, the inhibition of prostaglandin synthesis caused by aspirin is irreversible and prostaglandins can only be formed again as new enzyme is synthesised; thus aspirin-treated cells which are devoid of the biochemical machinery necessary to produce new protein (e.g. platelets) will be unable to synthesise prostaglandins for their entire life (8-11 days in the case of platelets). The dose required in man to inhibit platelet cyclo-oxygenase can be as little as 40 mg/day (Patrono, 1981). Other aspirin-like drugs have a different mode of action, but they all prevent the initial oxygen uptake and do not therefore, simply prevent the cyclization of an oxygenated intermediate. A model for the active site of the cyclo-oxygenase has been proposed (Gund and Shen, 1977) together with conformational analysis of indomethacin and other drugs which provide a stereo-specific structure-activity relationship of the enzyme, substrate and inhibitors. It has been established by the work of Lands and his co-workers (Smith and Lands, 1971; Lands et al, 1973) and Ku and Wasvary (1975)that the majority of non steroid anti-inflammatory drugs are "competitive, irreversible" inhibitors (see Flower, 1974; Lands and Rome, 1976). The inhibition is usually time dependent (Smith and Lands, 1971) and this appears to contradict the traditional concept of competitive inhibition. Several investigators have provided interpretations to reconcile this apparent paradox. For example, Lands and his co-workers (1973) have proposed that indomethacin binds to the enzyme not at the substrate site itself but rather at a position which reduces the affinity of the enzyme for the substrate.

Commonly used drugs which prevent prostaglandin synthesis by acting on the cyclo-oxygenase include aspirin, indomethacin, phenylbutazone, meclofenamic acid, ibuprofen and naproxen (see Nickander, McMahon and Ridolfo, 1979; Flower, Moncada and Vane, 1980).

Inhibition of Lipoxygenase

As information accumulates about the biological activities of the products of arachidonic acid metabolism via the lipoxygenase pathway, it is becoming increasingly clear that they probably play a role in the pathogenesis of several diseases. Leukotriene C_4 and LTD_4 (and possibly LTE_4) are the likely constituents of SRS-A (Murphy, Hammarstrøm and Samuelsson, 1979; Corey et al, 1980; Samuelsson, 1981). SRS-A causes prolonged contraction of bronchial smooth muscle and it has been suggested that it is an important mediator of symptoms in asthma and other hypersensitivity reactions (see Orange and Austen, 1969; Austen, 1978). The mono-hydroperoxy and hydroxy acids but especially the dihydroxy acid, LTB_4, are chemokinetic and chemotactic for leukocytes in vitro (Turner, Tainer and Lynn, 1975; Goetzl, Woods and Gorman, 1977; Goetzl and Sun, 1979; Ford-Hutchinson et al, 1980; Palmer et al, 1980) and in vivo (Carr et al, 1981; Smith, Ford-Hutchinson and Bray, 1980). Therefore these products may play a role in recruiting leukocytes to inflammatory sites. Indeed, some support for this hypothesis is provided by the finding that both 5-HETE and LTB_4 are present in high concentrations in synovial fluid from patients with rheumatoid arthritis (Klickstein, Shapleigh and Goetzl, 1980). Although the monohydroxy lipoxygenase products exhibit weaker chemokinetic activity they may still be of pathophysiological importance; for example 12-HETE has been detected in higher than normal levels in the psoriatic skin (Hammarstrøm et al, 1975). Therefore, inhibition of the synthesis of HPETE, HETE and the leukotrienes may be therapeutically advantageous and since all these products derive from lipoxygenase activity, it would seem desirable to inhibit this enzyme.

Highly specific inhibitors of the lipoxygenase are, as yet, unknown. Two compounds, the free radical scavenger nordihydroguaiaretic acid (Hamberg, 1976) and the substrate analogue 5,8,11-eicosatriynoic acid (Hammarstrøm, 1977) inhibit 12-HETE synthesis at doses lower than those required to inhibit the cyclo-oxygenase. A third compound, 15-HETE, which is itself formed from arachidonic acid by a lipoxygenase, has recently been claimed specifically to inhibit 12-HETE synthesis by platelets (Vanderhoek, Bryant and Bailey, 1980).

The foregoing data suggest that dual inhibitors of both cyclo-oxygenase and lipoxygenase would be valuable therapeutic agents. 5,8,11,14-eicosatetraynoic acid (ETYA) does block both enzymes with similar IC_{50} values (Hamberg and Samuelsson, 1974). However, its instability has precluded its use as an anti-inflammatory agent although it has been an effective experimental tool. A series of pyrazolidone derivatives inhibit both enzymes. The biochemical and biological properties of one, BW 755C (3-amino-1-,m-(trifluoromethyl)-phenyl.-2-pyrazoline), have been extensively investigated. It blocks the lipoxygenase of both platelets (Higgs, Flower and

Vane, 1979) and leukocytes (Radmark, Malmsten and Samuelsson, 1980; Randall et al, 1980) at similar doses to those required to inhibit the cyclo-oxygenase. Interestingly, Radmark et al (1980) demonstrated that the syntheses of 5-HETE, LTB_4 and SRS-A (all products of a "5-lipoxygenase") were more vulnerable to inhibition by BW 755C than was 15-HETE.

Using an animal model of inflammation (carrageenin-impregnated sponges implanted subcutaneously in rats) BW 755C was shown to be equi-active in reducing both the concentration of prostaglandins (measured as PGE_2) and the total number of leukocytes at the site of inflammation (Higgs, Flower and Vane, 1979). These activities were shared by a steroid, dexamethasone. However, although indomethacin selectively inhibited the production of prostaglandins it was subsequently shown to potentiate the cell numbers at low doses (Higgs et al, 1980). The interpretation of these data offered by the authors was that both dexamethasone and BW 755C inhibited production of both prostaglandins and lipoxygenase products (the decreased number of cells was presumed to be in part due to the reduction of chemotactic factors derived from lipoxygenase activity). It was suggested that low doses of indomethacin, which only blocked the cyclo-oxygenase, diverted substrate towards formation of chemotactic lipoxygenase products which accounted for the increased cell migration (Higgs, Flower and Vane, 1979). The simultaneous inhibition of both pathways achieved by BW 755C may provide a more effective type of anti-inflammatory drug without the complicating side effects exhibited by steroids. Such a drug would have advantages over the aspirin-like drugs in the treatment of chronic inflammation by having a greater effect on leukocyte migration.

The formation of SRS-A was also suppressed by BW 755C (Burka and Flower, 1979) which supported the then unproven hypothesis that SRS-A was a lipoxygenase product. As noted earlier, SRS-A causes prolonged contraction of bronchial smooth muscle and therefore may be a mediator of the symptoms associated with asthma and similar hypersensitivity reactions. Therefore, BW 755C may also provide an effective alternative to steroids in the treatment of asthma and already it has been shown to inhibit anaphylactic bronchoconstriction in guinea pigs (Nijkamp and Ramakers, 1980) and monkeys (Patterson, Pruzansky and Harris, 1981).

It has been claimed that other drugs may also be dual inhibitors of lipoxygenase and cyclo-oxygenase and these include benoxaprofen (Walker and Dawson, 1979).

Inhibition of Thromboxane Synthetase

Thromboxane A_2 is a powerful stimulant of platelet aggregation and indeed platelet aggregation is induced by agents such as collagen at least in part, through the formation of TXA_2 (see Moncada and Vane, 1978). On the other hand prostacyclin is the most potent, naturally occurring inhibitor of platelet aggregation yet discovered (Gryglewski et al, 1976; Moncada et al, 1976a). As both these compounds are derived by enzymic transformation of the prostaglandin endoperoxides (see Fig. 1) it follows that selective inhibition of the thromboxane synthetase may not only suppress the formation of TXA_2 but may also divert endoperoxide metabolism towards increased synthesis of prostacyclin. Theoretically, these properties should make specific inhibitors of thromboxane synthetase attractive as anti-thrombotic agents and consequently several groups of investigators have explored the possibility.

Various types of compound inhibit thromboxane synthetase. These include imidazole and 1-substituted analogues (Moncada et al, 1977; Blackwell et al, 1978b; Tai and Yuan, 1978), 2-iso-propyl-3-nicotyl indole (L8027) (Gryglewski et al, 1977), sodium p-benzyl-4,1-oxo-2-(4-chlorobenzyl)-3-propyl.phenyl phosphonate (N-0164) (Kulkarni and Eakins, 1976) and analogues of prostaglandin endoperoxides (for example, 9,11-iminoepoxyprosta-5,13-dienoic acid) (Fitzpatrick and Gorman, 1978; Fitzpatrick et al, 1979). However, several of these also inhibit cyclo-oxygenase and/or prostacyclin synthetase and would not, therefore, permit the augmentation of prostacyclin formation which is probably an important asset. Many analogues of imidazole are, however, both potent and selective inhibitors of thromboxane synthetase.

In a physiological situation, endoperoxide metabolism would be expected to be redirected towards prostacyclin. Indeed, such a diversion was observed in whole blood; a decreased amount of thromboxane but an increased synthesis of prostacyclin (analysed as its stable degradation product, 6-keto-$PGF_{1\alpha}$) was measured after addition of 1-n-butyl imidazole to blood in which aggregation of the platelets was induced with collagen or arachidonic acid (Blackwell et al, 1978c). In the latter experiments, prostacyclin was presumably formed by the leukocytes. Needleman, Wyche and Raz (1979) have demonstrated diversion of endoperoxide metabolism to prostacyclin when the TXA_2 formation by platelets in the presence of aortic microsomes (the latter being a source of prostacyclin synthetase) is prevented by imidazole.

Interestingly, Heersche and Jez (1981) have suggested, on the basis of the relative potencies of imidazole and two imidazole analogues on thromboxane synthetase, that bone resorption involves thromboxane A_2 formation.

Inhibition of Prostacyclin Synthetase

It is difficult to envisage situations in which it would be beneficial to inhibit prostacyclin synthesis although it could be useful to induce closure of the ductus arteriosus in premature infants, which may be kept patent by continuing prostacyclin synthesis. However, specific inhibitors are useful experimental tools in both biochemical and pharmacological investigations. Also, naturally occuring inhibitors may have a pathological relevance.

The 15-hydroperoxy derivative of arachidonic acid (initially called 15-HPAA although to retain a consistent nomenclature throughout this article, it will be abbreviated to 15-HPETE) inhibited prostacyclin synthesis (Moncada et al, 1976b) and thus provided an invaluable means of confirming the formation of prostacyclin in several in vitro experiments. Hydroperoxy derivatives of other fatty acids share the activity of 15-HPETE (Salmon et al, 1978) and since Harland et al (1972, 1973) have isolated cholesterol linoleate hydroperoxides from advanced atherosclerotic plaque it is attractive to speculate that the hydroperoxides in the plaque inhibit synthesis of prostacyclin, thereby giving rise to some of the symptoms (e.g. increased incidence of thrombosis) associated with atherosclerosis. This hypothesis also gives credence to the anti-thrombotic activity of vitamin E, an anti-oxidant, which would reduce lipid peroxidation thus permitting increased synthesis of prostacyclin.

Inhibition of Phospholipase Activity

The proposal that anti-inflammatory compounds exerted their effects by suppression of prostaglandin production (Vane, 1971) excluded anti-inflammatory steroids, for they did not affect the biosynthesis of prostaglandins by tissue homogenates or partially purified enzymes. This lack of effect initially hindered acceptance of the unifying simplistic concept that prostaglandins made an important contribution to the mediation of inflammation. However, in recent years, much data has been accumulated which demonstrates that glucocorticoids do, in fact, prevent the synthesis of prostaglandins but by a different mechanism from that of the non-steroid anti-inflammatory drugs.

Although steroids were ineffective in tissue homogenates, several groups of investigators demonstrated that prostaglandin biosynthesis was inhibited in whole animals, organs or tissues treated with steroids. Greaves and McDonald Gibson (1972) showed that steroids, albeit in high concentrations, inhibited prostaglandin biosynthesis in unseparated homogenates of rat skin and Eakins et al (1972) showed inhibition in ocular inflammation. This led to the suggestion that steroids somehow interfered with transport or release of prostaglandin precursors. Lewis and Piper (1975) proposed that steroids stopped the release of prostaglandins by preventing the transport from inside cells to the extracellular space but Herbaczynska-Cedro and Staszewska Barczak (1976) were the first to show in vivo that steroids inhibited prostaglandin generation, in this instance associated with muscular exercise in the hind legs of dogs.

Gryglewski and co-workers (1975) took up the story, using isolated mesenteric preparations. Hydrocortisone, dexamethasone and indomethacin inhibited the release of prostaglandins from the mesenteric bed following infusions of noradrenaline. Importantly, the inhibitory effects of hydrocortisone and dexamethasone but not of indomethacin were abolished if the preparation was supplemented by infusions of arachidonic acid. Gryglewski et al (1975) therefore concluded that the steroids owed their activity to limiting the availability of substrate, arachidonic acid, rather than affecting the release of prostaglandins. A similar explanation was proposed by Levine and co-workers (Kantrowitz et al, 1975; Tashjian et al, 1975; Hong and Levine, 1976; Tam, Hong and Levine, 1976) based on data derived from experiments using cell cultures. This implied that the effect of steroids may be directed at the phospholipase enzyme and this was confirmed by the finding that the rank order of potency of steroids as anti-inflammatory agents correlated well with their rank order as inhibitors of phospholipase activity whether the phospholipase activity was measured by bioassay (Nijkamp et al, 1976) or by a radiometric assay for phospholipase A_2 (Blackwell et al, 1978a).

How do corticosteroids inhibit phospholipase activity? Flower and Blackwell (1979) demonstrated that a "factor" was released from guinea pig lungs after treatment with steroids which could be transferred to a second lung made refractory to the actions of steroids by treatment with inhibitors of protein synthesis. The production of the "factor" was suppressed by treatment of the first "generator" lung with cycloheximide, puromycin (both inhibitors of protein synthesis) and/or actinomycin (an inhibitor of RNA synthesis). They concluded that the steroid-induced anti-phospholipase factor was probably due to induction of formation of a protein or peptide which exerted its action by a mechanism similar to that described for other effects of steroids (Thompson and Lippman, 1974). (Fig. 2). This mode of action was supported by similar data showing that the inhibition of prostaglandin synthesis caused by steroids could be markedly reduced by inhibitors of protein and/or RNA synthesis in rat renal papillary tissue (Danon and Assouline, 1978) rat reno-medullary interstitial cells grown in culture (Russo-Marie, Paing and Duval, 1979) and rat and rabbit leukocytes (Di Rosa and Persico, 1979; Hirata et al, 1980). Additional evidence is provided by the observation that the anti-inflammatory effects of steroids in vivo are also blocked by actinomycin D (Tsurufuji, Sugio and Takemasa, 1979).

Figure 2

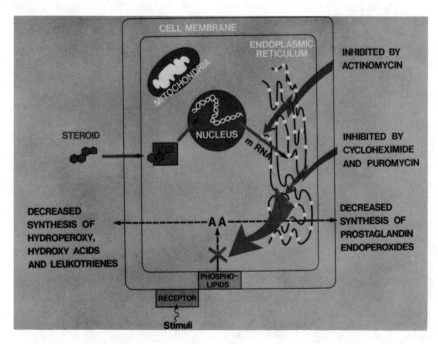

Mode of anti-inflammatory action of steroids.

The anti-inflammatory effects (e.g. inhibition of prostaglandin synthesis) of steroids can certainly be achieved at concentrations at which an action via specific steroid receptors is a feasible mechanism but it should be noted that some investigators have employed high doses of steroids to block prostaglandin synthesis in which case other effects on membrane function cannot be ignored.

The hypothesis that steroids exert their activity via the synthesis of a specific peptide also offers an explanation for the following: 1) the majority of investigators have reported a latency period after addition of steroid before prostaglandin production is affected (time is required for synthesis and/or release of the peptide factor through gene expression); 2) biosynthesis of prostaglandins in platelets, tissue homogenates or purified enzyme preparations is not blocked by steroids (the synthesis of new specific protein is not possible in these situations).

Blackwell et al (1980) have purified the factor (which they call macrocortin, and they have estimated that the molecular weight is approximately 15,000 although Hirata and co-workers (1980) have suggested a higher figure, 40,000 for a similar protein which they call lipomodulin. The latter group has demonstrated that the factor readily binds to serum albumin and concanavalin A resin, suggesting that it is a glycoprotein.

The effects of steroids cited above have, in most cases, been assessed by monitoring their ability to limit phospholipase A_2 activity, an enzyme which directly cleaves arachidonic acid from membrane phospholipids. However, there is some evidence (Bell et al, 1979; Billah, Lapetina and Cuatrecasas, 1979; Lapetina and Cuatrecasas, 1979; Rittenhouse-Simmons, 1979) that arachidonic acid may also be released by the combined action of phospholipase C and a diglyceride lipase. The effect of steroids on these latter enzymes is currently unknown although several serine esterase inhibitors do prevent mobilization of arachidonic acid and release of phosphatidic acid (i.e. inhibit phospholipase C activity) (Walenga, Vanderhoek and Feinstein, 1980). Also, the effect of steroids on other acylhydrolases which may liberate arachidonic acid from ester pools other than phospholipids has not been investigated.

The importance of the discovery that the anti-phospholipase activity of steroids is mediated by a soluble 'second messenger' is clear, for macrocortin or an active fragment may provide the anti-inflammatory (and indeed other activities mediated by inhibition of arachidonic acid metabolism) effects of steroids without the associated side effects of steroids.

There are relatively few reports of other inhibitors of phospholipase. Vargaftig and Dao Hai (1972) found that the release of rabbit aorta contracting substance (RCS; subsequently RCS was shown to be mainly comprised of thromboxane A_2) from lung tissue by bradykinin was diminished by mepacrine and inhibition of phospholipase A_2 was proposed as the underlying mechanism. The anti-phospholipase activity has been confirmed on isolated enzymes and mepacrine has therefore been used extensively as an experimental tool. Another anti-malarial, chloroquine, has a similar activity. p-bromophenacyl bromide and some local anaesthetics have also been reported to prevent fatty acid release via inhibition of phospholipase A_2 (Scherphof, Scarpa and Van Toorenenbergen, 1972; Waite and Sisson, 1972).

Finally, it should be emphasised that any interference with phospholipase activity will limit the synthesis of all metabolites of arachidonic acid (prostaglandins, prostacylin, thromboxane, HPETE, HETE and leukotrienes; see Fig. 1).

Summary

In this paper, the mechanisms by which drugs can inhibit the various enzymic reactions involved in the release and metabolism of arachidonic acid have been reviewed. The discovery that aspirin, indomethacin and other non-steroidal anti-inflammatory drugs inhibited the fatty acid cyclo-oxygenase and thereby suppressed the formation of prostaglandins provided an explanation for the anti-inflammatory acivities of these drugs. Inhibition of the cyclo-oxygenase was subsequently employed as the basis of developing other anti-inflammatory agents. Similarly, the mode of action of steroids could be explained by their ability to interfere with arachidonic acid metabolism; steroids induce the synthesis of an "anti-phospholipase" peptide which prevents the release of arachidonic acid from phospholipid stores and consequently inhibits the formation of arachidonic acid metabolites via both cyclo-oxygenase (prostacyclin, thromboxane, prostaglandins) and lipoxygenase (hydroperoxy and hydroxy acids, leukotrienes).

However, recent discoveries have extended our understanding of arachidonic acid metabolism which should now stimulate the development of new and improved therapeutic agents. For example, a "steroid-like" anti-inflammatory activity may be possible without the associated side effects of the steroids by "direct" inhibition of the cyclo-oxygenase and lipoxygenase (e.g. with BW 755C). Additionally, specific inhibition of thromboxane synthetase, allowing diversion of prostaglandin endoperoxide metabolism towards increased synthesis of prostacyclin, could form the basis of a screen for potential anti-thrombotic compounds.

REFERENCES

Austen KF (1978). Homeostasis effector systems which can also be recruited for immunologic reactions. J. Immunol 121:793-805.

Bell, RL, Kennerly DA, Stanford N, Majerus PW (1979). Diglyceride lipase: A pathway for arachidonate release from human platelets. In Samuelsson B, Ramwell P, Paoletti R (eds): "Advances in Prostaglandin and Thromboxane Research," Vol. 8. New York, Raven Press, p 219.

Bergström S (1966). The prostaglandins. Recent Prog Horm Res 22:153.

Billah MM, Lapetina EG, Cuatrecasas P (1979). Phosphatidylinositol-specific phospholipase C of platelets: association with 1,2-diacylglycerol-kinase and inhibition by cyclic AMP. Biochem Biophys Commun 90:92.

Blackwell GJ, Carnuccio R, Di Rosa M, Flower RJ, Parente L, Persico P (1980). Macrocortin: a polypeptide causing the anti-phospholipase effect of glucocorticoids. Nature 287:147.

Blackwell GJ, Duncombe WG, Flower RJ, Parsons MF, Vane JR (1977). The distribution and metabolism of arachidonic acid in rabbit platelets during aggregation and its modification by drugs. Br J Pharmac 59:353.

Blackwell GJ, Flower RJ (1978). 1-Phenyl-3-pyrazolidone: an inhibitor of cyclo-oxygenase and lipoxygenase pathways in lungs and platelets. Prostaglandins 16:417.

Blackwell GJ, Flower RJ, Nijkamp FP, Vane JR (1978a). Phospholipase A_2 activity of guinea pig isolated perfused lungs: stimulation, and inhibition by anti-inflammatory steroids. Br J Pharmacol 62:79.

Blackwell GJ, Flower RJ, Russell-Smith N, Salmon JA, Thorogood PB, Vane JR (1978b). 1-n-Butylimidazole: a potent and selective inhibitor of "thromboxane synthetase". Br J Pharmacol 64:435P.

Blackwell GJ, Flower RJ, Russell-Smith N, Salmon JA, Thorogood PB, Vane JR (1978c). Prostacyclin is produced in whole blood. Br J Pharmacol 64:436P.

Burka JF, Flower RJ (1979). Effects of modulators of arachidonic acid metabolism on the synthesis and release of slow-reacting substance of anaphylaxis. Br J Pharmacol 65:35.

Carr, SC, Higgs, GA, Salmon JA, Spayne JA (1981). The effects of arachidonate lipoxygenase products on leukocyte migration in rabbit skin. Br J Pharmacol 73:253P.

Corey EJ, Clark DA, Goto G, Marfat A, Mioskowski C, Samuelsson B, Hammarström S (1980). Stereospecific total synthesis of a slow reacting substance of anaphylaxis, leukotriene C-1. J Am Chem Soc 102:1436.

Danon A, Assouline G (1978). Inhibition of prostaglandin biosynthesis by corticosteroids requires RNA and protein synthesis. Nature 273:552.

Di Rosa M, Persico P (1979). Mechanism of inhibition of prostaglandin biosynthesis by hydrocortisone in rat leukocytes. Br J Pharmacol 66:161.

Eakins KE, Whitelocke RA, Bennett A, Martenet AC (1972). Prostaglandin-like activity in ocular inflammation. Br Med J 3:452.

Euler US von (1936). On the specific vasodilating and plain muscle stimulating substances from accessory glands in man and certain animals (prostaglandin and vesiglandin). J. Physiol (Lond) 88:213.

Ferreira SH, Moncada S, Vane JR (1971). Indomethacin and aspirin abolish prostaglandin release from the spleen. Nature New Biol 231:237.

Ferreira SH, Vane JR (1974). New aspects of the mode of action of non-steroid anti-inflammatory drugs. Ann Rev Pharmac 14:57.

Ferreira SH, Vane JR (1979). Mode of action of anti-inflammatory agents which are prostaglandin synthetase inhibitors. In Vane JR, Ferreira SH (eds): "Anti-inflammatory Drugs," Berlin: Springer-Verlag, p 348.

Fitzpatrick FA, Gorman RR (1978). A comparison of imidazole and 9,11-azoprosta-5,13-dienoic acid. Two selective thromboxane synthetase inhibitors. Biochim Biophys Acta 539:162.

Fitzpatrick FA, Gorman R, Bundy G, Honohan T, McGuire J, Sun, F (1979). 9,11-iminoepoxyprosta-5,13-dienoic acid is a selective thromboxane A_2 synthetase inhibitor. Biochim Biophys Acta 573:238.

Flower RJ (1974). Drugs which inhibit prostaglandin biosynthesis. Pharmac Revs 26:33.

Flower RJ, Blackwell GJ (1976). The importance of phospholipase A_2 in prostaglandin biosynthesis. Biochem Pharmac 25:285.

Flower RJ, Blackwell GJ (1979). Anti-inflammatory steroids induce biosynthesis of a phospholipase A_2 inhibitor which prevents prostaglandin generation. Nature 278:456.

Flower RJ, Moncada S, Vane JR (1980). Analgesic-antipyretics and anti-inflammatory agents; drugs employed in the treatment of gout. In Gilman AG, Goodman LS, Gilman A (eds): "Pharmacological Basis of Therapeutics," 6th Edition, New York: Macmillan Publishing Co, p 682.

Flower RJ, Vane JR (1972). Inhibition of prostaglandin synthetase in brain explains the anti-pyretic activity of paracetamol (4-acetamidophenol). Nature 240:410.

Flower RJ, Vane JR (1974). Inhibition of prostaglandin biosynthesis. Biochem Pharmacol 23:1439.

Ford-Hutchinson AW, Bray MA, Doig MV, Shipley ME, Smith MJH (1980). Leukotriene B, a potent chemokinetic and aggregating substance released from polymorphonuclear leukocytes. Nature 286:264.

Goetzl E, Sun FF (1979). Generation of unique mono-hydroxy eicosatetraenoic acids from arachidonic acid by human neutrophils. J Exp Med 150:406.

Goetzl EJ, Woods JM, Gorman RR (1977). Stimulation of human eosinophil and neutrophil polymorphonuclear leukocyte chemotaxis and random migration by 12-L-Hydroxy-5,8,10,14-eicosatetraenoic acid. J Clin Invest 59:179.

Goldblatt MW (1935). Properties of human seminal plasma. J Physiol (Lond) 84:208.

Graf P, Glatt M, Brune K (1975). Acidic nonsteroid anti-inflammatory drugs accumulating in inflamed tissue. Experientia 31:951.

Greaves MW, McDonald Gibson W (1972). Inhibition of prostaglandin biosynthesis by corticosteroids. Br Med J 2:83.

Gryglewski RJ, Bunting S, Moncada S, Flower RJ, Vane JR (1976). Arterial walls are protected against deposition of platelet thrombi by a substance (Prostaglandin X) which they make from prostaglandin endoperoxides. Prostaglandins 12:685.

Gryglewski RJ, Panczenko B, Korbut R, Grodzinska L, Ocetkiewicz A (1975). Corticosteroids inhibit prostaglandin release from perfused mesenteric blood vessels of rabbit and from perfused lungs of sensitized guinea pig. Prostaglandins 10:343.

Gryglewski RJ, Zmuda A, Korbut R, Krecioch E, Beiron K (1977). Selective inhibition of thromboxane A_2 biosynthesis in blood platelets. Nature 267:627.

Gund P, Shen TY (1977). A model for the prostaglandin synthetase cyclo-oxygenation site and its inhibition by anti-inflammatory arylacetic acids. J Med Chem 20:1146.

Ham EA, Cirillo VJ, Zanetti M, Shen TY, Kuehl FA Jr (1972). Studies on the mode of action of non-steroidal anti-inflammatory agents. In Ramwell PW, Phariss, BB (eds): " Prostaglandins in Cellular Biology," New York: Plenum Press p 343.

Hamberg M (1972). Inhibition of prostaglandin synthesis in man. Biochem Biophys Res Comm 49:720.

Hamberg M (1976). On the formation of thromboxane B_2 and 12L-hydroxy 5,8,10,14-eicosatetraenoic acid (12-ho-20:4) in tissues from the guinea pig. Biochim Biophys Acta 431:651.

Hamberg M, Samuelsson B (1974). Prostaglandin endoperoxides. Novel transformation of arachidonic acid in human platelets. Proc Natl Acad Sci USA 71:3400.

Hammarström S (1977). Selective inhibition of platelet n-8 lipoxygenase by 5,8,11-eicosatriynoic acid. Biochim Biophys Acta 487:517.

Hammarström S, Hamberg M, Samuelsson B, Duells EA, Stawski M, Voorhees JJ (1975). Increased concentrations of non-esterified arachidonic acid, 12L-hydroxy, 5,8,10,14-eicosatetraenoic acid, prostaglandin E_2 and prostaglandin $F_{2\alpha}$ in epidermis of psoriasis. Proc Natl Acad Sci USA 72:5130.

Harland WA, Gilbert JD, Brooks CJW (1973). Lipids of human atheroma VIII. Oxidised derivatives of cholesterol linoleate. Biochim Biophys Acta 316:378.

Harland WA, Gilbert JD, Steel G, Brooks CJW (1972). Lipids of human atheroma. Part 5. The occurance of a new group of polar sterol esters in various stages of human atherosclerosis. Atherosclerosis 13:239.

Heersche JNM, Jez DH (1981). The effect of imidazole and imidazole-analogues on bone resorption in vitro: a suggested role for thromboxane A_2. Prostaglandins 21:401.

Herbaczynska-Cedro K, Staszewska-Barczak J (1976).
Adrenocortical hormones and the release of prostaglandin-
like substances. Second Congress of the Hungarian
Pharmacological Society, Budapest, October 1976. Akademiai
Kiado, Budapest (Publishing House of the Hungarian Academy
of Sciences, p 157.
Higgs GA, Eakins KE, Mugridge KG, Moncada S, Vane JR (1980).
The effects of non-steroid anti-inflammatory drugs on
leukocyte migration in carrageenin-induced inflammation.
Eur J Pharmacol 66:81.
Higgs GA, Flower RJ, Vane JR (1979). A new approach to anti-
inflammatory drugs. Biochem Pharmac 28:1959.
Hirata F, Schiffmann E, Venkatasubramanian K, Salomon D,
Axelrod J (1980). A phospholipase A_2 inhibitory protein
in rabbit neutrophils induced by glucocorticoids. Proc
Natl Acad Sci USA 77:2533.
Hong SL, Levine L (1976). Inhibition of arachidonic acid
release from cells as the biochemical action of anti-
inflammatory corticosteroids. Proc Natl Acad Sci USA
73:1720.
Kantrowitz F, Robinson DR, McGuire MB, Levine L (1975).
Corticosteroids inhibit prostaglandin production by
rheumatoid synovia. Nature 258:737.
Klickstein LB, Shapleigh T, Goetzl EJ (1980). Unique
products of the oxygenation of arachidonic acid in synovial
fluid in rheumatoid arthritis and spondylarthritis. Arth
Rheum 23:704.
Ku EC, Wasvary JM (1975). Inhibition of prostaglandin
synthetase by piroprofen: studies with sheep vesicle
enzyme. Biochim Biophys Acta 384:360.
Kulkarni PS, Eakins KE (1976). N-0164 inhibits generation of
thromboxane A_2-like activity from prostaglandin
endoperoxides by human platelet microsomes. Prostaglandins
12: 465.
Kunze H, Vogt W (1971). Significance of phospholipase A for
prostaglandin formation. Ann NY Acad Sci 180:123.
Lands WEM, Rome LH (1976). Inhibition of prostaglandin
biosynthesis. In Karim SMM (ed): "Prostaglandins: Chemical
and Biochemical Aspects," Lancaster: MTP Press, p 87.
Lands WEM, Samuelsson B (1968). Phospholipid precursors of
prostaglandins. Biochim Biophys Acta 164:426.
Lands WEM LeTellier PR Rome LH Vanderhoek JY (1973).
Inhibition of prostaglandin biosynthesis. In Bergström S,
Bernhard S (eds): "Advances in the Biosciences," Vol. 9,
Oxford: Pergamon Press, p 15.

Lapetina EG, Cuatrecasas P (1979). Stimulation of phosphatidic acid production in platelets precedes the formation of arachidonate and parallels the release of serotonin. Biochim Biophys Acta 573:394.

Lewis GP, Piper PJ (1975). Inhibition of release of prostaglandins as an explanation of some of the actions of anti-inflammatory corticosteroids. Nature 254:308.

Moncada S, Bunting S, Mullane KM, Thorogood P, Vane JR (1977). Imidazole: a selective potent antagonist of thromboxane synthetase. Prostaglandins 13:611.

Moncada S, Gryglewski RJ, Bunting S, Vane JR (1976a). An enzyme isolated from arteries transforms prostaglandin endoperoxides to an unstable substance that inhibits platelet aggregation. Nature 263:663.

Moncada S, Gryglewski RJ, Bunting S, Vane JR (1976b). A lipid peroxide inhibits the enzyme in blood vessel microsomes that generates from prostaglandin endoperoxides the substance (Prostaglandin X) which prevents platelet aggregation. Prostaglandins 12:715.

Moncada S, Vane JR (1978) Unstable metabolites of arachidonic acid and their role in haemostasis and thrombosis. Brit Med Bull 34:129.

Moncada S, Vane JR (1979). Mode of action of aspirin-like drugs. In Stollerman GH (ed): "Advances in Internal Medicine," vol. 24, Memphis: Year Book Medical Publishers Inc, p 1.

Murphy RC, Hammarström S, Samuelsson B (1979). Leukotriene C: a slow reacting substance from murine mastocytoma cells. Proc Natl Acad Sci USA 76:4275.

Needleman P, Wyche A, Raz A (1979). Platelet and blood vessel arachidonate metabolism and interactions. J Clin Invest 63:345.

Nickander R, McMahon FG, Ridolfo AS (1979). Nonsteroidal anti-inflammatory agents. Ann Rev Pharmac Toxicol 19:469.

Nijkamp FP, Flower RJ, Moncada S, Vane JR (1976). Partial purification of rabbit aorta contracting substance releasing factor and inhibition of its activity by anti-inflammatory steroids. Nature 263:479.

Nijkamp FP, Ramakers AGM (1980). Prevention of anaphylactic bronchoconstriction by a lipoxygenase inhibitor. Eur J Pharmacol 62:121.

Orange RP, Austen KF (1969): Slow-reacting substance of anaphylaxis. Adv Immunol 10:105.

Palmer RJ, Stepney R, Higgs GA, Eakins KE (1980): Chemokinetic activity of arachidonic acid lipoxygenase products on leukocytes from different species. Prostaglandins 20:411.

Patrono C (1981). Personal communication.
Patterson R, Pruzansky JJ, Harris KE (1981). An agent which releases basophil and mast cell histamine but blocks cyclo-oxygenase and lipoxygenase metabolism of arachidonic acid inhibits IgE mediated asthma in rhesus monkeys. J Allergy Clin Immunol. (In press).
Radmark O, Malmsten C, Samuelsson B (1980). The inhibitory effects of BW755C on arachidonic acid metabolism in human polymorphonuclear leukocytes. FEBS Lett 110:213.
Ramwell P (1980). "Prostaglandin Synthetase Inhibitors: New Clinical Applications," New York: Alan R Liss Inc.
Randall RW, Eakins KE, Higgs GA, Salmon JA, Tateson JE (1980). Inhibition of arachidonic acid cyclo-oxygenase and lipoxygenase activities of leukocytes by indomethacin and compound BW755C. Agents and Actions 10:553.
Rittenhouse-Simmons J (1979). Production of diglyceride from phosphatidylinositol in activated human platlets. J Clin Invest 63:580.
Robinson HJ, Vane JR (1974). "Prostaglandin Synthetase Inhibitors: their Effects on Physiological Function and Pathological States," New York: Raven Press.
Roth GJ, Majerus PW (1975). The mechanism of the effect of aspirin on human platelets. J Clin Invest 56:624.
Roth GJ, Stanford N, Majerus PW (1975). Acetylation of prostaglandin synthetase by aspirin. Proc Natl Acad Sci USA 72:3073.
Russo-Marie F, Paing M, Duval D (1979). Involvement of glucocorticoid receptors in steroid-induced inhibition of prostaglandin secretion. J Biol Chem 254:8498.
Salmon JA, Smith DR, Flower RJ, Moncada S, Vane JR (1978). Further studies on the enzymatic conversion of prostaglandin endoperoxides into prostacyclin by porcine aorta microsomes. Biochim Biophys Acta 523:250.
Samuelsson B (1972). Biosynthesis of prostaglandins. Fed Proc 31:1442.
Samuelsson B (1981). See this volume.
Scherphof GL, Scarpa A, Van Toorenenbergen A (1972). The effect of local anaesthetics on the hydrolysis of free and membrane-bound phospholipids catalyzed by various phospholipases. Biochim Biophys Acta 270:226.
Smith JB, Willis AL (1971). Aspirin selectively inhibits prostaglandin production in human platelets. Nature (New Biol) 231:235.
Smith, MJH, Ford-Hutchinson AW, Bray MA (1980). Leukotriene B: a potent mediator of inflammation. J Pharm Pharmacol 32:517.

Smith WL, Lands WEM (1971). Stimulation and blockade of the prostaglandin biosynthesis. J Biol Chem 246:6700.

Tai H-H, Yuan B (1978). On the inhibitory potency of imidazole and its derivatives on thromboxane synthetase. Biochim Biophys Acta 80:236.

Tam S, Hong S-C, Levine L (1976). Inhibition of arachidonic acid release from cells as the biochemical action of anti-inflammatory corticosteroids. Proc Natl Acad Sci USA 73:1730.

Tashjian AH, Voelkel EF, McDonough J, Levine L (1975): Hydrocortisone inhibits prostaglandin production by mouse fibrosarcoma cells. Nature 258:739.

Thompson EB, Lippman ME (1974). Mechanism of action of glucocorticoids. Metabolism 23:159.

Tomlinson RV, Ringold HJ, Qureshi MC, Forchielli E (1972). Relationship between inhibitors of prostaglandin synthesis and drug efficacy: support for the current theory on mode of action of aspirin-like drugs. Biochem Biophys Res Commun 46:552.

Tsurufuji S, Sugio K, Takemasa F (1979). The role of glucocorticoid receptor and gene expression in the anti-inflammatory action of dexamethasone. Nature 280:408.

Turner SR, Tainer JA, Lynn WS (1975). Biogenesis of chemotactic molecules by the arachidonate lipoxygenase system of platelets. Nature 257:680.

Vanderhoek JY, Bryant RW, Bailey JM (1980). 15-Hydroxy-5,8,11,13-eicosatetraenoic acid. A potent and selective inhibitor of platelet lipoxygenase. J Biol Chem 255:5996.

Vane JR (1971). Inhibition of prostaglandin synthesis as a mechanism of action for aspirin-like drugs. Nature New Biol 231:232.

Vargaftig BB, Dao Hai N (1972). Selective inhibition by mepacrine of the release of rabbit aorta contracting substance evoked by the administration of bradykinin. J Pharm (Lond) 24:159.

Vonkeman H, Van Dorp DA (1968). The action of prostaglandin synthetase on 2-arachidonyl lecithin. Biochim Biophys Acta 164:430.

Waite M, Sisson P (1972). Effect of local anaesthetics on phospholipases from mitochondria and lysosomes. A probe into the role of calcium ion in phospholipid hydrolysis. Biochemistry 11:3098.

Walenga R, Vanderhoek JY, Feinstein MB (1980). Serine esterase inhibitors block stimulus-induced mobilization of arachidonic acid and phosphatidylinsitide-specific phospholipase C activity in platelets. J Biol Chem 255:6024.

Walker JR, Dawson W (1979). Inhibition of rabbit PMN lipoxygenase activity by benoxaprofen. J Pharm Pharmacol 31:778.

Whittle BJR, Higgs GA, Eakins KE, Moncada S, Vane JR (1980). Selective inhibition of prostaglandin production in inflammatory exudates and gastric mucosa. Nature 284:271.

Prostaglandins and Cancer: First International Conference, pages 47–65
© 1982 Alan R. Liss, Inc., 150 Fifth Avenue, New York, NY 10011

THE MOLECULAR BASIS OF THE PHARMACOLOGY OF THE ARACHIDONATE METABOLITES

P.W. Ramwell, J.W. Karanian and M.L. Foegh

Departments of Physiology and Biophysics
and of Medicine
Georgetown University Medical Center
Washington, DC 20007 USA

INTRODUCTION

The objective of this chapter is to attempt to provide for members of the Conference a simplified working concept of the pharmacology of the prostaglandins and their associated arachidonate metabolites. This objective was first attempted in 1966 by Horton and Main who studied seven prostaglandins of which three were PGE and four were PGF compounds. At that time they focussed on the structure activity relationships. In particular they studied the effects of and isomerism of the PGF compounds at C-9, different degrees of unsaturation at C-5,6, C-13,14 and C-17,18, and finally the differences between the 9-keto and the 9-hydroxy function which differentiates the prostaglandins of the E from the F series. Attempts to classify prostaglandin effects based on two receptors proved to be premature due to the rapid discovery of more natural products and the description of many more analogs. Moreover, as the primary prostaglandins were made more available, an incredible range of effects began to be described in the literature.

Now we are reconciled to the knowledge that few if any cells are unaffected by prostaglandins and that arachidonic acid yields many more other oxygenated products in addition to the prostaglandins. However, it was against the earlier background that in 1969, at the Laurentian Hormone Conference, we showed it was possible to classify the action of nearly all the prostaglandins then known, as falling into two categories. These categories are those pharmacological effects which relate to adenylate cyclase and those which involve calcium influx (Ramwell and Shaw, 1970).

Paradoxically, the discovery of so many new arachidonate products as the thromboxanes (TX), prostacyclins (PGI) and the complex family of leukotrienes (LT) which have an even more extensive range of activity, has made the situation more understandable since the trends can now be readily perceived. Thus it is possible to extend this concept of a dual mechanism of action to the whole range of arachidonate products and to make the idea more comprehensive.

DUAL MECHANISM OF ACTION OF ARACHIDONATE PRODUCTS

Many of the effects of prostaglandins on the function of transporting epithelia, gastric secretion, lipolysis, anterior pituitary hormone release and other endocrine systems have been documented as being related to the generation of cyclic AMP. For example, PGE_2 mimicks the effects of both TSH on the thyroid and LH on the corpus luteum. These aspects have been appraised elsewhere (Flack et al, 1971; Ramwell and Rabinowitz, 1971). Similarly, the relaxation of the four types of smooth muscle eg. airway, vascular, alimentary and reproductive is also related to adenylate cyclase activation and the resulting intracellular accumulation of cyclic AMP. The order of effectiveness of the arachidonate metabolites to activate adenylate cyclase and relax smooth muscle in general appears can be ranked as follows:
$$PGI_2 : PGE_2 : PGD_2 : PGF_{2a} : TXA_2 : LT_4.$$
This is also the order of increasing effectiveness of these compounds as contractile agonists. TXA_2 and LT do not have an appreciable effect in promoting relaxation of smooth muscle as far as we are aware.

PGI_2 possesses the unusual property of relaxing most types of smooth muscle with only few exceptions. These exceptions are so few as to be remarkable and are delineated in table 1. PGI_2 is a powerful activator of adenylate cyclase and presumably this and or a reduction in intracellular calcium is the mechanism leading to relaxation (Greenberg, 1981). However the contraction of

TABLE I

PARADOXICAL EFFECTS OF PROSTACYCLIN IN VASCULAR SMOOTH MUSCLE

PREPARATION	SPECIES	EFFECT (UG/ML)	REFERENCE
CORONARY ARTERY	MAN	RELAXATION (<0.3) CONTRACTION (>0.3)	1
"	PIG	CONTRACTION (>0.4)	2
AORTA	RAT	CONTRACTION (>0.5)	3
"	RABBIT	CONTRACTION (>1.0)	4
UMBILICAL ARTERY	MAN	RELAXATION (<0.3) CONTRACTION (>0.3)	5
PULMONARY ARTERY	RABBIT	VARIABLE (0.01-1.0)	6
BASILAR ARTERY	DOG	RELAXATION (<0.03) CONTRACTION (>3.0)	7
PORTAL VEIN	RAT	CONTRACTION (>0.1)	8
VENA CAVA	RAT	CONTRACTION (>0.5)	8

1. Ginsburg, R., Bristow, M.R., Harrison, D., Stinson, E.B.,; Studies With Isolated Human Coronary Arteries; Chest, 78:1 Supplement 1980, p. 180-186. 2. Dusting, G., Moncada, S. and Vane J.R.; Prostacyclin (PGI_2) is a weak contractor of coronary arteries of the pig, Europ. J. Pharmacol. 45:301, 1977. 3. Levy, J.V.; Prostacyclin-Induced Contraction of Isolated Aortic Strips From Normal and Spontaneously Hypertensive Rats (SHR); Prostaglandins, 19:4, 517-529,1980 4. Omini, G., Moncada, S. and Vane, J.R.; The Effects of Prostacyclin (PGI_2) on Tissues Which Detect Prostaglandins (Pgs). Prostaglandins 14:625, 1977. 5. Pomerantz, Sintetos, A., and Ramwell, P.W.; The Effect of Prostacyclin on the Human Umbilical Artery. Prostaglandins 15:6, 1035-1044, 1978. 6. Salzman, P.M., Salman, J.A. and Moncada, S.. Prostacyclin and Thromboxane A_2 Synthesis by Pulmonary Artery. J. Pharmacol. Exp. Ther. 215:240-247, 1980. 7. Chapleau, C. and White R.; Effects of Prostacyclin on the Canine Isolated Basilar Artery. Prostaglandins 17:573, 1979. 8. Levy, J.V.: Contractile Response of Human Saphenous and Rat Venous Tissue. Prostaglandins 16:93, 1978.

venous tissue, pulmonary and some coronary arteries at very high doses of PGI_2 is presumably due to calcium influx resulting from PGI_2 binding to a low affinity receptor of another arachidonate product.

In marked contrast, at the opposite end of the sequence, is thromboxane and its stable analog mimics such as 9a ,11a-epoxymethanoprostaglandin H_2 which contract nearly all types of smooth muscle. We think that this general spasmogemic property of TXA_2 is shared also by the leukotrienes. We have summarized the published data for vascular (table 2), airway (table 3) and alimentary smooth muscle (table 4). Some of the effects of leukotrienes are mediated by release of cyclo-oxygenase products. Consequently to determine the effects of the leukotrienes per se it is necessary to employ a cyclo-oxygenase inhibitor such as indomethacin as shown in tables 2-4. Confirmation of the action of leukotrienes is obtained with the FPL receptor antagonists or by interdicting thromboxane release by imidazoles. Figure 1 illustrates the effect of leukotrienes LTC_4 and LTD_4 on the release of cyclo-oxygenase products from rat peritoneal macrophages (Feuerstein et al, 1981).

The intermediate members of the arachidonate product sequence, such as PGE_2, contract or relax smooth muscle depending upon the nature of the tissue and on the circumstances. One of the circumstances, as Vogt (1963) originally suspected involves the pool of loosely bound extracellular calcium and its subsequent influx. Paton and Daniel (1967) were some of the first to show the unusual dependence of prostaglandins, as a class of oxytoxic agents, on extracellular calcium. The wide-ranging effectiveness of prostaglandins and the thromboxane-mimics such as 9a ,11a-epoxymethanoprostaglandin H_2 in contracting vascular tissue appears to be related to their effectiveness to use this extracellular calcium pool (Loutzenhizer and Van Breemen, 1980). This dependence is in sharp contrast to other agonists such as norepinephrine, which uses mainly the intracellular calcium pool. It seems likely that this finding may also apply to intestinal, reproductive and possibly airway muscle. The effectiveness of thromboxane and its mimics in permitting influx from the loosely bound extracellular calcium has lead to use of the term "calcium ionophore" to describe the actions of these compounds on platelets and other cells (Gerrard et al, 1978).

There is in fact some evidence that TXA_2 mimics inhibit adenylate cyclase in platelets by permitting calcium influx. We have alluded to this potential role of calcium in inhibiting adenylate cyclase in another situation namely epinephrine stimulated lipolysis and the antidiuretic effects of vasopressin both of which are mediated by cyclic-AMP (Ramwell and Shaw, 1970). In both circumstances PGE_1 has the unusual action of inhibiting the hormonally-elicited increase in cyclic-AMP. We suggest that PGE_1 in these tissues increases calcium influx as it might in eliciting a contractile response from smooth muscle. PGE_1 does not inhibit adenylate cyclase in adipocyte cell membrane preparations which suggests it may indeed be acting by promoting calcium influx.

One approach to the problem was made by Kury et al, (1974 and 1975) who studied the effect of PGE_1 and PGE_2 on the fluidity of human erythrocytes by using a spin-label fatty acid probe and measuring changes in electron paramagnetic resonance. PGE_1 and PGE_2 (10^{11}M) had opposite effects on the fluidity of the membrane and both required external calcium. It was concluded that PGE_1 and PGE_2 differentially affected the ratio of bound and free calcium which modifies the phosphorylation of the erythrocyte cytoskeletal protein, spectrin. These experiments demonstrate in a cell deficient of adenylate cyclase that prostaglandins influence intracellular calcium.

STEREOISOMERISM AND MOLECULAR CONFORMATION

The prostaglandin and leukotriene molecules are exceptional in possessing many assymmetric centers which permits the synthesis of an unusually large number of stereoismers. Chemical reduction of PGE_2 produces PGF_{1a} together with its C-9-epimer, PGF_{1b}. The C-9 epimer shows about 5% of the potency of the natural isomer. Figure 1 shows the C-9 and the other four asymmetric centers at C-8, C-11, C-12 and C-15); thus even in this simple prostaglandin, 32 isomers are possible, excluding the double-bound isomerizations. The success in the total synthesis of prostaglandins by E.J. Corey and his colleagues and the further developments by N. Andersen allowed us to test a large number of diastereomers and formulate the hair-pin conformation hypothesis (Rabinowitz et al, 1971). This chiral conformation provides a rationale for the diasteromer structure activity data (Ramwell and Rabinowitz, 1972). The hair-pin conformation is shown in figure 2 where it will be seen that the three

TABLE 2

VASCULAR SMOOTH MUSCLE RESPONSE TO LEUKOTRIENE AND ITS INHIBITION

PREPARATION	SPECIES	LEUKOTRIENE	EFFECT	INHIBITION	REFERENCE
PERFUSED LUNG	GP	B4,C4	PROSTAGLANDIN + TXA$_2$ RELEASE	FPL55712* INDOMETHACIN †	1
SKIN MICROVASCULATURE	GP	SRS-A B4,C4	CONSTRICTION	INDOMETHACIN	2,3,4,5
"	GP	C1,D	CONSTRICTION		6
"	RAT,RABBIT	C4	CONSTRICTION		4
(CHEEK POUCH)	GP	A4,B4	CONSTRICTION		7
"	HAMSTER	C4,D4	CONSTRICTION		7,8
PULMONARY ARTERY	MAN	C4,D4	CONTRACTION		9
(ARTERY)	GP	C4,D4	CONTRACTION		10
CORONARY FLOW	GP	SRS-A C4,D4	DECREASE	FPL55712 (D4)§ INDOMETHACIN IMIDAZOLE¶(C4)§	3,11,12
PRE-CONTRACTED (K$^+$) CORONARY ARTERY	GP	C4,D4	RELAXATION	INDOMETHACIN	12
BLOOD PRESSURE	GP	C4	INCREASE→DECREASE	FPL55712 INDOMETHACIN	13
"	GP	C1,D4	INCREASE→DECREASE W/OUT ANESTHESIA DECREASE W/ANESTHESIA		6
"	RABBIT	C4,D4	DECREASE		4
"	MONKEY	C4,D4	DECREASE		14

*LEUKOTRIENE RECEPTOR ANTAGONIST †CYCLO-OXYGENASE INHIBITOR ¶THROMBOXANE SYNTHETASE INHIBITOR
§INHIBITION WAS LIMITED TO THE DESIGNATED LEUKOTRIENE

1. Sirois, P., Borgeat, P., Jeanson, A., Roy, S. and Girard, G.; The Action of Leukotriene B$_4$ (LTB$_4$) on the Lung. Prostaglandins and Medicine 5, 429-444, 1980. 2. Deck, M.J., Piper, P.J., and Williams, T.J.; The Effect of Leukotrienes C$_4$ and D$_4$ on the Microvasculature of Guinea Pig Skin. Prostaglandins 21(2), 315-321, 1981. 3. Letts, L.G., Piper, P.J.; Cardiac Actions of Leukotrienes C$_4$ and D$_4$; International Symposium on Leukotrienes and other Lypoxygenase Products: Florence, Italy, 1981 *. 4. Katori, M., Akinori, U. and Tanaka, K.; Negligable Response of Rabbit Skin in Increased Vascular Permeability to Synthetic Leukotrienes *. 5. Piper, P.J.; Pharmacological Actions of SRS-A and the Leukotrienes *. 6. Drazen, J.M., Austen, K.E., Lewis, R.A., Clark, D.A., Goto, G., Marafat, A. and Corey, E.J.; Comparative Airway and Vascular Activities of Leukotrienes C-1 and D in vivo and in vitro. Proc. Natl. Acad. Sci. USA 77(7), 4354-8, 1980. 7. Hedquist, P.; Pulmonary and Microvascular Effects of the Leukotrienes *. 8. Bjork, J., Pahlen, S., Hedquist, P. and Arfors, K.; Microvascular Effects of Leukotrienes *. 9. Hanna, C.J., Bach, M.K., Pars, P.J. and Schellenberg, R.R.; Slow Reacting Substances (Leukotrienes) Contract Human Airway and Vascular Smooth Muscle in vitro. Nature 290, 343-4, 1981. 10. Gleason, J.G., Krell, R.D., Ali, F.E., Veichman, B.M. and Berkowitz, B.; Synthesis and Comparative Pharmacology of Leukotrienes C$_4$ and D$_4$ on Airway and Vascular Smooth Muscle: Antagonism by a Novel Leukotriene Antagonist *. 11. Levi, R.; SRS-A, Leukotrienes and Immediate Hypersensitivity Reaction of the Heart *. 12. Burke, J.A., Levi, R., Rouzer, C.A., Scott, W.A. and Corey, E.J.; Cardiovascular Effects of "Slow Reacting Substances" derived from Anaphylactic Guinea Pig Lung and Resident Mouse Peritoneal Macrophages: Comparison with Effects of Pure Synthetic Leukotrienes C & D *. 13. Omini, C., Rossoni, G., Folco, G.C. and Berti, F.; Leukotriene C$_4$ causes Cardiovascular and Respiratory Effects in Guinea Pig that are dependent on PGI$_2$ and TXA$_2$ Formation *. 14. Casey, L., Clark, J., Ramwell, P.W. and Fletcher, J.; Cardiovascular and Respiratory Effect of Intravenous Leukotrienes in Primates *.
* International Symposium on Leukotrienes and Other Lipoxygenase Products: Florence, Italy, 1981.

TABLE 3

AIRWAY SMOOTH MUSCLE RESPONSE TO LEUKOTRIENE AND ITS INHIBITION

PREPARATION	SPECIES	LEUKOTRIENE	EFFECT	INHIBITION	REFERENCE
PARENCHYMAL STRIP	GP	B4	CONTRACTION	INDOMETHACIN[*] IMIDAZOLE [†]	1,15,16,17
"	GP	C1,D	CONTRACTION	FPL55712[¶](D)[§]	6
"	GP	C4,D4,E4	CONTRACTION	SK+F88046[¶](D4)[§] FPL55712 INDOMETHACIN ASPIRIN (C4,D4)	9,10,16
"	GP	A4	CONTRACTION		16
"	MAN	C4,D4	CONTRACTION		5,9,18,19
BRONCHI	GP,RAT	E4	CONTRACTION	FPL55712 INDOMETHACIN	21
"	GP	C4,D4	CONTRACTION	FPL55712 INDOMETHACIN ASPIRIN	7,10,16,21
"	MAN	C4,D4	CONTRACTION	FPL55712 FPL59257	7,9,16,18,19,22,23
TRACHEA	GP	C1,D	CONTRACTION	FPL55712	6,19,22,24
"	GP	C4,D4	CONTRACTION	FPL55712 INDOMETHACIN	5,9,10,18,20
"	GP	E4	CONTRACTION		20

[*]CYCLO-OXYGENASE INHIBITOR, [†]THROMBOXANE SYNTHETASE INHIBITOR, [¶]LEUKOTRIENE RECEPTOR ANTAGONIST, [§]INHIBITION WAS LIMITED TO THE DESIGNATED LEUKOTRIENE.

1. Sirois, P., Borgeat, P., Jeanson, A., Roy, S. and Girard, G.; The Action of Leukotriene B_4 (LTB$_4$) on the Lung. Prostaglandins and Medicine 5, 429-444, 1980. 5. Piper, P.J.; Pharmacological Actions of SRS-A & the Leukotrienes. International Syposium on Leukotrienes and other Lypoxygenase Products: Florence, Italy, 1981*. 6. Drazen, J.M., Austen, K.E., Lewis, R.A., Clark, D.A., Goto, G., Marafat, A. and Corey, E.J.; Comparative Airway and Vascular Activities of Leukotrienes C-1 and D in vivo and in vitro. Proc. Natl. Acad. Sci. USA 77(7), 4354-8, 1980. 7. Hedquist, P.; Pulmonary and Microvascular Effects of the Leukotrienes *. 9. Hanna, C.J., Bach, M.K., Pars, P.J. and Schellenberg, R.R.; Slow Reacting Substances (Leukotrienes) Contract Human Airway and Vascular Smooth Muscle in vitro. Nature 290, 343-4, 1981. 10. Gleason,J.G., Krell, R.D.; Ali, F.E., Veichman, B.M. and Berkowitz, B.; Synthesis and Comparative Pharmacology of Leukotrienes C_4 and D_4 on Airway and Vascular Smooth Muscle: Antagonism by a Novel Leukotriene Antagonist *. 15. Sirois,P., Sylvain, R., Borgeat, P., Pichard, S. and Corey, E.J.; Structural Requirement for the Action of Leukotriene on the Guinea Pig Lung: Importance of the Double Bond Geometry in the 6,8,10-Triene Unit. Biochem Biophys Res Comm 99(2), 385-90, 1981. 16. Dahlen, S.E., Hedquist, P.; Leukotriene-induced Bronchoconstriction: Structure-activity Requirements and Mode of action *. 17. Sirois, P., Roy, S. and Borgeat, P.; Potency and Specificity of Action of Leukotriene B_4 (LTB$_4$) on the Guinea Pig Lung *. 18. Hedquist, P., Dahlen, S.E., Gustafsun, L., Hammarstrom, S. and Samuelsson, B.; Biological Profile of Leukotrienes C_4 and D_4. Acta Physiol Scand., 110, 331-337, 1980. 19. Schellenberg, R.R., Nicholls, I., Bach, M.K., Rokach, J. and Hanna, C.J.; Leukotriene C and D Responses on Human Lung Smooth Muscle *. 20. Welton, A.F., Crowley, H.J., Miller, P.A., Yaremko, B.; Biological Activities of a Chemically Synthesized form of Leukotriene E_4 *. 21. Vargaftig, B.B., Lefurt, J. and Murphy, R.C.; Inhibition by Non-steroidal anti-inflammatory Drugs of the Effect of Leukotrienes on the Guinea Pig *. 22. Dahlen, S.E., Hedquist, P., Hammarstrom, S. and Samuelsson, B.; Leukotrienes are Potent Constrictors of Human Bronchi. Nature 288, 484-6, 1980. 23. Hulroyde, M.C., Altounyan, R.C., Cole, M., Dixon, M. and Elliott, E.V.; Bronchoconstriction Produced in man by Leukotrienes C & D. Lancet 2:8236, 17-18, 1981. 24. Holme, G., Piechuta, H., Massun, P., Girard, Y. and Rokach, T.; The Activity of Synthetic Leukotriene C_1 (LTC-1) on Guinea Pig Trachea and Ileum. Prostaglandins 20(4), 717-78, 1980.
* International Symposium on Leukotrienes and Other Lipoxygenase Products: Florence, Italy, 1981.

TABLE 4

VISCERAL (GI) SMOOTH MUSCLE RESPONSE TO LEUKOTRIENE AND ITS INHIBITION

PREPARATION	SPECIES	LEUKOTRIENE	EFFECT	INHIBITION	REFERENCE
ILEUM	GP,RAT	E4	CONTRACTION	FPL55712*	20
"	GP	C4,D4	CONTRACTION		5,25
"	GP	C1	CONTRACTION	FPL55712	24,26
"	GP	C5	CONTRACTION		27
"	GP	C3	CONTRACTION		28
"	GP	D3	CONTRACTION		28
"	RAT	SRS-A,C,D	NO EFFECT		29
FUNDUS	RAT	C4,D4	CONTRACTION	FPL55712	29
DUODENUM	RAT	C4,D4	NO EFFECT		29
COLON	RAT	C4,D4	CONTRACTION	FPL55712	29
GASTRIC(MOTILITY	GP	C4,D4	CONTRACTION		29

*LEUKOTRIENE RECEPTOR ANTAGONIST.

5. Piper, P.J.; Pharmacological Actions of SRS-A and the Leukotrienes. International Symposium on Leukotrienes and Other Lipoxygenase Products: Florence, Italy, 1981 *. 20. Welton, A.F., Crowley, H.J., Miller, P.A. and Yaremko, B.; Biological Activities of a chemically Synthesized Form of Leukotriene E_4 *. 24. Holme, G., Brunet, G., Piechuta, H., Massun, P., Girard, Y. and Rokach, J.; The Activity of synthetic Leukotriene C_1 (LTC-1) on Guinea Pig Trachea and Ileum. Prostaglandins 20 (4), 717-78, 1980. 25. Orning, L., Hammerstrom, S. and Samuelsson, B.; Leukotriene D: A Slow React- ing Substance from Rat Basophilic Leukemia Cells. Proc. Natl. Acad. Sci.; 77(4), 2014-7, 1979. 26. Murphy, R.C., Hammarstrom, S. and Samuelsson, B.; Leukotriene C: A Slow Reacting Substance from Murine Mastoma Cells. Proc. Natl. Acad. Sci. USA 76(9), 4275-4279, 1979. 27. Hammarstrom, S.; LTC_5: A Slow Reacting Substance Derived from Eicosapentaenoic Acid. J. Biol. Chem., 255(15), 7039-4, 1980. 28. Hammarstrom, S.; Conversion of 5,8,11-Eicosatrienoic Acid to Leukotrienes C_3 and D_3. J. Biol. Chem.; 256(5), 2275-9, 1981. 29. Goldberg, M.N. and Subeis, E.M.; Effect of Synthetic Leukotriene C (LTC_4) and Leukotriene D (LTD_4) on Isolated Gastrointestinal Tissues of the Rat *.
* International Symposium on Leukotrienes and Other Lipoxygenase Products: Florence, Italy, 1981.

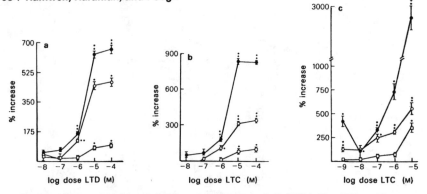

Figure 1 (a) Effect of leukotriene D_4 (LTD) on release of prostaglandin E_2 (PGE$_2$), 6-keto-PGF$_{1\alpha}$ and thromboxane B_2 (TxB$_2$) from rat peritoneal macrophages in suspension. Peritoneal cells (1×10^6) were incubated for 3 h with various doses of LTD. PGE$_2$ (●); 6-keto-PGF$_{1\alpha}$ (O); TxB$_2$ (□). Points show means; vertical lines indicate s.e. mean. $n=4$. *$P<0.01$; **$P<0.001$. (b) Effect of leukotriene C_4 (LTC) on release of PGE$_2$, 6-keto-PGF$_{1\alpha}$ and TxB$_2$ from rat peritoneal macrophages in suspension. Peritoneal cells (1×10^6) were incubated for 3 h with various doses of LTC. Symbols as in (a). Points show means; vertical lines indicate s.e. mean. $n=4$. *$P<0.01$; **$P<0.001$. (c) Effect of LTC on release of PGE$_2$, 6-keto-PGF$_{1\alpha}$ and TxB$_2$ from rat peritoneal macrophages in monolayer. Peritoneal cells (3×10^6) were adhered for 4 h. Thereafter the non-adherent cells were removed and the adherent cells were incubated for 20 h with various doses of LTC. Symbols as in (a). Points show means; vertical lines indicate s.e. mean. $n=4$. *$P<0.05$; **$P<0.01$.

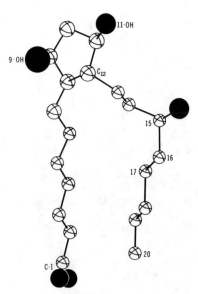

Fig 2   –Hairpin conformation of PGF$_{1\alpha}$.

hydroxyl groups at C-9, 11 and 15 are all on top and facing the viewer so as to form a chiral or right hand wedge. Any change from this hair-pin conformation or changes in chirality or inversion of any one of the hydroxyl groups leads to loss of biological activity (Andersen and Ramwell, 1974; Andersen et al, 1976). These diastereomers provides an unusual opportunity for definitive studies on binding and receptor activation. Recently Andersen et al. (1981) has constrained the analogs of PGF_{2a} to the "hair-pin" alignment by covalent bonding between the terminal portions of the side chains and confirmed the validity of this model in a series of new PGF syntheses.

The question arises as to how prostaglandins and the other arachidonate products may exert at 10^{11}M, a cooperative effect on the cell membrane. The biologically active prostaglandins appear to be amphipathic molecules of novel design in that their hydrophilic groups lie on one side of the molecule and the other side is hydrophobic, while both ends are hydrophilic. These molecules in fact possess many of the requisites set out by Onsager (1970) for cation-transporting molecules at a pore: they are (i) partially lipid soluble, (ii) can hold a stable conformation as calculations indicate, and (iii) may relieve internal electrostatic repulsive forces by forming a cation complex. More attractive to us, in the light of our considerations of the conformational energies of these molecules, is a view of the prostaglandins as effector molecules in a cooperative membrane. The general scheme would involve (i) a change in the molecular environment of the prostaglandin, (ii) succeeded by a conformational change of the prostaglandin (iii) followed by an interphase action of the prostaglandin to (iv) act on an enzyme system such as adenylate cyclase or an ion channel, such as calcium.

Structure activity studies for the leukotrienes have been performed now by Drazen et al (1981). It is of particular interest that recently LTB_4 was found to promote calcium influx in the rabbit polymorphnuclear leukocyte (Naccache et al, 1981). Although similar studies have not been described for TXA_2 or its mimics, the latter are known to promote both aggregation of both PMN and platelets – a process involving calcium influx.

BINDING AND RECEPTOR ACTIVATION

If these two postulated mechanisms are born in mind namely activation of adenylate cyclase and opening of calcium channels, then we can more effectively scrutinize the recent developments in binding of prostaglandins and receptor activation. The effect of a wide variety of prostaglandins may in fact be mediated by a more limited number of receptors. This certainly is the case in the human platelet receptor which is coupled to adenylate cyclase. An early and important discovery was by Kloeze (1967) who showed that PGE_1 inhibited the aggregation of platelets.Since then other prostaglandins which promote cyclic-AMP formation have been shown to stabilize platelets. Platelets appear to contain two high affinity receptors. The anti-aggregating effects of PGE_1, PGE_2, 6-keto-PGE_1 and PGI_2 may be mediated primarily by the PGI_2 receptor and PGD_1 and PGD_2 by the PGD receptor. There are also low affinity binding sites on the plasma membrane and these may be involved in the differences between the cyclic-AMP kinetics observed with PGE_1, PGD_2 and PGI_2. Thus, the more prominent effect on cyclic-AMP formation seen with PGI_2 may be due to binding to both the high PGI_2 receptor and a low affinity PGD_2 receptor (Harris et al, 1979).

Although these types of binding and receptor studies help to clarify the situation, there is a problem when two very closely related prostaglandins have opposite effects.For example duodenal circular muscle of the rat and toad is relaxed by PGE_1 but contracted by PGE_2. The possibility that these differential effects may be mediated by other mechanisms such as the release of 5HT by PGE_2 has been ruled out (Main, 1973). The idea of a separate PGE_1 and PGE_2 receptor in these preparations is not necessarily far fetched since the high affinity PGF_{2a} binding site in corpora lutea membranes is surprisingly specific for only PGF_{2a} and its immediate metabolites and not for PGF_{1a} (Hammarstrom et al, 1976; Rao, 1976). Consequently in duodenal circular muscle we might expect PGE_1 to increase cyclic AMP and induce relaxation and PGE_2 to bind to a separate receptor which leads to an increase in calcium influx with consequent contraction.

A relevant situation occurs in rat myometrium where both PGE_2 and PGF_2 are oxytocic. However PGE_2 has also been shown to increase cyclic AMP (Harbon and Clauser 1971). We suggest that the calcium influx resulting from

PGE_2 binding to a spasmogenic receptor overwhelms the cyclic-AMP mediated mechanism for reducing intracellular calcium which would normally lead to relaxation. In other words rat myometrium may contain both a PGE_2-adenylate cyclase and a PGE_2-calcium receptor. This may also be the case in the duodenal circular muscle experiments referred to above i.e. both PGE_1 and PGE_2 may increase cyclic-AMP but PGE_2 is also linked to a calcium channel. The availability of extracellular calcium and intracellular calcium and calcium antagonists such as nifedipine and TMB8 respectively allows these possibilities to be explored. Greenberg (1981) has studied the effect of PGI_2 and a thromboxane mimic on magnesium as well as on calcium influx; he concludes that relaxation induced by PGI_2 in pulmonary vessels is due to inhibition of calcium influx.

A more difficult problem is encountered where there is a biphasic response by a tissue to different doses of a prostaglandin. This is seen in the human umbilical artery preparation which relaxes to low doses of PGI_2 and contracts to higher doses (Pomerantz et al, 1978). This is a more general phenomenon in that other prostaglandins have this effect in the umbilical artery preparation and also in other vessels such as the human coronary artery (table 1) Since a comprehensive drug antagonist cocktail was used in the umbilical artery studies we conclude that it is unlikely for the prostaglandins to be mediating a biphasic effects by differential release of endogenous substances. The data are consistent as indicated earlier with the idea of receptors with a high and low affinity binding sites coupled to adenylate cyclase on the one hand and to the opening of a calcium channel on the other.

RECEPTOR ANTAGONISM

This classical approach to establishing the identity of receptors has developed only slowly in the prostaglandin field since the main organic synthetic effort has been devoted to the development of long acting PGE, PGF and PGI analogs. Nevertheless there are specific and competitive inhibitors of PGF and PGE which can be used in vivo (Fitzpatrick et al, 1981). Although there is good discrimination between the PGE and PGF series there is poor discrimination between the prostaglandins of both series containing the C5 and C13 double bonds. The same strategy, namely synthesis of the C-1 dimethylamine or dimethylamide which was used for developing the PGF_2 antagonist, was also used for PGI_2 but without success. This is interesting since the strategy has been successfully extended to PGE.

Because TXA_2 is regard as a pathogenic mediator there has been more incentive by industry to develop an antagonist. Recently a specific thromboxane receptor antagonist from Squibb has been described. The same reasoning also was behind the development of an SRS-A antagonist by Fisons which proved effective against synthetic LTC_4 and LTD_4 (see tables 2-4). However these receptor antagonists are not generally available and consequently the systematic studies have yet to be performed which will evaluate the relationship between receptors which mediate the activation of adenylate cyclase, smooth muscle relaxation and contraction.

CONCLUSIONS

1.   A simplistic but useful working concept of the pharmacological effects of prostaglandins and other arachidonate products is based on the idea that there are two mechanisms involving adenylate cyclase and calcium, respectively.

2.   The rank order of pharmacological effectiveness of arachidonate products appears to be:
PGI_2 : PGE_2 : PGD_2 : PGF_{2a} : TXA_2 : LT_4.

3.   The complexity of the pharmacology of the arachidonate products is contributed to by the release of other active substances.

4.   The products themselves can promote release of further arachidonate metabolites.

5.   Consequently enzyme inhibitors and receptor antagonists are mandatory in defining the pharmacology of arachidonate products.

6.   The specific membrane domains of the molecular site of action of arachidonate products are likely to be universal features of all cells since few cells if any are unresponsive.

Acknowledgement: We thank NIH and ONR for their support.

REFERENCES

Andersen NH, Ramwell PW (1974). Biological aspects of prostaglandins. Archiv Int Med 133:30-50.

Andersen NH, Ramwell PW, Loevey EMK, Johnson M (1976). Biological consequences of prostaglandin molecular conformation. Adv Prost Thrombox Res 1:271-288.

Andersen NH, Imamoto S, Subramanian N, Picker DH et al. (1981). Molecular basis for prostaglandin potency. III. Tests of the significance of the "hairpin conformation"in biorecognition phenomena. Prostaglandins 22:841-856.

Drazen JM, Lewis RA, Austen KF, Toda M, Brion F, Marfat A, Corey EJ (1981). Contractile activities of structural analogs of leukotriene C and D: Necessity of a hydrophobic region. Proc Natl Acad Sci 78:3195-3198.

Flack JD, Ramwell PW, Shaw JE (1971). Endocrinological implications of the prostaglandins. In "Current Topics in Experimental Endocrinology" Academic Press NY p 199-228.

Fitzpatrick TM, Stinger RB, Ramwell PW, Kot PA (1981). Prostaglandin analogs that antagonize the vascular responses to particular prostaglandins. In Berti F, Velo GP (Eds.): The Prostaglandin System. Plenum NY p 283-290.

Feuerstein N, Bash JA, Woody JN, Ramwell PW (1981). Leukotriene C stimulates prostaglandin release from rat peritoneal macrophages. Biochem Biophys Res Comm 100:1085-1090.

Feuerstein N, Foegh M, Ramwell PW (1981). Leukotrienes C_4 and D_4 induce prostaglandin and thromboxane release from rat peritoneal macrophages. Br J Pharmac 72:389-391.

Gerrard JM, Butler AM, Graff G, Stoddard SF, White JG (1978). Prostaglandin endoperoxides promote calcium release from a platelet membrane fraction in vitro. Prostaglandins Med 1:373-385.

Greenberg S (1981). Effect of prostacyclin and 9,11-epoxymethanoprostaglandin H_2 on calcium and magnesium fluxes and tension development in canine intralobar arteries and veins. J Pharm Exp Therap 219:326-337.

Hammarstrom S, Powell WS, Kylden U, Samuelsson B (1976). Some properties of a prostaglandin F_2 receptor in corpora lutea. Adv Prost Thrombox Res 1:235-246.

Harbon S, Clauser H (1971). Cyclic adenosine 3,5 monophosphate levels in rat myometrium under the influence of epinephrine, prostaglandins and oxytocin correlations with uterus motility. Biochem Biophys Res Comm 44:1496-1503.

Harris RH, Ramwell PW, Gilmer PJ (1979). Cellular mechanisms of prostaglandin action. Ann Rev Physiol 41:653-658.

Kury PG, McConnell HM (1975). Regulation of membrane flexibility in human erythrocytes. Biochemistry 14:2798-2803.

Kury PG, Ramwell PW, McConnell HM (1974). The effect of prostaglandins E_1 and E_2 on the human erythrocyte as monitored by spin labels. Biochem Biophys Res Comm 56:478-483.

Loutzenhizer R, van Breemen C (1981). The mechanism of activation of isolated rabbit aorta by the PGH_2 analog, U44069. Am J Phys In press.

Main IHM (1973). Prostaglandins and the gastrointestinal tract In Cuthbert MF (Ed) "The Prostaglandins" Heinemann London p 287-323.

Naccache PH, Sha'afi RI, Borget P, Goetzl E.J. (1981) Mono-and dihydroxyeicosatetraenoic acids alter calcium homeostasis in rabbit neutrophils J Clin Invest 67:1584-1587

Onsager L (1970). In Snell F et al (Eds)"The Physical Principles of Biological Membranes" Gordon & Breach NY p 137.

Paton DM, Daniels EE (1967). On the contractile response of the isolated rat uterus to PGE_1. Can J Physiol Pharmacol. 45 795-800

Pomerantz K, Sintetos A, Ramwell PW (1978). The effect of prostacyclin on the human umbilical artery. Prostaglandins 15:1035-1044.

Rabinowitz I, Ramwell PW, Davison P (1971). The Conformation of prostaglandins. Nature 233:88-89.

Ramwell PW, Shaw JE (1970)Biological significance of the prostaglandins. Recent Prog Hormone Res 26:139-187.

Ramwell PW, Rabinowitz I (1971). Interaction of prostaglandins and cyclic AMP. In Rabin BR and Feedman RB (Eds.) "Effects of Drugs on Cellular Control Mechanism. Macmillan Press NY p 207-235.

Rao CV (1976). Discrete prostaglandin receptors in the outer cell membranes of bovine corpora lutea. Adv Prost Thrombox Res 1:247-258.

Vogt W (1963). Pharmacologically active acidic phospholipids and glycolipids. Biochem Pharmcol 12:415-420.

**Prostaglandins and Cancer: First
International Conference, pages 67-77**
© 1982 Alan R. Liss, Inc., 150 Fifth Avenue, New York, NY 10011

PROSTAGLANDIN ANALOGUES

J.E. Pike and G.L. Bundy

Research Laboratories
The Upjohn Company
Kalamazoo, Michigan 49001 USA

Soon after the first members of the prostaglandin family were characterized chemically by Bergström and his associates (Bergström, S., 1967), and pure materials were available for biological studies, the preparation of chemically modified prostaglandins or analogues began. About 15 years ago at the Nobel Symposium held in Stockholm in 1966 some structural variations of PGE_1 and $PGF_2\alpha$ were described, made either by total synthesis or by modifications of the natural products (Pike, J.E., 1967). Since then a very large number of analogues have been made by many research groups, and this paper is an attempt to review why they have been made, rather than to give a comprehensive listing of all the structural variations reported. Examples of analogues which have been devised for particular purposes will be chosen mainly from Upjohn research since these are best known to me, but this selection is not to be interpreted as any judgement as to the relative merits of the analogues made by other laboratories.

The types of analogues synthesized have expanded as the number of arachidonic acid metabolites formed from the cyclooxygenase have grown to include the endoperoxides, the thromboxanes, and prostacyclins. More recently the lipoxygenase pathway has been further characterized to cover the hydroperoxy and hydroxy fatty acids and the leukotrienes (Piper, P.J., 1981). However complex the transformation products based on arachidonic acid oxygenation, the reasons for preparing the analogues have remained essentially the same. It became apparent very early that these fatty acid-based autacoids were usually quite short-lived in vivo

(Samuelsson, B., 1971), although the half-life of the endo-peroxides (5 minutes) and thromboxane A$_2$ (30 seconds) were especially noteworthy (Hamberg, M., 1976). The 15-hydroxy prostaglandin dehydrogenase which is the metabolic enzyme which degrades the prostaglandins to the relatively inactive 15-keto derivatives is widespread and largely responsible for the short-lived effects (Änggård, E., 1966). If the various pharmacologic end points associated with the various prosta-glandins were to have some practical value then clearly for most purposes one needed longer-lasting compounds which would escape the rapid inactivation in the circulation, or would enable one to find orally active compounds which es-caped breakdown in absorption through the gastric mucosa. So, the first reason for analogue synthesis was to provide increased metabolic stability and consequently longer bio-logical half-life in vivo (Fig. 1). A second main reason

WHY SYNTHESIZE "PROSTAGLANDIN" ANALOGUES?

1. To provide increased *metabolic stability.*

2. To give greater *chemical stability.*

3. To improve *biological selectivity.*

4. To provide *enzyme inhibitors* and *antagonists.*

Fig. 1

for analogue modifications is an attempt to overcome the intrinsic chemical instability of many of the arachidonic acid metabolites. Here the object could be to prepare a modification of an agent such as prostacyclin, thought to have valuable pharmacologic properties, but which would not be unstable at low pH; or it could be to study stable agonists and to see if structural modifications lead to antagonism of the natural hormone. With the wide range of biological end points affected by exogenous prostaglandins from uterine stimulation to blood pressure regulation and the inhibition of gastric secretion another hope in analogue design was to find agents with greater selectivity, for example in causing uterine stimulation without affecting gastric motility.

Before discussing in more detail examples of each of these four reasons for analogue synthesis it might be help-ful to give the historical sequence in this area and the chemical methods which have been used at Upjohn over the years to obtain the compounds (Fig. 2). It is clear that

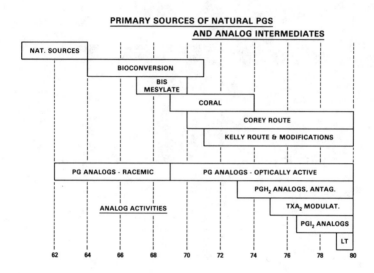

Fig. 2

we are only at the beginning of the "analogue" phase in the leukotriene area. As chemical nomenclature is essential to an understanding of the various analogues I have included a listing of key references (Nelson, N.A., 1974; Johnson, R.A., 1978; Samuelsson, B., 1978) which describe the correct nomen-clature for the prostaglandins, the thromboxanes and the prostacyclins (Fig. 3).

Soon after the characterization of the first metabolites of the prostaglandins resulting from oxidation of the 15-hydroxyl to a 15-ketone by the dehydrogenase (Ånggård, E., 1966) it was decided to look at the effect of introduction of a 15-methyl group to prevent this oxidation (Fig. 4). These compounds were synthesized and proved to have full agonist activity but with an increased biological half-life because they could not be oxidized to the corresponding 15-ketone (Bundy, G., 1971). Subsequently several of these

NOMENCLATURE IN THE PG AREA

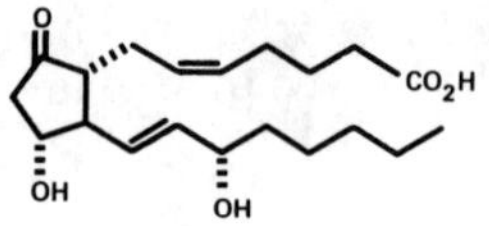
O
CO_2H
OH
OH

PROSTAGLANDINS: N.A. Nelson, J. Med. Chem. 17, 911 (1974).

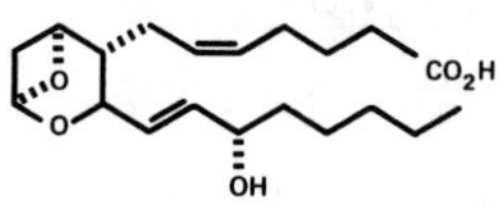
O
O
CO_2H
OH

THROMBOXANES: B. Samuelsson, M. Hamberg, L.J. Roberts III, J.A. Oates, N.A. Nelson, Prostaglandins 16 (6), 857 (1978).

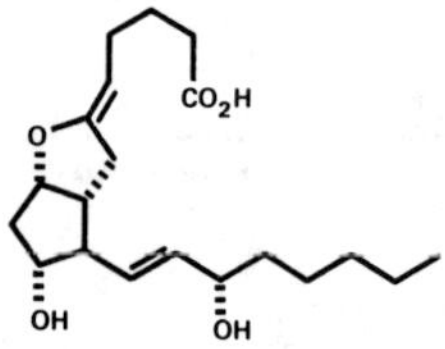
CO_2H
O
OH
OH

PROSTACYCLINS: R.A. Johnson, D.R. Morton, N.A. Nelson, Prostaglandins 15 (5), 737 (1978).

Fig. 3

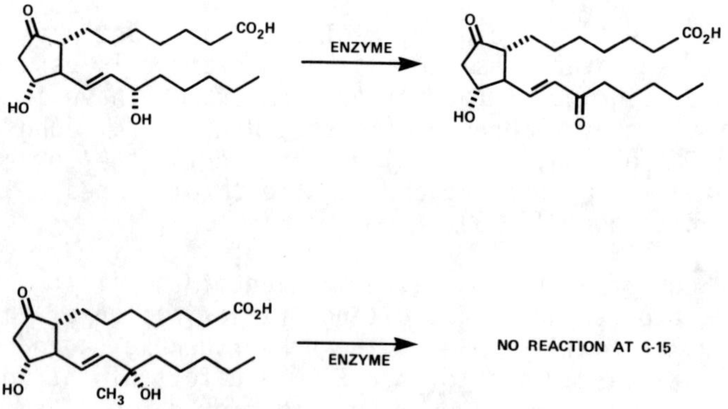
ENZYME
ENZYME
NO REACTION AT C-15
CH_3 OH

Fig. 4

15-methyl analogues have provided valuable therapeutic agents for pregnancy termination (Karim, S.M.M., 1975), menstrual induction (Bygdeman, M., 1980) and for the treatment of gastric and duodenal ulcers (Robert, A., 1980). Other strategies have been used to prevent the metabolic inactivation of the lower side chain by the 15-hydroxydehydrogenase. These have involved the concept of steric crowding close to the 15 position by the synthesis of 16,16-dimethyl analogues such as 16,16-dimethyl-PGE$_2$ (Magerlein, B.J., 1973) which are again not substrates for the enzyme and maintain agonist activity (Fig. 5). Another tactic has been to substitute

PG ANALOGS···INCREASED METABOLIC STABILITY

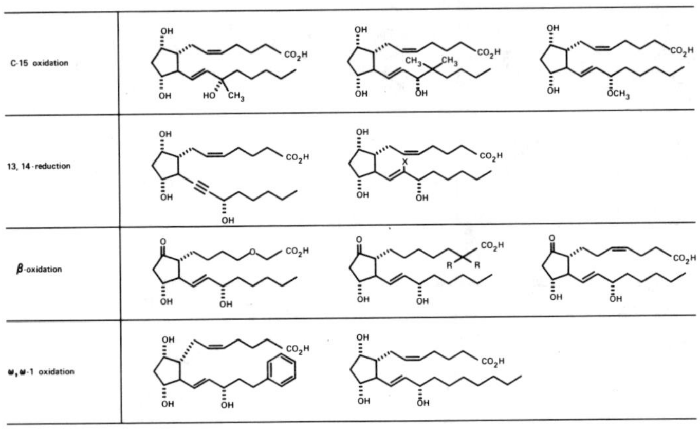

Fig. 5

the alkyl lower side chain with aromatic rings such as phenyl or phenoxy residues (Magerlein, B.J., 1975; Crossley, N.S., 1976) and this has again led to useful analogues of PGF$_2\alpha$ probably by an effect on the prevention of ω-hydroxylation and on the dehydrogenase. The metabolism of prostaglandins continues beyond the initial oxidation at C-15 to produce dicarboxylic acids and this suggested that chemical modifications, for example, of the carboxy side chain could also provide compounds with increased metabolic stability. One example of variations with decreased propensity to undergo β-oxidation of the carboxy chain are the Δ^4-prostanoids

(Green, K., 1978) such as cis-Δ^4-PGF$_1\alpha$ and the interphenylene prostaglandins (Nelson, N.A., 1975).

The second main theme in analogue synthesis has been to design compounds which overcome intrinsic chemical instability (Fig. 6). Prostaglandins of the E series are very

PG ANALOGS • • • INCREASED CHEMICAL STABILITY

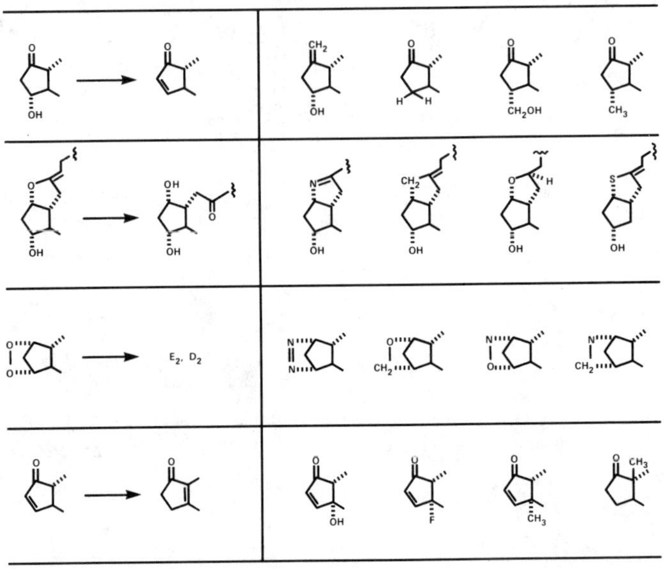

Fig. 6

unstable in acidic or basic solutions or on prolonged storage, and this presents a serious problem in designing effective practical agents for therapeutic use. Prostacyclin is also an unstable material, because of the acid-labile enol ether functionality (Vane, J.R., 1979), and the endoperoxides also decompose readily on standing (Samuelsson, B., 1977). Examples are shown in Fig. 6 of modifications which have been designed to overcome these chemical degradations. For instance the 9-deoxy-9-methylene analogs were synthesized in part because this removed the tendency of the molecule to undergo dehydration to a PGA ($\Delta^{10(11)}$) structure. The hydrolysis of the enol ether in prostacyclin could be

prevented by substituting the oxygen of the 5-membered ring
with nitrogen (Bundy, G.L., 1978), sulphur (Nicolaou, K.C.,
1977) or carbon (Morton, D.R., 1979) or by a reduction of
the enol ether double bond (Johnson, R.A., 1979). The cyclic
endoperoxides are unstable and undergo a breakdown by cleavage
of the -O-O- bond. This has been overcome by replacing each
or both of the oxygen atoms by carbon (Bundy, G.L., 1975;
Corey, E.J., 1976) or nitrogen (Bundy, G.L., 1978; Pike, J.E.,
1979) to give chemically stable analogues with interesting
biological properties (Corey, E.J., 1975), especially when
combined with a removal of the 15 hydroxy group (Gorman, R.R.,
1977). One of the 9-methylene analogues is undergoing clinical
trials for cervical dilatation and menses induction. Note
that this particular compound 9-deoxo-9-methylene-16,16-
dimethyl PGE_2 (Bundy, G.L., 1980) exemplified two design
aspects, the substitution of two methyl groups at C-16 to
increase metabolic stability and the 9 methylene feature to
provide chemical stability for the 5-membered ring.

With prostacyclin there is both enzymatic and non-
enzymatic breakdown and analogues have been prepared which
combine the stabilizing features mentioned above with substitution in the lower side chain to prevent the enzymatic oxidation at C-15. Examples are the carbacyclin analogues which
also incorporate geminal substitution with fluorine at C-16
(Aiken, J.W., 1981). The 16,16-difluoro function like the
16,16-dimethyl substitution acts as a steric barrier to
operation of the enzymatic oxidation at C-15.

As mentioned chemical analogues of the endoperoxides have
been synthesized and these have shown activities similar to
those of the natural endoperoxides and thromboxane A_2
(Coleman, R.A., 1980; Coleman, R.A., 1981). It is somewhat
unexpected that while chemically these analogues, for example
the 9,11-methanoepoxy analogue, mimic the endoperoxides their
biological properties are believed to be thromboxane A_2-like.
In synthesizing a variety of structural variants of the
'stable' endoperoxides it was discovered that the 15-deoxy
analogues had properties as thromboxane synthetase inhibitors
and thromboxane antagonists. This was especially true in
those 15-deoxy analogues where each of the oxygens has been
replaced by an NH group as for instance 11α, 9α-(epoxyimino)-
prosta-5Z, 13E-dienoic acid a thromboxane synthetase inhibitor and 9α, 11α-(epoxyimino) prosta-5Z, 13E-dienoic acid a
thromboxane antagonist.

The synthesis of several stable thromboxane A_2 analogues has been described (Nicolaou, K.C., 1979; Lefer, A.M., 1980; Maxey, K.M., 1980; Corey, E.J., 1980; Ohuchida, S., 1981) and only in one case (Ohuchida, S., 1981) has the structure synthesized been associated with agonist activity comparable to that expected based on the biological properties of the natural product. For example three 11a-carba-thromboxane A_2 analogues were reported to be both receptor level antagonists of thromboxane A_2 or thromboxane synthetase inhibitors (Gorman R.R., 1981). Equally these compounds were lacking agonist or antagonist activity on rat aortic strip implying different receptor characteristics in platelets and vascular smooth muscle.

The other main goal of imparting greater pharmacological selectivity to prostaglandin analogues has been achieved in part with some compounds showing 'splits' for example between various types of biological activity. In general this remains a major objective and will doubtless justify a substantial effort in analogue synthesis for some time to come. The final table (Fig. 7) lists those compounds, both natural prostaglandins and their analogues, which are in clinical trials or are marketed either in the U.S. or outside. Certainly in the next several years this list can be expected to grow as we continue to meet the objectives outlined here for analogue design.

PROSTAGLANDIN ANALOGUES EITHER MARKETED OR IN CLINICAL TRIAL (U.S. OR FOREIGN)

Trivial Name	Generic Name	Trademark	Clinical Application
15-methyl-$PGF_{2\alpha}$	carboprost	Prostin/15M	Abortion, menstrual induction, cervical dilatation
15-methyl-PGE_2	—	—	Postpartum hemorrhage
(15R)-15-methyl-PGE_2	arbaprostil	—	Gastric antisecretory, anti-ulcer
trans-Δ^2-16,16-dimethyl-PGE_2 methyl ester	gemeprost	—	Abortion, menstrual induction, cervical dilatation
9-deoxy-9-methylene-16,16-dimethyl-PGE_2	meteneprost	—	Menstrual induction, cervical dilatation
N-methanesulfonyl-16-phenoxy-ω-tetranor-PGE_2 carboxamide	sulprostone	Sulglandin	Abortion, menstrual induction
16-[m-(trifluormethyl)-phenoxy]-ω-tetranor-$PGF_{2\alpha}$	fluprostenol	Equimate	Estrus induction in horses
16-m-chlorophenoxy-tetranor-$PGF_{2\alpha}$	cloprostenol	Estrumate	Estrus synchronization

Fig. 7

References

Aiken JW (1981). Presented at International Pharmacology Congress. Tokyo, Japan (July).

Anggård E, Samuelsson B (1966). Purification and properties of a 15-hydroxy-prostaglandin dehydrogenase from swine lung. Ark Kemi 25:293.

Bergstrom S (1967). Isolation, structure and action of the prostaglandins. In Bergstrom S, Samuelsson B (eds): "Prostaglandins," Nobel Symposium 2, Stockholm: Almquist and Wiksell, p 21.

Bundy G, Lincoln F, Nelson N, Pike J, Schneider W (1971). Novel prostaglandin synthesis. In Ramwell P, Shaw J (eds): "Annals of New York Academy of Sciences" 180, New York: NY Academy of Sciences, p 76.

Bundy GL (1975). The synthesis of prostaglandin endoperoxide analogs. Tetrahedron Letters, p 1957.

Bundy GL, Baldwin JM (1978). The synthesis of nitrogen-containing prostacyclin analogs. Tetrahedron Letters, p 1371.

Bundy GL, Peterson D (1978). The synthesis of 15-deoxy-9,11-epoxymino prostaglandins - potent thromboxane synthetase inhibitors. Tetrahedron Letters, p 41.

Bundy GL, Kimball FA, Robert A, Aiken JW, Maxey KM, Sebek OK, Nelson NA, Sih JC, Miller WL, Hsi RSP (1980). Synthesis and biological activity of 9-deoxo-9-methylene and related prostaglandins. In Samuelsson B, Paoletti R (eds): "Advances in Prostaglandin and Thromboxane Research" Vol. 6, New York: Raven Press, p 355.

Bygdeman M, Bremme K, Cristensen N, Lundstrom V, Greén K (1980). A comparison of 2 stable prostaglandin E analogues for termination of early pregnancy and for cervical dilatation. Contraception 22:471.

Coleman RA, Humphrey DDA, Kennedy I, Levy GP, Lumley P (1980). U-46619, a selective thromboxane A_2-like agonist? Br J Pharmac 69:265.

Coleman RA, Humphrey DDA, Kennedy I, Levy GP, Lumley P (1981). Comparison of the actions of U-46619, a prostaglandin H_2 analogue, with those of prostaglandin H_2 and thromboxane A_2 on some isolated smooth muscle preparations. Br J Pharmac 73:773.

Corey EJ, Nicolaou KC, Machida Y, Malmsten CL, Samuelsson B (1975). Synthesis and biological properties of a 9,11-azo-prostanoid: highly active biochemical mimic of prostaglandin endoperoxides. Proc Natl Acad Sci USA 72:3355.

Corey EJ, Shibasaki M, Nicolaou KC, Malmsten CL, Samuelsson B (1976). Simple stereocontrolled total synthesis of a biologically active analog of the endoperoxides (PGH$_2$, PGG$_2$). Tetrahedron Letters, p 737.

Corey EJ, Ponder JW, Ulrich P (1980). Synthesis of a stable analog of thromboxane A$_2$ with methylene replacing the 9,11-bridging oxygen. Tetrahedron Letters, p 137.

Crossley NS (1976). Prostaglandins. Chemistry and Industry, p 334.

Gorman RR, Bundy GL, Peterson DC, Sun FF, Miller OV, Fitzpatrick FA (1977). Inhibition of human platelet thromboxane synthetase by 9,11-azoprosta-5,13-dienoic acid. Proc Natl Acad Sci USA 74:4007.

Gorman RR, Maxey KM, Bundy GL (1981). Inhibition of human platelet thromboxane synthetase by 11a-carba-thromboxane A$_2$ analogs. Biochem Biophys Res Commun 100(1):184.

Greén K (1978). Metabolism of Δ^4-cis PGF$_1\alpha$ in the monkey. Prostaglandins 15:813.

Hamberg M, Svensson J, Samuelsson B (1976). Novel Transformations of Prostaglandin Endoperoxides: Formation of thromboxanes. In Samuelsson B, Paoletti R (eds): "Advances in Prostaglandin and Thromboxane Research" Vol. 1, New York: Raven Press, p 19.

Johnson RA, Morton DR, Nelson NA (1978). Nomenclature for analogs of prostacyclin (PGI$_2$). Prostaglandins 15(5):737.

Johnson RA, Lincoln FH, Smith HW, Ayer DE, Nidy E, Thompson JL, Axen U, Aiken JW, Gorman RR, Nishizawa EE, Honohan T (1979). In Vane JR, Bergstrom S (eds): "Prostacyclin," New York: Raven Press, p 17.

Karim SMM, Amy JJ (1975). Interruption of pregnancy with prostaglandins. In Karim SMM (ed): "Prostaglandins and Reproduction," Lancaster UK: MTP Press, p 77.

Lefer AM, Smith EF, Araki H, Smith JB, Aharony D, Claremon DA, Magolda RL, Nicolaou KC (1980). Dissociation of vasoconstrictor and platelet aggregatory activities of thromboxane by carbocyclic thromboxane A$_2$, a stable analog of thromboxane A$_2$. Proc Natl Acad Sci USA 77:1706.

Magerlein BJ, DuCharme DW, Magee WE, Miller WL, Robert A, Weeks JR (1973). Synthesis and biological properties of 16-alkyl prostaglandins. Prostaglandins 4(1):143.

Magerlein BJ, Bundy GL, Lincoln FH, Youngdale GA (1975). Synthesis of 17-phenyl-18,19,20-trinor prostaglandins II. PG$_2$ Series. Prostaglandins 9:5.

Maxey KM, Bundy GL (1980). The synthesis of 11a-carbathromboxane A$_2$. Tetrahedron Letters, p 445.

Morton DR, Bundy GL, Nishizawa EE (1979). Five-membered

ring-modified prostacyclin analogs. In Vane JR, Bergstrom S (eds): "Prostacyclin," New York: Raven Press, p 31.

Nelson NA (1974). Prostaglandin nomenclature. J Med Chem 17:911.

Nelson NA, Jackson RW, Au AT, Wynalda DJ, Nishizawa EE (1975). Synthesis of dℓ-4,5,6-trinor-3,7-inter-$\underline{m}$-phenylene-3-oxa prostaglandins including one which inhibits platelet aggregation. Prostaglandins 10(5):795.

Nicolaou KC, Barnette WE, Gasic GP, Magolda RL (1977). 6,9-Thiaprostacyclin. A stable and biologically potent analogue of prostacyclin (PGI$_2$). J Am Chem Soc 99:7736.

Nicolaou KC, Magolda RL, Smith JB, Aharony D, Smith EF, Lefer AM (1979). Synthesis and biological properties of pinane thromboxane A$_2$ a selective inhibitor of coronary artery constriction, platelet aggregation and thromboxane formation. Proc Natl Acad Sci USA 76:2566.

Ohuchida S, Hamanaka N, Hayashi M (1981). Synthesis of thromboxane A$_2$ analogues: DL-9,11:11,12-dideoxa-9,11:11,12-diepithio thromboxane A$_2$. J Am Chem Soc 103:4597.

Pike JE, Kupiecki FP, Weeks JR (1967). Biological activity of the prostaglandins and related analogs. In Bergstrom S, Samuelsson B (eds): "Prostaglandins," Nobel Symposium 2, Stockholm: Almquist and Wiksell, p 161.

Pike JE, Bundy GL, Fitzpatrick FA, Gorman RR (1979). The synthesis of compounds formed in the arachidonic acid cascade and agents which modulate their production. In Roberts SM, Scheinman F (eds): "Chemistry Biochemistry and Pharmacological Activity of Prostanoids," Oxford: Pergamon Press, p 115.

Piper PJ (1981). "SRS-A and Leukotrienes," New York: John Wiley and Sons.

Robert A (1980). Prostaglandins and digestive diseases. In Samuelsson B, Paoletti R (eds): "Advances in Prostaglandin and Thromboxane Research" Vol. 8, New York: Raven Press, p 1533.

Samuelsson B, Granstrom E, Greén K, Hamberg M (1971). Metabolism of Prostaglandins. In Ramwell P, Shaw J (eds): "Annals of New York Academy of Sciences" 180, New York: NY Acad of Sciences, p 138.

Samuelsson B (1977). Prostaglandin Endoperoxide and Thromboxanes: Short-lived bioregulators. In Crabbé P (ed): "Prostaglandin Research," New York: Academic Press, p 17.

Samuelsson B, Hamberg M, Roberts LJ, Oates JA, Nelson NA (1978). Nomenclature for thromboxanes. Prostaglandin 16(6):857.

Vane JR, Bergstrom S (1979). "Prostacyclin," New York: Raven Press.

CARCINOGENESIS-INITIATION

**Prostaglandins and Cancer: First
International Conference, pages 81-96**
© **1982 Alan R. Liss, Inc., 150 Fifth Avenue, New York, NY 10011**

THE INITIATION STAGE OF CHEMICAL CARCINOGENESIS: AN
INTRODUCTORY OVERVIEW

James A. Miller and Elizabeth C. Miller

McArdle Laboratory for Cancer Research
The University of Wisconsin Medical School
Madison, Wisconsin   53706

INTRODUCTION

Chemical carcinogenesis became an experimental science
in 1915 when it was reported that tumors of the rabbit skin
could be induced by the repetitive application of coal tar
(Yamagiwa and Ichikawa, 1918).   Subsequent to this seminal
finding, several workers showed that the process of skin
carcinogenesis in the rabbit and mouse could be either
enhanced or inhibited by various non-carcinogenic treatments
(reviewed in Miller, E.C. and Miller, J.A., 1979a).
Following these suggestive findings, Rous and his associates
(Rous and Kidd, 1941; MacKenzie and Rous, 1941) demonstrated
that papillomas, which had been induced on the ears of
rabbits by limited doses of tar and which had then
regressed, could reappear after subsequent applications of
turpentine or after wounding.   In the same year Berenblum
(1941) reported that topical treatments with the irritant
croton oil greatly increased the incidence of papillomas in
mouse skin simultaneously treated with benzo(a)pyrene.   The
significance of these findings in rabbit and mouse skin was
suggested by Mottram (1944) who found that repetitive applications of croton oil to mouse skin subsequent to a single
non-carcinogenic dose of benzo(a)pyrene yielded a high
incidence of papillomas.   In the same year, Friedewald and
Rous (1944) proposed the concept that skin carcinogenesis
could be divided into an initiating process, which was
responsible for the conversion of normal cells into
initiated or latent tumor cells, and a promoting process,
which caused the initiated cells to progress to gross
tumors.   From this background of data, Berenblum and Shubik

(1947) devised the now common two-stage assay for assessing the initiating and promoting activities of chemicals for mouse skin. Other evidence for the occurrence of initiation and promotion stages in chemically induced skin carcinogenesis came from the work of Tannenbaum, Rusch, and Boutwell and their associates (Tannenbaum, 1944; Boutwell, 1964) and from the demonstration of the pure initiating activity of ethyl carbamate for mouse skin (Salaman and Roe, 1953). The initial studies of Berenblum and Shubik (1947, 1949), as well as subsequent work by other investigators, especially by Boutwell (1964) and by Van Duuren and his associates (1969,1975,1978), demonstrated that in mouse skin initiation occurs rapidly, is essentially irreversible, and must precede the promotion stage. Promotion, on the other hand, appears to be reversible, at least in the early phases, and requires repetitive doses over a long period (Boutwell, 1964).

For some time these basic observations on initiation and promotion were regarded as relatively unique for skin carcinogenesis and were not applied to studies on chemical carcinogenesis in other tissues. However, particularly in the past decade, initiation and promotion stages have been established for chemical carcinogenesis in the liver, mammary gland, urinary bladder, lung, intestinal epithelium, and thyroid (Hall and Bielschowsky, 1949; Peraino et al., 1971; Berenblum, 1974; Armuth and Berenblum, 1972,1974 ; Hicks et al., 1975; Slaga et al., 1978; Kitagawa et al., 1979). The two stages of initiation and promotion have also been demonstrated in cultures of rat and mouse fibroblasts (Lasne et al., 1974; Mondal et al., 1976).

STRUCTURAL FEATURES OF CHEMICAL CARCINOGENS

The early findings on the biology of chemical carcinogenesis were paralleled by initial studies on the chemistry, biochemistry, and metabolism of pure chemical carcinogens (Miller, E.C. and Miller, J.A. 1979a). In 1930 Kennaway and Hieger in England discovered the first pure chemical carcinogen, the synthetic polycyclic aromatic hydrocarbon dibenz(a,h)anthracene. This advance was soon followed by the isolation, characterization, and synthesis of benzo(a)-pyrene, a coal tar constituent (Cook, Hewitt, and Hieger, 1933; Haddow and Kon, 1947). Organic chemists have since provided many analogous synthetic hydrocarbons for oncologic studies. At about the same time, hepatocarcinogenic aminoazo dyes were discovered in Japan (Yoshida, 1933; Kinosita, 1937), and the carcinogenicity of 2-naphthylamine in the dog urinary bladder was demonstrated in the United States (Hueper et al., 1938). From 1940 on, a great number and variety of chemical carcinogens were discovered by accident and by design (Miller, E.C., 1978).

As the discovery of new chemical carcinogens proceeded it became evident that these agents belong to many classes of chemicals that share no common structural features. This lack of common structure among the chemical carcinogens can be noted among representative synthetic carcinogens such as benzo(a)pyrene, 2-acetylaminofluorene, N-methyl-4-aminoazo-benzene, 4-nitroquinoline-1-oxide, 3-hydroxyxanthine, dimethylnitrosamine, carbon tetrachloride, ethyl carbamate, and ethionine (Miller, J.A. and Miller, E.C., 1966). Likewise, the 30 or more naturally occurring metabolites of fungi and green plants, such as aflatoxin B_1, mitomycin C, the toxic pyrrolizidine alkaloids, cycasin, and safrole share no common structural groups (Miller, E.C. and Miller, J.A., 1979b). This is also true of the synthetic carcinogenic alkylating agents, such as certain N-mustards, alkyl-methane sulfonates, epoxides, and β-propiolactone (Miller, J.A. and Miller, E.C., 1966). However, the common electrophilic reactivities of these latter agents contrast with the non-reactive natures of the synthetic and naturally occurring chemical carcinogens which form the majority of the known carcinogenic compounds. For many years it was not recognized that the carcinogenic alkylating agents are prototypes of the reactive forms of the other chemical carcinogens (see below).

THE METABOLISM OF CHEMICAL CARCINOGENS

It was early recognized that some carcinogens produced tumors at various sites of application (e.g., the polycyclic aromatic hydrocarbons), and it was suggested that these might be active in the forms administered. Other carcinogens induced tumors only in specific organs regardless of the site of application (e.g., the hepatocarcinogenic aminoazo dyes), and this finding suggested that specific metabolism might be required for their activity. Nevertheless the early studies on the metabolism of the chemical carcinogens revealed only metabolites which had no carcinogenic activity (Miller, E.C. and Miller, J.A., 1966).

The first evidence for the chemical alteration of cellular components in vivo by a chemical carcinogen was noted in the covalent binding of metabolite(s) of N,N-dimethyl-4-aminoazobenzene to protein in the liver of the rat (Miller, E.C. and Miller, J.A., 1947). Subsequently, the availability of carcinogens labelled with ^{14}C and ^{3}H permitted the demonstration of covalently bound residues of chemical carcinogens to DNA, RNA, and protein in vivo, especially in target tissues, as a general property of carcinogenic compounds (Miller, E.C. and Miller, J.A., 1966). These data implied that reactive forms of unreactive carcinogens were generated in vivo and that metabolites of some carcinogens might be found that would be more carcinogenic than their parent compounds. Evidence for this idea was first obtained with the isolation of the N-hydroxy metabolite of 2-acetylaminofluorene and the demonstration that it is a stronger carcinogen than the parent compound (Cramer et al., 1960; Miller, E.C. et al., 1961). Since this metabolite was not reactive with tissue constituents, it was regarded as a proximate carcinogen and as a precursor of reactive form(s) in vivo (see below).

The realization that the reactive forms of chemical carcinogens are electrophiles (i.e., electron-deficient species) was first noted in the metabolism in vitro and in vivo of N-methyl-4-aminoazobenzene and 2-acetylaminofluorene (Lotlikar et al., 1966; Miller, E.C. et al., 1966; Poirier et al., 1967; Kriek et al., 1967; DeBaun et al., 1968; King and Phillips, 1968). Subsequent work with many carcinogens has extended this concept that the reactive forms of most, if not all, chemical carcinogens are strong electrophilic reactants (Miller, J.A. and Miller, E.C., 1969; Miller, J.A., 1970; Miller, E.C. and Miller, J.A., 1981). Thus, the majority of chemical carcinogens must be metabolized to a common electronic form, i.e., reactive electrophiles, before they can react with cellular components and act as carcinogens. The great variety of chemical carcinogens, both non-reactive and reactive, without common structural features is explained on this basis. Likewise, it became evident that the covalent binding of chemical carcinogens in vivo was the result of reactions between these reactive electrophiles and nucleophilic sites in cellular components, especially the informational macromolecules DNA, RNA, and protein. The view thus developed that the initiating activity of chemical carcinogens resided in their electrophilic reactive forms (Figure 1). Not surprisingly, these reactive forms proved to be mutagenic (Maher et al., 1968; Miller, E.C. and Miller, J.A., 1971; Ames et al., 1973). The general correlations between the mutagenicity and carcinogenicity of chemicals (McCann et al., 1976; Sugimura et al., 1976), despite poor correlations with specific groups of compounds (Rinkus and Legator, 1979), suggests a genetic or genetic-viral mechanism of initiation (Figure 1).

It is not clear whether the promoting activities of complete chemical carcinogens are due to some of their electrophilic or non-electrophilic metabolites or to both (Figure 1). However, studies with "pure" promoters for skin and liver carcinogenesis strongly suggest that their active forms are not electrophilic (e.g., they are not mutagenic and do not bind covalently to nucleic acids).

Electrophiles involving electrophilic carbon atoms are generated in the metabolism of the majority of chemical carcinogens (Figure 2). The carcinogenic alkylating agents, which are electrophiles as such, also contain electrophilic carbon atoms. A few classes of carcinogens involve electrophilic nitrogen atoms. The carcinogenic metal ions (Figure

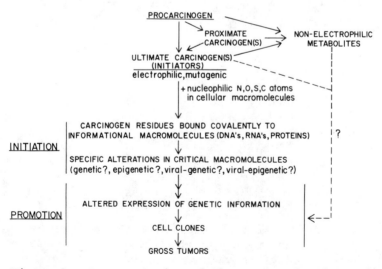

Figure 1. A current view of the gross molecular and cellular events in chemical carcinogenesis.

2) are electrophilic as such and form electrostatic bonds with nucleophiles in protein and nucleic acids. The association of these ions with nucleotides, polynucleotides, and polymerases results in miscoding and infidelity in the replication of DNA (Loeb and Zakour, 1980).

The great variety of the known nucleophilic targets in DNA, RNA, and proteins for the electrophilic metabolites of chemical carcinogens in vivo are also shown in Figure 2. The problem of identifying targets critical to the initiation of carcinogenesis by specific electrophiles is a task that is far from completion. The available evidence points to DNA as the major critical target for initiation, although the possibility that specific proteins or RNA's may be involved in initiation by some carcinogens under some conditions can not be ignored. The most detailed studies have been carried out with the methylating and ethylating agents. In these agents, the levels, persistence, and repair of the 0^6-alkyl-guanyl adducts in DNA appear to be much better correlated with carcinogenesis than are similar parameters for N-7 alkylation of guanyl residues (O'Connor et al., 1979).

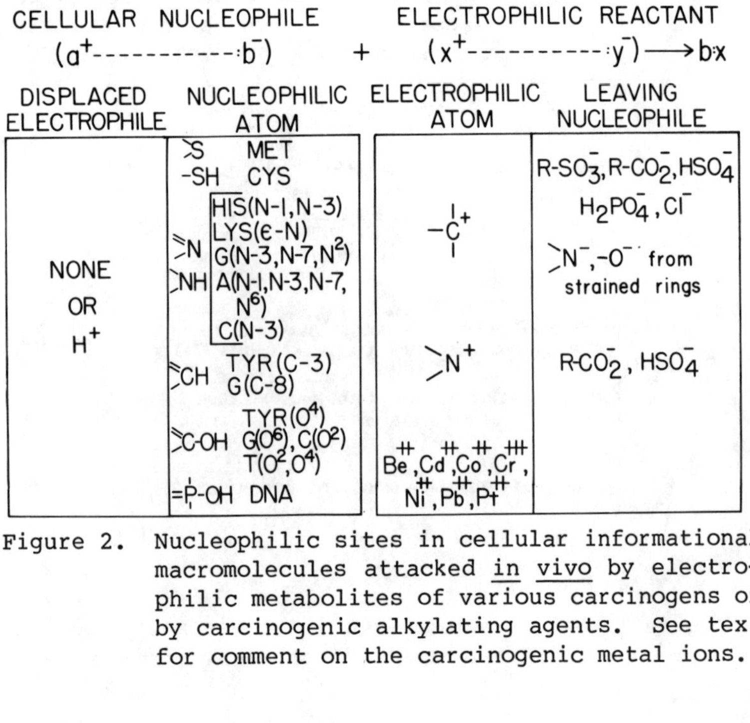

Figure 2. Nucleophilic sites in cellular informational macromolecules attacked in vivo by electrophilic metabolites of various carcinogens or by carcinogenic alkylating agents. See text for comment on the carcinogenic metal ions.

However, the possible roles of other adducts in DNA (especially the 0-alkyl pyrimidines) and the importance of alterations of specific sites in DNA are also important problems that need much further study.

The problems are even more complex with chemical carcinogens that require metabolism to proximate and ultimate metabolites. Their metabolism may involve a number of enzyme systems and may involve more than one intermediate and/or more than one ultimate metabolite. Furthermore, like the direct alkylating agents reaction may occur at various sites on DNA (and other nucleophilic targets in the cell), and the persistence and biological effects of these adducts may be quite different.

The systems that appear to be most frequently responsible for metabolic activation, as well as for inactivation, are the microsomal cytochrome P-450 monooxygenases outlined in Figure 3 (Testa and Jenner, 1976; Estabrook and Werringloer, 1979; Coon et al., 1979). Examples of the role of these enzymes in the metabolic activation of a nitrosamine, an aromatic amide, and a polycyclic aromatic hydro-

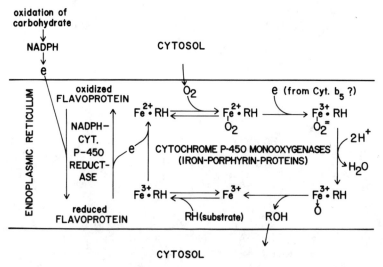

Figure 3. The mechanism of action of the microsomal cytochrome P-450 monooxygenases, which are involved in the metabolism of chemical carcinogens, drugs, and other foreign molecules.

carbon are shown in Figures 4-6. Figures 5 and 6 also exemplify the importance of other enzymes, in these cases epoxide hydratase and cytosolic transferases, in the activation of some carcinogens. As will be discussed in this symposium, cooxidative metabolism of chemical carcinogens by microsomal prostaglandin synthetase has recently been found to give rise to electrophiles that bind to cellular nucleophiles and that may be important in the initiation of carcinogenesis. In a few cases the electrophilic intermediate that reacts with DNA or other cellular constituents may not be derived directly from the carcinogen. Thus, for example, recent studies implicate free hydroxyl radicals as being responsible for the NADPH-cytochrome-P-450-dependent cleavage of DNA on incubation with adriamycin (Berlin and Haseltine, 1981).

SOME PERSPECTIVES

Although much has been learned during the past few decades about the events that occur in chemical carcino-

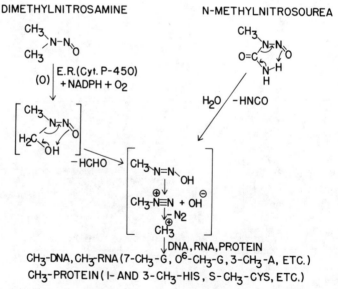

Figure 4.   The metabolic activation of dimethylnitrosamine and the decomposition of N-methyl-N-nitrosourea in water to yield methylating species (see O'Connor and Margison, 1979).

genesis, the molecular mechanisms involved in both the initiation and promotion stages are not yet evident. As noted above, the binding of carcinogen residues to DNA has been associated with the primary events in initiation [Grover (ed.), 1979]. Replication of DNA containing carcinogen adducts appears to be a requirement for "fixing" the carcinogen-induced changes in the DNA as altered sequences of normal bases, i.e., mutations. While the biologic and biochemical data suggest nuclear DNA as the critical target, the findings that N-nitroso derivatives, polycyclic hydrocarbons, and $7\alpha,8\beta$-dihydroxy-$9\beta,10\beta$-epoxy-7,8,9,10-tetrahydrobenzo(a)pyrene bind at higher levels to mitochondrial DNA than to nuclear DNA (Wunderlich et al., 1970,1971/72; Allen and Coombs, 1980; Backer and Weinstein, 1980) necessitate further study of mitochondrial DNA in relation to carcinogenesis.

Since changes in DNA appear to be essential to initiation, more study is needed to elucidate the nature of

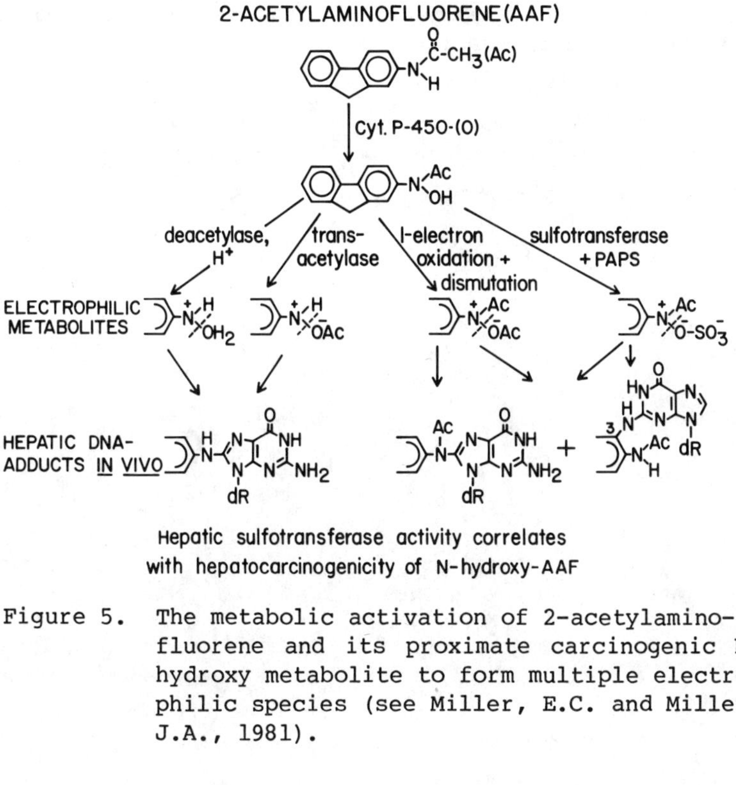

Hepatic sulfotransferase activity correlates
with hepatocarcinogenicity of N-hydroxy-AAF

Figure 5.   The metabolic activation of 2-acetylamino-fluorene and its proximate carcinogenic N-hydroxy metabolite to form multiple electrophilic species (see Miller, E.C. and Miller, J.A., 1981).

the changes. Carcinogens can cause point mutations, frame-shift mutations, and deletions of various sizes; some car-cinogens are most effective at causing one type of mutation, while others are most effective in causing another type. Are some types of mutations more likely than others to initiate a neoplastic event, and are there "hot-spots" for initiation in the DNA? In addition to sites made especially liable to mutation by their base sequences, one can envision that mutations in certain "promoter" regions for transcrip-tion of DNA, especially promoters for genes that are involved in the control of cell replication, might be much more effective for initiation than are mutations at other sites. Likewise, the possible effects of carcinogen modifi-cation of DNA on the movement of and control of genetic elements, such as transposons, may become a critical issue in chemical carcinogenesis as more is learned of the roles of these genetic elements in normal differentiation, cellular control, and viral carcinogenesis in animal cells (McKay, 1980; Cairns, 1981; Marx, 1981; Rigby, 1981; Wyke, 1981). However, it is not unlikely that transposition may be a more critical component of promotion than of the initiation phase of carcinogenesis.

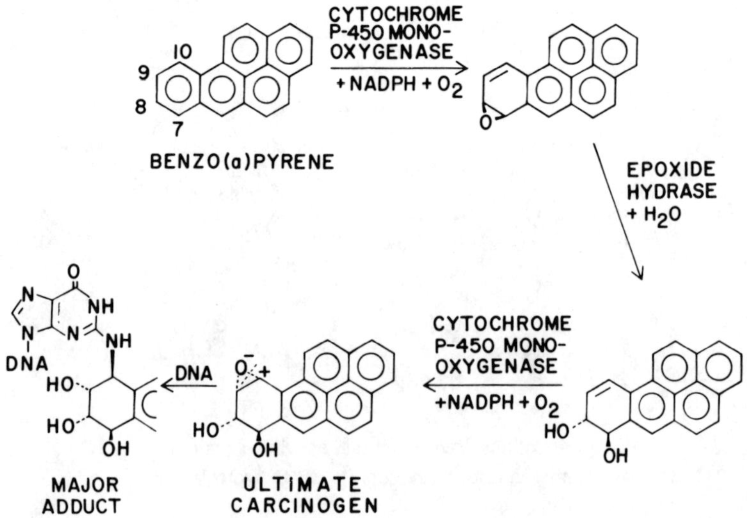

Figure 6. A major route for the metabolic activation of benzo(a)pyrene. See references in Miller, E.C. and Miller, J.A., 1981 and in Harvey, 1981.

REFERENCES

Allen JA, Coombs MM (1980). Covalent binding of polycyclic aromatic compounds to mitochondrial and nuclear DNA. Nature 287:244

Ames BN, Durston WE, Yamasaki E, Lee FD (1973). Carcinogens are mutagens: A simple test system combining liver homogenates for activation and bacteria for detection. Proc Natl Acad Sci USA 70:2281.

Armuth V, Berenblum I (1972). Systemic promoting action of phorbol in liver and lung carcinogenesis in AKR mice. Cancer Res 32:2259.

Armuth, V, Berenblum I (1974). Promotion of mammary carcinogenesis and leukemogenic action by phorbol in virgin female Wistar rats. Cancer Res 34:2704.

Backer J, Weinstein IB (1980). Mitochondrial DNA is a major cellular target for a dihydrodiol-epoxide derivative of benzo(a)pyrene. Science 209:297.

Berenblum I (1941). The cocarcinogenic action of croton resin. Cancer Res 1:44.

Berenblum I (1974). "Carcinogenesis as a Biological Problem." Amsterdam/Oxford: Raven, p. 122.

Berenblum I, Shubik P (1947). A new quantitative approach to the study of the stages of chemical carcinogenesis in the mouse's skin. Br J Cancer 1:383.

Berenblum I, Shubik P (1949). The persistence of latent tumor cells induced in the mouse's skin by a single application of 9,10-dimethyl-1,2-benzanthracene. Br J Cancer 3:384.

Berlin V, Haseltine WA (1981). Reduction of adriamycin to a semiquinone-free radical by NADPH cytochrome P-450 reductase produces DNA cleavage in a reaction mediated by molecular oxygen. J Biol Chem 256:4747.

Boutwell RK (1964). Some biological aspects of skin carcinogenesis. Prog Exp Tumor Res 4:207.

Cairns J (1981). The origin of human cancers. Nature 289:353.

Cook JW, Hewett CL, Hieger I (1933). The isolation of a cancer-producing hydrocarbon from coal tar (Parts I, II, and III). J Chem Soc p 395.

Coon MJ, Chiang YL, French JS (1979). Chemical characterization of the enzymes involved in drug metabolism. In Estabrook RW, Lindenlaub E (eds): "The Induction of Drug Metabolism," Stuttgart/New York: Schattauer Verlag, p 201.

Cramer JW, Miller JA, Miller EC (1960). N-Hydroxylation: A

new metabolic reaction observed in the rat with the carcinogen 2-acetylaminofluorene. J Biol Chem 235:885.

DeBaun JR, Rowley JY, Miller EC, Miller JA (1968). Sulfotransferase activities of N-hydroxy-2-acetylaminofluorene in rodent livers susceptible and resistant to this carcinogen. Proc Soc Exp Biol Med 129:273.

Estabrook RW, Werringloer J (1979). The microsomal enzyme system responsible for the oxidative metabolism of many drugs. In Estabrook RW, Lindenlaub E (eds): "The Induction of Drug Metabolism," Stuttgart/New York: Schattauer Verlag, p 187.

Friedewald WF, Rous P (1944). The initiating and promoting elements in tumor production. An analysis of the effects of tar, benzpyrene, and methylcholanthrene on rabbit skin. J Exp Med 80:101.

Grover PL (ed) (1979). "Chemical Carcinogens and DNA." Vols I, II. Boca Raton, Florida: CRC Press, 236 pp, 210 pp.

Haddow A, Kon GAR (1947). Chemistry of carcinogenic compounds. Br Med Bull 4:314.

Hall, WH, Bielschowsky, F (1949). The development of malignancy in experimental induced adenomata of the thyroid. Br J Cancer 3:534.

Harvey RG (1981). Activated metabolites of carcinogenic hydrocarbons. Acc Chem Res 14:218.

Hicks RM, Wakefield J StJ, Chowaniec J (1975). Evaluation of a new model to detect bladder carcinogens or cocarcinogens; results obtained with saccharin, cyclamate, and cyclophosphamide. Chem Biol Interact 11:225.

Hueper WC, Wiley FH, Wolfe HD (1938). Experimental production of bladder tumors in dogs by administration of beta-naphthylamine. J Ind Hygiene Toxicol 20:46.

Kennaway EL, Hieger I (1930). Carcinogenic substances and their fluorescence spectra. Br Med J 1:1044.

King CM, Phillips B (1968). Enzyme catalyzed reactions of the carcinogen N-hydroxy-2-fluorenylacetamide with nucleic acid. Science 159:1351.

Kinosita R (1937). Studies on the cancerogenic chemical substances. Trans Jap Path Soc 27:665.

Kitagawa T, Pitot HC, Miller EC, Miller JA (1979). Promotion by dietary phenobarbital of hepatocarcinogenesis by 2-methyl-N,N-dimethyl-4-aminoazobenzene in the rat. Cancer Res 39:112.

Kriek E, Miller JA, Juhl U, Miller EC (1967). 8(N-2-fluorenylacetamido)-guanosine, an arylamidation reaction product of guanosine and the carcinogen N-acetoxy-N-2-

fluorenylacetamide in neutral solution. Biochemistry 6:177.

Lasne C, Gentil A, Chouroulinkow I (1974). Two-stage malignant transformation of rat fibroblasts in tissue culture. Nature 247:490.

Loeb LA, Zakour RA (1980). Metals and genetic miscoding. In Spiro GT (ed): "Nucleic Acid-Metal Ion Interactions," New York: Wiley, p 115.

Lotlikar PD, Scribner JD, Miller JA, Miller EC (1966). Reactions of esters of aromatic N-hydroxy amines and amides with methionine in vitro: A model for in vivo binding of amine carcinogens to protein. Life Sci 5:1263.

MacKenzie I, Rous P (1941). The experimental disclosure of latent neoplastic changes in tarred skin. J Exp Med 73:391.

Maher VM, Miller EC, Miller JA, Szybalski W (1968). Mutations and decreases in density of transforming DNA produced by derivatives of the carcinogens 2-acetylamino-fluorene and N-methyl-4-aminoazobenzene. Mol Pharmacol 4:411.

Marx JL (1981). Tumors viruses and the kinase connection. Science 211:1336.

McCann J, Ames BN (1976). Detection of carcinogens as mutagens in the Salmonella/microsome test: Assay of 300 chemicals: Discussion. Proc Natl Acad Sci USA 73:950.

McKay R (1980). Movable genes. Nature 287:188.

Miller EC (1978). Some current perspectives on chemical carcinogenesis in humans and experimental animals: Presidential address. Cancer Res 38:1479.

Miller EC, Juhl U, Miller JA (1966). Nucleic acid guanine: Reaction with the carcinogen N-acetoxy-2-acetylamino-fluorene. Science 153:1125.

Miller EC, Miller JA (1947). The presence and significance of bound aminoazo dyes in the livers of rats fed p-dimethylaminoazobenzene. Cancer Res 7:468.

Miller EC, Miller JA (1966). Mechanisms of chemical car-cinogenesis: Nature of proximate carcinogens and inter-actions with macromolecules. Pharmacol Rev 18:805.

Miller EC, Miller JA (1971). The mutagenicity of chemical carcinogens: Correlations, problems, and interpreta-tions. In Hollaender A (ed): "Chemical Mutagens - Principles and Methods for their Detection, vol 1." New York/London: Plenum, p 83.

Miller EC, Miller JA (1979a). Milestones in chemical car-cinogenesis. Sem Oncol 6:445.

Miller EC, Miller JA (1979b). Naturally occurring chemical

carcinogens that may be present in foods. In Neuberger A, Jukes TH (eds): "Biochemistry of Nutrition" 1A, Vol 27, Baltimore: University Park Press, p 123.

Miller EC, Miller JA (1981). Searches for ultimate chemical carcinogens and their reactions with cellular macromolecules. Cancer 47:2327.

Miller EC, Miller JA, Hartmann, HA (1961). N-Hydroxy-2-acetylaminofluorene: A metabolite of 2-acetylaminofluorene with increased carcinogenic activity in the rat. Cancer Res 21:815.

Miller JA (1970). Carcinogenesis by chemicals: An overview - GHA Clowes memorial lecture. Cancer Res 30:559.

Miller JA, Miller EC (1966). A survey of molecular aspects of chemical carcinogenesis. Lab Invest 15:217.

Miller JA, Miller EC (1969). Metabolic activation of carcinogenic aromatic amines and amides via N-hydroxylation and N-hydroxy esterification and its relationship to ultimate carcinogens as electrophilic reactants. In Bergmann E, Pullman B (eds): "Physiochemical Mechanisms of Carcinogenesis, Vol 1, The Jerusalem Symposia on Quantum Chemistry and Biochemistry." Jerusalem: The Israel Academy of Sciences and Humanities, p 237.

Mondal S, Brankow DW, Heidelberger C (1976). Two-stage chemical oncogenesis in cultures of C3H/10Tl/2 cells. Cancer Res 36:2254.

Mottram JC (1944). A developing factor in experimental blastogenesis. J Path Bact 56:181.

O'Connor PJ, Saffhill R, Margison GP (1979). N-nitroso compounds: Biochemical mechanisms of action. In Emmelot P, Kriek E (eds): "Environmental Carcinogenesis: Occurrence, Risk Evaluation and Mechanisms," Amsterdam/New York: Elsevier/North-Holland, p 73.

Peraino C, Fry RJM, Staffeldt E (1971). Reduction and enhancement by phenobarbital of hepatocarcinogenesis induced in the rat by 2-acetylaminofluorene. Cancer Res 31:1506.

Poirier LA, Miller JA, Miller EC, Sato K (1967). N-Benzoyloxy-N-methyl-4-aminoazobenzene: Its carcinogenic activity in the rat and its reactions with proteins and nucleic acids and their constituents in vitro. Cancer Res 27:1600.

Rigby PWJ (1981). The detection of cellular transforming genes. Nature 290:186.

Rinkus SJ, Legator MS (1979). Chemical characterization of 465 known or suspected carcinogens and their correlation with mutagenic activity in the Salmonella typhimurium system. Cancer Res 39:3289.

Rous P, Kidd JG (1941). Conditional neoplasms and sub-threshold neoplastic states: A study of the tar tumors of rabbits. J Exp Med 73:365.

Salaman MH, Roe FJC (1953). Incomplete carcinogens: Ethyl carbamate (urethane) as an initiator of skin tumor formation in the mouse. Br J Cancer 7:472.

Slaga TJ, Sivak A, Boutwell RK (Eds) (1978). "Carcino-genesis: A Comprehensive Survey." New York: Raven, p 421.

Sugimura T, Sato S, Nagao M, Yahagi T, Matsushima T, Seino Y, Takeuchi M, Kawachi T (1976). Overlapping of carcinogens and mutagens. In Magee PN, Takayama S, Sugimura T, Matsushima T (eds): "Fundamentals in Cancer Prevention," Baltimore: University Park Press, p 191.

Tannenbaum A (1944). a. The dependence of the genesis of induced skin tumors on the caloric intake during different stages of carcinogenesis. b. The importance of dif-ferential consideration of the stages of carcinogenesis in the evaluation of carcinogenic and anticarcinogenic effects. c. The dependence of the genesis of induced skin tumors on the fat content of the diet during different stages of carcinogenesis. Cancer Res 4:673, 678, 683.

Testa B, Jenner P (1976). "Drug Metabolism: Chemical and Biochemical Aspects," New York/Basel: Dekker, p 273.

Van Duuren BL (1969). Tumor-promoting agents in two-stage carcinogenesis. Prog Exp Tumor Res 11:31.

Van Duuren BL, Sivak A, Katz C, Seidman I, Melchionne S (1975). The effect of aging and interval between primary and secondary treatment in two-stage carcinogenesis on mouse skin. Cancer Res 35:502.

Van Duuren BL, Smith AC, Melchionne SM (1978). Effect of aging in two-stage carcinogenesis on mouse skin with phorbol myristate acetate as promoting agent. Cancer Res 38:865.

Wunderlich V, Schütt M, Böttger M, Graffi A (1970). Preferential alkylation of mitochondrial deoxyribonucleic acid by N-methyl-N-nitrosourea. Biochem J 118:99.

Wunderlich, V, Tetzlaff I, Graffi A (1971/72). Studies on nitrosodimethylamine: Preferential methylation of mito-chondrial DNA in rats and hamsters. Chem Biol Interact 4:81.

Wyke J (1981). Strategies of viral oncogenesis. Nature 290:629.

Yamagiwa K, Ichikawa K (1918). Experimental study of the pathogenesis of carcinoma. J Cancer Res 3:1.

Yoshida T (1933). Uber die serienweise Verfolgung der Veränderungen der Leber dei der experimentellen Hepatomerzeugung durch o-Amidoazotoluol. Trans Jap Path Soc 23:636.

**Prostaglandins and Cancer: First
International Conference, pages 97–111**
© **1982 Alan R. Liss, Inc., 150 Fifth Avenue, New York, NY 10011**

PROSTAGLANDIN SYNTHETASE-DEPENDENT COOXYGENATION

Lawrence J. Marnett, Michael J. Bienkowski, Marie
Leithauser, William R. Pagels, Augustine
Panthananickal, and Gregory A. Reed
Department of Chemistry
Wayne State University
Detroit, Michigan 48202

The first stage in the biosynthesis of prostaglandins
is the oxygenation of polyunsaturated fatty acids such as
arachidonic acid to the hydroperoxy endoperoxide, PGG_2,
which is then reduced to the hydroxy endoperoxide, PGH_2
(Hamberg et al, 1974; Nugteren and Hazelhof, 1973). During
the reduction of PGG_2, an oxidizing agent is generated which
oxygenates or oxidizes xenobiotics Scheme 1 (Marnett et
al, 1975).

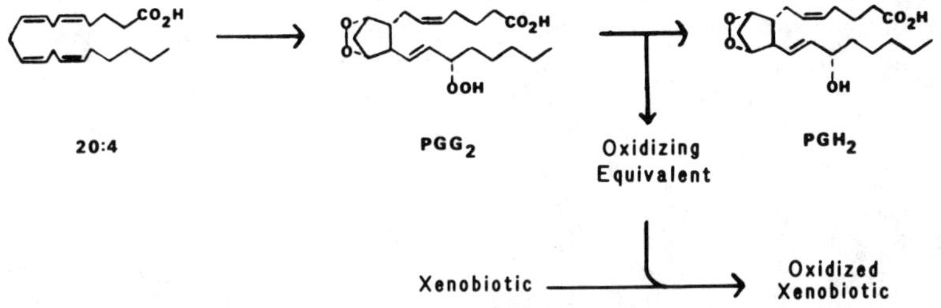

Scheme 1

Since oxygenation is important in the activation of compounds to toxic and/or carcinogenic derivatives (Miller,
1970), it occurred to us that prostaglandin synthetase might
participate in the oxidative activation of xenobiotics.
This has provided the driving force behind our attempts to
answer the following questions:
    1. Can prostaglandin synthetase trigger the cooxygena-
tion of non-carcinogenic compounds to carcinogenic derivatives?
    2. What is the identity of the peroxidase which inter-

acts with PGG$_2$ to trigger cooxygenation?
   3.   What are the mechanisms of the hydroperoxide-dependent cooxygenations?

Our results are outlined below.

METABOLISM AND ACTIVATION OF POLYCYCLIC HYDROCARBONS DURING PROSTAGLANDIN BIOSYNTHESIS

Benzo[a]pyrene

   The polycyclic hydrocarbon benzo[a]pyrene (BP) was chosen for our initial attempts to detect metabolic activation because a great deal is known about the metabolism and carcinogenicity of BP and its derivatives, and because we had shown earlier that BP is metabolized to unidentified products during prostaglandin biosynthesis (Sims and Grover, 1974; Levin et al, 1977; Jerina et al, 1977; Harvey, 1981; Marnett et al, 1975). The incubation of [^{14}C]-BP with ram seminal vesicle microsomes (RSVM), which contains a highly active prostaglandin synthetase, in the presence of arachidonic acid followed by HPLC analysis of the organic extract, indicates that three [^{14}C]-labeled products are formed (Marnett et al, 1977). Spectral analysis of the isolated products indicates that they are the 1,6-,3,6-, and 6,12-quinone derivatives of BP. The time course of their formation parallels the time course of the conversion of arachidonic acid to PGH$_2$ and in the absence of arachidonate, quinone formation is supported by PGG$_2$ or by a hydroperoxide analog 15-hydroperoxy-5,8,11,13-eicosatetraenoic acid, 15-HPETE. Indomethacin (10 µM) completely inhibits arachidonate-dependent quinone formation. Literature precedents suggest that the quinones are formed by the air oxidation of the initial BP metabolite, 6-hydroxy-BP (Lesko et al, 1975; Nagata et al, 1974). The latter compound is formed directly from BP without epoxide intermediates (eq 1). We have found no evidence for the prostaglandin synthetase-dependent oxidation of BP to epoxides.

   Inclusion of t-RNA in incubations containing BP, RSVM, and arachidonate leads to the formation of covalent adducts between a derivative of BP and the t-RNA (31 pmol/mg t-RNA) (Marnett and Reed, 1979). Despite this fact, no mutagenic derivatives can be detected following the incubation of BP, RSVM, and arachidonate with <u>Salmonella</u> <u>typhimurium</u> strains

eq 1

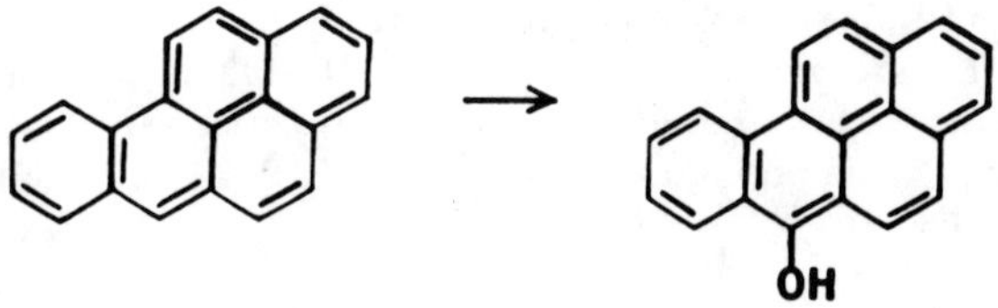

TA 98 or TA 100. This is true even though controls indicate that the bacteria do not inhibit BP metabolism to quinones or t-RNA binding derivatives by RSVM. The obvious interpretation is that even though covalent binding of BP to Salmonella DNA may occur, it does not lead to mutation. Alternatively, it is possible that the electrophilic derivatives of BP are too unstable under the conditions of their generation to diffuse into the bacteria and bind to DNA.

7,8-Dihydroxy-7,8-dihydrobenzo[a]pyrene.

There is a tremendous amount of evidence which indicates that the most mutagenic metabolites of BP are 7,8-diol-9, 10-epoxide derivatives (Levin et al, 1977; Jerina et al, 1977; Harvey, 1981). In liver, these compounds are formed by the sequential action of a mixed-function oxidase, epoxide hydrase, and a mixed-function oxidase (Levin et al, 1977; Huberman et al, 1976). The 7,8-dihydrodiol is an inactive precarcinogen which is oxygenated at the 9,10 position to form the ultimate carcinogen, the diolepoxide (Kapitulnik et al, 1978). For simplicity, equation 2 shows only the isomer of the diolepoxide in which the epoxide oxygen and the 7-hydroxyl oxygen are on opposite sides of the tetrahydrobenzo ring (anti-). Another isomer exists in which the epoxide oxygen and the 7-hydroxyl oxygen are

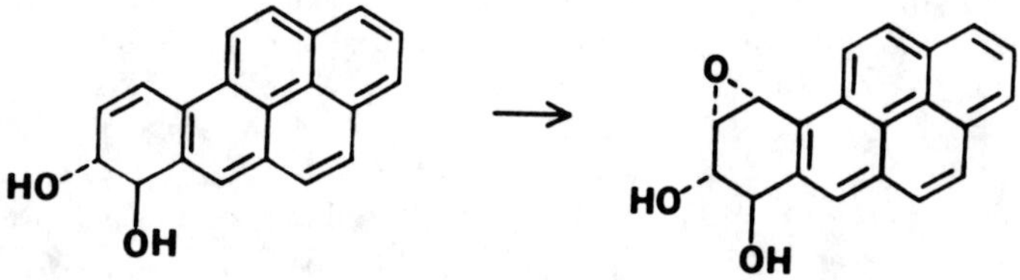

eq 2

on the same side of the molecule (syn-)(Wislocki et al, 1976). Evidence for the formation of both isomers, although in different amounts, has been acquired using microsomal and

nuclear mixed-function oxidases and purified cytochrome
P-450. It should also be pointed out that both the anti
and syn-diolepoxides can have enantiomers so that, in fact,
there are four possible 7,8-diol-9,10-epoxides which can be
formed from BP.

Arachidonate-dependent metabolism of BP-7,8-diol by a
Tween 20-solubilized preparation from RSVM results in the
formation of a derivative strongly mutagenic to Salmonella
typhimurium strains TA 98 and TA 100 (Marnett et al, 1978).
Linear dose-response is observed at BP-7,8-diol concentration of 1 to 20 μM. Stimulation of the formation of a mutagen requires BP-7,8-diol, 20:4, and enzyme and is inhibited by indomethacin. This metabolic activation is specific
to BP-7,8-diol. Under identical conditions, no increase in
the number of revertants of TA 98 to histidine independence
is observed with BP-4,5-diol or BP-9,10-diol (Marnett et al,
1978).

Incubation of $[^{14}C]$ BP-7,8-diol with 20:4 and RSVM
leads to the formation of two products which we have identified as 7,8,9,10-tetrahydroxy-7,8,9,10-tetrahydro BP's
(Marnett et al, 1979). These two tetraols are the non-
enzymatic hydrolysis products of the anti-diolepoxide (eq 3)
(Keller et al, 1976). It is suggested that the BP-7,8-diol
is initially oxidized to the anti-diolepoxide which undergoes spontaneous hydrolysis to the mixture of tetraols.

eq 3

Formation of both tetraols is inhibited by heat-inactivation
of the microsomes, omission of 20:4, or inclusion of indomethacin in the incubation mixture (Marnett et al, 1979).
The time course of the formation of the tetraols parallels
the time course of the oxygenation of 20:4 by prostaglandin
synthetase. Oxygenation of BP-7,8-diol can also be effected by the addition of 15-HPETE to RSVM. The product profile is identical to that observed when oxidation is triggered by the addition of 20:4. Heat inactivation of the
microsomes inhibits the 15-HPETE-dependent oxidation by 45%,
which indicates that an appreciable non-enzymatic hydro-

peroxide-dependent oxygenation occurs.

The inclusion of polyguanylic acid, poly (G), in incubations containing [^{3}H]-BP-7,8-diol, arachidonate, and RSVM results in covalent attachment of radioactivity to poly (G) (940 pmol/mg/nucleic acid) (Panthananickal and Marnett, 1981). Covalent binding requires arachidonate and RSVM and is inhibited by indomethacin. Digestion of the poly (G) adducts to nucleoside adducts followed by reversed-phase HPLC indicates that the principal adducts cochromatograph with adducts formed by the cis and trans addition of the exocyclic amino group of guanine to the (±)-anti-diolepoxide (Moore et al, 1977). Integration of the peak areas of the adduct HPLC profile suggests that both enantiomers of the diolepoxide are formed in equal amounts. The obvious corollary of this observation is that both enantiomers of BP-7,8-diol are oxidized to enantiomers of the anti-diolepoxide to equal extents.

Experiments similar to these, performed with DNA rather than poly (G), provide further evidence for the formation of the anti-diolepoxide from BP-7,8-diol during prostaglandin biosynthesis. Figure 1 is a comparison of the HPLC profile of the deoxynucleoside adducts isolated following the reaction of (±)-anti-diolepoxide with DNA with the profile determined following the incubation of (±)-BP-7,8-diol with arachidonate and RSVM in the presence of DNA. The profiles are virtually identical, providing further evidence for the metabolism of (±)-BP-7,8-diol to (±)-anti-diolepoxide during prostaglandin biosynthesis.

The product studies, nucleic acid binding studies, and mutagenicity studies provide strong evidence for the arachidonic acid-dependent cooxygenation of BP-7,8-diol to the anti-diolepoxide. Since the anti-diolepoxide is believed to represent the ultimate carcinogenic form of BP, our studies suggest that prostaglandin synthetase can participate in the metabolic activation of non-carcinogenic compounds to carcinogenic derivatives. It is interesting that prostaglandin synthetase metabolizes BP to quinones but BP-7,8-diol to an epoxide. This implies that if prostaglandin synthetase plays a role in BP carcinogenesis, it can only act after BP is converted to BP-7,8-diol by the sequential action of a mixed-function oxidase and epoxide hydrase.

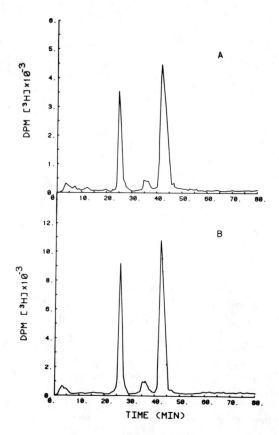

Figure 1. HPLC profile of deoxynucleoside adducts formed by reaction of rat liver DNA with [^{3}H]-BP-7,8-diol, RSVM, and arachidonic acid (A) or with [^{3}H]-diolepoxide 2 (B).

7,8-Dihydrobenzo[a]pyrene.

Neither of the diolepoxide isomers of BP are substrates for epoxide hydrase. This is apparently due to the presence of the hydroxyl groups at C-7 and C-8 since the epoxide derivative of 7,8-dihydrobenzo[a]pyrene (7,8-DHBP) (eq 4) is a substrate for rat liver microsomal epoxide hydrase (Waterfall and Sims, 1972).

The relative amounts of epoxide hydrolysis products differ depending on whether the reaction is spontaneous or

eq 4

epoxide hydrase–catalyzed (eq 5). Since epoxide hydrase

eq 5

activity can be manipulated by the use of inhibitors, this
provides a probe for the involvement of epoxides in the
metabolism of 7,8-DHBP. We have synthesized [^{14}C]-DHBP and
authentic standards of the epoxide, ketone, and dihydrodiol
hydrolysis products. The stereochemistry of the dihydrodiols was assigned on the basis of chemical methods.

Incubation of [^{14}C]-DHBP with RSVM and arachidonic
acid leads to the production of all three labeled solvolysis products plus a small amount of BP by dehydrogena-
tion of DHBP. The percentage yields of the solvolysis
products are given in Table 1. The major product is the
cis-diol with nearly an equivalent amount of the trans-diol.
When the incubations are performed in the presence of the
epoxide hydrase inhibitor, trichloropropylene oxide, the
ratio of the cis to trans-diol doubles, and when a purified
prostaglandin synthetase preparation is used, the ratio
nearly triples. Epoxide hydrase catalyzes the trans hydra-
tion of epoxides and the decreased yields of the trans-diol
in the presence of the epoxide hydrase inhibitor or in the
absence of epoxide hydrase suggests that an epoxide is
formed as an intermediate in the metabolism of 7,8-DHBP.

TABLE 1. Product ratios from 7,8-DHBP metabolism by prostaglandin synthetase.

Conditions	Trans	Cis	Ketone
RSVM[a]	1	1.2±0.2	0.4±0.5
RSVM + TCPO[b]	1	2.3±0.4	1.2±0.4
Purified Enzyme[c]	1	2.8±0.6	0.7±0.2

a) [Arachidonate] = 100 µM, [7,8-DHBP]= 10 µM, [Protein] =
1 mg/ml
b) [TCPO] = 5 mM
c) [Hematin] = 1 µM, [Protein]= 3 µg/ml, [15-HPETE] = 50 µM

IDENTIFICATION OF THE PEROXIDASE IN RAM SEMINAL VESICLE MI-
CROSOMES RESPONSIBLE FOR XENOBIOTIC COOXYGENATION

Arachidonic acid-dependent cooxygenation is peroxidatic and utilizes PGG_2 as the hydroperoxide substrate
(Marnett et al, 1975). Until recently, the peroxidase responsible for the cooxygenations had not been unequivocally
identified although it had been suggested that it is the
hydroperoxidase component of PES (Zenser et al, 1980). We
have attempted to identify the peroxidase utilizing two complementary approaches.

We have purified prostaglandin synthetase from the seminal vesicles to apparent electrophoretic homogeneity by
using detergent solubilization, gel filtration, and ion-ex-
change chromatography. Upon reconstitution with hematin,
the purified protein exhibits a peroxidase activity toward
phenylbutazone, epinephrine, guiaicol, and BP-7,8-diol. Reconstitution of cyclooxygenase and peroxidase activities requires exactly 1 heme per subunit. The overall yield of PES
and peroxidase is approximately 20%, the purified protein
represents the major peroxidase activity in the microsomal
fraction and is the sole peroxidase eluting from the ion-
exchange column (the principal purification step). Subsequent chromatography of the purified protein on an ion-
exchange column at a different pH, on hydroxylapatite, on
gel filtration, and on a chromatofocusing column does not
resolve the cyclooxygenase from the peroxidase activity.
The enzyme isolated following chromatofocusing exhibits a
single zone on two dimensional isoelectricfocusing-SDS-poly-
acrylamide gel electrophoresis. These data indicate that
the peroxidase purified to homogeneity from ram seminal
vesicles is a component of prostaglandin synthetase.

The above studies indicate that PES purified to homogeneity has a reconstitutable peroxidase activity which will
cooxygenate xenobiotics. We have also used an immunochemical method to identify the peroxidase present in crude
preparations from ram seminal vesicles. Dr. William Smith
of the Biochemistry Department of Michigan State University
has provided us with a monoclonal antibody which he has
raised against purified prostaglandin synthetase. This antibody can be coated on attenuated Staphylococcus aureus
cells or protein A-Sepharose beads to render it precipitat-
ing and it is then incubated for 5 minutes with Tween 20-
solubilized preparations from RSVM. The cells or beads are

pelleted and the supernatant is assayed for cyclooxygenase
and peroxidase activity. Controls are run using media in
which no cells were grown. Table 2 lists the percentage of
peroxidase activity which remains in the supernatant following incubation with the antibody and the control preparation. The first two columns represent the percentage of
peroxidase activity which remains in the supernatant following incubation with the antibody and the control preparation. The third column represents the percentage of peroxidase activity precipitated by the antibody relative to controls (the control really measures inactivation rather than
precipitation).

TABLE 2. Immunoprecipitation of peroxidase activity in
Tween 20-solubilized ram seminal vesicle microsomes by anti-PES.

Compound	Activity in Supernatant		% Precipitated
	Immune	Non-Immune	
DPBF	31	72	57
Phenylbutazone	17	100	83
Epinephrine	32	62	49

The cyclooxygenase and peroxidase activities are not
inactivated by the antibody so that it is possible to re-
suspend the pellet following incubation with the protein
preparation and assay it for both activities. This has
been done for the PES and DPBF-peroxidase activities and
the results indicate that both activities are actually precipitated by the antibody. This rules out the possibility
that the antibody is causing disappearance of activity from
the supernatant by a process unrelated to immunoprecipitation. As a control for the specificity of the antibody, we
have iodinated the proteins in the solubilized preparation
with the Bolton-Hunter reagent and treated them with the
antibody-coated S. aureus cells. The precipitated proteins
were analyzed by SDS-acrylamide gel electrophoresis and exhibited a single radioactive protein which comigrates with
authentic prostaglandin synthetase. This verifies that the
antibody is monospecific for prostaglandin synthetase.

The purification and immunochemical experiments provide complementary data which suggest that prostaglandin
synthetase is the major if not the sole peroxidase responsible for arachidonic acid-dependent cooxygenation in ram
seminal vesicles. Extrapolation of these results to other

tissues may not be possible. Although the ram seminal vesicle has levels of cytochrome P-450 which are below the limit of detection by conventional spectral and enzymatic
assays (Marnett et al, 1979; Sivarajah et al, 1979), this
tissue has one of the highest levels of prostaglandin synthetase of any mammalian tissue (Christ and Van Dorp, 1972).
It is, therefore, expected that the major peroxidase in
RSVM is the peroxidase of prostaglandin synthetase and that
other peroxidases such as cytochrome P-450 do not contribute significantly to hydroperoxide-dependent oxygenation.
Most other tissues have significant levels of other peroxidases such as cytochrome P-450 and much lower levels of
prostaglandin synthetase. Thus, it will be necessary to
employ methods similar to the above to determine the relative contribution of arachidonic acid-dependent xenobiotic
cooxygenation in these tissues. Of particular interest will
be tissues which are target organs for drug toxicity and
chemical carcinogenesis such as lung, skin, kidney, colon,
bladder, and brain.

MECHANISM OF ARACHIDONIC ACID-DEPENDENT COOXYGENATION

As discussed above, the oxidation of BP to quinones is
likely to proceed through the intermediacy of 6-OH-BP, although this has not been proven. Substantial literature
precedents suggest that the formation of 6-OH-BP and its
subsequent decomposition occur by free radical mechanisms
(Lesko et al, 1975; Nagata et al, 1974). This is consistent with the chemistry observed for other compounds co-
oxygenated during PGH_2 biosynthesis. For the compounds
where product studies are available, the cooxygenation
products are the same as the radical oxidation products.
Further support for radical oxidation mechanisms is provided by the observation of inhibition of cooxygenation by
a variety of antioxidants. BP cooxygenation is inhibited
in a dose-response fashion by BHA, BHT, Vitamin E, or
Vitamin C at concentrations ranging from 50 to 55 µM
(Marnett et al, 1977).

An important piece of mechanistic information is the
source of the oxygen incorporated into the oxidized substrate. Since arachidonic acid-dependent cooxygenation is
actually a hydroperoxide-dependent cooxygenation, the oxygen could derive from the hydroperoxide oxygen, molecular
oxygen, or water. We have tested this by incubating

various oxidizable substrates with RSVM and various $[^{18}O]$-labeled oxygen sources. Our studies indicate that the oxygen incorporated into diphenylisobenzofuran, phenylbutazone, and BP-7,8-diol is molecular oxygen (Figure 2) (Marnett et al, 1979a; Marnett et al, 1980; Marnett and Bienkowski, 1980). For example, incubation of BP-7,8-diol and RSVM with 15-HPETE labeled with ^{18}O in both peroxide oxygens (91 atom % excess) leads to incorporation of 5 atom % excess ^{18}O into the product tetraols. When similar incubations are conducted with ^{16}O-labeled 15-HPETE under an $^{18}O_2$ atmosphere (98 atom % excess), 90 atom % excess ^{18}O (one atom) is incorporated into tetraols.

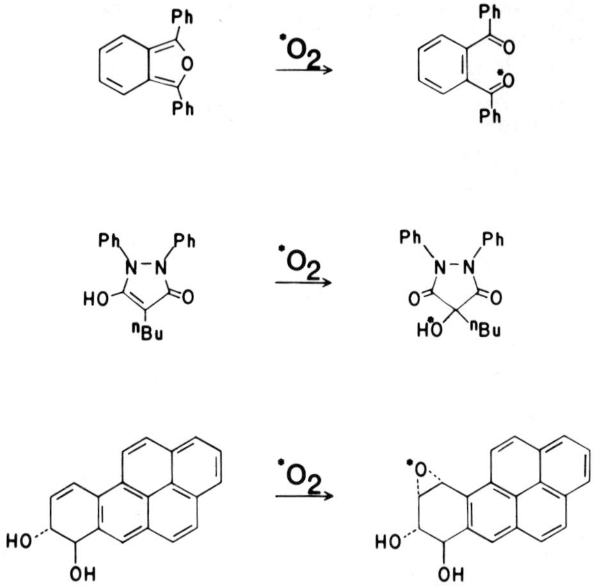

Figure 2

Finally, we have found that the stoichiometry of diphenylisobenzofuran oxidized to hydroperoxide added varies from 2:1 to 3000:1 indicative of the operation of a chain process (Marnett et al, 1979a). Taken with the source of the oxygen and the inhibition by antioxidants, this suggests that the hydroperoxide-dependent oxidation of BP and the compounds listed in Figure 2 occurs by free radical mechanisms. We have proposed that the interaction of PGG_2 with the peroxidase component of prostaglandin synthetase triggers the release of an oxidizing radical which reacts with the cosubstrate (Marnett et al, 1979a). The identity of the oxidizing radical is unknown; experiments indicate that it is not superoxide anion, hydroxyl radical, or hydrogen peroxide. The difference in the cooxygenation products are probably due to the unique chemistry of each of the oxidizable cosubstrates in the presence of radical oxidants.

Figure 3 displays a model for prostaglandin synthetase-dependent cooxygenation which encompasses our findings and those of other investigators. A stimulus interacts with the plasma membrane of a particular cell resulting in the release of arachidonate and subsequent PGG_2 biosynthesis. The PGG_2 interacts with a peroxidase (prostaglandin synthetase or another peroxidase) and releases oxidizing radicals which oxidize endogenous substrates or xenobiotics. The oxidized xenobiotic may be toxic and/or mutagenic; the latter would result in tumor initiation. Recent evidence suggests oxidizing radicals may play an important role in tumor promotion by unknown mechanisms (Goldstein et al, 1979). Since tumor promoters are among the agents which trigger the formation of oxidizing radicals from arachidonic acid, it is possible that prostaglandin synthetase-dependent cooxidation plays a role in tumor promotion as well as tumor initiation.

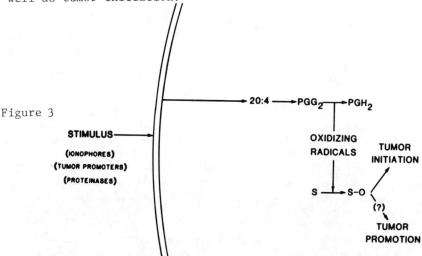

Figure 3

The present report describes the results of our research on arachidonate-dependent cooxygenation in vitro. Other laboratories, particularly those of Eling and Zenser, have made significant contributions to this field and their results are described in this volume and in a recent review (Marnett, 1981).

ACKNOWLEDGEMENTS

We are grateful to the National Institutes of Health (GM 23642) and the American Cancer Society (BC 244) for financial support.

REFERENCES

Christ E J, Van Dorp D A (1972) Comparative aspects of prostaglandin biosynthesis in animal tissues. Biochim Biophys Acta 270:537-545.

Goldstein B D, Witz G, Amoruso M, Troll W (1979) Protease inhibitors antagonize the activation of polymorphonuclear leukocyte oxygen consumption. Biochem Biophys Res Comm 88:854-860.

Hamberg M, Svensson J, Wakabayashi T, Samuelsson B (1974) Isolation and structure of two prostaglandin endoperoxides that cause platelet aggregation. Proc Natl Acad Sci USA 71:345-349.

Harvey R (1981) Activated metabolites of carcinogenic hydrocarbons. Acc Chem Res 14:218-226.

Huberman E, Sachs L, Yang S K, Gelboin H V (1976) Identification of mutagenic metabolites of benzo[a]pyrene in mammalian cells. Proc Natl Acad Sci USA 73:607-611.

Jerina D M, Lehr R, Schaefer-Ridder M, Yagi H, Karle J M, Thakker D R, Wood A W, Lu A Y H, Ryan D, West S, Levin W, Conney A H (1977) Bay-region epoxides of dihydrodiols: a concept explaining the mutagenic and carcinogenic activity of benzo[a]pyrene and benzo[a]anthracene. In Hiatt H H, Watson J D, Winsten J A (eds): "Origins of Human Cancer," Cold Spring Harbor, Cold Spring Harbor Laboratory, p 639-658.

Kapitulnik J, Wislocki P G, Levin W, Yagi H, Jerina D M, Conney A H (1978) Tumorigenicity studies with diolepoxides of benzo[a]pyrene which indicate that (±)-trans-$7\beta,8\alpha$-dihydroxy-$9\alpha,10\alpha$-epoxy-7,8,9,10-tetrahydrobenzo[a]pyrene is an ultimate carcinogen in newborn mice. Cancer Res 38:354-358.

Keller J W, Heidelberger C, Beland F A, Harvey R G (1976) Hydrolysis of syn-and anti-benzo[a]pyrene diol epoxides: stereochemistry, kinetics, and the effect of an intramolecular hydrogen bond on the rate of syn-diol epoxide solvolysis. J Amer Chem Soc 98:8276-8277.

Lesko S, Caspary W, Lorentzen R, Ts'o POP (1975) Enzymic formation of 6-oxobenzo[a]pyrene radical in rat liver homogenates from carcinogenic benzo[a]pyrene. Biochemistry 14:3978-3984.

Levin W, Lu A Y H, Ryan D, Wood A W, Kapitulnik J, West S, Huang M-T, Conney A H, Thakker D R, Holder G, Yagi H, Jerina D M (1977) Properties of the liver microsomal monoxygenase system and epoxide hydrase: factors influencing the metabolism and mutagenicity of benzo[a]pyrene. In Hiatt H H, Watson J D, Winsten J A (eds): "Origins of Human Cancer," Cold Spring Harbor, Cold Spring Harbor Laboratory, p 659-682.

Marnett L J, Wlodawer P, Samuelsson B (1975) Cooxygenation of organic substrates by the prostaglandin synthetase of sheep vesicular gland. J Biol Chem 250:8510-8517.

Marnett L J, Reed G A, Johnson J T (1977) Prostaglandin synthetase dependent benzo[a]pyrene oxidation: products of the oxidation and inhibition of their formation by antioxidants. Biochem Biophys Res Comm 79:569-576.

Marnett L J, Reed G A, Denison D J (1978) Prostaglandin synthetase dependent activation of 7,8-dihydro-7,8-dihydroxy-benzo[a]pyrene to mutagenic derivatives. Biochem Biophys Res Comm 82:210-216.

Marnett L J, Johnson J T, Bienkowski M J (1979) Arachidonic acid dependent metabolism of 7,8-dihydroxy-7,8-dihydrobenzo[a]pyrene by ram seminal vesicles. FEBS Letters 106: 13-16.

Marnett L J, Reed G A (1979) Peroxidatic oxidation of benzo[a]pyrene and prostaglandin biosynthesis. Biochemistry 18:2923-2929.

Marnett L J, Bienkowski M J, Pagels W R (1979a) Oxygen-18 investigation of the prostaglandin synthetase dependent cooxidation of diphenylisobenzofuran. J Biol Chem 254: 5077-5082.

Marnett L J, Bienkowski M J, Pagels W R, Reed G A (1980) Mechanism of xenobiotic cooxygenation coupled to prostaglandin H_2 biosynthesis. In Samuelsson B, Ramwell P W, Paoletti R (eds): "Advances in Prostaglandin and Thromboxane Research, Vol 6" New York: Raven Press p 149-151.

Marnett L J (1981) Polycyclic aromatic hydrocarbon oxidation during prostaglandin biosynthesis. Life Sciences 29: 531-546.

Miller J A (1970) Carcinogenesis by chemicals: an overview-GHA Clowes memorial lecture. Cancer Res 30:559-576.

Moore P D, Koreeda M, Wislocki P G, Levin W, Conney A H, Yagi H, Jerina D M (1977) In vitro reactions of the diastereomeric 9,10-epoxides of (+)- and (-)-trans-7,8-dihydroxy-7,8-dihydrobenzo[a]pyrene with polyguanylic acid and evidence for the formation of an enantiomer of each diastereomeric 9,10-epoxide from benzo[a]pyrene in mouse skin. In Jerina D M (ed): "Drug Metabolism Concepts," Vol 44 Washington DC: American Chemical Society, p 127-154.

Nagata C, Tagashira Y, Kodama M (1974) Metabolic activation of benzo[a]pyrene: significance of the free radical. In "The Biochemistry of Disease Vol 4. Chemical Carcinogenesis" (Ts'o POP, Dipaolo J A, eds) New York: Marcel Dekker Inc. p 87-111.

Nugteren D H, Hazelhof E (1973) Isolation and properties of intermediates in prostaglandin biosynthesis. Biochim Biophys Acta 326:448-461.

Panthananickal A, Marnett L J (1981) Arachidonic acid-dependent metabolism of (±)-7,8-dihydroxy-7,8-dihydrobenzo-[a]pyrene to polyguanylic acid-binding derivatives. Chem Biol Interactions 33:239-252.

Sims P, Grover P L (1974) Epoxides in polycyclic aromatic hydrocarbon metabolism and carcinogenesis. Adv. Cancer Res 20:166-274.

Sivarajah K, Mukhtar H, Eling T (1979) Arachidonic acid-dependent metabolism of (±) trans-7,8-dihydroxy-7,8-di-hydro-benzo[a]pyrene (BP-7,8-diol) to 7,10/8,9 tetrols. FEBS Letters 106:17-20.

Waterfall J F, Sims P (1972) Epoxy derivatives of aromatic polycyclic hydrocarbons. The preparation and metabolism of epoxides related to benzo[a]pyrene and to 7,8-and 9,10-dihydrobenzo[a]pyrene. Biochem J 128:265-277.

Wislocki P G, Wood A W, Chang R L, Levin W, Yagi H, Hernandez O, Jerina D M, Conney A H (1976) High mutagenicity and toxicity of a diol-epoxide derived from benzo-[a]pyrene. Biochem Biophys Res Comm 68:1006-1012.

Zenser T V, Mattammal M B, Davis B B (1980) Mechanism of FANFT cooxidation by prostaglandin endoperoxide synthetase. J Pharmacol Exp Ther 214:312-317.

**Prostaglandins and Cancer: First
International Conference, pages 113–122**
© **1982 Alan R. Liss, Inc., 150 Fifth Avenue, New York, NY 10011**

OXIDATION OF CHEMICAL CARCINOGENS
BY PROSTAGLANDIN SYNTHETASE

Thomas Eling, Jeff Boyd and K. Sivarajah

Laboratory of Pulmonary Function and Toxicology
National Institute of Environmental Health Sciences
P.O. Box 12233, Research Triangle Park, NC 27709

Prostaglandin endoperoxide synthetase (PGS) catalyzes
the conversion of polyunsaturated fatty acids, particularly
arachidonic acid (AA), to the endoperoxide PGH_2. PGH_2 is
the pivotal point from which prostaglandins (PGs), thromboxane A_2 (TXA_2) and prostacyclin (PGI_2) arise. PGS consists of two components: the first, fatty acid cyclo-
oxygenase, converts AA to the hydroperoxide PGG_2; the
second, hydroperoxidase, converts PGG_2 to the corresponding
alcohol, PGH_2. Both the cyclooxygenase and hydroperoxidase
activity co-purify (Ogino, Miyamato, Yamamoto, Hayaishi,
1977; Ohki, Ogino, Yamamoto, Hayaishi, 1979; Van der Ouderaa,
Buytenhek, Nugteren, Van Dorp, 1977). Metabolism or co-
oxidation of chemicals (Marnett, Wlodawer, Samuelsson,
1975) is catalyzed by the hydroperoxidase activity of PGS
and is dependent on the presence of the hydroperoxide PGG_2.
A large number of chemical substrates can serve as co-
factors for hydroperoxides (Marnett, 1981; Sivarajah,
Lasker, Abou-Donia, Eling, 1981; Lasker, Sivarajah, Mason,
Kalyanaraman, Abou-Donia, Eling, 1981). However, other
peroxides may also serve as a substrate for this peroxidase
activity (Marnett, Reed, 1979).
    Many carcinogenic chemicals are not themselves carcino-
genic but must be metabolized by the animal to a carcinogenic
metabolite(s) (Gelboin, 1980). The cytochrome P-450 mixed
function oxidase system (MFO) oxidizes chemicals to reactive
metabolites that bind covalently with DNA and produce
cellular damage. Many extra-hepatic tissues, like the lung,
have low MFO activity and yet are targets for the induction
of tumors by exposure to chemicals. Since the lung has
relatively high PGS activity, the possibility exists that

chemicals could also be oxidized to carcinogenic metabolites by PGS. To investigate the problem, we chose the polycyclic aromatic hydrocarbon benzo(a)pyrene (BP), which induces pulmonary tumors, as a model substrate for co-oxidation by PGS.

Extensive studies showed that BP is oxidized by the MFO system to <u>trans</u>-7,8-dihydroxy-7,8-dihydrobenzo(a)pyrene (BP-7,8-diol), the proximate carcinogen, and is further oxidized to BP diol-epoxides (BPDE), the ultimate carcinogenic metabolites of BP (Gelboin, 1980). As seen in Fig. 1, two diol-epoxides are formed by the MFO system. The epoxides are unstable and break down to stable tetrols which can be isolated and estimated after separation by HPLC.

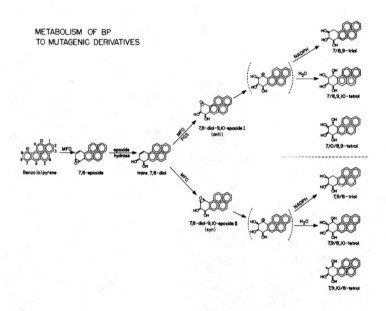

METABOLISM OF BP
TO MUTAGENIC DERIVATIVES

Preliminary experiments used ram seminal vesicle microsomes (RSV) as a source of PGS. On addition of AA to RSV, ^{3}H-BP-7,8-diol was oxidized by PGS to the tetrols produced from diol-epoxide I. No tetrols formed from diol-epoxide II were detected (Sivarajah, Mukhtar, Eling, 1979; Marnett, Johnson, Bienkowski, 1979). Furthermore, metabolism of BP-7,8-diol by PGS produced a reactive metabolite(s),

since radioactivity remained covalently bound to RSV.
These results suggest that BP-7,8-diol was oxidized to diol-
epoxide I by PGS (Fig. 1). A modified Ames assay system
was developed using RSV as the activating enzyme system.
BP-7,8-diol was converted to mutagenic metabolites by the
RSV system in the presence of AA. Indomethacin, a PGS
inhibitor, inhibited the formation of mutagenic metabolites
(Guthrie, Robertson, Zeiger, Boyd, Eling, 1981). This is
in agreement with results of Reed and Marnett (Marnett,
Reed, 1979). These results support the hypothesis that
during the oxidation of AA to PGs, BP-7,8-diol is oxidized
to diol-epoxide I.

RSV have exceptionally high PGS activity, while target
organs, lung for example, possess approximately 1-2% of the
activity of RSV (Sivarajah, Lasker, Eling, 1981). Furthermore, these target organs also have MFO activity. Thus,
two questions arise: (1) Will PGS-dependent oxidation of
BP-7,8-diol occur in target organs? (2) How does PGS-
dependent oxidation compare to MFO-dependent oxidation of
BP-7,8-diol? We determined the rate of oxidation by the
MFO and PGS system in a number of tissues as seen in Table 1.

In the presence of NADPH, rat lung microsomes oxidized
BP-7,8-diol at a rate which was almost 10 times faster than
in the presence of AA (Table 1). In the case of guinea pig
lung microsomes, however, the rates of BP-7,8-diol oxidation to tetrols were about equal when these different
cofactors were used. Human lung microsomes exhibited more
variability. Lung microsomes from one patient did not
oxidize BP-7,8-diol at all in the presence of NADPH, although a significant AA-dependent rate was observed. In two
other cases, the rates of pulmonary microsomal prostaglandin
synthetase dependent BP-7,8-diol oxidation were 52% and 67%
of the cytochrome P-450 MFO-dependent rates. For comparison,
BP-7,8-diol metabolism by these 2 enzymatic systems was
also determined with rat liver microsomes. While the rate
of NADPH dependent metabolism was the highest in this
tissue of all those examined, AA-dependent BP-7,8-diol
oxidation was not detectable. Under the conditions used,
rat liver microsomes have very low prostaglandin synthetase activity (Murota, Mouta, 1980). Indomethacin (100 μM)
inhibited AA-dependent oxidation but did not alter
NADPH-dependent oxidation.

Human lung, guinea pig lung, and rat lung microsomes
all metabolized BP-7,8-diol in the presence of NADPH to
diol-epoxides I and II. In contrast, these tissues formed

only diol-epoxide I in the presence of AA. These results indicate that the prostaglandin synthetase-dependent oxidation of BP-7,8-diol in human, rat and guinea pig lung proceeds via BP-diol-epoxide I, while the cytochrome P-450 dependent oxidation pathway in these tissues proceeds via both BP-diol-epoxide I and BP-diol-epoxide II. These results suggest that co-oxidation of BP-diol could play a role in development of human pulmonary tumors after exposure to BP.

TABLE 1. COMPARISON OF THE IN VITRO METABOLISM OF BP-7,8-DIOL BY AA AND NADPH IN VARIOUS TISSUES

	Tetrols (pmole/ml/min)	BPDE I (%)	BPDE II	Unknown
Ram Seminal Vesicles				
NADPH	ND	-	-	-
AA	411 ± 41	100	0	-
Rat Lung				
NADPH	167 ± 15	96	4	0
AA	17 ± 3	98	0	2
Guinea Pig Lung				
NADPH	190 ± 23	99	1	0
AA	175 ± 20	97	0	3
Rat Liver				
NADPH	342 ± 20	72	28	0
AA	ND	-	-	-
Human Lung				
Patient A				
NADPH	ND	-	-	-
AA	42 ± 5	A		
Patient B				
NADPH	77 ± 7	82	18	0
AA	52 ± 9	87	0	13
Patient C				
NADPH	83 ± 8	92	8	0
AA	43 ± 3	88	0	12

A = Not determined; ND = Not detectable; Values are mean ± S.D.; N=4 determinations.

The co-oxidation of BP-diol was shown using an in vitro microsomal system only. This raises three questions: (1) Does co-oxidation of BP-7,8-diol occur in an intact cell? (2) Can co-oxidation of BP-7,8-diol lead to an alteration in cellular DNA? (3) How does NADPH dependent compare to the AA-dependent oxidation in an intact cell? To answer these questions, we studied the metabolism of BP-7,8-diol in C3H 10T1/2 mouse embryo fibroblasts. This system was chosen since the cells have both MFO (Nesnow, Heidelberger, 1976) and PGS activity (Ali, Barrett, Eling, 1980), the cells transform after exposure to carcinogens (Ali, Barrett, Eling, 1980), and PGS activity is well characterized (Nesnow, Heidelberger, 1976).

BP-diol-epoxide I was the major organic extractable metabolite of BP-7,8-diol produced by the 10T1/2 confluent monolayers (Fig. 2). Major water soluble metabolites were glucuronides of BP-7,8-diol. These oxidations appear to be mediated via the MFO system since the formation of PGs is low in confluent monolayers (Ali, Barrett, Eling, 1980), and addition of indomethacin, an inhibitor of PGS but not MFO, to the cells, did not inhibit the metabolism. Stimulation of PGS by the addition of AA to the cells produced a 2-3 fold increase in diol-epoxide I formation (Fig. 2).

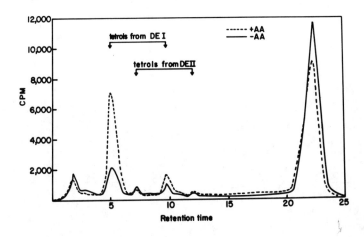

The addition of indomethacin reduced the stimulation of diol-epoxide I formation observed on addition of AA. These results suggest that co-oxidation by PGS can occur in an intact cell that has MFO activity, and produce an increase in BP-7,8-diol metabolism to the diol-epoxide I.

Metabolism in the presence and absence of AA was studied over a range of BP-7,8-diol concentrations. As seen in Table 2, an increase on the formation of diol-epoxide I on the addition of AA was dependent on the concentration of the diol. At low BP-7,8-diol concentration, no stimulation was observed while at 5 and 20 μM, a significant increase in metabolism occurred. At 50 μM BP-7,8-diol, the addition of AA did not alter the metabolism of the BP-7,8-diol by the 10T1/2 cells. The addition of indomethacin inhibits the AA-dependent increase in BP-7,8-diol metabolism. Thus, co-oxidation of BP-7,8-diol in these cells was dependent on the concentration of BP-7,8-diol. Moreover, this dose-dependent relationship varied from experiment to experiment. AA addition did not alter the formation of diol-epoxide II.

TABLE 2. BP-7,8-DIOL METABOLISM BY 10T1/2 CELLS

BP-diol	AA[a]	Indo[b]	BPDE 1[c]	BPDE II[d]
			(nmoles/dish)	
1 μM	-	-	1.1	0.09
	-	+	1.1	0.
	+	-	1.2	0.09
	+	+	1.3	0.1
5 μM	-	-	2.8	0.6
	-	+	2.7	0.6
	+	-	7.1	0.6
	+	+	1.6	0.4
20 μM	-	-	10.0	3.3
	-	+	9.9	2.6
	+	-	17.6	4.3
	+	+	8.9	2.6

[a] Arachidonic acid - 100 μM.
[b] Indomethacin - 100 μM.
[c] BP-diol-epoxide I
[d] BP-diol-epoxide II
Values are mean of two measurements. BPDE's estimated from total organic extractable tetrols. Dishes contained 10^6 cells.

The increased diol-epoxide I formation observed on addition of AA to the cells should also result in an increase in cell transformation. We therefore examined the effect of AA and indomethacin on cell transformation induced by various concentrations of BP-7,8-diol. As seen in Table 3, AA and indomethacin of 100 μM did not produce an increased number of foci (transformed cells). At 1 μM BP-7,8-diol, the addition of AA increased the number of foci from 1 to 11. Indomethacin addition reduced the increased transformation to 3 foci. At 5 μM BP-7,8-diol, the AA and indomethacin had little or no effect on the number of foci. At higher doses of BP-7,8-diol, cell toxicity was observed. Thus, over this narrow concentration range, stimulation of BP-7,8-diol co-oxidation by PGS can result in an increase in cell transformations. This concentration dependence also varied from experiment to experiment.

TABLE 3. TRANSFORMATION OF 10T1/2 FIBROBLASTS BY BP-7,8-DIOL

BP-diol	AA[a]	Indo[b]	Foci
0	-	-	0
	-	+	0
	+	-	0
	+	+	0
1 μM	-	-	1
	-	+	1
	+	-	11
	+	+	3
5 μM	-	-	5
	-	+	6
	+	-	5
	+	+	5

[a] 100 μM arachidonic acid
[b] 100 μM indomethacin

These results demonstrate that co-oxidation does occur
in an intact cell and increases the formation of diol-
epoxide I, leading to increase in cell transformation.
In the presence of the MFO system, co-oxidation does occur
producing an increase in metabolism. One can envision a
model for the oxidation of BP by intact cells as seen in
Fig. 3. BP is metabolized by the MFO and epoxide hydrase
system to BP-7,8-diol, which in turn is oxidized by P-450
to BP-7,8-diol epoxide I, the ultimate carcinogen of BP.
Stimulation of PG formation by various mechanisms increases the formation of BPDE-I by PGS-dependent co-oxidation. This leads to increased cell transformation. The
relative contribution of MFO and PGS systems depend, in
part, on the concentrations of the BP-7,8-diol and turnover
of AA. Our results suggest a possible role for co-oxidation
in the development of pulmonary tumors in vivo after exposure
to BP. Confirmation of this hypothesis requires further
investigation.

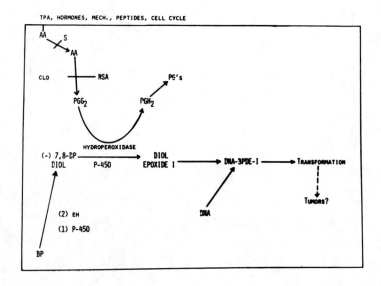

REFERENCES

Ali A, Barrett C, Eling T (1980). Prostaglandin and thromboxane production by vascular endothelial cells and
fibroblasts. Prostaglandins 20:667.
Gelboin H (1980). Benzo(a)pyrene metabolism, activation,
and carcinogenesis: Role of and regulation of mixed-
function oxidases and related enzymes. Phys. Rev.
60:1107.
Guthrie J, Robertson F, Zeiger E, Boyd J, Eling T
(1981). Activation and selective metabolism of bay
region dihydrodiols of several polycyclic aromatic
hydrocarbons to mutagenic products by prostaglandin
synthetase. Cancer Res. In press, 1981.
Lasker J, Sivarajah K, Mason R, Kalyanaraman B, Abou-Donia
M, Eling T (1981). A free radical mechanism of
prostaglandin synthetase-dependent aminopyrene demethy-
lation. J. Biol. Chem. 256:7764.
Marnett L (1981). Polycyclic aromatic hydrocarbon oxidation
during prostaglandin biosynthesis. Life Sci. 29:531.
Marnett L, Johnson J, Bienkowski M (1979). Arachidonic acid
dependent metabolism of 7,8-dihydroxy-7,8-dihydro-benzo
(a)pyrene by ram seminal vesicles. FEBS Lett. 106:13.
Marnett L, Reed G (1979). Peroxidatic oxidation of benzo(a)
pyrene and prostaglandin biosynthesis. Biochem. 18:2923.
Marnett L, Reed G, Dennison D (1978). Prostaglandin synthetase-dependent activation of 7,8-dihydro-7,8-dihydroxy
benzo(a)pyrene to mutagenic derivatives. Biochem. Biophys. Res. Comm. 82:210.
Marnett L, Wlodawer P, Samuelsson B (1975). Co-oxygenation
of organic substances by prostaglandin synthetase of
sheep vesicular gland. J. Biol. Chem. 250:8510.
Murota S, Mouta I (1980). Prostaglandin synthesizing system
in rat liver: changes with aging and various stimulation.
Adv. Prost. Thromb. Res. 8:1495.
Nesnow S, Heidelberger C (1976). The effect of modifiers
of microsomal enzymes in chemical oncogenesis in cultures of C3H mouse cell lines. Cancer Res. 36:1801.
Ogino N, Miyamato T, Yamamoto S, Hayaishi O (1977).
Prostaglandin endoperoxide E isomerase from bovine
vesicular gland microsomes, a glutathione-requiring
enzyme. J. Biol. Chem. 252:890.
Ohki S, Ogino N, Yamamoto S, Hayaishi O (1979). Prostaglandin hydroperoxidase, an integral part of prostaglandin endoperoxide synthetase from bovine vesicular gland
microsomes. J. Biol. Chem. 254:829.

Sivarajah K, Lasker J, Abou-Donia M, Eling T. Metabolism
    of N-alkyl compounds during prostaglandin synthesis.
    Mol. Pharm. In press, 1981.
Sivarajah K, Mukhtar H, Eling T (1979). Arachidonic acid
    dependent metabolism of (±) trans -7,8-dihydroxy-7,8-
    dihydro-benzo(a)pyrene (BP-7,8-diol) to 7,10/8,9 tetrols
    FEBS Lett. 106:17.
Sivarajah K, Lasker J, Eling T (1981). Prostaglandin
    synthetase-dependent cooxidation of (±)-benzo(a)
    pyrene-7,8-dihydrodiol by human lung and other mamma-
    lian tissue. Cancer Res. 41:1834.
Van der Ouderaa F, Buytenhek M, Nugteren P, Van Dorp D
    (1977). Purification and characterization of prosta-
    glandin endoperoxide synthetase from sheep vesicular
    gland. Biochem. Biophys. Acta. 487:315.

ACKNOWLEDGMENTS

    The authors wish to thank Dr. Iain Robertson for
carrying out the mutagenic assay and Dr. Carl Barrett for
performing the cell transformation assay.

Prostaglandins and Cancer: First
International Conference, pages 123-141
Published by Alan R. Liss, Inc., 150 Fifth Avenue, New York, NY 10011

Role of Prostaglandin Endoperoxide Synthetase in Benzidine
and 5-Nitrofuran-Induced Kidney and Bladder Carcinogenesis

T.V. Zenser, S.M. Cohen, M.B. Mattammal,
G. Murasaki, and B.B. Davis
VA Medical Center and St. Louis University,
St. Louis, MO 63125 and University of Nebraska
Omaha, NE 68105

Chemical carcinogens frequently exhibit a high degree
of organ specificity in the manifestation of their
carcinogenic effects. Potential reasons for this
specificity are the unique physiologic, anatomic and
metabolic characteristics of the target organ. A variety
of chemical compounds are carcinogenic and/or toxic to the
kidney or urinary collecting system. Some of those
compounds are illustrated in Figure 1.

A number of unique physiologic and anatomic features
of the kidney and urinary collecting system might be
partially responsible for the effects of these compounds
on those organs (Maher, 1976). Renal blood flow is high,
25% of cardiac output, and thus the kidney is exposed to
relatively large amounts of circulating carcinogens. In
addition the renal cortex contains transport systems for a
number of organic compounds. Examples of such transport
systems are the organic anion and cation transport
systems, which are parts of the mechanism by which the
kidney functions as an excretory organ. Active secretion
combined with high rates of renal blood flow serve to
decrease circulating levels of compounds which are handled
by those renal mechanisms. On the other hand these renal
functions serve to increase the concentrations of
compounds in renal tissue and in the urinary space. Under
ordinary circumstances approximately 99% of the filtered
water is reabsorbed from the renal tubules. This process
of water extraction from the tubular urine effectively
increases the concentration of many solutes within the
urinary space. When combined with active tubular

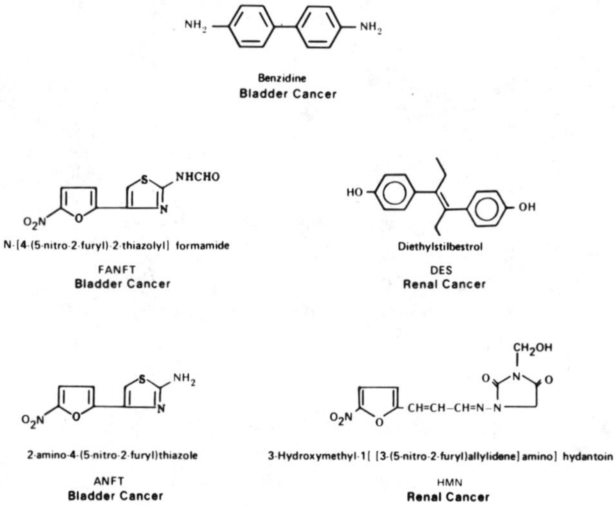

Figure 1. Structures of compounds metabolized by prostaglandin endoperoxide synthetase.

secretion, the processes of water extraction may result in very high concentrations of drugs and xenobiotics in the urinary space. Thus, there are a number of unique physiologic and anatomic characteristics of the kidney and urinary system which make these organs susceptible to adverse effects of certain carcinogens.

High concentrations of drugs and xenobiotics in urinary tissue would be of particular significance if the renal or urothelial tissue possessed the capacity to metabolically activate those compounds to more reactive forms. We have previously demonstrated three enzyme systems within the kidney and urinary tract with the potential to activate procarcinogens (Table 1). There was anaerobic nitroreductase activity which was similar in renal cortex, inner medulla and bladder transitional epithelial tissue, but very low in bladder non-epithelial tissue. Cytochrome P-450 was present in renal cortex and bladder transitional epithelial tissue but not detectable

Table 1

Distribution of Microsomal Nitroreductase, Cytochrome P-450
and Prostaglandin Endoperoxide Synthetase in Different
Areas of Rabbit Kidney and Bladder

	Nitroreductase	Cytochrome P-450	Prostaglandin Endoperoxide Synthetase
	nmol FANFT reduced/ mg/min	nmol/mg	nmol FANFT metabolized/ mg/min
Kidney			
Cortex	0.21 ± 0.01	0.07 ± 0.003	3.6 ± 0.5
Inner Medulla	0.27 ± 0.02	N.D.	15.8 ± 1.3
Bladder			
Transitional Epithelial	0.30 ± 0.02	0.09 ± 0.004	19.4 ± 1.3
Non-Epithelial	0.003 ± 0.002	N.D.	N.D.

N.D. = not detected.

in renal inner medulla or bladder non-epithelial tissue.
Each tissue except bladder non-epithelial contained
prostaglandin endoperoxide synthetase activity.
Prostaglandin endoperoxide synthetase-catalyzed metabolism
of FANFT was 64-fold greater than nitroreductase in
bladder transitional epithelial tissue. In this report we
will emphasize our investigations of the potential role of
prostaglandin endoperoxide synthetase in 5-nitrofuran and
benzidine-induced kidney and urothelial carcinomas.

Prostaglandin Endoperoxide Synthetase-Catalyzed Metabolism and Binding of 5-Nitrofurans and Benzidine with Microsomal Preparations

Prostaglandin endoperoxide synthetase-catalyzed
metabolism and subsequent binding of carcinogens to
proteins, RNA, and DNA was assessed since the initiation
of chemical carcinogenesis is thought to involve the
covalent binding of electrophilic carcinogens to
nucleophilic sites on macromolecules (Miller 1970; Miller
& Miller, 1977). In these experiments, metabolism of
^{14}C-FANFT was indicated by an increase in the amount of
radioactivity relative to the blank which did not contain
microsomes (Table 2). Values observed in the presence or
absence of microsomes were not measurably different. By
contrast, metabolism and binding of FANFT was observed
following arachidonic acid addition. The distribution of
FANFT products in the presence of arachidonic acid was
30%, 18%, 46% and 6% in the organic soluble, aqueous,
non-TCA precipitable, aqueous, TCA precipitable and t-RNA
bound fractions, respectively. Arachidonic acid-mediated
metabolism was completely inhibited by 0.05 mM
indomethacin and 1 mM aspirin. Prostaglandin E_2, NADPH,
and 11,14,17-eicosatrienoic acid did not initiate
metabolism of FANFT. With the addition of t-RNA at the
end of the incubation, there was no binding of FANFT to
t-RNA. The metabolism and binding of FANFT required
specific fatty acid substrates and was prevented by
specific inhibitors of prostaglandin endoperoxide
synthetase. The lack of effect of 11,14,17-eicosatrienoic
acid and NADPH in the presence of oxygen suggest that
lipoxygenases, lipid peroxidation, mixed-function
oxidases, and nitroreductases are not involved in
cooxidative metabolism of FANFT. The lack of covalent

Table 2
Characteristics of Solubilized Ram Seminal Vesicle Prostaglandin
Endoperoxide Synthetase-Catalyzed [14C]FANFT Metabolism and Covalent Binding

Additions	Concentration mM	Organic Soluble	Aqueous Non-TCA Precipitable	Aqueous TCA Precipitable	t-RNA Bound
			nmol/mg protein/5 min		
None	--	N.D.	N.D.	N.D.	N.D.
5,8,11,14-Eicosa-tetraenoic acid	0.06	1.2 ± 0.4	0.7 ± 0.1	1.9 ± 0.5	0.3 ± 0.05
+ Indomethacin	0.05	N.D.	N.D.	N.D.	N.D.
+ Aspirin	1.00	N.D.	N.D.	N.D.	N.D.
Prostaglandin E_2	0.06	N.D.	N.D.	N.D.	N.D.
11,14,17-Eicosa-trienoic acid	0.06	N.D.	N.D.	N.D.	N.D.
NADPH	1.0	N.D.	N.D.	N.D.	N.D.
5,8,11,14-Eicosa-tetraenoic acid[a]	0.06	1.4 ± 0.3	0.8 ± 0.1	1.8 ± 0.5	N.D.[a]

Reaction mixture contained 0.5 mg protein, 0.1 M phosphate buffer pH 7.8, 0.025 mM [14C]FANFT, 0.0012 mM methemoglobin and the indicated concentration of test substances. (N = 3 to 6). N.D. = not detected.
a t-RNA added at the end of the incubation.

binding to t-RNA following its addition after the reaction suggests that an activated metabolite is formed. These data support the conclusion that aerobic FANFT metabolism and subsequent binding to macromolecules is prostaglandin endoperoxide synthetase-catalyzed.

The organic soluble fraction following FANFT metabolism was further characterized by HPLC analysis (Figure 2). Panel A illustrates the HPLC profile of

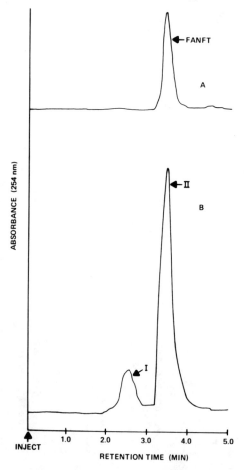

Figure 2. High-pressure liquid chromatographic elution profile. Panel A, authentic FANFT; Panel B, sample containing the complete reaction mixture plus 0.18 mM arachidonic acid.

authentic FANFT (Zenser et al., 1980b). In reaction
mixtures that contained arachidonic acid a new peak, peak
I, was observed (Panel B). The uv spectra of this
compound was also distinct from FANFT. Reaction mixtures
that contained indomethacin or aspirin exhibit HPLC
profiles identical to that observed in panel A. That is,
only FANFT was observed. Therefore, this visible
demonstration of product formation is consistent with the
radiochemical data (Table 2). Product formation depends
upon prostaglandin endoperoxide synthetase.

The metabolism and binding of ^{14}C-ANFT to protein,
t-RNA, and DNA was examined (Table 3). In these
experiments, metabolism of ^{14}C-ANFT was indicated by an
increase in the amount of radioactivity relative to the
blank which did not contain arachidonic acid. Values
determined in the absence of arachidonic acid or in the
absence of microsomes were not significantly different.
Indomethacin inhibited binding. Not shown here, when
t-RNA or DNA are added at the end of a 5 min incubation,
no binding occurs. This suggests that a reactive
intermediate is formed. In addition to arachidonic acid,
the organic hydroperoxide -- 15-HPETE -- also initiates
metabolism and binding but its effect was not inhibited by
indomethacin. The metabolism of ANFT was also shown to
require ferric heme and not protoporphyrin IX or manganese
heme. Similar results have been observed with ^{14}C-FANFT,
^{14}C-benzidine (Zenser et al., 1979; Zenser et al., 1980),
and ^{14}C-diethylstilbestrol (Davis et al., 1981). These
results are consistent with the hydroperoxidase activity
of prostaglandin endoperoxide synthetase mediating
metabolism (Zenser et al., 1980a) and with metabolism
resulting in the formation of an activated metabolite
which covalently binds macromolecules such as DNA (Zenser
et al., 1980; Davis et al., 1981).

To further investigate the relationships between
prostaglandin endoperoxide synthetase and drug metabolism,
the dose response relationships between indomethacin
inhibition of PGE$_2$ synthesis and benzidine metabolism
were examined (Figure 3). Benzidine metabolism was
assessed by the incorporation of 30 µM ^{14}C-benzidine
into TCA precipitable material in the presence of 50 µM
unlabeled arachidonic acid (Zenser et al., 1979). PGE$_2$
synthesis was assessed by the conversion of ^{14}C-

Table 3

Covalent Binding of $[^{14}C]$ANFT to Protein, DNA, and t-RNA-Catalyzed by Prostaglandin Endoperoxide Synthetase Prepared from Rabbit Bladder Transitional Epithelial Microsomes

Conditions	Aqueous, TCA-Precipitable	DNA Bound	t-RNA Bound
	nmol/mg protein/5 min		
Complete system			
– Arachidonic Acid	0.16 ± 0.02	0.014 ± 0.002	0.020 ± 0.003
– Microsomes	N.D.	N.D.	N.D.
+ Indomethacin (50 µM)	0.002 ± 0.002	0.003 ± 0.002	0.002 ± 0.001
	N.D.	N.D.	N.D.
15–HPETE (30 µM)	0.23 ± 0.02	0.026 ± 0.003	0.034 ± 0.005
+ Indomethacin (100 µM)	0.23 ± 0.004	0.024 ± 0.005	0.031 ± 0.004
+ Vitamin E (50 µM)	N.D.	N.D.	N.D.

The complete system consists of 0.5 mg proteins, 0.024 mM $[^{14}C]$ANFT, 0.0012 mM methemoglobin, 0.06 mM arachidonic acid and the indicated concentration of test agents in a total volume of 0.25 ml. Where indicated, 15-HPETE was used instead of arachidonic acid. All inhibitors were preincubated for two minutes at 25°C. The amount of radioactive product bound to nucleic acid was 14 pmol/mg DNA and 20 pmol/mg t-RNA, respectively.

N.D. = not detected.

arachidonic acid to ^{14}C-PGE$_2$ in the presence of 30 μM unlabeled benzidine. The similarity of the indomethacin ID$_{50}$ values is consistent with prostaglandin endoperoxide synthetase-catalyzed PGE$_2$ synthesis and covalent binding of benzidine to protein.

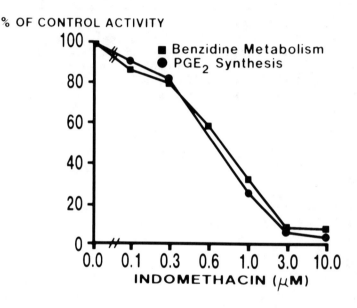

Figure 3. Dose-response effects of indomethacin on PGE$_2$ synthesis and benzidine metabolism with rabbit inner medullary microsomes.

To further investigate the role of prostaglandin endoperoxide synthetase in aromatic amine metabolism, we have examined the metabolism of o-dianisidine, o-tolidine, and o-toluidine. Each of these compounds exhibited spectral changes consistent with metabolism by prostaglandin endoperoxide synthetase. Of particular interest was the similarity of the spectral changes catalyzed by horseradish peroxidase and prostaglandin endoperoxide synthetase. These results are consistent with the prostaglandin hydroperoxidase component of prostaglandin endoperoxide synthetase catalyzing the metabolism of a variety of aromatic amines.

Proposed Mechanism of Prostaglandin Hydroperoxidase-Catalyzed Metabolism of Chemical Compounds

A wide range of structurally diverse renal and bladder carcinogens are metabolized by prostaglandin hydroperoxidase (Figure 1). The precise mechanism by which prostaglandin hydroperoxidase metabolizes drugs and xenobiotics is not known. Peroxidase reactions are generally characterized as two-electron oxidation-reduction reactions which require electron donors (Poulos & Kraut, 1980). An oxidant has been shown to be released from prostaglandin hydroperoxidase which is capable of inactivating prostacyclin synthetase (Ham et al., 1979). This oxidant would also be available for the oxidation of procarcinogens. Prostaglandin hydroperoxidase is a component of prostaglandin endoperoxide synthetase (Ohki et al., 1979). Prostaglandin hydroperoxidase-catalyzed metabolism has been shown to correlate with prostaglandin synthetic activity (Zenser et al., 1980a; Zenser et al., 1980b). Therefore, we propose that this overall reaction (Figure 4) results in the formation of an activated enzyme complex (E (IV)) and release of an oxidant ($[O_x]\cdot$). Depending upon its structure, the carcinogen (A) may react with either the enzyme complex (i.e., aromatic amines) or the oxidant (i.e., polyaromatic hydrocarbons). Either reaction would result in the formation of an activated carcinogen.

Prostaglandin Endoperoxide Synthetase-Catalyzed Metabolism and Binding of Benzidine with Intact Tissue

It is critical to demonstrate prostaglandin endoperoxide synthetase-mediated metabolism in intact tissue. Renal inner medullary slices were used for this purpose (Figure 5). Slices were subjected to two successive incubations in Krebs-Ringer bicarbonate buffer with 1 mg/ml each of glucose and BSA (Rapp et al., 1980). Both 150 μM arachidonic acid and 25 μM ^{14}C-benzidine were present in only the second incubation. Other test agents were present during both incubations. Binding was assessed in TCA precipitable material. Arachidonic acid increased ^{14}C-benzidine binding. This increase was prevented by indomethacin, aspirin, and meclofenamic acid. Mixed-function oxidase inhibitors -- metyrapone and

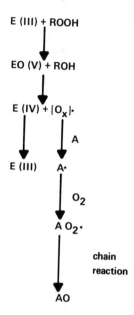

E (III) + ROOH

EO (V) + ROH

E (IV) + $[O_x]$·

E (III)   A·

A

O_2

$A O_2$·

chain
reaction

AO

Figure 4. Proposed mechanism of prostaglandin hydroperoxidase--catalyzed oxidations.

SKF-525A -- did not inhibit arachidonic acid-mediated increases in benzidine metabolism. Therefore, we have successfully demonstrated covalent binding of renal and bladder carcinogens by prostaglandin endoperoxide synthetase using both microsomes and intact tissue preparations. This covalent binding is a necessary step in the carcinogenic process.

Facilitated Transport of Renal and Bladder Carcinogens by the Kidney

We propose that the specificity of these carcinogens for producing tumors in the kidney and bladder is due to the specific transport characteristics of the kidney. Therefore, we assessed the possibility that the 5-nitrofuran carcinogens enter the kidney and bladder by facilitated transport (Zenser et al., 1981). Hippuran is a model compound used to demonstrate organic anion transport. Shown in Figure 6 is the effect of HMN on

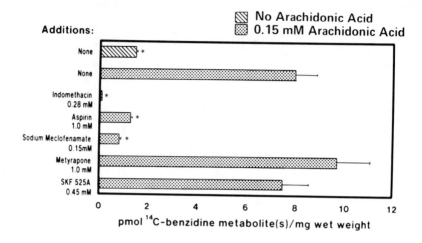

Figure 5. Effects of different agents on ^{14}C-benzidine binding in rabbit renal inner medullary slices.

^{131}I-hippuran uptake. Incubations were for 60 min at 37°C. HMN exhibited a dose-dependent inhibition of hippuran uptake. This inhibition by HMN was reversible. In separate experiments, ANFT and FANFT were also shown to inhibit hippuran uptake. By contrast, the aromatic amine -- benzidine -- did not alter hippuran transport but is transported by the organic cation system in the kidney. These results indicate that both anionic and cationic carcinogens are transported by the kidney. They suggest that because of that transport the renal and urothelial tissue would be subjected to high concentrations of those carcinogens.

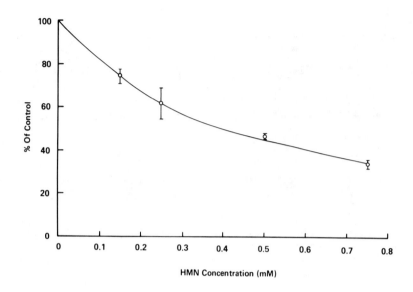

Figure 6. Concentration-dependent inhibition of rabbit cortical slice ^{131}I-hippuran accumulation by HMN.

Evidence for Prostaglandin Endoperoxide Synthetase Initiation of FANFT-Induced Bladder Cancer in Whole Animal Feeding Study

If prostaglandin endoperoxide synthetase is involved in the initiation of FANFT carcinogenesis, we propose that aspirin could prevent FANFT-induced bladder lesions. The protocol for such a study is illustrated in Figure 7.

The in vivo model for studying FANFT-induced bladder carcinogenesis has been well characterized. Rats fed a 0.2% or 0.1% diet of FANFT for just 12 weeks develop a 100% incidence of bladder cancer by one year. Evidence of urothelial malignancy can be observed after 12 weeks of FANFT treatment (Jacobs et al., 1977; Arai et al., 1979). Rat bladder PGE_2 content at weeks 1, 2, 6, and 13 of aspirin treatment were one-tenth to one-fourth that observed in controls.

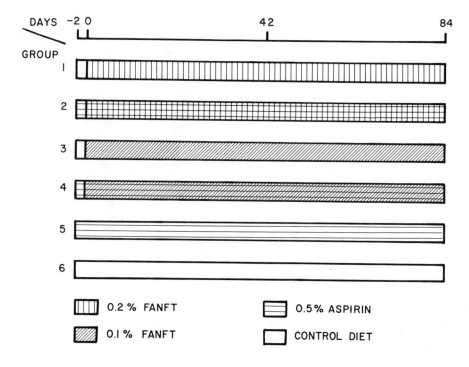

Figure 7. Experimental design for 12 week FANFT feeding study.

The effects of feeding aspirin on development of bladder lesions induced by 12 weeks of feeding FANFT are shown in Table 4. The dose of aspirin was as high as possible to provide adequate urinary levels. No bladder lesions were observed in aspirin fed rats and 1 out of 12 control rats had minimal hyperplasia. In several hundred control rats previously examined, hyperplasia and ropy microridges have been observed in less than 1% of these rats. By contrast, 80 to 100% of the rats fed 0.2% or 0.1% FANFT for 12 weeks had hyperplasia, ropy microridges and uniform microvilli. These lesions are thought to represent early stages during urothelial carcinogenesis and the hyperplasia was usually more marked than that seen in control rats. Aspirin produced a dose-dependent inhibition of these lesions. Aspirin completely inhibited lesions induced by 0.1% FANFT and partially prevented

Table 4

Effect of Aspirin on Bladder Lesions Induced by Twelve Weeks of Feeding FANFT

Group	Chemicals	No. of Rats	Hyperplasia[a]	Ropy Microridges[b]	Uniform Microvilli[b]	Pleomorphic Microvilli[b]
1	0.2% FANFT	9	9	9	7	5
2	0.2% FANFT 0.5% Aspirin	10	2[c]	5[d]	2[d]	2[d]
3	0.1% FANFT	9	4	8	7	1
4	0.1% FANFT 0.5% Aspirin	10	1	0[e]	0[e]	0
5	0.5% Aspirin	8	0	0	0	0
6	Control	12	1	1	0	0

[a] By light microscopy
[b] By scanning electron microscopy
[c] $p < 0.001$, Group 2 vs. Group 1
[d] $p < 0.05$, Group 2 vs. Group 1
[e] $p < 0.001$, Group 4 vs. Group 3

lesions induced by 0.2% FANFT. With rat transitional
epithelial microsomes, metabolism was observed only after
addition of 0.1 mM arachidonic acid (2.5 $\pm$ 0.2 nmol/mg
protein/min). Aspirin at 0.1 mM and 1.0 mM caused 60% and
100% inhibition, respectively, of rat microsomal FANFT
metabolism. These results are consistent with
prostaglandin endoperoxide synthetase-catalyzed initiation
of FANFT-induced bladder cancer. Since previous studies
have shown that FANFT is not immunosuppressive (Headley et
al., 1981; Johansson et al., 1978), it is unlikely that
this effect of aspirin is mediated through the immune
system. However, it is difficult to rule out an effect of
aspirin on promotion. The present study shows inhibition
only of early lesions. A long-term study is underway to
determine if the formation of carcinoma is also inhibited.

Summary

A scheme depicting 5-nitrofuran-induced cancer and
nephrotoxicity is illustrated in Figure 8. A salient
feature of our model is target tissue metabolism of these
carcinogens. Therefore, we propose that transport of
these carcinogens into the kidney and bladder is
facilitated by the organic acid transport system. This
transport feature may also explain the tissue specificity
of these carcinogens. That is, why they cause cancer in
the kidney and bladder but not liver. Carcinogens are
activated by the hydroperoxidase activity of prostaglandin
endoperoxide synthetase to electrophiles which covalently
bind to macromolecules such as DNA. This results in the
initiation of the carcinogenic process and nephrotoxicity.
We have experimental evidence to support each step in this
model: 1) organic acid transport of 5-nitrofurans; 2)
prostaglandin hydroperoxidase-catalyzed covalent binding
of carcinogens to tissue macromolecules and 3) prevention
of the expression of FANFT-induced lesions by aspirin in
whole animal feeding studies.

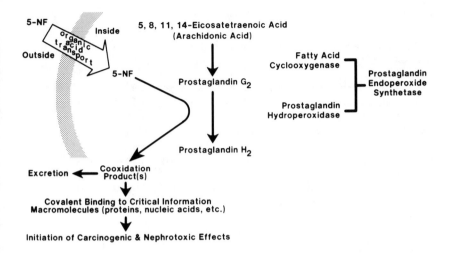

Figure 8. Model describing initial steps in 5-nitrofuran (5-NF)-induced bladder cancer.

References

Arai M, Cohen SM, Jacobs JB, Friedell GH (1979). Effect of dose on urinary bladder carcinogenesis induced in F344 rats by N-[4-(5-nitro-2-furyl)-2-thiazolyl]-formamide. J Natl Cancer Inst 62:1013.

Cohen SM, Zenser TV, Murasaki G, Fukushima S, Mattammal MB, Rapp NS, Davis BB (1981). Aspirin inhibition of N-[4-(5-nitro-2-furyl)-2-thiazolyl]-formamide-induced lesions of the urinary bladder correlated with inhibition of metabolism by bladder prostaglandin endoperoxide synthetase. Cancer Res 41:3355.

Davis BB, Mattammal MB, Zenser TV (1981). Renal metabolism of drugs and xenobiotics. Nephron 27:187.

Ham EA, Egan RW, Soderman DD, Gale PH, Kuehl Jr FA (1979). Peroxidase-dependent deactivation of prostacyclin synthetase. J Biol Chem 254:2191.

Headley DB, Klopp RG, Michie PM, Erturk E, Bryan GT (1981).
Temporal comparisons of immune status and target organ
histology in mice fed carcinogenic 5-nitrofurans and
their nornitro analogs. Cancer Res 41:1397.

Jacobs JB, Arai M, Cohen SM, Friedell GH (1977). A long-
term study of reversible and progressive urinary
bladder cancer lesions in rats fed N-[4-(5-nitro-2-
furyl)-2-thiazolyl]formamide. Cancer Res 37:2817.

Johansson S, Cohen SM, Yang JPS, Arai M, Friedell GH
(1978). The influence of N-[4-(5-nitro-2-furyl)-2-
thiazolyl]formamide and phenacetin on the immune
status in male Fischer rats. Invest Urol 15:308.

Maher JF (1976). Toxic nephropathy. In Brenner B,
Rector F (eds): "The Kidney", Philadelphia: W.B.
Saunders Co., p 1355.

Miller JA (1970). Carcinogenesis by chemicals: An
overview — GHA Clowes memorial lecture. Cancer Res
30:559.

Miller JA, Miller EC (1977). The concept of reactive
electrophilic metabolites in chemical carcinogenesis:
Recent results with aromatic amines, safrole, and
aflatoxin B. In Jollow DJ, Kocsis JJ, Synder R,
Vainio H (eds): "Biological Reactive Intermediates,"
New York: Plenum Press, p 6.

Ohki S, Ogino N, Yamamoto S, Hayaishi O (1979).
Prostaglandin hydroperoxidase, an integral part of
prostaglandin endoperoxide synthetase from bovine
vesicular gland microsomes. J Biol Chem 254:829.

Poulos TL, Kraut J (1980). The stereochemistry of
peroxidase catalysis. J Biol Chem 255:8199.

Rapp NS, Zenser TV, Brown WW, Davis BB (1980). Metabolism
of benzidine by a prostaglandin-mediated process in
renal inner medullary slices. J Pharmacol Exp Ther
215:401.

Zenser TV, Balasubramanian TM, Mattammal MB, Davis BB (1981). Transport of the renal carcinogen 3-hydroxy-methyl-1-[(3-(5-nitro-2-furyl)-allydidene)amino]-hydantoin (HMN) by renal cortex and cooxidative metabolism by renal prostaglandin endoperoxide synthetase. Cancer Res 41:2032.

Zenser TV, Mattammal MB, Armbrecht HJ, Davis BB (1980). Benzidine binding to nucleic acids mediated by the peroxidative activity of prostaglandin endoperoxide synthetase. Cancer Res 40:2839.

Zenser TV, Mattammal MB, Davis BB (1979). Cooxidation of benzidine by renal medullary prostaglandin cyclooxy-genase. J Pharmacol Exp Ther 211:460.

Zenser TV, Mattammal MB, Davis BB (1980a). Mechanism of FANFT cooxidation by prostaglandin endoperoxide synthetase. J Pharmacol Exp Ther 214:312.

Zenser TV, Mattammal MB, Davis BB (1980b). Metabolism of N-[4-(5-nitro-2-furyl)-2-thiazolyl]formamide by prostaglandin endoperoxide synthetase. Cancer Res 40:114.

Investigations were supported by the National Institute of Health Grant No. CA28015, the American Cancer Society, Missouri Chapter, and EPA Contract No. ES8071.

**Prostaglandins and Cancer: First
International Conference, pages 143–148
© 1982 Alan R. Liss, Inc., 150 Fifth Avenue, New York, NY 10011**

METABOLIC ACTIVATION OF DIETHYLSTILBESTROL BY PROSTAGLANDIN
SYNTHETASE AS A MECHANISM FOR ITS CARCINOGENICITY

Sharon Bennett, Wayne Marshall and Peter J. O'Brien

Dept. of Biochemistry, Memorial University of
Newfoundland, St. John's, Newfoundland

The synthetic oestrogen diethylstilbestrol (DES) induces
kidney tumors in hamsters and genital tract tumors in rodents (1) Cervicovaginal alterations including carcinoma
were also observed in the female offspring of DES treated
women, as were certain teratogenic changes in the genital
tract of their male progeny as a result of its transplacental
toxicity. Metzler et al. have suggested that peroxidases of
oestrogens target organs are responsible by catalysing DES
oxidation to intermediates that bind to nucleic acids and
other cellular macromolecules (2). Our research shows that
prostaglandin synthetase in these organs could also be a
catalyst.

The three hormones estrone, estradiol -17B, ethnyl
estradiol also induce tumors in two or more animal species
and there is epidemiological evidence inferring oestrones are
carcinogenic in man (IARC 1979). However the mechanisms by
which these compounds are carcinogenic is not known. The
liver microsomal mixed function oxygenase has been shown to
catalyse the oxidation of diethylstilbestrol (3,4) or
estradiol -17B (5,6) to reactive metabolites which bind to
cellular macromolecules or exogenous DNA (7-9). The majority
of carcinogens seem to act by forming metabolites which
react covalently with DNA and cause mutations. These hormones are not however mutagenic (10).

METHODS

(Monoethyl-^{3}H) diethylstilbestrol (116Ci/mole) and (^{3}H)
Estradiol (53Ci/nmole)were purchase from Amersham and New
England Nuclear respectively. Unlabelled Diethylstilbestrol
and Estradiol were obtained from Sigma.

   Incubations with sheep seminal vesicular gland microsomes or rat liver or uterine microsomes (2-3 mgs of protein/
assay) were carried out with 90 nmoles of Diethylstilbestrol
or 140 nmoles of Estradiol, 200 nmoles of Arachidonic Acid,
2-3 mgs of calf thymus DNA in a total volume of 2 mls of
0.1 M Phosphate Buffer (pH = 7.5), at 37°C with shaking for
1 hour. Unchanged Diethylstilbestrol was obtained by
4 x 2 ml ether extractions of the aqueous incubation mixture. The ether was evaporated and the residue counted in
Aquasol (or Omniflor in Dioxane). Protein and DNA were
isolated in separate experiments. Protein was isolated
simply by precipitation with 10% trichloroacetic acid. DNA
was isolated by the addition of 0.40 mls of 10% sodium
dodecyl sulfate, and 2 mls of buffer saturated phenol to
the aqueous layer. The solution was then chilled in ice
with frequent shaking for 15-30 minutes before adding 4
volumes of cold 95% ethanol to precipitate the DNA. The
isolated macromolecules were washed with ethanol and then
ether before adding scintillation fluid and counting in a
scintillation counter. Aliquots of the aqueous layer were
also counted.

Table 1   MICROSOMAL CATALYSED DIETHYLSTILBESTROL AND
          ESTRADIOL BINDING TO PROTEIN AND EXOGENOUS DNA.

Experiment	Diethylstilbestrol nmoles bound/mgm		Estradiol nmoles bound/mgm	
	DNA	Protein	DNA	Protein
SVG + Arachidonate	0.34	0.68	0.70	0.19
RLM + Arachidonate	0.00	0.00	0.00	0.00
RLM + NADPH	0.96	0.00	0.50	1.17
RLM + Hydroperoxide	2.5	0.84	2.15	0.11
RLM + Lipoxygenase	0.18	0.00		
UM + Arachidonate	0.15		0.12	
UM + NADPH	0.00		0.00	
UM + H_2O_2	0.32		0.25	

Rat liver microsomes (RLM) or sheep vesicular gland microsomes (SVG) or uterine microsomes (UM) at 1 mgm protein/ml in 0.1 M phosphate buffer pH 7.5 were incubated with 45μM diethylstilbestrol or 70μM estradiol, and either arachidonate (0.1 mM), NADPH (1.0mM), cumene hydroperoxide (1.0 mM), H_2O_2 (35μM) or lipoxygenase (1 unit) in the presence of calf thymus DNA (1 mgm/ml) at 37°C for 1 hour. The isolation of DNA and protein was carried out as described in methods.

Table 2   INDUCTION OF ENZYMES INVOLVED IN CATALYSING THE BINDING OF DIETHYLSTILBESTROL TO DNA.

IN VIVO INDUCER	SYSTEM (Rat Microsomes)	DNA binding nmoles/mgm
3 Methylcholanthrene	Liver-NADPH	2.8 ± 0.3
None	Liver-NADPH	1.3 ± 0.11
3 Methylcholanthrene	Liver-Cumene hydroperoxide	4.8 ± 0.5
None	Liver-Cumene hydroperoxide	2.9 ± 0.3
Oestradiol	Immature uterus-H_2O_2	0.44
None	Immature uterus-H_2O_2	0.12
Oestradiol	Immature uterus-arachidonate	0.28
None	Immature uterus-arachidonate	0.09

RESULTS & DISCUSSION

From Table 1 it can be seen that sheep vesicular gland microsomes-arachidonate readily catalysed the binding of C^{14} diethylstilbestrol to exogenous DNA. Binding also occurred to the microsomal protein. Some binding also occurred in the absence of arachidonate and could indicate binding by **autooxidation products of diethylstilbestrol. The purity of** the diethylstilbestrol was checked by HPLC and found to be **91% pure. Indomethacin (50μM) and glutathione (1 nM) pre-** vented the binding catalysed by arachidonate. Prostaglandin synthetase can therefore catalyse the binding of diethylstilbestrol to DNA. The responsible intermediates also readily react with glutathione.

Liver microsomal mixed function oxidase also catalysed the binding to DNA but not to protein. As can also be seen from Table 1 a twofold greater binding was obtained with cumene hydroperoxide than with NADPH. The extent of binding was similar for the range of cumene hydroperoxide concentrations of 0.2 mM -5 mM. Cumene hydroperoxide has previously been shown to replace NADPH, O_2, and reductase in cytochrome P450 catalysed reactions (11). This indicates that cytochrome P450 is the catalyst for the liver microsomal catalysed binding. The greater activity with cumene hydroperoxide also may indicate that the binding intermediates are reduced by the NADPH-cytochrome P450 reductase. However microsomal lipid peroxidation is induced by cumene hydroperoxide (11) and lipoxygenase can also catalyse some binding as a result of lipid peroxidation oxidising the diethylstilbestrol to binding intermediates.

Prostaglandin synthetase and mixed function oxidase also catalysed the binding of oestradiol to DNA and protein. However as can be seen from Table 1, oestradiol differed from diethylstilbestrol in that liver microsomal protein binding occurred with the mixed function oxidase catalysed system whereas no binding occurred with diethylstilbestrol. Uterine microsomes prepared from 200 gm rats were also active in catalysing the binding of diethylstilbestrol or oestradiol to DNA in the presence of arachidonate. However as can be seen from Table 1 there was no mixed function oxidase activity. The arachidonate catalysed reaction was inhibited by indomethacin and indicates that prostaglandin synthetase catalysed this reaction. It has previously been shown that PFG$_{2\alpha}$ is the principal product when arachidonate is incubated with uterine microsomes (12). Uterine microsomes also contain peroxidase activity and hydrogen peroxide was also effective at catalysing the binding.

The enzymes catalysing the binding seem to be induced in vivo. As shown in Table 2, 3 methylcholanthrene induced the liver mixed function oxidase catalysed reaction indicating that cytochrome P448 is more effective than cytochrome P450. 5 rats were used and the different results are shown. The activity of uterine microsomes prepared from 25 immature rats (50 gms) was much lower than that from mature rats. However oestradiol (20 hrs. s.c. inj. 4 μgms) markedly induced the protaglandin synthetase catalysed reaction as well as the peroxidase catalysed reaction. Other investigators have shown that oestradiol induces peroxidase (13) whilst others have shown that prostaglandin synthetase activity varies with the oestrus cycle (12).

High pressure liquid chromatography was used to measure the diethylstilbestrol products and in the case of uterine microsomes and H_2O_2 or arachidonate, the principal product was Z,A dienestrol. Presumably a free radical mechamism was involved so that the semiquinone or quinones were responsible for the binding (14).

In conclusion the liver microsomes can catalyse the binding of diethylstilbestrol or estradiol to exogenous DNA via either a mixed function oxidase or to a lesser extent via lipid peroxidation. This effect may contribute to the liver necrosis induced by diethylstilbestrol. Uterine microsomes on the other hand have no mixed function oxidase acitivity but catalyse this binding using either a peroxidase or prostaglandin synthetase activity. Oestradiol markedly induces both activities. This binding may contribute to the association of oestrogens and cancers of tissues whose growth is effected by oestrogen.

ACKNOWLEDGMENTS

This work was supported by the National Cancer Institute of Canada.

Blackburn GM, Flavell AJ and Thompson MH. Cancer Res 34:2015.
Blackburn GM, Thompson MH and Keng HWS (1976). Biochem J 158:643.
Drevon C, Piccoli C and Montesans R (1981). Mutation Research 89:83-90.
Jellinek PH and Fletcher R (1970). Can J Biochem 48:1192-1198.
Kirkman H and Bacon RL (1950). Cancer Res 10:122-123.
Lyttle CR and DeSonbre ER (1974). Proc Nat Acad Sci 74: 3162-3166.
Marks F and Hecker E (1969). Biochem Biophys Acta 187: 250-265.
Metzler M (1975). Biochem Pharmacol 24:1449-1453.
Metzler M (1976). J Toxicol Environ Health Suppl 1:21-35.
Metzler M and MacLachlan JA (1978). Biochem Pharmacol 27:1087-1094.

Metzler M, and MacLachlan JA (1978). Biochem Biophys Res
  Comm 85:874-884.
O'Brien PJ (1978).   Pharmacology and Therapeutics 2A:517-536.
Tsibris JCM, and McGuire PM (1977). Biochem Biophys Res
  Comm 78:411-417.
Wlodaiver P, Kindahl H, Hamberg M (1976). Biochem Biophys
  Acta 431:603-614.

Prostaglandins and Cancer: First
International Conference, pages 149-154
© 1982 Alan R. Liss, Inc., 150 Fifth Avenue, New York, NY 10011

THE EFFECTS OF VITAMIN E AND/OR SELENIUM DEFICIENCY ON
ENZYMES INVOLVED IN THE BIOSYNTHESIS AND DEGRADATION OF
PROSTANOIDS IN RAT TISSUES

C. C. Reddy, T. L. Grasso, R. W. Scholz,
T. J. Labosh, C. E. Thomas, and E. J. Massaro

Center for Air Environment Studies and
Department of Veterinary Science
The Pennsylvania State University
University Park, Pennsylvania 16802

Dietary vitamin E (vit E) and selenium (Se) have been
implicated in the protection of cell membranes from
peroxidative damage (McCay, King 1980; Tappel 1980). Vitamin
E as an integral part of membranes functions as a biological
antioxidant, preventing the formation of lipid hydroperoxides
by scavenging free radicals involved in the propagation of
lipid peroxidation (McCay, King 1980). Selenium, as an
essential component of Se-dependent glutathione peroxidase
(Se GSH-Px), acts to reduce hydroperoxides formed via lipid
peroxidation to less reactive alcohols (Tappel 1980).
Recently, another enzyme, Se-independent GSH-Px (non-Se
GSH-Px), has been implicated in the protection of membranes
from oxidative attack (Burk et al. 1980; Reddy et al. 1981).

Certain lipid hydroperoxides and cyclic endoperoxides
which are intermediates in the biosynthesis of prostaglandins
(PGs), thromboxanes (TXs), prostacyclins (PGIs), and
leukotrienes (LTs), affect the catalytic activities of PGI_2
synthetase and cyclooxygenase (Ham et al. 1979; Hemler et al.
1979). Also, free radicals generated during prostanoid
biosynthesis may inactivate cyclooxygenase and PGI_2 synthetase
(Egan et al. 1976; Ham et al. 1979). In addition, peroxyl,
alkoxy, and hydroxyl radicals, produced by autooxidation of
lipid hydroperoxides, may exert deleterious effects on these
enzymes. Therefore, vit E and Se GSH-Px have the potential
to modulate the activities of enzymes involved in the turnover
of arachidonic acid (AA) and the profile of intermediates/
products of the AA cascade. Accordingly, we investigated the

effects of vit E and Se deficiency on selected enzymes of AA
metabolism in tissues of the Long-Evans Hooded rat maintained
on chemically defined diets containing adequate or documented
deficiencies of vit E, Se or both (diets: +E, +Se; -E, +Se;
+E, -Se; -E, -Se).

Effect of Vit E and/or Se Deficiency on PG Synthetase and
Prostaglandin Dehydrogenase Activity:

The effect of vit E and Se deficiency on the rate of PG
biosynthesis and metabolism was assessed by measuring the
activity of microsomal PG synthetase and cytosolic (105,000xg)
PG dehydrogenase (PGDH), respectively. PG synthetase activity
was elevated in liver and lung microsomes from vit E deficient
animals (Table 1) as reported by Hope et al. (1975) for rat

TABLE 1

PG Synthetase

	+E, +Se	-E, +Se	+E, -Se	-E, -Se
Liver Microsomes	94.8±12.0	138.6±19.0	99.0±18.0	139.8±19.0
Lung Microsomes	201.0±24.6	234.0±32.0	141.0±13.8	297.6±35.0
Kidney Microsomes	49.8±12.6	53.4± 6.6	42.0± 9.0	59.0± 1.0

Enzyme activity was assayed polarographically as described by Hemler
et al. (1976) and is expressed as nmoles of O_2 consumed per min. per
mg protein (means ± SE of 6-8 observations).

sera. In contrast, Chan et al. (1979) reported severely
impaired PG synthesis in vit E deficient rabbit skeletal
muscle. Such discrepancies may be due to tissue differences
in response to vit E status. These observations suggest that
vit E may play a regulatory role in PG biosynthesis by
controlling the formation of key lipid hydroperoxides and
cyclic endoperoxides.

Lung PGDH activity is unaffected in vit E status, but
is elevated in Se deficiency (Table 2). Neither vit E nor
Se status had any significant effect on kidney and liver
PGDH activity (Table 2). Likewise, Chan et al. (1980)
reported no effect of vit E deficiency on the PGDH activity
of rabbit kidney and heart. It is of interest to note that,
in vit E deficiency, PG synthetase activity is elevated while
PGDH activity is not affected whereas in Se deficiency, PG
synthetase activity is unaltered while PGDH activity is

increased. Presently, we have no satisfactory explanation for these observations.

TABLE 2

PG Dehydrogenase

	+E, +Se	-E, +Se	+E, -Se	-E, -Se
Liver	11.8± 2.2	11.2± 2.5	16.3± 2.2	18.0± 2.3
Kidney	40.1± 4.5	29.9± 6.5	47.0± 9.8	52.1±12.4
Lung	70.0±24.0	61.0±16.0	106.0±20.0	123.0±18.0

Enzyme activity was assayed by the method of Anggard and Samuelsson (1966) and is expressed as pmoles of chromophore formed per min. per mg protein (means ± SE of 6-8 observations).

Effect of Vit E and/or Se Deficiency on Glutathione-S-Transferase and Epoxide Hydratase Activity:

Glutathione transferase (GSH-Tr) activity was increased in the cytosolic fraction of liver, lung, and kidney of Se deficient animals (Table 3). Similar results were obtained

TABLE 3

Glutathione-S-Transferase

	+E, +Se	-E, +Se	+E, -Se	-E, -Se
Liver	1722.3±84.4	1709.6±243.3	3116.4±296.8	2330.1±151.8
Lung	107.3± 7.2	102.1± 6.2	137.7± 13.9	124.5± 11.0
Kidney	62.7± 7.2	64.5± 6.1	141.7± 7.7	109.3± 7.9
Testis	658.5±45.0	783.0± 31.0	687.0± 16.0	730.0± 28.0
Spleen	39.5± 3.2	40.8± 2.1	32.7± 4.0	31.0± 4.1

Enzyme activity of the 105,000g supernatants was monitored spectro-photometrically as previously described (Reddy et al. 1981) and is expressed as nmoles per min. per mg protein (means ± SE of 6-9 observations).

for liver and brain microsomes (data not shown). Vitamin E deficiency had no effect on these enzymes. Because the multifunctional GSH-Trs appear to be involved in the synthesis of leukotriene C_4 and some prostaglandins (Murphy et al. 1979; Samuelsson et al. 1978), these results suggest that Se deficiency may exacerbate the hyperallergic condition and other related processes mediated through LTs. However, certain GSH-Trs also exhibit Se-independent GSH-Px activity (Burk et al. 1980; Reddy et al. 1981). The increased levels of non-Se GSH-Px activity found in the lung in Se deficiency (Table 4) could accelerate the conversion of highly reactive 5-hydroperoxy eicosatetraenoic acid (5-HPETE), the precursor of LTA_4 which is a precursor of LTC_4, to less reactive 5-hydroxy ETE and, thereby, moderate the LT mediated pathological conditions.

TABLE 4

Non-Se-Glutathione Peroxidase

	+E, +Se	-E, +Se	+E, -Se	-E, -Se
Liver	135.6+19.6	230.3+12.8	189.6+9.9	173.2+7.8
Lung	17.0+ 3.1	16.6+ 3.2	25.3+3.0	21.4+2.1
Kidney	7.5+ 1.3	6.1+ 1.6	58.3+4.8	43.9+5.4
Stomach	7.4+ 4.0	8.9+ 2.0	4.2+2.3	6.2+1.4
Brain	49.3+ 3.2	48.1+ 7.6	50.5+1.4	41.3+0.9

Non-Se GSH-Px activity of the 105,000xg supernatants was determined by a modification of the method of Paglia and Valentine as described by Reddy et al. (1981) and is expressed nmoles of product formed per min. per mg protein (means + SE of 6-8 animals).

In addition to the GSH-Trs, epoxide hydratase (EH) also can act on lipid epoxides such as LTA_4 converting them to diols and limiting the precursor source for the synthesis of LTC_4. However, in Se deficient state, EH activity was increased (2x) only in liver microsomes.

Effect of Vit E and/or Se Deficiency on GSH and Cytochrome P-450 Peroxidase Activity:

Recently Hemler et al. reported that Se GSH-Px may play an important role in regulation of the rate of prostanoid formation by controlling the hydroperoxide tone of the cell (Hemler et al. 1979). We have investigated the effect of vit E and/or Se deficiency on Se-dependent and non-Se GSH-Pxs and cytochrome P-450 (cyt P-450) peroxidase to assess the capacity of tissues to metabolise hydroperoxides. It was observed that Se GSH-Px activity was greatly reduced in Se deficiency (Table 5). In contrast, non-Se GSH-Px activity was increased in the cytosolic fraction of liver and kidney (Table 4). This suggests that, at least in some tissues, non-Se GSH-Px may partially compensate for the decreased Se

TABLE 5

Se-Dependent Glutathione Peroxidase

	+E, +Se	-E, +Se	+E, -Se	-E, -Se
Blood	97.8+ 8.5*	89.6+ 9.8	14.5+2.4	18.1+3.0
Liver	347.4+18.9	348.0+13.5	3.2+0.3	3.5+0.3
Lung	103.4+ 6.6	101.1+ 6.2	7.7+0.9	8.3+0.7
Kidney	39.0+ 1.9	39.8+ 1.6	4.5+0.6	6.9+0.7
Heart	257.0+14.4	247.4+12.1	10.0+3.4	11.6+1.5
Brain	66.8+ 5.6	64.9+ 3.9	7.2+0.7	6.6+0.6

The activity of Se GSH-Px in blood and in the 105,000xg supernatants of
the tissues was determined by the procedure of Paglia and Valentine (1967)
with hydrogen peroxide as substrate and is expressed as nmoles of
product formed per min. per mg protein (means $\pm$ SE of 6-8 animals).

* nmoles of product formed per min. per mg Hb for blood.

GSH-Px activity observed in Se deficiency. In addition, we
have observed that the activity of cyt P-450 peroxidase, an
enzyme capable of decomposing both organic hydroperoxides and
H_2O_2, increased slightly in Se deficiency, but was markedly
reduced in vit E deficiency.

Since non-Se GSH-Px acts only on organic hydroperoxides,
and catalase, which is localized primarily in peroxisomes,
has a high Km value for H_2O_2, drastic reduction in Se GSH-Px
activity could severely impair H_2O_2 metabolism. H_2O_2 can
readily react with superoxide anion (O_2^-) to generate highly
reactive hydroxyl radicals which may affect vital cellular
processes including PG synthesis deleteriously. The foregoing results suggest that vit E and/or Se deficiency may
severely impair hydroperoxide metabolism and, thereby, alter
PG biosynthesis.

Anggard E, Samuelsson B (1966). Purification and properties
    of a 15-hydroxy prostaglandin dehydrogenase from swine
    lung. Arkiv for Kemi 25:293.
Burk RF, Trumble NJ, Lawrence RA (1980). Rat hepatic
    cytosolic glutathione-dependent enzyme protection against
    lipid peroxidation in the NADPH-microsomal lipid peroxida-
    tion system. Biochim Biophys Acta 618:35.
Chan AC, Allen CE, Hegarty PVJ (1980). The effects of
    vitamin E depletion and repletion on prostaglandin synthesis
    in semitendinosus muscle of young rabbits. J Nutr 110:66.

Chan AC, Hegarty PVJ, Allen CE (1980). The effects of vitamin E depletion and repletion on prostaglandin dehydrogenase activity in tissues of young rabbits. J Nutr 110:74.

Egan RW, Paxton J, Kuehl FA Jr (1976). Mechanism for irreversible self-deactivation of prostaglandin synthetase. J Biol Chem 251:7329.

Ham EA, Egan RW, Soderman DD, Gale PH, Kuehl FA Jr (1979). Peroxidase-dependent deactivation of prostacyclin synthetase. J Biol Chem 254:2191.

Hemler ME, Lands WEM, Smith WL (1976). Purification of the cyclooxygenase that forms prostaglandins. J Biol Chem 251:5575.

Hemler ME, Cook HW, Lands WEM (1979). Prostaglandin biosynthesis can be triggered by lipid peroxides. Arch Biochem Biophys 193:340.

Hope WC, Dalton C, Machlin LJ, Filipski, RJ, Vane FM (1975). Influence of dietary vitamin E on prostaglandin biosynthesis in rat blood. Prostaglandins 10:557.

McCay PB, King MM (1980). Vitamin E: its role as a biological free radical scavenger and its relationship to the microsomal mixed function oxidase system. In Machlin LJ (ed): "Vitamin E", New York: Marcel Dekker Inc., p. 289.

Murphy RC, Hammarstrom S, Samuelsson B (1979). Leukotriene C: a slow-reacting substance from murine mastocytoma cells. Proc Natl Acad Sci USA 76:4275.

Paglia DE, Valentine WN (1967). Studies on the quantitative and qualitative characterization of erythrocyte glutathione peroxidase. J Lab Clin Med 70:158.

Reddy CC, Tu C-PD, Burgess JR, Ho C-Y, Scholz RW, Massaro EJ (1981). Evidence for the occurrence of selenium-independent glutathione peroxidase activity in rat liver microsomes. Biochem Biophys Res Comm 101:970.

Samuelsson B, Goldyne M, Granstrom E, Hamberg M, Hammarstrom S, Malmsten C (1978). Prostaglandins and thromboxanes. Ann Rev Biochem 47:997.

Tappel AL (1980). Vitamin E and selenium protection from in vivo lipid peroxidation. Ann NY Acad Sci 355:18.

**Prostaglandins and Cancer: First
International Conference, pages 155-158
© 1982 Alan R. Liss, Inc., 150 Fifth Avenue, New York, NY 10011**

PROSTAGLANDIN SYNTHETASE MEDIATED ACTIVATION OF p-DIMETHYL-
AMINOAZOBENZENE (BUTTER YELLOW)

S. Vasdev, Y. Tsuruta, and P.J. O'Brien

Dept. of Biochemistry, Memorial University of
Newfoundland
St. John's, Newfoundland, Canada A1B 3X9

Whilst much emphasis has been placed in chemical carcinogenesis on the 2e oxidation catalytic activity of mixed
function oxidases, it is clear that 1e oxidation pathways
mediated by prostaglandin synthetase, lipid peroxidation or
mixed function oxidase activity can also form metabolites
which readily bind to the informational macromolecules and
could be a critical step in the initiation of neoplasia.
The 1e oxidation pathway is more active in catalysing this
binding with phenols, amines and hydrazines and free radicals
rather than electrophiles could explain the necrosis or carcinogenesis induced by acetaminophen, diethylstilbestrol,
methylhydrazine, benzidine, hair dyes, cyclophosphamide (1).

p-Dimethylaminoazobenzene is one of the most extensively studied chemical carcinogens and induces lung tumors in
mice, liver tumors in rats and bladder tumors in dogs (IARC
1976). It is widely held that the metabolic N-hydroxylation
of carcinogenic arylamines and arylamides are an obligatory
step in the activation of these compounds to carcinogenic
derivatives and that subsequent esterification, catalysed by
a liver sulfotransferase, leads to the formation of the ultimate carcinogen in the liver. Liver DNA adducts following
in vivo administration of N-methyl-4-aminoazobenzene (MAB)
could be explained this way (2,3). However in other tissues
the lack of sulfotransferase makes this pathway less attractive.

C^{14} MAB BINDING

MAB-(ring C^{14}) was synthesized (4) and had a specific activity of 0.54 mCi/mmole and purity of > 99%. The incubation mixture contained in a final volume of 2 ml: Tris-HCl buffer 0.1 M (pH 7.4), microsomal protein (2 mgm), NADPH (0.4 mM) or cumene hydroperoxide (1.5 mM) or arachidonate (100 µM). When binding to DNA was studied, 2 mgm of DNA was added to the incubation mixture. Following incubation in a metabolic shaker for 15 mins at $37^\circ C$, four extractions with 5 ml of diethyl ether were carried out. The precipitation and purification of protein or DNA was carried out as described (5).

PRODUCT ANALYSIS

The ether extracts were evaporated, dissolved in ethanol and analysed by high performance liquid chromatography monitored at 254 nm on a µ Bondapak C18 reverse phase column using a 50-100% methanol linear gradient at a flow rate of 1 ml/min at 20°C.

As can be seen from the Table pig bladder microsomes or sheep vesicular gland microsomes readily catalysed the binding of methylaminoazobenzene to exogenous DNA and microsomal protein with arachidonate. Little binding was observed in the absence of microsomes or if the microsomes were kept at 90°C for 5 mins. Similar results were observed with rat lung microsomes. Some mixed function oxidase activity with NADPH was apparent with pig bladder or rat lung microsomes but not vesicular gland microsomes, and this was considerably less effective than arachidonate. Hydroperoxides have previously been shown to catalyse cytochrome P450 function and can substitute for NADPH, O_2 and reductase in the mixed function oxidase activity (6). Hydroperoxide was two or three orders more effective than NADPH in catalysing this binding. Little binding occurred in the absence of microsomes. This suggests that NADPH/reductase inactivates the radical species by reduction. Hydroperoxides were also found to be more effective than NADPH even in the presence of cytosolic sulfotransferase, ATP, and sulfate (7).

THE *IN VITRO* COVALENT BINDING OF (C^{14})-MAB METABOLITES TO
EXOGENOUS DNA CATALYSED BY PROSTAGLANDIN SYNTHETASE

	PIG BLADDER Microsomes nmole/g		SHEEP VESICULAR Microsomes nmole/g	
	DNA	Protein	DNA	Protein
Microsomes + NADPH	60	100	8	7
Microsomes Only	3	10	8	7
Microsomes + Hydroperoxide	430	1,390		
Microsomes + Arachidonate	800	1,380	4,110	4,320
Ht. Denat. Microsomes + Arachidonate	20	80	7	7

Bladder microsomes and vesicular gland microsomes and
arachidonate oxidised methylaminoazobenzene to aminoazobenzene. In contrast liver microsomal mixed function oxidase
formed aminoazobenzene, 4-OH-methylaminoazobenzene and a
trace of 4-OH-aminoazobenzene. N-OH-methylaminoazobenzene
was also formed with NADPH. Hydroperoxide was equally effective as NADPH in catalysing the oxidation of MAB and the
products were similar except that no N-OH-methylaminoazobenzene was formed (8). This indicates that cytochrome P450
catalyses both N-demethylation and ring hydroxylation of methylaminoazobenzene and that the N-hydroxylation is catalysed by microsomal amine oxidase. Furthermore the binding of
MAB to exogenous DNA and protein catalysed by the prostaglandin synthetase-arachidonate or cytochrome P450-hydroperoxide
system clearly does not involve N-OH-MAB as an intermediate
and it is likely that amine radical is responsible for the
DNA/protein binding formed by the amine acting as a peroxidase donor. The prostaglandin synthetase or mixed function
oxidase activity of the bladder or lung could be responsible
for the bladder or lung carcinogenesis. In the case of liver
carcinogenesis the presence of cytosolic sulfotransferase
makes N-OH-MAB an alternative carcinogenic pathway to the le

oxidation pathway of the mixed function oxidase or those mediated by lipid peroxidation.

ACKNOWLEDGEMENT

This work was supported by the National Cancer Institute of Canada.

REFERENCES

1. O'Brien, P.J. (in Press) "Lipid Peroxides in Biology and Medicine", Ed. K. Yagi, Academic Press, N.Y.
2. W.G. Tarpley, J.A. Miller, and E.C. Miller (1980) Cancer Res. 40, 2493-2499.
3. Beland, F.A., D.L. Tullis, F.F. Kadlubar, K.M. Straub and F.E. Evans (1980) Chem. Biol. Interactions 31, 1-17.
4. Meunier, I. and Chaveau, J. (1970) Int. J. Cancer 6 463-469.
5. Sivarajah, K., Anderson, M.W. and Eling, T.E. (1978) Life Science 23, 2571-2578.
6. O'Brien, P.J. (1978) Pharm. Ther. 2A 517-536.
7. Labuc, G.E. and Blunck, J.M. (1979) Biochemical Pharm. 28, 2367-2373.
8. Kadlubar, F.F., Miller, J.A. and Miller, E.C. (1976) Cancer Res. 36, 1196-1206.

**Prostaglandins and Cancer: First
International Conference, pages 159–162**
© **1982 Alan R. Liss, Inc., 150 Fifth Avenue, New York, NY 10011**

PROSTAGLANDIN SYNTHETASE CATALYZED DNA STRAND BREAKS BY
AROMATIC AMINES

A. Rahimtula[1], P. Moldeus, B. Andersson, and
M. Nordenskjöld
[1]Biochemistry Dept., Memorial University, St.
John's, Nfld., Canada and the Departments of
Forensic Medicine and Clinical Genetics,
Karolinska Institute, Stockholm, Sweden

Aromatic amines are compounds of considerable indus-
trial and commercial importance. Some of them have potent
toxicological properties. Benzidine, 2-naphthylamine, 4-
aminobiphenyl, etc. are potent bladder carcinogens in
several animal species and man (Radomski, 1979). Several
other amines like p-aminophenol, p-phenetidine, etc. are
also renal medullary toxins (Hook et al., 1979). The
mechanism for the nephrotoxicity of the various amines is
not likely to be dependent on cytochrome P450 catalyzed
activation, since the concentration of this enzyme is very
low in the kidney. A likely catalyst, primarily located in
the inner medulla where the toxicity occurs, is prostaglandin synthetase. Several workers have demonstrated that
prostaglandin synthetase present in sheep seminal vesicles
(SSV), rabbit kidney medulla, guinea pig lung, etc. can
carry out the arachidonic acid dependent cooxidation of a
variety of xenobiotics including carcinogens (Marnett et al.
1978; Zenser et al., 1979; Sivarajah et al., 1981). In this
paper we show that prostaglandin synthetase can carry out
the metabolic activation of several aromatic amines to
products or intermediates that cause DNA strand breaks in
cultured human fibroblasts.

Human fibroblasts from healthy donors were grown on
glass plates and the DNA labelled by adding [^{3}H]-thymidine
(2μCi/ml medium). Fibroblasts were preincubated for 10 min
with 100μM cytosine-1-β-D-arabinoside (Ara C) before addition of SSV microsomes (1 mg/ml) arachidonic acid (100μM)
and substrate. Incubations were carried out in 1.5 ml of
Dulbecco's phosphate-buffered saline pH 7.6 at 37°C for

30 min. The reaction was terminated by washing the cells twice in ice-cold Dulbecco's phosphate buffered saline pH 7.4. DNA strand breaks were determined by alkali treatment and hydroxylapatite chromatography (Nordenskjöld et al., 1979). Paracetamol glutathione conjugate formation and binding of [3H] paracetamol to microsomal proteins was carried out as described previously (Moldeus, Rahimtula, 1980; Moldeus et al., 1981). Glutathione conjugate formation was carried out in 1 ml of 0.1 M phosphate buffer pH 8.0 containing 200 μM paracetamol, 1 mg SSV microsomes, 2.5 mM glutathione and the desired concentration of the amine in 5-10μl of DMSO. Reactions were initiated with 0.2 mM arachidonic acid. For covalent binding studies [3H]paracetamol was used and glutathione was omitted.

Table 1. Effect of Aromatic Amines on the Induction of DNA-Strand Breaks in Human Fibroblasts in the Presence of SSV Microsomes and Arachidonic Acid.

Additions	Concentration μM	Change in % single stranded DNA from control
DMSO		0.0 ± 3.1
2,4-Diaminotoluene	50	13.3 ± 6.9
2-Naphthylamine	50	16.5 ± 6.0
Aminoazobenzene	50	3.9 ± 1.3
Benzidine	50	1.2 ± 3.4
Phenylhydrazine	100	8.6 ± 0.3
p-Phenetidine	50	21.7 ± 10.1
p-Aminophenol	50	19.4 ± 12.4

Table 2. Effect of Aromatic Amines on Arachidonic Acid Dependent Paracetamol Glutathione Conjugate Formation and Irreversible Binding to Proteins Catalyzed by SSV Microsomes.

Additions	GSH Conjugate nmoles/min/mg protein	Protein Binding
Paracetamol	29.3 (200μM)*	2.30 (200μM)
+ 2,4-Diaminotoluene	9.3 (100μM)	1.50 (50μM)
+ 2-Naphthylamine	2.4 (100μM)	0.96 (50μM)
+ Aminoazobenzene	8.1 (100μM)	1.50 (50μM)
+ Phenylhydrazine	3.3 (50μM)	0.27 (50μM)
+ p-Phenetidine	6.7 (50μM)	1.22 (50μM)
+ p-Aminophenol	14.9 (50μM)	0.23 (50μM)

*Values in parentheses represent amine concentrations

RESULTS AND DISCUSSION

SSV microsomes have the ability to catalyze the arachidonic acid dependent activation of several aromatic amines including 2,4-diaminotoluene, 2-naphthylamine, aminoazobenetidine and p-aminophenol. When coincubated with cultured human fibroblasts, these activated intermediates caused an increase in single stranded DNA formation (Table 1). Indomethacin inhibited this reaction indicating the involvement of prostaglandin synthetase. This is also evident from the ability of these amines to compete with and inhibit another prostaglandin synthetase catalyzed reaction – the activation of paracetamol detected both as paracetamol glutathione conjugate formation and irreversible binding to protein (Table 2). Addition of 50 µM amines inhibited both glutathione conjugate formation and irreversible protein binding of paracetamol by 30-90%.

Metabolic N-hydroxylation of aromatic amines is believed to be an obligatory step in the activation of these compounds to carcinogenic derivatives and that subsequent esterification, catalyzed by a liver sulfotransferase, leads to the formation of the ultimate carcinogen in the liver (Miller, Miller, 1981). However, in other tissues the lack of sulfotransferase makes this hypothesis less attractive. In Fig. 1 we propose an alternate mechanism for the activation of aromatic amines. PGG2 formed from arachidonic acid via the cyclooxygenase catalyzes the 1e peroxidatic cooxidation of the aromatic amine to a free radical intermediate(s) which then causes DNA strand breaks. Other hydroperoxides can replace PGG2 and the antioxidant butylated hydroxyanisole inhibits the peroxidase reaction. A 3-4 fold increase in oxidation of GSH to GSSG occured in the presence of the amine indicating that the amine radical intermediate can be reduced back to the free amine at the expense of GSH.

Dr. A. Rahimtula thanks MRC Canada for financial support. Dr. Peter Moldeus, B. Andersson and M. Nordenskjöld thank MRC Sweden for financial support.

REFERENCES

Marnett LJ, Reed GA, Dennison DJ (1978). Prostaglandin synthetase dependent activation of 7,8-dihydro-7,8-dihydroxy-benzo(a)pyrene to mutagenic derivatives. Biochem Biophys

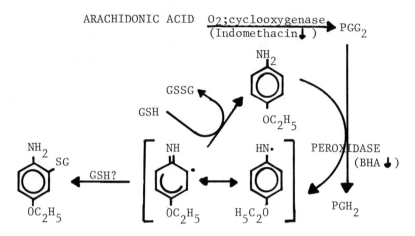

Figure 1.   Possible Mechanism for Arylamine Activation

Res Commun 82:210.

Miller EC, Miller JA (1981). Searches for ultimate chemical carcinogens and their reactions with cellular macromolecules. Cancer 47:2327.

Moldeus P, Rahimtula AD (1980). Metabolism of paracetamol to a glutathione conjugate catalyzed by prostaglandin synthetase. Biochem Biophys Res Commun 96:469.

Moldeus P, Andersson B, Rahimtula AD, Berggren M (1981). Prostaglandin synthetase catalyzed activation of paracetamol. Submitted to Biochem Pharmacol.

Nordenskjöld M, Söderhäll S, Moldeus P (1979). Studies of DNA strand breaks induced in human fibroblasts by chemical mutagens/carcinogens. Mutat Res 63:393.

Sivarajah K, Lasker JM, Eling TE (1981). Prostaglandin synthetase dependent cooxidation of (±)-benzo(a)pyrene-7,8-dihydrodiol by human lung and other mammalian tissues. Cancer Res 41:1834.

Zenser TV, Mattramal MB, Davis BB (1979). Cooxidation of benzidine by renal medullary prostaglandin cyclooxygenase. J Pharmacol Exp Ther 211:460.

**Prostaglandins and Cancer: First
International Conference, pages 163-166
© 1982 Alan R. Liss, Inc., 150 Fifth Avenue, New York, NY 10011**

THE INVOLVEMENT OF PROSTAGLANDIN INTERMEDIATES IN COVALENT
BINDING TO NUCLEIC ACIDS AND IN AGEING PIGMENT FORMATION

Sudesh Vasdev and Peter J. O'Brien

Dept. of Biochemistry, Memorial University of
Newfoundland
St. John's, Newfoundland, Canada A1B 3X9

In lipid peroxidation, the unsaturated fatty acid moiety
of phospholipids is broken down giving rise to the formation
of peroxidised fatty acids and malonaldehyde. The latter a-
gent can bind the amino groups of phosphatidylethanolamine,
amino groups of proteins or nucleic acids leading to the formation of fluorescent chromolipids. During ageing there is
an increase in tissue chromolipid or lipofuscin (1).

Enzymic microsomal lipid peroxidation is mediated by
NADPH: cyt. P450 reductase (2). Lipofuscin pigment however
has been found in tissues which have a low activity of the
reductase but have high prostaglandin synthetase activity
(1). Labelled arachidonic acid is covalently bound to microsomal protein in tissues having prostaglandin synthetase
activity (3-5). PGG_2 was also rapidly bound (5).

Arachidonic acid (AA), DNA (calf thymus), indomethacin,
glutathione (GSH) and NADPH were purchased from Sigma Chemical Co. (St. Louis, Mo, U.S.A.). $(1-C^{14})$ arachidonic acid
(sp. act. 56 ci. mol^{-1}) was purchased from Amersham/Searle
(Des Plaines, Il., U.S.A.). Male Sprague-Dawley Rats weigh-
ing 175-200 g were used. Microsomes from human platelets
were prepared as described by Needleman et al. (6). Protein
was determined by the method of Lowry et al. (7). Incubation
mixtures consisted of the following: microsomal protein, 2
mg; Tris-HCl buffer 0.1 M, pH 7.0; arachidonic acid (100 μM)
in a total volume of 2 ml. The reaction was initiated by the
addition of $(1-C^{14})$ arachidonic acid in ethanol. Incubation
at 37°C was performed for 60 min. When binding to DNA was

studied, 2 mgm DNA was added. The reaction was terminated by four extractions with 5 ml of ethyl acetate/acetone (2:1). DNA and protein was precipitated and purified and arachidonate binding was determined as described (8).

Fluorescence analysis of chloroform-methanol extracts of microsomes were carried out as described (9). For measurements of fluorescence bound to DNA, the incubation mixture was centrifuged at 105,000 x g for 1 hour and the supernatant was dialysed against sucrose-tris-buffer (pH 7.0) in a cold room for 24 hours and fluorescence measured.

Proteins were separated by sodium dodecyl sulfate (SDS)-polyacrylamide gel electrophoresis, as described by Koster and Slee (9).

RESULTS

Incubation of arachidonate with sheep seminal vesicle microsomes (SVM) for 60 minutes led to covalent binding of arachidonic acid metabolites to microsomal protein and also exogenous DNA (Table 1). Addition of glutathione (GSH) or indomethacin decreased this binding. This system, also led to the production of chloroform, methanol soluble (lipofuscin) and DNA bound fluorescence material (Table 1). SDS polyacrylamide gel electrophoresis of the proteins showed the disappearance of some bands and appearance of higher MW proteins indicating polymerisation.

Incubation of arachidonate with microsomes from rat tissues having prostaglandin synthetase activity, such as lung, kidney, brain, and testes, led to the binding of labelled arachidonate metabolites to microsomal protein and lipofuscin formation. This was inhibited by indomethacin. With the microsomes from spleen, liver, aorta, and heart which have very low activity of PG synthetase, there was little or no binding and lipofuscin formation (Table 2). Incubation of human platelet microsomes and rat heart microsomes with arachidonate led to increased production of lipofuscin as well as binding of arachidonate metabolites to protein compared to platelets or heart microsomes alone.

Table 1 THE INVOLVEMENT OF PROSTAGLANDIN SYNTHETASE IN COVALENT BINDING OF (^{14}C)-ARACHIDONATE INTERMEDIATES TO LIPOFUSCIN FORMATION.

ADDITION	MICROSOMES FLUORES. U/mg/Prot.	PROTEIN BINDING	DNA FLUORES. U/mg/DNA	DNA BINDING
Complete System	292 ± 16	1448 ± 35	382 ± 19	296 ± 12
+GSH (5 mM)	--	825 ± 25	--	90 ± 18
+Indo. (100 μM)	--	758 ± 32	--	75 ± 12
Ht. Den. Microsomes	25 ± 8	18 ± 3	32 ± 6	11 ± 2
Microsomes	29 ± 5	--	28 ± 3	--

Values are mean ± SE of four observations. Fluorescence (Fluores.) was measured at excitation 348 nm and emission 454 nm. Binding values indicate nmole Arachidonate intermediates bound per mg protein or DNA. Indo=Indomethacin.

Table 2 THE INVOLVEMENT OF PROSTAGLANDIN SYNTHETASE IN "LIPOFUSCIN" FORMATION AND PROTEIN BINDING.

MICROSOMES	PROTEIN BINDING nmole A.A. bound/mg			FLUORESCENCE UNITS Excit. 350 nm Emission 430 nm	
		+Ht.	+Indo.		+Ht.
Lung	150 ± 9	6 ± 2	90 ± 4	300 ± 18	40 ± 5
Kidney	130 ± 20	11 ± 2	85 ± 7	160 ± 23	30 ± 3
Brain	99 ± 19	6 ± 1	36 + 4		
Testes	93 ± 11	8 ± 1	40 ± 6	100 ± 18	40 ± 5
Heart	6 ± 1	6 ± 1	6 ± 1	45 ± 4	44 ± 4
Platelets	70 ± 6	16 ± 2	30 ± 5	130 ± 15	
Heart + Plateltes	191 ± 22		102 ± 10	360 ± 21	

Values are mean ± SE of four observations. Ht.=Heat.

DISCUSSION

The data presented demonstrate that prostaglandin synthetase activity can lead to lipofuscin formation, binding
of arachidonate metabolites to microsomal protein and exogenous DNA, and polymerisation of microsomal protein in the
tissues involved in prostaglandin synthesis. This activity
is very low in heart and aorta but when human platelets which
have high activity were added to the heart microsomes, increased binding of arachidonate metabolites and lipofuscin
formation occurred when compared with platelets alone. This
suggests that prostaglandin could be involved in lipofuscin
formation, ageing process and heart damage. It has been
suggested that the polymerisation and the fluorescence produced are due to the formation of malonaldehyde (10) but another aldehyde may be involved (11), as the excitation and
emission spectra of malonaldehyde are different from that o-
bserved (12). The binding could also be due to the fatty
acid free radical.
This work was supported by the Canadian Heart Foundation.

REFERENCES

1. Pyror, W.A. (1977) in Free Radicals in Biology (Miavel,
   J. Bensch, K.G. and Johnson, Jr. J.E.). Vol III, p 133-
   182. Academic Press, New York.
2. Orrenius, S., Dallner, G. and Ernster, C. (1964). Biochem.
   Biophys. Res. Commun. 141 139.
3. Anderson, M.W., Crutchley, D.J., Chudhari, A. and Wilson,
   A.G.E. (1978). Biochem. Biophys. Acta 573, 40-50.
4. Eling, T.E., Wilson, A.G.E., Chudhuor, A. and Anderson,
   M.W. (1979). Life Sciences 21, 245-252.
5. Crutchley, D.J., Hawkins, H.J., Eling, T.E. and Anderson,
   M.W. (1979). Biochem. Pharmacol. 28, 1519-1523.
6. Needleman, P. Moncada, S., Bunting, S., Vane, J.R. Hamburg
   M. and Samuelson, B. (1976). Nature (London), 261, 558-560.
7. Lowry, D.H., Rosebrough, N.J., Farr, A.L. and Randall, R.R.
   (1951). J. Biol. Chem. 193, 265-275.
8. Sivarajah, K., Anderson, M.W. and Eling, T.E. (1978). Life
   Sciences 23, 1571-2578.
9. Koster, J.F. and Slee, R.G. (1980). Biochem. Biophys.
   Acta 620, 489-499.
10. Chio, K.S. and Tappel, A.L. (1969). Biochemistry 8, 2821.
11. Benedetti, A. Comporti, M. and Esterbauer, H. (1980).
    Biochem. Biophys. Acta 620, 281-296.
12. Reiss, U. and Tappel, A.L. (1973). Lipids 8, 199-202.

Prostaglandins and Cancer: First
International Conference, pages 167–179
© 1982 Alan R. Liss, Inc., 150 Fifth Avenue, New York, NY 10011

EVIDENCE FOR LIPOXYGENASE-PEROXIDASE ACTIVATION OF N-HYDROXY-
-2-ACETYLAMINOFLUORENE BY RAT MAMMARY GLAND PARENCHYMAL CELLS

Peter K. Wong, Ph.D., M. J. Hampton
and Robert A. Floyd, Ph.D.

Oklahoma Medical Research Foundation
Biomembrane Research Laboratory
Oklahoma City, Oklahoma   73104

ABSTRACT

Rat mammary gland parenchymal cells activate N-hydroxy-
2-acetylaminofluorene (N-OH-AAF) to 2-nitrosofluorene (NOF)
and N-acetoxy-2-acetylaminofluorene (N-OAc-AAF) via a nitroxyl free radical form of the carcinogen. Prostaglandin
synthetase has a peroxidase activity and hence we have examined parenchymal cells to determine if the activation of N-
OH-AAF in these cells occurs by this route. Freshly isolated cells activate N-OH-AAF to NOF as detected by high pressure liquid chromatography (HPLC). Cells frozen at -60°C
are more active. N-OH-AAF activation appears to be peroxidative since ascorbate and ρ-aminophenol completely inhibit
NOF formation. The deacylase route does not occur to any
appreciable extent in the cells. Exogenously added arachidonate enhances N-OH-AAF activation and the inhibitor 5,8,-
11,14-eicosatetraynoic acid (ETYA) considerably decreased N-
OH-AAF activation while indomethacin or aspirin were not
effective. Ram seminal vesicle microsomes activate N-OH-AAF
by the prostaglandin synthetase route. Our work indicates
that N-OH-AAF was activated by lipoxygenase pathway in these
cells. The 12L-hydroperoxy-5,8,10,14-eicosatetraenoic acid
(12-HPETE) generated through endogenous or exogenous arachidonate sources probably is the hydroperoxide substrate
for the peroxidase. Platelets which are rich in lipoxygenase also activate N-OH-AAF. Since 12-HPETE is one of the
three hydroperoxides found in the animal kingdom, the peroxidase activation may have significant importance in mammary
gland carcinogenesis.

INTRODUCTION

AAF (2-acetylaminofluorene) induces liver tumors in male rats and mammary gland tumors in female rats. AAF is one of a large class of carcinogens, the arylamine carcinogens, and has been studied extensively with respect to the mechanism of xenobiotic metabolism. A first necessary step in the metabolic activation of AAF is N-hydroxylation to form N-hydroxy-2-acetylaminofluorene (N-OH-AAF). Although N-OH-AAF is a more active carcinogen than AAF (Miller, 1966), it is not the ultimate reactive species. Further activation is required for this compound to exert its carcinogenic potential (Miller, 1970). Bartsch et al. (1971) and Floyd et al. (1976, 1977) showed that N-OH-AAF can be activated into two more potent carcinogens, 2-nitrosofluorene (NOF) and N-acetoxy-2-acetylaminofluorene (N-OAc-AAF) via a free radical route (peroxidative route) as indicated in the following equation:

Equation 1

Enzymatic deacetylation of N-OH-AAF is another activation route for N-OH-AAF (Irving, 1966) producing N-hydroxy-amino-fluorene and after oxidation, NOF. The acyltransferase mechanism is still another possible route by which N-OH-AAF is activated into NOF. Of all these activation routes, only the peroxidative route will produce N-OAc-AAF in addition to NOF formation. We report here the results of a study demonstrating that peroxidative activation of N-OH-AAF occurs in rat mammary cells leading to NOF formation. The nature of the processes involved and possible correlation between mammary gland carcinogenesis and the activation process were investigated.

MAMMARY CELL PEROXIDATIVE ACTIVATION OF N-OH-AAF

We have found that incubating N-OH-AAF with mammary gland epithelial cells in the presence of arachidonic acid would produce NOF and N-OAc-AAF as detected by high pressure liquid chromatography (HPLC). The chromatogram in Fig. 1 (right side) demonstrating formation of NOF and NO-OAc-AAF in mammary cells is similar to the chromatogram

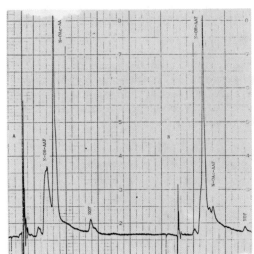

Figure 1. Activation products of N-hydroxy-2-acetylaminofluorene (N-OH-AAF) by horseradish peroxidase/H_2O_2 system and rat mammary gland cells. A = reaction products by horseradish peroxidase/H_2O_2 system; B = reaction products by rat mammary gland cells. Chromatographic conditions: column C_{18} (4.6 X 30 cm); mobile phase: methanol/acetate buffer (60:40); flow rate: 0.8 ml/min; detector: uv 285 nm.

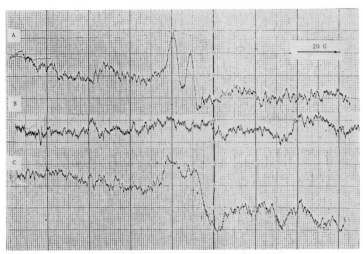

Figure 2. Electron spin resonance spectrum during activation of N-hydroxy-2-acetylaminofluorene (N-OH-AAF) by horseradish peroxidase/H_2O_2 system and rat mammary gland cells.

in Figure 1 (left side) which was obtained by using the
model peroxidase system: horseradish peroxidase/hydrogen
peroxide (HRP/H_2O_2) catalyzed oxidation of N-OH-AAF. We
have also found that during the incubation process, free
radicals are produced which have similar spectral characteristics for both systems as detected by EPR at room temperature (Reigh and Floyd, 1977) and at -140°C as indicated
in traces A and C of Figure 2.

ESR spectrum was obtained utilizing a Varian E-9 X-band
spectrophotometer. The instrument settings were scan range
200 gauss, modulation amplitude 10 gauss, time constant 3
sec, scan time 8 min, modulation frequency 100 kHz, 24 mW
microwave power and temperature -140°C.

EFFECT OF VARIOUS TREATMENTS UPON ACTIVATION OF N-OH-AAF BY RAT MAMMARY CELLS

ADDITIVE	CONCENTRATION (mM)	FUNCTION	NOF FORMED (p.mole/10^5 cells/30 min)
Control	---	---	3.8
Boiling (5 min)	---	Denatured	N.D.
Butylated Hydroxy-toulene (BHT)	1.0	Antioxidant	N.D.
Ascorbate	1.0	Antioxidant	N.D.
Diethyl p-nitrophenyl phosphate	0.5	Esterase inhibitor	16.8
Control	---	---	19.0
p-Aminophenol	1.0	Peroxidase inhibitor	2.9
Control	---	---	54.3
Sonicated (control)	3 sec		14.2
Unsonicated	3 sec		5.1

Each sample contained 0.1 mM N-OH-AAF and about 10^5 mammary cells suspended in phosphate buffer (0.15 M, pH 7.4) and was incubated at 37°C for 30
min. NOF is extracted with hexane and quantitated by HPLC.

N.D. = not detected

Table 1

Table 1 is a summary of results obtained where various treatments have been imposed on the activation of N-
OH-AAF by mammary cells. The amount of NOF formed was
estimated from the height of the peak in the chromatogram.
Antioxidants, butylated hydroxytoluene and ascorbate, as
well as nordihydroguiaric acid (data not shown), completely inhibited the formation of NOF. ρ-Aminophenol, which
inhibited NOF formation in the HRP/H_2O_2 activation system,
was also effective in the inhibition of NOF production in
the mammary cell system. The known esterase inhibitor,

diethyl-ρ-nitro-phenylphosphate (Schut, 1978) has little, if any, effect upon the formation of NOF. This ruled out, as a major pathway, the deacetylase route N-OH-AAF activation by mammary cells. ρ-Aminophenol which inhibits the acyltransferase mediated formation of the N-acetoxy-2-aminofluorene-t-RNA adduct from N-OH-AAF (King, 1974) by competing with the initial deacetylation product of N-OH-AAF, N-OH-AF, as an acetyl acceptor, should actually cause an increase in NOF formation if the acyltransferase pathway occurs. The fact that ρ-aminophenol does inhibit NOF formation as in the case of the HRP/H$_2$O$_2$ peroxidative activation system further suggested that peroxidative activation predominates in the mammary cell activation process and that the acyltransferase pathway may not be operating as effectively in this system.

INVOLVEMENT OF LIPOXYGENASE IN THE MAMMARY CELL ACTIVATION OF N-OH-AAF

The hydroperoxides required in the peroxidative mechanism are believed to be generated by lipoxygenase present in the mammary cells. Arachidonate metabolism via the lipoxygenase pathway provides the hydroperoxide, 12L-hydroperoxy-5,8,10,14-eicosatetraenoic acid (12-HPETE), as

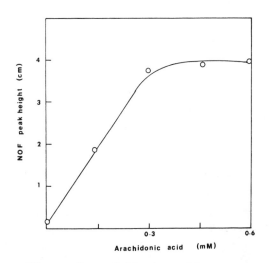

Figure 3. Effect of arachidonic acid on mammary cell activity towards NOF formation

the possible substrate for the peroxidase. This is supported by the fact that formation of NOF is dependent on
the exogenously added arachidonic acid. Figure 3 shows
the relationship between the amount of arachidonic added
and the amount of NOF formed during incubation.

Table 2 is a summary of results obtained where various
treatments have been imposed on the reaction of N-OH-AAF
with mammary cell. The anti-inflammatory, analgesic and
antipyretic drugs, aspirin and indomethacin, which inhibit
prostaglandin cyclooxygenase, have essentially no effect
on the generation of NOF through mammary cell activation.
The lipoxygenase inhibitor, 5,8,11,14-eicosatetraynoic
acid (ETYA) does have a much greater effect in inhibiting
NOF formation. Platelets, rich in lipoxygenase activity,
activated N-OH-AAF in the presence of added arachidonate
(data not shown). Ram seminal vesicle microsomes (RSVM),
which have a high prostaglandin biosynthetic capacity,
activate N-OH-AAF to NOF through the cyclooxygenase and
hydroperoxidase activities.

EFFECT OF ETYA, ASPIRIN AND INDOMETHACIN ON MAMMARY CELL ACTIVATION OF N-OH-AAF

Additive	Concentration (mM)	Function	NOF formed (p.mole/10^5 cell/30 min)
Control	--	--	2.53
Aspirin	1.0	Prostaglandin synthetase inhibitor	2.66
BHA	1.0	Antioxidant	0.39
ETYA	0.3	Lipoxygenase & prostaglandin synthe-tase inhibitor	0.53
Indomethacin	0.15	Prostaglandin synthe-tase inhibitor	2.39

Each sample contained 0.1 mM N-OH-AAF and about 10^5 mammary cell suspended in
phosphate buffer (0.15 M pH 7.4) and was incubated at 37°C for 30 min after preincubating the enzyme with additives for 5 min. NOF formed is extracted with
hexane and quantitated by HPLC.

ETYA = eicosatetraynoic acid
BHA = butylated hydroxyanisole

Table 2

Table 3 is a summary of results obtained where various
treatments have been imposed on the reaction of N-OH-AAF
with RSVM. ETYA, aspirin and indomethacin all exhibit considerable inhibitory effects on the activation of N-OH-AAF
by this enzyme. These inhibitors prevent the formation of
prostaglandin G_2 which would act as a hydroperoxide sub-

strate for the peroxidase portion of prostaglandin synthetase to activate N-OH-AAF via the mechanisms demonstrated in
Figure 4.

EFFECT OF ETYA, ASPIRIN INDOMETHACIN ON RAM SEMINAL VESICLE MICROSOMES ACTIVATION
OF N-OH-AAF

ADDITIVE	CONCENTRATION (mM)	FUNCTION	NOF FORMED p.mole/mg protein/15 min
Aspirin	1.0	Prostaglandin synthetase inhibitor	291
ETYA	0.3	Lipoxygenase & prostaglandin synthetase inhibitor	N.D.
Indomethacin	0.15	Prostaglandin synthetase inhibitor	194
Boiling		Denatured	N.D.
Control	-	-	874

Each sample contained 0.1 mM N-OH-AAF, 0.3 mM arachidonic acid, and ram seminal
vesicle microsomes (0.008 mg protein) suspended in phosphate buffer (0.15 M, pH 7.4)
and was incubated at 37°C for 15 min after preincubating the enzyme with additives
for 5 min. NOF formed is extracted with hexane and quantitated by HPLC.

ETYA = eicosatetraynoic acid

N.D. = not detected

Table 3

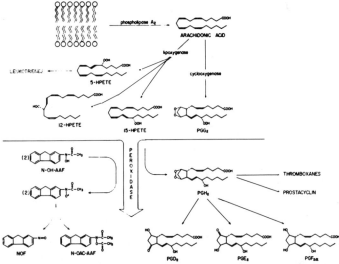

Figure 4. Activation of N-OH-AAF via the prostaglandin
synthetase route

ETYA, aspirin and indomethacin all exhibit considerable inhibitory effects on the activation of N-OH-AAF by this en-zyme. These inhibitors prevent the formation of prostaglan-din G_2 which would act as a hydroperoxide substrate for the peroxidase portion of prostaglandin synthetase to activate N-OH-AAF via the mechanisms demonstrated in Figure 4.

SOME CHARACTERISTICS OF N-OH-AAF ACTIVATION BY MAMMARY CELLS

It was found that the activity of the mammary cell pre-paration is dependent on the duration of freezing at about -10°C. Freshly prepared cells usually have less activity than those frozen for a longer period of time. Cells fro-zen for longer periods of time required less incubation time to reach maximum activity. Figure 5 summarized our results.

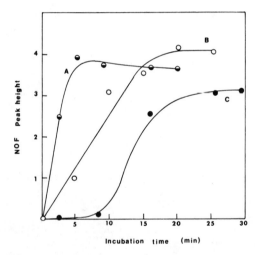

Incubation time (min)

Figure 5. Effect of freezing on mammary cell activity to-wards NOF formation. A = Cells frozen for 30 days; B = Cells frozen for 5 days; C = Cells frozen for 1 day.

As indicated previously, cell activity also depends on exogenously added arachidonate (Fig. 3). A linear rela-tionship exists up to arachidonate concentrations of about 0.3 mM. The increased activity of aged cell may be due to

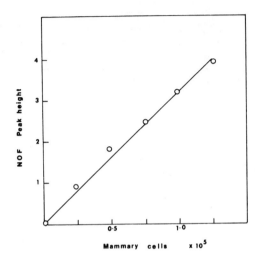

Figure 6. NOF formation as a function of mammary cell number

slow release of arachidonate from endogenous sources by the action of phospholipases. Cells sonicated briefly give higher activity than unsonicated cell preparations (Table 1). Linear relationship between NOF formation and the amount of cells can also be obtained up to 10^5 cells (Fig. 6).

TREATMENTS AND CONDITIONS OF ANIMALS ON MAMMARY CELL ACTIVITY

Figure 7 summarizes the results obtained on the mammary cell activity when various treatments have been imposed on the animals. Rats fed a selenium-deficient diet yielded mammary gland cells which activated N-OH-AAF much more readily than those animals that had been fed the selenium-deficient diet but to which selenium had been added.

Clayton and Baumann (1949) observed that cancer induction by arylamine carcinogens was decreased by a diet containing selenium. Our results seem to indicate that it is in the metabolism of the carcinogen where selenium (Se) exerts its suppressive effect. The selenium effect is most likely manifested through its effect on glutathione peroxidase but this remains to be proven. Se is an essential component of glutathione peroxidase (Rotruck, 1973), an enzyme that would be expected to compete for hydroperoxides formed, thus, in effect, lowering the potential for peroxidative activation of the carcinogens.

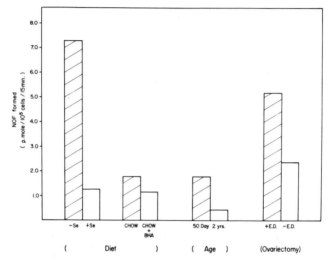

Figure 7. Mammary gland peroxidative activity: effect of dietary selenium, butylated hydroxyanisole and treatment of animals. BHA = butylated hydroxyanisole; +Se = animals on selenium supplement diet; -Se = animals on selenium deficient diet; +E.D. = ovariectomized animal at 50 days old were injected estradiol (10 µg) 20 hr before sacrifice; -E.D. = untreated ovariectomized animals

It has also been shown that antioxidant such as butylated hydroxytoulene (BHT) is effective in suppressing N-OH-AAF induced hepatoma and mammary tumors in rats (Ulland, 1973). This is in agreement with our in vitro finding that mammary cells from animals fed BHA are less active toward N-OH-AAF oxidation.

It has been shown that administration of estradiol to immature rats causes substantial increase in the peroxidase enzyme activity of the uterus (Lucas, 1955). Histochemical

studies suggested that estrogen-induced peroxidase increases only in those tissues susceptible to this hormone
such as uterus, vagina, and carcinogen-induced mammary
tumor (DeSombre, 1975). Mammary cells from rats at reproductive age injected with estradiol would be expected to
have higher peroxidase activity than those not injected
with this hormone. The results shown in Figure 7 are in
good agreement with this prediction. Mammary cells from
ovariectomized rats showed less activity toward NOF formation than those from estradiol injected ovariectomized
rats. In addition, we have found that mammary cells from
animals at 50 days old activate N-OH-AAF much more readily
than older animals. This is consistent with the fact that
animals at or about 50 days old are more susceptible to
mammary tumor formation from other carcinogens such as
dimethylbenzanthracene.

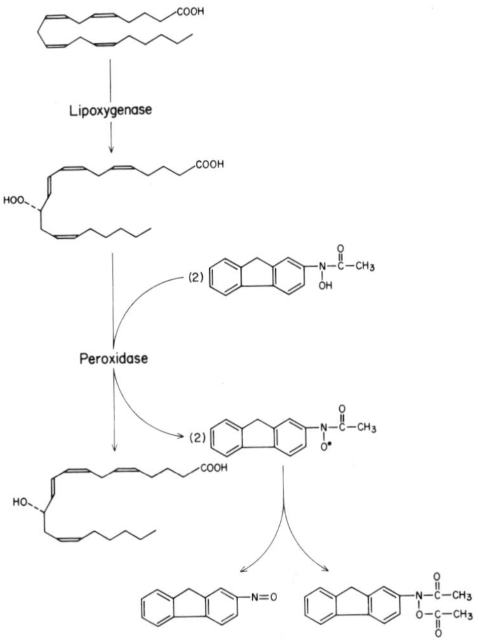

Figure 8. Activation of N-OH-AAF by the lipoxygenase peroxidase route

CONCLUSIONS

By comparing EPR spectrum and activation products as detected by HPLC with model HRP/H_2O_2 peroxidase system as well as the studies of the effect of various inhibitors upon the activation pathway, we concluded that mammary cell activation of N-OH-AAF is peroxidative and that the lipoxygenase pathway is responsible for providing hydroperoxide substrate from endogenously and exogenously added arachidonate sources (Fig. 8).

Studies on the effect of antioxidant diet and estrogen injection all appear to indicate the probable connection between mammary cell peroxidase and lipoxygenase activities and mammary gland carcinogenesis.

ACKNOWLEDGMENTS

This study was supported in part by NIH research grant R01-CA18591. We thank Ms. E. Miser for excellent secretarial assistance and Dr. R. Sridhar for beneficial discussion of the research results.

REFERENCES

Bartsch H, Traut M, Hecker E (1971). On the metabolic activation of N-hydroxy-N-2-acetylaminofluorene II. Simultaneous formation of 2-nitrosofluorene and N-acetoxy-N-2-acetyl-aminofluorene from N-hydroxy-2-acetylaminofluorene via a free radical intermediate. Biochim Biophys Acta 237:556.
Bartsch H, Hecker H (1971). On the metabolic activation of N-hydroxy-N-acetylaminofluorene. III. Oxidation with horseradish peroxidase to yield 2-nitrosofluorene and N-acetoxy-N-2-acetylaminofluorene. Biochim Biophys Acta 237:567.
Clayton CC, Baumann CA (1949). Diet and azo dye tumor: effect of diet during a period when the dye is not fed. Cancer Res 9:575.
DeSombre ER, Anderson WA, Kang Y-H (1975). Identification, subcellular localization and estrogen regulation of peroxidase in 7,12-dimethylbenz(a)anthracene-induced rat mammary tumors. Cancer Res 35:172.

Floyd RA, Soong LM, Walker RN, Stuart M (1976). Lipid
hydroperoxide activation of N-hydroxy-N-acetylaminofluorene via a free radical route. Cancer Res 36:2761.
Floyd RA, Soong LM (1977). Obligatory free radical intermediate in the oxidation activation of carcinogen N-
hydroxy-2-acetylaminofluorene. Biochim Biophys Acta
498:244.
Irving CC (1966). Enzymatic deacetylation of N-hydroxy-2-
acetylaminofluorene by liver microsomes. Cancer Res
26:1390.
King CM (1974). Mechanism of reaction, tissue distribution and inhibition of arylhydroxamic acid acyltransferase. Cancer Res 34:1503.
Lucas FV, Neufeld HA, Utterback JG, Martin AP, Stotz E
(1955). The effect of estrogen on the production of a
peroxidase in the rat uterus. J Biol Chem 214:775.
Miller EC, Miller JA, Hartman HA (1961). N-hydroxy-2-ace-
tylaminofluorene: a metabolite of 2-acetylaminofluorene
with increased carcinogenic activity in the rat. Cancer
Res 21:815.
Miller JA (1970). Carcinogenesis by chemicals: an overview - G.H.A. Clowes memorial lecture. Cancer Res
30:559.
Reigh DL, Stuart M, Floyd RA (1978). Activation of the
carcinogen N-hydroxy-2-acetylaminofluorene by rat mammary peroxidase. Experientia 34:107.
Rotruck JT, Pope AL, Ganther HE, Swanson AB, Hafeman DG,
Hockstra WG (1973). Selenium: biochemical role as a
component of glutathione peroxidase. Science 179:588.
Ulland BM, Weisburger JH, Yamamoto RS, Weisburger EK (1973).
Antioxidants and carcinogenesis: butylated hydroxytoluene,
but not diphenyl-p-phenylenediamine, inhibits cancer induction by N-2-fluorenylacetamide and by N-hydroxy-N-2-
fluorenylacetamide in rats. Food Cosmet Toxicol 11:199.

CARCINOGENESIS-PROMOTION

Prostaglandins and Cancer: First
International Conference, pages 183–188
© 1982 Alan R. Liss, Inc., 150 Fifth Avenue, New York, NY 10011

OVERVIEW OF TUMOR PROMOTION

R. K. Boutwell

McArdle Laboratory for Cancer Research
University of Wisconsin
Madison, Wisconsin 53706

To be understood, tumor promotion must be presented in
the context of the two-stage model for the production of
experimental neoplasia. To accomplish this, the historical
events which set the stage for current research will be
discussed. Next, the biology of the two-stage system in
mouse skin will be presented, which is the best understood
model, and then two-step models in other tissues will be
briefly described. Finally, the biochemistry of tumor
promotion will be reviewed in order to provide background
information for the papers to follow which will be concerned
with prostaglandins and tumor promotion.

A simple but basic premise is that dividing the carcinogenic process into its components facilitates elucidation
of its mechanism. And secondly, an understanding of the
molecular changes essential to these components allows
rational measures for the prevention of carcinogenesis.
This is now being accomplished in experimental carcinogenesis.

The earliest pioneers in studies of experimental carcinogenesis in mouse and rabbit skin using coal tar
emphasized the irritation that accompanied the process and
so as early as 1924 Deelman showed that wounding mouse skin
in conjunction with tar applications hastened the appearance
of tumors. Berenblum through the deacde of the 30's pursued
the issue and found that croton oil applied to mouse skin in
conjunction with multiple applications of benzpyrene was an
unusually effective regimen for tumor formation (Berenblum,
1978).

Data from an experiment based on Berenblum's original model are presented in Fig. 1. The incidence of papilloma-bearing mice treated once weekly at four dose levels of 7,12-dimethylbenz[a]anthracene is shown with and without mid-week treatment with croton oil. At the highest dose, 1200 µg, of carcinogen applied once each week, tumor incidence of 100% was achieved at 20 weeks regardless of whether croton oil treatments were made at mid-week or not. In the absence of the croton oil treatments, tumor incidence remained high at weekly doses of 400 µg of carcinogen, but fell to very low levels at doses of 40 and 4 µg each week. In contrast, mice that were treated in the middle of each week with croton oil attained a high incidence of tumors.

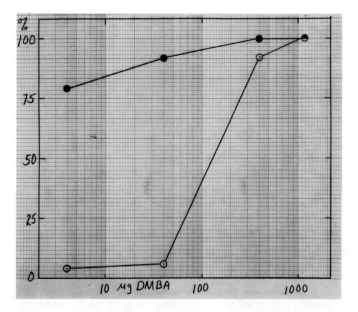

Figure 1.   The tumor incidence (expressed as percent of mice with one or more papillomas) treated once each week with either 4, 40, 400 or 1200 µg of 7,12-dimethylbenz[a]anthracene to the skin of the back (O).   Other groups were treated similarly (●) except that an optimal dose of croton oil was applied to the same area of the back in the middle of each week. Data at 20 weeks.

Two conclusions from this experiment should be pointed out. First, there is apparently a component of the carcinogenic activity of dimethylbenzanthracene that is lost at low levels and this component can be supplied by croton oil. Using current terminology, the initiating component is retained at lower dose levels at which the promoting component is lost. Secondly, and very important, the two-stage model for carcinogenesis is entirely dependent on the dose of the initiating and promoting components; dose is the important determining factor although, more commonly, dose of the initiator is in part controlled by utilizing a single application of the initiator according to the model developed by Mottram (Mottram, 1944).

The latter model is commonly used in two-stage carcinogenesis (Slaga et al., 1978). Thus a single application of the initiator, most commonly 7,12-dimethylbenz[a]anthracene, is applied to mouse skin in a dose that causes no tumors during the period of observation and for all practical purposes during the animal's life. After an interval of a week or two, repetitive treatment with a tumor promoter elicits benign and malignant tumors. The tumor promoter does not cause neoplasia if applied to the skin of uninitiated control mice during the time required for a maximal incidence of benign tumors but a very low incidence of tumors may result from life-time exposure to the promoting stimulus. It is likely that this is a manifestation of cells initiated by events outside the control of the experimentalist (Van Duuren, 1969), but it is possible that promoting agents may be inefficient initiators.

The most effective and commonly used promoting agent is 12-0-tetradecanoylphorbol-13-acetate (TPA , also known as PMA), the compound responsible for the promoting activity of croton oil (Slaga et al., 1978).

The remarkable synergism observed on application of the initiator followed by the promoter is lost if the agents are applied in the reverse order; the response is no greater than that observed in the controls treated with either agent alone. Further evidence for qualitative differences in the action of initiators and promoters arises from the fact that the action of initiators is essentially irreversible; mice given a promoting stimulus after an interval of as long as a year develop many tumors. In contrast, intervals of 4 weeks between application of a promoting stimulus to initiated mouse skin reduces the promoting efficacy to near zero.

Both initiation and promotion are dose-dependent and it is important to recognize the pharmacological truism that treatments on the dose-response curve are essential for properly designed experiments in order to properly evaluate modifying factors.

The volume and nature of the solvent used to apply agents to mouse skin must be specified because these factors determine the spread of the agents and their deposition in contact with the skin. Although acetone is toxic to cells, it remains the solvent of choice becuase it spreads readily over the shaved skin of mice and evaporates rapidly leaving the solute in intimate contact with the skin. Thus the amount of material potentially available to a cell depends not only on the amount of material applied but also the volume and nature of the solvent. A volume of 0.2 ml of acetone has proven useful; it is desirable to cover a large area of the skin of the back and then count the number of benign tumors per mouse as the best quantitative measure of the effectiveness of the experimental regimen.

The phenomenon of promotion has been further subdivided into at least two additional components (Slaga, 1980), and this is proving to be a very useful model for further specifying the changes that are essential for accomplishing neoplasia.

Following the report of Peraino defining a two-step procedure for the production of liver tumors, there has been widespread recognition that tumors arising in many organs including the bladder, mammary gland, and others may be elicited by a two-step procedure (Pitot and Sirica, 1980).

However, the two-stage model of mouse skin has a number of advantages for studies on the mechanism of carcinogenesis exemplified by the data on prostaglandins being presented at this conference. The clear-cut division of carcinogenesis into discrete, qualitatively different components is of basic importance and can not be overemphasized. Furthermore, by the use of the optimal conditions for maximal initiation and promotion including susceptible mice, the benign tumors arise rapidly in all mice and their incidence is readily quantitated. The benign tumor incidence is indicative of the ultimate yield of malignant tumors, and the incidence is dependent on the dose of the initiator and the promoter as well as on modifying factors (e.g., inhibitors of prostaglandin synthesis). The complications inherent in systemically administered agents are eliminated since the gastrointestinal tract, liver, etc. are not exposed to the agents. Technics for biochemical and enzymatic analyses of all sorts are possible on the epidermal tissue from which the tumors arise. Thus by the imposition of variables such as dose, structure, and modifying factors, the molecular responses can be directly correlated with the tumor response. This allows reasonably sound conclusions to be drawn about the relevance of the observed molecular change to the appearance of tumors.

The remainder of this discussion is based on studies using the potent promoting phorbol ester, TPA. Its predominant characteristic is its pleiotypic effect on cultured cells as well as on the skin of intact mice (Hecker et al., 1982). It is highly effective; responses are observed in cultured cells at concentrations as low as 10^{-10} M and it causes metabolic changes in mouse skin at doses of a few tenths of a nmol to 10 nmol when administered in 0.2 ml of acetone. Responses are observed as early as 2 min after exposure. It appears to be active in the form administered and membrane receptors exist (Ashendel and Boutwell, 1981).

Some of the biochemical responses to TPA treatment of mouse skin include increased levels of cyclic GMP and cyclic AMP, increased phosphatidyl choline turnover and increased synthesis of prostaglandins E and F, phosphorylation of certain histones, increased RNA turnover, induction of ornithine decarboxylase activity and resultant transient elevation of polyamines, and the culminating events of pleiotypic action, namely, increased DNA synthesis followed by cell division (Hecker et al., 1982). These responses correlate with tumor formation, but the essential nature of some of these effects in tumor formation is yet to be proven.

Circumstantial evidence linking some of these effects to the mechanism of tumor formation has come from inhibitor studies. Thus inhibitors of prostaglandin synthesis not only prevent the increased synthesis of prostaglandins in response to TPA treatment, indomethacin is also capable of inhibiting the induction of ornithine decarboxylase by TPA and, in addition, indomethacin also inhibits tumor promotion by TPA. Both inhibitions are overcome by specific prostaglandins, and these facts will be dealt with in detail in the chapters that follow.

Other inhibitors of tumor promotion with specific effects at the molecular level include protease inhibitors, retinoids, and corticosteroids (Hecker et al., 1982). Our increasing knowledge of pleiotypic effects of promoters is progressing rapidly and in parallel with the rational development of inhibitors of the components of the processes of promotion. It is not unreasonable to hope that this research will lead to practical methods to inhibit the development of cancer. It is particularly encouraging that combinations, each of which is capable of inhibiting a specific molecular effect of TPA, add or synergise in their ability to inhibit the promotion of tumors by TPA. It appears that combinations of inhibitors are effective at lowered levels of each component of the combination.

REFERENCES

Ashendel CL, Boutwell RK (1981). Direct measurement of specific binding of highly lipophilic phorbol diester to mouse epidermal membranes using cold acetone. Biochem Biophys Res Commun 99:543.
Berenblum I (1978). Historical perspective. In Slaga TJ, Sivak A, Boutwell RK (eds): "Carcinogenesis, a Comprehensive Survey," Vol. 2, New York: Raven Press, p. 2.
Hecker EH, Fusenig NE, Kunz W, Marks F (1982). "Carcinogenesis, A Comprehensive Survey," Vol. 7, New York: Raven Press.
Mottram JC (1944). A developing factor in experimental blastogenesis. J Path Bact 56:181.
Pitot HC, Sirica AE (1980). The stages of initiation and promotion in hepatocarcinogenesis. Biochim Biophys Acta 605:191.
Slaga TJ, Fischer SH, Nelson K, Gleason GL (1980). Studies on the mechanism of skin tumor promotion: evidence for several stages in promotion. Proc Nat Acad Sci USA 77:3659.
Slaga TJ, Sivak A, Boutwell RK (1978). "Mechanisms of Tumor Promotion and Cocarcinogenesis." New York: Raven Press.
Van Duuren BL (1969). Tumor promoting agents in two-stage carcinogenesis. Prog Exptl Tumor Res 11:31.

Prostaglandins and Cancer: First
International Conference, pages 189-204
© 1982 Alan R. Liss, Inc., 150 Fifth Avenue, New York, NY 10011

STIMULATION OF CELLULAR PROSTAGLANDIN PRODUCTION BY PHORBOL-
ESTERS AND GROWTH FACTORS AND INHIBITION BY CANCER CHEMO-
PREVENTIVE AGENTS

Lawrence Levine

Department of Biochemistry
Brandeis University
Waltham, Massachusetts 02254

Carcinogenesis appears to be a multistep process (Boutwell, 1974; Slaga et al., 1980), and it is probable that
various environmental factors act at different steps in
this process. In one of the best-studied models, i.e. the
"two-stage carcinogenesis" system in mouse skin (Berenblum,
1969), two distinct stages designated "initiation" and "promotion" have been identified. Additional stages and cofactors may play a role in cancer induction in tissues and
species other than mouse skin. The interaction of multiple
factors probably is required for the induction of many human
cancers. In the simple two-stage model in mouse skin,
croton oil prepared from the seeds of Croton tiglium was the
promoting agent. The fractions from the croton oil responsible for the activity have been purified and characterized
by Hecker (1968) and van Duuren (1969) and their colleagues.
The most active tumor-promoting phorbol diester was 12-0-
tetradecanoyl-phorbol-13-acetate (TPA). TPA stimulated
several types of cells to produce prostaglandins (Table 1).
The two most responsive cells were the canine kidney cell
line (MDCK) and smooth muscle cells derived from bovine
aorta; as little as 10^{-9} M TPA was sufficient to stimulate
prostaglandin production. Phorbol-12,13-didecanoate (PDD)
at 10^{-9} M also stimulated prostaglandin production by MDCK
cells, but the non-tumor-producing phorbol diester 4α-
phorbol-12,13-didecanoate (4α-PDD) was inactive even at
10^{-7} M (Levine and Hassid, 1977a; Ohuchi and Levine, 1978a).

When MDCK cells, prelabelled with arachidonic acid,
were cultured in serum-supplemented medium in the presence
of TPA, increased quantities of radiolabelled compounds

TABLE 1

CELLS IN WHICH ARACHIDONIC ACID TRANSFORMATION IS STIMULATED BY TPA

Cell	Source	Reference
MDCK	Dog kidney	Levine and Hassid, 1977a
WEHI-5	Mouse lymphoma	Levine et al., 1979
HSDM$_1$	Mouse fibrosarcoma	Levine, unpublished data
LC-540	Rat Leydig	Levine, unpublished data
Smooth muscle	Bovine aorta	Levine, unpublished data
WI-38	Human embryonic lung	Levine et al., 1979
D-550	Human foreskin	Levine et al., 1979
MC5-5	Transformed mouse fibroblast	Levine et al., 1979
Macrophages	Mouse peritoneum	Brune et al., 1978
Osteosarcoma	Human bone	Shupnik and Tashjian, unpub. data
Y-1	Mouse adrenal	Levine, unpublished data
HEL/30	Mouse epidermis	Fürstenberger and Marks, 1979
Fibroblasts	Chick embryo	Mufson et al., 1979
HeLa		Crutchley et al., 1980

were found in the conditioned medium, even at a concentration of 2×10^{-10} M TPA. The identified radioactive materials that were released corresponded to arachidonic acid, $PGF_{2\alpha}$ and PGE_2. After 20 hours of incubation in the presence of TPA (250 pg/ml) or PDD (1.0 ng/ml), the released radioactivity was increased around 4-fold, whereas that released by cells incubated in the presence of 4α-PDD (10 ng/ml) was equal to that of the control serum-supplemented medium (Table 2). The TPA and PDD-stimulated radioactivity in the conditioned medium was due mainly to increased levels of prostaglandins E_2 and $F_{2\alpha}$ (14.5-fold with TPA and 10.6-fold with PDD). Treatment with TPA and PDD apparently perturbs the plasma membrane (Sivak et al., 1972; Sivak and van Duuren, 1967; Rohrschneider and Boutwell, 1973) in such a way that acylhydrolase and cyclooxygenase activities are more tightly coupled (Levine and Hassid, 1977a). TPA treatment did not release radioactive materials from [^{14}C]linoleic acid labelled MDCK cells (Ohuchi and Levine, 1978b). TPA probably stimulated specific phospholipases; alternatively, phospholipid pools, because of heterogeneous positioning within the lipid membrane, may have had different activities with respect to deacylation and reacylation cycles.

STIMULATION OF PROSTAGLANDIN PRODUCTION BY GROWTH FACTORS

A variety of growth factors enhance prostaglandin synthesis in cultured cells; these include epidermal growth factor (Levine and Hassid, 1977b; Tashjian and Levine, 1978), serum (Hong et al., 1976), platelet derived growth factor (Shier, 1980; Coughlin et al., 1980; Coughlin et al., 1981; Hohmann et al., 1981), several transforming growth factors (Levine, 1981) recently characterized (DeLarco and Todaro, 1978; Roberts et al., 1980), monoleukin 1 (Mizel et al., 1981; Dayer et al., 1977), interleukin 2 (Levine, unpublished data), human synovium factor (Meats et al., 1980), and colony stimulating factors (Kurland et al., 1978; Kurland et al., 1979). Several of these growth factors stimulated prostaglandin production in cells being cultured in our laboratory (Table 3). It would not be surprising if many more growth factors were found to enhance prostaglandin production by certain cells and it is possible that some of the biological activities of growth factors, such as osteoclast activating factor, are causally related to this enhancement.

TABLE 2

RADIOACTIVE COMPOUNDS IN CONDITIONED MEDIA OF RADIOACTIVELY
LABELLED MDCK CELLS AND PHORBOL DIESTERS (Levine and Hassid, 1977a)

Compound	MEM (+)[b]	Radioactivity (cpm)[a]		
		MEM (+) with TPA (0.25 ng/ml)	MEM (+) with PDD (1.0 ng/ml)	MEM (+) with 4α-PDD (10 ng/ml)
Phospholipids	281	718	457	144
Prostaglandin $F_{2\alpha}$	568	7088	5224	528
Prostaglandin E_2	300	5507	3996	302
Arachidonic acid	3429	4725	6387	3922
Triglycerides	122	214	241	33
Unidentified*	1508	8170	5781	1018
TOTAL	6208**	26422**	22086**	5947**

[a] 1.6 ml radioactive medium (out of a total of 2 ml) was extracted and chromatographed as described by Hassid and Levine, 1977. Incubation was for 20 hours.

[b] MEM (+) represents serum-supplemented medium.

* Scatter throughout TLC.

** Cell number initially was 0.64 x 10^6/60 mm dish but cells were not counted after the 20 hour incubation.

TABLE 3

GROWTH FACTORS THAT STIMULATE ARACHIDONIC ACID
METABOLISM IN CELLS

Epidermal Growth Factor
Serum
Platelet Derived Growth Factor
Sarcoma Transforming Growth Factor
Kidney Transforming Factor
Bladder Carcinoma Transforming Growth Factor
Monoleukin 1
Interleukin 2

Treatment of smooth muscle cells or human fibroblasts
with platelet derived growth factor (PDGF) increases the
expression of low density lipoprotein receptors (Chait et
al., 1980; Witte and Cornicelli, 1980); increases the expression of luteinizing hormone receptors on granulosa
cells in response to follicle stimulating hormone (Mondschein
and Schomberg, 1981); modulates the receptors for epidermal
growth factor (EGF) on 3T3 cells (Wrann et al., 1980) and
increases the number of serotonin receptors or the efficiency of coupling between the serotonin receptor and prostaglandin production in smooth muscle cells (Coughlin et
al., 1981). In addition, stimulation of prostaglandin
production in smooth muscle and MDCK cells by PDGF is dependent on its presence in the medium (Coughlin et al.,
1980). It appears that the cytological target for PDGF,
and most likely all of the growth factors, is the cell membrane.

Weinstein and his colleagues have shown that TPA alters
membrane receptors to several biologically active ligands
(Weinstein et al., 1980). TPA blocks binding of EGF to its
receptor (Lee and Weinstein, 1978; Osborne et al., 1981)
although such inhibition may be indirect (Osborne et al.,
1981). Thus it was not surprising to find that the effects
of TPA and EGF on smooth muscle cells with respect to prostaglandin production were not additive. Their combined
effects were synergistic (Table 4). A synergistic response
also was found after treatment with PDGF and TPA. However,
the combined effect of TPA and another factor, interleukin
2, on prostaglandin production by smooth muscle cells was
not synergistic; and in a methylcholanthrene-transformed
mouse fibroblast cell line (MC5-5), the combined effect of

TABLE 4

EFFECT OF TPA AND EGF OR TPA AND INTERLEUKIN 2
ON ARACHIDONIC ACID METABOLISM IN SMOOTH MUSCLE CELLS

Stimulant	6-keto-PGF$_{1\alpha}$* ng/ml
Control	0.04 ± 0.01 (6)
EGF, 0.2 µg/ml	0.11 ± 0.01 (3)
TPA, 5 ng/ml	6.2 ± 0.6 (3)
EGF (0.2 µg) and TPA (5 ng)	32.0 ± 0.0 (3)
Control	0.12 ± 0.03 (8)
Rat interleukin 2 (10 ½max. units/ml)	0.27 ± 0.04 (3)
TPA, 2 ng/ml	6.4 ± 0.01 (3)
Interleukin 2 (10 ½max. units/ml) and TPA, 2 ng/ml	4.4 ± 0.8 (3)

* Average value ± standard deviation; ( ) = number of
culture dishes.

PDGF and TPA was less than additive. Thus, TPA's perturbation of the membrane can result in enhanced, inhibited or
unaffected stimulation of prostaglandin production by growth
factors depending on the growth factor and/or the cells.
TPA's regulation of stimulation of prostaglandin production
by growth factors probably reflects the biochemical composition proximate to the particular growth factor's receptor.

EFFECT OF INHIBITORS OF TUMOR PRODUCTION ON TPA'S STIMULA-
TION OF CELLULAR ARACHIDONIC ACID FORMATION

The retinoids are a class of inhibitors that block
tumor promotion (Sporn et al., 1976; Sporn and Newton,
1979). Retinoids inhibit promoter-induced ornithine decarboxylase (ODC) activity in mouse epidermis (Verma and Boutwell, 1977; Verma et al., 1978). Those retinoids that inhibit TPA-induced ODC activity in mouse epidermis also
inhibit TPA-induced ODC activity in phytohemagglutinin-
treated bovine lymphocytes (Kensler et al., 1978) and TPA's
comitogenic activity in these lectin-treated cells (Kensler
and Mueller, 1978). Retinoids, at low concentrations, stimulate plasminogen-activator synthesis in chick-embryo fibroblasts, and at suboptimal levels of TPA, the effects of
retinoic acid and TPA are synergistic (Wilson and Reich,

TABLE 5. 13-trans-RETINOIC ACID INHIBITS TPA-STIMULATED PROSTAGLANDIN PRODUCTION IN SMOOTH MUSCLE BUT NOT IN MDCK CELLS

	MDCK PGE$_2$ ng/ml*	Bovine Aorta Smooth Muscle Cells 6-keto-PGF$_{1\alpha}$ ng/ml*
Control	0.92 ± 0.15 (3)	0.14 ± 0.03 (3)
TPA, 0.4 ng/ml	10.23 ± 0.62 (3)	
+ Retinoic acid, 0.5 µg/ml	13.6 ± 0.3 (3)	
TPA, 5.0 ng/ml		5.67 ± 0.57 (3)
+ Retinoic acid, 0.5 µg/ml		0.52 ± 0.01 (3)

* Average value ± standard deviation; ( ) = number of culture dishes.

TABLE 6. LEUPEPTIN INHIBITS TPA-STIMULATED PROSTAGLANDIN PRODUCTION IN SMOOTH MUSCLE BUT NOT IN MDCK CELLS

	MDCK PGE$_2$ ng/ml*	Bovine Aorta Smooth Muscle Cells 6-keto-PGF$_{1\alpha}$ ng/ml*
Control	0.92 ± 0.16 (6)	0.099 ± 0.032 (4)
TPA, 0.4 ng/ml	13.3 ± 0.4 (6)	
+ Leupeptin, 10 µg/ml	12.8 ± 0.4 (6)	
TPA, 2.0 ng/ml		3.4 ± 1.2 (6)
+ Leupeptin, 10 µg/ml		0.67 ± 0.15 (6)

* Average value ± standard deviation; ( ) = number of culture dishes.

1978). In MDCK cells the retinoids, cis retinoic acid, trans retinoic acid, retinyl acetate, retinol, retinal, retinyl palmitate and trimethylmethoxyphenyl retinoic acid do not affect deacylation of phospholipids or prostaglandin production and, at relatively high concentrations, even enhance them (Levine and Ohuchi, 1978a). However, in chick embryo fibroblasts trans retinoic acid (10^{-5} to 10^{-6} M) inhibits TPA-induced arachidonic acid release and prostaglandin production (Mufson et al., 1979). Smooth muscle cells obtained from bovine aorta are also stimulated by TPA to metabolize arachidonic acid (Table 1); and retinoic acid does inhibit the TPA-stimulated prostaglandin synthesis in these cells. Of the total cyclooxygenase products made in culture by smooth muscle cells, 70-90% is PGI_2, 5-15% $PGF_{2\alpha}$ and about 5% is PGE_2 (Coughlin et al., 1980). As can be seen in Table 5, 13-trans-retinoic acid (1.7 x 10^{-6} M) inhibited 90% of the production of PGI_2 (measured as 6-keto-$PGF_{1\alpha}$) stimulated by 8 x 10^{-9} M TPA. TPA's stimulation of prostaglandin production in the MDCK cells was not inhibited by the trans retinoic acid.

Among the pleiotypic effects of TPA is the induction of proteases. Protease inhibitors, such as leupeptin, block tumor promotion in mouse skin (Troll et al., 1970; Hozumi, et al., 1972). Only at relatively high levels (1.5 x 10^{-4} M) does pepstatin, antipain and leupeptin inhibit TPA-stimulated prostaglandin production in MDCK cells; about 25% (Levine, 1981). However, even at the 1 x 10^{-5} M level, leupeptin inhibited the TPA-stimulated arachidonic acid metabolism by smooth muscle cells 80% (Table 6).

Several agents that affect tumor growth are listed in Table 7. Natural and synthetic glucocorticoids inhibit tumor promotion (Belman and Troll, 1972; Ghadially and Green, 1954; Schwartz et al., 1977). Topical application of dexamethasone inhibits TPA-mediated tumor promotion (Scribner and Slaga, 1973). Fluocinolone acitonide is as effective as dexamethasone at lower dose levels and also blocks promoter-induced hyperplasia and DNA synthesis. Glucocorticoids inhibit expression of acylhydrolase activity and consequently prostaglandin production in some cells (Hong and Levine, 1976; Blackwell et al., 1980) and tissues. Indomethacin, a more potent inhibitor of prostaglandin production but a weak inhibitor of acylhydrolase activity at low doses, is only a weak inhibitor of TPA-induced tumor-promotion (Viaje et al., 1977) but at high doses is an

TABLE 7

TUMOR CHEMOPREVENTION AND ARACHIDONIC ACID METABOLISM

Agent	Arachidonic Acid Metabolism	Tumor Growth
Anti-inflammatory steroids Dexamethasone	↓ →	↓
Retinoids 13-trans-retinoic acid	↓ ↗ *	↓↑
Non-steroidal anti-inflam- matory agents Indomethacin	↓	↓
Phenolic inhibitors Butylated hydroxyanisol (BHA)	↓	↓
Protease inhibitors Leupeptin	↓ → *	↓
Flavinoids--natural & synthetic α-Naphthoflavone Quercetin	↓ →	↓↑
Miscellaneous products of plant origin Gossypol Nordihydroguaiaretic acid	↓ **	?
Diterpine tumor promoters TPA	↑	↑
Growth factors EGF	↑	↑

*/ Effect after TPA stimulation
** Effect after A23187 stimulation

effective inhibitor of TPA-induced biochemical effects.
Indomethacin (100 to 125 µg) administered to mice daily with
their food, reduces the weights of the $HSDM_1$ fibrosarcoma 27%
(Tashjian, Jr. et al., 1973). Indomethacin (50 µg administered subcutaneously on alternate days) reduces the size
of Maloney sarcoma virus-induced tumors in 20 day old BALB/c
mice and delays the onset of tumor growth. In older mice
(6-week-old), the same dose of indomethacin is much more
effective at reducing the size of the Maloney sarcoma virus-
induced tumors (Strausser and Humes, 1975). Bone destruction by the virus-induced tumor is also inhibited by this
indomethacin treatment. The growth of a transplanted
methylcholanthrene-induced mouse fibrosarcoma is reduced in

mice given indomethacin (125 μg/day) interperitoneally for
the first 10 or 14 days (Plescia et al., 1975). Treatment
of mice with aspirin is effective at reducing the growth of
tumors; aspirin (150 mg/kg administered twice daily by
mouth) inhibits the growth of the transplanted mast-cell
ascites tumor (P185) and Lewis lung carcinoma. Indomethacin
(3 to 5 mg/kg) is even more effective (Hial et al., 1976).
In C3H mice bearing a transplantable methylcholanthrene-
induced fibrosarcoma, indomethacin or aspirin (administered
by way of drinking water from day 7 to 49 after tumor transplantation) reduces the tumor size measured at day 46 (Lynch
et al., 1978). Indomethacin, aspirin or hydrocortisone also
increases survival time of the mice. Indomethacin treatment
inhibits the development of methylnitrosourea-induced rat
colon tumors (Pollard and Luckert, 1981) and 1,2-dimethyl-
hydrazine or methylazoxymethanol acetate-induced intestinal
tumors in rats (Narisawa et al., 1981). The non-steroidal
anti-inflammatory drug, flurbiprofen, an effective inhibitor
of prostaglandin production, in combination with chemotherapy
or radiotherapy reduces tumor growth in mice, when compared
to the treatment by chemotherapy and/or radiotherapy alone
(Bennett et al., 1979). In addition, flurbiprofen, given
with methotrexate in mice following removal of the primary
tumor, prolongs survival and reduces the incidence of local
recurrence (Berstock et al., 1980). Indomethacin inhibits
growth of fibrosarcoma in mice and potentiates immunotherapy
(Lynch and Salomon, 1979). Administration of indomethacin
to rats with Yoshida hepatoma cells reduces tumors (Trevisani
et al., 1980). N-(4-hydroxyphenyl)retinamide, an effective
inhibitor of prostaglandin production (Levine, 1979), inhibits the development of breast cancer induced in rats by
N-nitroso-N-methylurea when fed orally to rats over a 2 week
or 6 month period (Moon et al., 1979).

Anti-oxidants, especially butylated hydroxyanisol (BHA),
have been found to be effective inhibitors of tumor production in mice and rats (Wattenberg, 1978); and flavones, such
as α-napthoflavone, inhibit tumor production (Gelboin et al.,
1970; Slaga and Bracken, 1977). Polyphenols, such as gossypol and nordihydroguaiaretic acid, are potent inhibitors of
the lipoxygenase pathways of arachidonic acid metabolism.
Gossypol (1,1', 6,6', 7,7'-hexahydroxy-5,5'-diosopropyl-
3,3'-dimethyl[2,2'-binapthalene]-8,8'-dicarboxaldehyde) is
a polyphenol found in certain species of cotton plant (Adams
et al., 1960). Studies, mostly by Chinese investigators,
suggest that it is an effective antifertility agent for

males (National Coordinating Group on Male Fertility, 1978). Gossypol is a potent inhibitor of leukotriene production (Levine, unpublished data). Nordihydroguaiaretic acid, also a product of plants, had previously been shown to be a potent inhibitor of lipoxygenases (Goetzl et al., 1980). Both are relatively weak inhibitors of the cyclooxygenase pathway. Inhibition of tumor production by gossypol or nordihydroguaiaretic acid would suggest that tumor production and lipoxygenase pathways are related.

A causal relationship between arachidonic acid transformation and cancer has yet to be demonstrated. At least three steps in the arachidonic acid transformation scheme (Fig. 1) can be considered as being responsible for any such

FIGURE 1

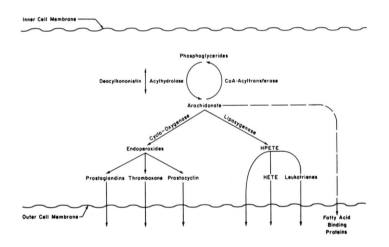

Arachidonate Metabolism

association: (1) Acylhydrolase activity can lead to production of lysophospholipids and alteration of membrane fluidity (Hirata and Axelrod, 1980) (TPA treatment alters membrane fluidity [Castagna et al., 1979; Weinstein et al., 1979]). The expression of acylhydrolase activity may be mediated by deacylkanonistin, a polypeptide whose activity is altered by anti-inflammatory steroids (Hong and Levine, 1976; Tam et al., 1977; Blackwell et al., 1980; Hirata and

Axelrod, 1980). (2) Cyclooxygenase activity leads to production of the prostaglandins, prostacyclins and thromboxanes; and (3) lipoxygenase activity leads to formation of the hydroxyfatty acids and the leukotrienes. Inhibitors of cyclooxygenase activity are only partially effective, at best, at reducing tumors, whereas inhibitors of acylhydrolase activities such as glucocorticoids, which also block reactions (2) and (3), are more effective. Thus, acylhydrolase activity, or possibly lipoxygenase activity, is more likely to be causally related to cancer than cyclooxygenase activity. It is possible that all three activities combine to give the tumor cell a favorable advantage for growth; i.e., the altered fluidity increases growth potential and differentiation properties of the cell and at the same time the cell is stimulated to synthesize products that inhibit the immune response.

SUMMARY

1. TPA stimulates many cells to deacylate membrane phospholipids and to metabolize arachidonic acid.

2. Growth factors stimulate many cells to produce prostaglandins.

3. Depending on the cell and/or the growth factor, TPA enhances, inhibits, or has no effect on the growth factor's stimulation of prostaglandin production.

4. Many agents that affect tumor production in vivo, affect arachidonic acid transformation in cell culture: Agents that inhibit tumor growth, inhibit arachidonic acid metabolism in cell culture; Agents that enhance tumor growth, stimulate arachidonic acid metabolism in cell culture.

ACKNOWLEDGMENTS

The author's research is supported by Grants GM-27256 and CA-17309 from the National Institutes of Health. He is an American Cancer Society Research Professor of Biochemistry (Award PRP-21).

REFERENCES

Adams R, Geissman TA, Edwards JD (1960). Chem Rev 60:555-574.
Belman S, Troll W (1972). Cancer Res 32:450-454.
Bennett A (1979). In Karim SMM (ed): "Practical Applications of Prostaglandins and their Synthesis Inhibitors," Lancaster: MTP Press Ltd., pp 149-188.
Berenblum I (1969). Prog Exp Tumor Res 11:21-30.
Berstock DA, Houghton J, Bennett A (1980). Adv Prostaglandins and Thromboxane Res 6:567-569.
Blackwell GJ, Carnuccio R, DiRosa M, Flower RJ, Parente L, Persico P (1980). Nature 287:147-149.
Boutwell RK (1974). CRC Crit Rev Toxicol 2:419-443.
Brune K, Kaun H, Schmidt R, Hecker E (1978). Cancer Lett 4:333-342.
Castagna M, Rochette-Egly C, Rosenfeld C, Mishal C (1979). FEBS Lett 100:62-66.
Chait A, Ross R, Albers J, Bierman E (1980). Proc Natl Acad Sci USA 77:4084-4088.
Coughlin SR, Moskowitz MA, Zetter BR, Antoniades HN, Levine L (1980). Nature 288:600-602.
Coughlin SR, Moskowitz MA, Antoniades HN, Levine L. Serotonin receptor-mediated stimulation of smooth muscle cell prostacyclin synthesis and its modulation by platelet-derived growth factor. Proc Natl Acad Sci USA, in press.
Crutchley DJ, Cohanan LB, Maynard JR (1980). Cancer Res 40:849-852.
Dayer J, Robinson DR, Krane SM (1977). J Exp Med 145:1399-1404.
DeLarco JE, Todara GJ (1978). Proc Natl Acad Sci USA 75:4001-4005.
Fürstenberger G, Marks F (1979). Biochem Biophys Res Comm 92:749-756.
Gelboin HV, Wiebel F, Diamond L (1970). Science 170:169-171.
Ghadially FN, Green HN (1954). Br J Cancer 8:291-295.
Goetzl EJ, Weller PF, Sun FF (1980). J Immunol 124:926-933.
Hassid A, Levine L (1977). J Biol Chem 252:6591-6593.
Hecker E (1968). Cancer Res 28:2338-2349.
Hial V, Horakova Z, Shalf RE, Beaven MA (1976). Eur J Pharmacol 37:367-376.
Hirata F, Axelrod J (1980). Science 209:1082-1090.
Hohmann E, Levine L, Antoniades HN, Tashjian AH Jr (1981). Prog 63rd Ann Meeting of the Endocrine Society, p 237, Abstract no. 619.

Hong SL, Polsky-Cynkin R, Levine L (1976). J Biol Chem 251: 776-780.

Hong SL, Levine L (1976). Proc Natl Acad Sci USA 73:1730-1734.

Hozumi M, Ogawa M, Suginmura T, Takeuchi T, Umezawa H (1972). Cancer Res 32:1725.

Kensler TW, Mueller GC (1978). Cancer Res 38:771-775.

Kensler TW, Verma AK, Boutwell RK, Mueller GC (1978). Cancer Res 38:2896-2899.

Kurland J, Broxmeyer H, Bockman RS, Pelus L, Moore MAS (1978). Blood 52:388-407.

Kurland JI, Pelus L, Ralph P, Bockman RS, Moore MAS (1979). Proc Natl Acad Sci USA 76:2326-2330.

Lee LS, Weinstein IB (1978). Science 202:313-315.

Levine L (1979). Prostaglandins and Medicine 4:285-296.

Levine L (1981). In Hecker E (ed): "Cocarcinogenesis and Biological Effects of Tumor Promoters," New York: Raven Press, in press.

Levine L, Alam I, Langone J (1979). Prostaglandins and Medicine 2:177-189.

Levine L, Hassid A (1977a). Biochem Biophys Res Commun 76: 1181-1187.

Levine L, Hassid A (1977b). Biochem Biophys Res Commun 79: 477-484.

Lynch NR, Castes M, Astoin M, Salomon JC (1978). Br J Cancer 38:503-512.

Lynch NR, Salomon JC (1979). J Nat Cancer Inst 62:117-121.

Meats JE, McGuire MB, Russell RGG (1980). Nature 286:891-892.

Mizel SB, Dayer J-M, Krane SM, Mergenhagen SE (1981). Stimulation of rheumatoid synovial cell collagenase and prostaglandin production by partially purified lymphocyte activating factor (interleukin 1). Proc Natl Acad Sci USA, in press.

Mondschein JS, Schomberg DW (1981). Science 211:1179-1180.

Moon RC, Thompson HJ, Becci PJ, Grubbs CJ, Gander RJ, Newton DL, Smith JM, Phillips SL, Henderson WR, Mullen LT, Brown CC, Sporn MB (1979). Cancer Res 39:1339-1346.

Mufson RA, DeFoe D, Weinstein IB (1979). Mol Pharm 16:569-578.

Narisawa T, Sato M, Tani M, Kudo T, Takahashi T, Goto A (1981). Cancer Res 41:1954-1957.

National Coordinating Group on Male Fertility (1978). Chinese Med J 4:417-428.

Ohuchi K, Levine L (1978a). J Biol Chem 253:4783-4790.

Ohuchi I, Levine L (1978b). Prostaglandins and Medicine 1: 421-431.
Osborne CK, Hamilton B, Nover M, Ziegler J (1981). J Clin Invest 67:943-951.
Plescia OJ, Smith AH, Grinwich K (1975). Proc Natl Acad Sci USA 72:1848-1851.
Pollard M, Luckert PH (1981). Proc Soc Exp Biol Med 167: 161-164.
Roberts AB, Lamb LC, Newton DL, Sporn MB, DeLarco JE, Todaro GJ (1980). Proc Natl Acad Sci USA 76:195-199.
Rohrschneider LR, Boutwell RK (1973). Cancer Res 33:1945-1952.
Schwarz JA, Viaje A, Slaga TJ, Yuspa SH, Hennings H, Lichti U (1977). Chem Biol Interact 17:331-347.
Scribner JD, Slaga TJ (1973). Cancer Res 33:542-546.
Shier WT (1980). Proc Natl Acad Sci USA 77:137-141.
Sivak A, Mossman BT, van Duuren BL (1972). Biochem Biophys Res Commun 46:605-609.
Sivak A, van Duuren BL (1967). Science 157:1443-1444.
Slaga TJ, Fischer SM, Nelson K, Gleason GL (1980). Proc Natl Acad Sci USA 77:3659-3663.
Slaga TJ, Bracken WM (1977). Cancer Res 37:1631-1635.
Sporn MB, Dunlop NM, Newton DL, Smith JM (1976). Fed Proc 35:1332-1338.
Sporn MB, Newton DL (1979). Fed Proc 38:2528-2534.
Strausser H, Humes J (1975). Int J Cancer 15:724-730.
Tam S, Hong SL, Levine L (1977). J Pharmacol Exp Ther 203: 162-168.
Tashjian Jr AH, Levine L (1978). Biochem Biophys Res Commun 85:966-975.
Tashjian Jr AH, Voelkel EF, Goldhaber P, Levine L (1973). Prostaglandins 3:515-524.
Troll W, Klassen A, Janoff A (1970). Science 169:1211-1213.
Trevisani A, Ferretti E, Capuzzo A, Tomasi V (1980). Br J Cancer 41:341-347.
van Duuren BL (1969). Prog Exp Tumor Res 11:31-68.
Verma AK, Boutwell RK (1977). Cancer Res 37:2196-2201.
Verma AK, Rice HM, Shapas BG, Boutwell RK (1978). Cancer Res 38:793-801.
Viaje A, Slaga TJ, Wigler M, Weinstein IB (1977). Cancer Res 37:1530-1536.
Weinstein IB, Mufson RA, Lee L-S, Fisher PB, Laskin J, Horowitz AD, Ivanovic V (1980). In Pullman B, Tsa POP, Gelboin H (eds): 13th Jerusalem Symposium, "Carcinogenesis: Fundamental Mechanisms and Environmental Effects," Amsterdam, Holland: R. Reidel Publishing Co.

Weinstein IB, Yamasaki H, Wigler M, Lee L-S, Fisher PB, Jeffrey A, Grunberger D (1979). In Griffin AC, Shaw CR (eds): "Carcinogens and Mechanisms of Action," New York: Raven Press, pp 399–418.
Wattenberg LW (1978). Adv Cancer Res 26:197–226.
Wilson EL, Reich E (1978). Cell 15:385–392.
Witte LD, Cornicelli JA (1980). Proc Natl Acad Sci USA 77: 5962–5966.
Wrann M, Fox CF, Ross R (1980). Science 210:1363–1364.

Prostaglandins and Cancer: First
International Conference, pages 205-215
© 1982 Alan R. Liss, Inc., 150 Fifth Avenue, New York, NY 10011

PROSTAGLANDIN RESPONSE IN MOUSE SKIN TO TUMOR PROMOTERS

Edward Bresnick

Department of Biochemistry, University of Vermont

Burlington, Vermont 05405

The formation of a neoplasm is believed to involve the cooperative action of an initiator and a promoter, in the classical 2-stage mechanism of carcinogenesis. Considerable effort has been devoted to developing a rationale through which the mechanism of action of an initiator might be understood and much progress has evolved. Unfortunately, we have little knowledge of the fundamental events responsible for the promotion effect.

The application of tumor promoters such as 12-0-tetradecanoylphorbol-13-acetate (TPA) to shaved mouse skin or its addition to cell culture systems results in a number of biochemical changes and ultimately leads to alterations in cell function (reviewed in Boutwell 1978, Blumberg 1981). Virtually all the biochemical responses appear associated with interaction of the promoter with a component of the plasma membrane, i.e., a receptor. The initial evidence for this hypothesis was provided by VanDuuren et al (1976) with the observation that interaction of TPA with cell membranes was accompanied by fluorescence changes.

TPA has striking properties as an irritant, and indeed, several investigators have attributed its promoter activity to this property. In view of the well-known inflammatory action of a number of the prostaglandins (Ferriera and Vane 1974), these substances have been implicated in the action of promoters (Karim and Rao 1976, Brune et al 1978). More circumstantial evidence is provided by the localization of the precursor for the prostaglandins, i.e., arachidonic acid, which is stored in the form of phospholipids and

triglycerides in the plasma cell membrane. In addition,
Boutwell's laboratory (Verma et al 1977) have reported
that indomethacin, an inhibitor of prostaglandin synthesis,
blocked the TPA-mediated increase in ornithine decarboxylase in epidermal cells. The blockade was prevented by
prostaglandins of the E series (PGE).

We set about to investigate the effects of certain
tumor promoters as well as of a complete carcinogen, 3-
methylcholanthrene (MC) upon a) the levels of PGE_2 and $PGF_{2\alpha}$
in epidermis b) the anabolism of exogenous arachidonic acid
and c) the activity of a major enzyme responsible for the
generation of intracellular arachidonic acid, phospholipase
A_2. The results of these studies are reported in this
manuscript.

EXPERIMENTAL

Male CD-1 mice, 8-10 wk of age, were used in the
experiments described below. The mice were fed Purina Lab
Chow and water ad libitum. They were maintained on a constant light-dark cycle.

Preparation of Epidermis and Chemical Determinations

The backs of the mice were shaved 24 hr before topical
administration of the TPA (10 μg in 0.1 ml acetone) or of
acetone alone. At various times after topical administration, the mice were killed by cervical dislocation, the
shaved 2 x 2 cm area of skin was removed, and epidermis was
isolated as described previously (Bresnick et al 1979). DNA
and protein in the epidermis were determined by the methods
of Burton (1956) or Zubroff and Sarma (1976) and Lowry et al
(1951), respectively. Prostaglandins were extracted into
ethylacetate and were quantitated after silicic acid chromatography as described previously (Bresnick et al 1979). The
separated PGE and PGF were dried under a N_2 stream, redissolved in ethanol and subjected to radioimmunoassay as
reported by Jaffe and Behrman (1974).

^{3}H-Arachidonate Incorporation Into Mouse Skin

The treated mouse skin was cut into 5 x 10 mm pieces,
and the latter was incubated at 37° for various periods of

time in Waymouth's medium which contained in addition 10 μCi of [5,6,8,9,11,12,14,15-^{3}H]-arachidonic acid (80 Ci/mmol). The skin was removed, washed and homogenized at 4° in 0.9% NaCl. The homogenate was extracted 3 x with CHCl$_3$:CH$_3$OH (4:1, v/v), the organic layer was evaporated under a N2 stream and redissolved in this CHCl3:CH$_3$OH. The extract was subjected to thin layer chromatographic analysis with CHCl3:-CH$_3$OH:CH$_3$COOH:H$_2$0 (50:30:4:1, v/v/v/v) as the developing solvent. After visualization with I$_2$ vapor, the phospholipid, triglyceride and arachidonate areas were scraped into vials, scintillation fluid was added and the amount of ^{3}H was determined.

Phospholipase Assay

The substrate for the phospholipase A2 assay was prepared from the phospholipid components of L-cell membranes after these components had been radioactively labeled with ^{3}H-arachidonic acid. The phospholipid fraction consisted by 60% phosphatidylcholine and 25% phosphatidylethanolamine and its specific activity was 10^4 dpm/mmol. This substrate was dispersed by evaporating 80 nmol in a conical centrifuge tube, adding 0.8 ml H$_2$0 and sonicating for 3 x 60 sec with 30 sec intervals.

Sonicated epidermal cells were centrifuged at 1000 g for 5 min, and the resultant supernate was used as the enzyme source. Phospholipase activity was measured at pH 4.5 in the presence of EDTA and at pH 8.5 in the presence of Ca^{+2} (phospholipase A2). The experimental conditions are as have recently been published (Bresnick et al in press). After incubation of the labelled substrate with the enzyme preparation, the reaction was stopped with CH$_3$OH:CHCl3 (2:1) and additional CHCl3 was added. The mixtures were vortexed, and the organic phase was evaporated under N2, redisssolved in CH$_3$OH and subjected to thin layer chromatography with CHCl3:CH$_3$OH:acetic acid:water (90:8:1:0.8) as the developing solvent. The arachidonic acid area was scraped into a vial, counted and the amount of this fatty acid produced during the enzymatic reaction was calculated.

RESULTS

The effects of topical administration of TPA upon epidermal cell prostaglandins are indicated in Table 1.

Table 1

Epidermal Prostaglandins After Topical Administration of TPA

	Treated/Control		
Treatment	PGE_2	$PGF_{2\alpha}$	$PGE_2/PGF_{2\alpha}$
TPA, 1 hr	1.8	1.5	1.2
, 12 hr	6.5	3.2	2.0
, 24 hr	9.5	2.7	3.6
, 48 hr	6.5	1.2	5.4

TPA (10 μg) was applied to shaved backs of CD-1 mice and the mice were killed at the times indicated. The mouse skin was removed, epidermis was isolated and the prostaglandins were determined by radioimmunoassay. The control $PGE_2/PGF_{2\alpha}$ = 3.8. Each value represents the average of at least 3 separate determinations.

TPA caused an immediate increase in the PGE_2 level which reached a maximum value by 24 hr; PGE_2 was still elevated by 48 hr. $PGF_{2\alpha}$ levels were increased but to a much lesser extent; control values were reached by 48 hr after topical administration.

In view of this dramatic change in epidermal PGE_2, we turned our attention to arachidonate metabolism. In the first phase of this study, we investigated the incorporation of exogenous ^{3}H-arachidonic assay into mouse skin organ cultures. The results indicate a very rapid conversion of arachidonate into phospholipids and triglycerides (Table 2).

We then determined the effect of TPA administration upon the conversion of arachidonate to phospholipids and to triglycerides (Table 3).

Table 2

In vitro Incorporation of ^{3}H-Arachidonate into Mouse Skin

Compound	% Incorporation Time of Incubation (hr)		
	0.5	1	3
Arachidonate	79.0	62.9	42.0
Phospholipids	4.5	9.2	15.7
Triglycerides	14.2	21.7	37.6

The total amount of radioactivity incorporated into mouse skin organ cultures was 9,000, 16,000 and 29,000 cpm at 0.5, 1 and 2 hr, respectively.

Table 3

Effect of TPA Administration upon Arachidonate Incorporation into Phospholipids of Mouse Skin Organ Cultures

Condition	Treated/Control
Control	1.0
TPA, 1 hr	0.93
, 3 hr	1.60
, 6 hr	1.63
, 15 hr	1.67

Male CD-1 mice were topically treated with 10 μg TPA or with acetone. At the times indicated in the Table, mouse skin organ cultures were prepared and ^{3}H-arachidonate incorporation into phospholipids and triglycerides were determined. The % incorporation/g wet wt/hr for control mouse skin was 8.7 ± 1.0 (8 determinations).

As is apparent from the data of Table 3, TPA treatment of mouse skin resulted in an increase in incorporation of ^{3}H-arachidonate into the phospholipid components. This increase was manifested at 3 hr after treatment and persisted for at least 15 hr.

We next investigated the effects of the tumor promoter upon the system responsible for the generation of intracellular arachidonate, phospholipase A2. This enzyme is a component of plasma membranes and requires Ca^{+2} for activation at pH 8.5. As a control experiment, we also determined the effects of topical administration of TPA upon acid phospholipase activity, presumably present within lysosomes; the latter has a pH optimum of 4.5 and does not require calcium ions. We have found that expressing the specific activity per unit of epidermal DNA was considerably better than per unit of protein and accordingly, all the data are presented in that manner. Acid phospholipase and phospholipase A2 activities in epidermis were linear to 2.3 µg of DNA and up to 60 min of incubation at 37°.

The results of our studies are presented in Table 4.

Table 4

Phospholipase Activity in Mouse Epidermis:
The Effect of TPA

% Arachidonic Acid Formed/µg DNA/hr

Conditions (no. of Groups)	pH 8.5	pH 4.5
Control (15)	1.01 ± 0.08	0.76 ± 0.05
TPA, 1 hr (4)	2.51	0.90
, 6 hr (2)	3.12	0.68
, 12 hr (4)	5.10	0.95
, 24 hr (2)	2.78	0.76
, 72 hr (3)	2.70	0.98

The significant values are underlined.

Phospholipase A2 activity was 30% greater than acid phospholipase in control epidermis. Topical administration of TPA exerted little significant effect upon the latter while producing a marked elevation in the specific activity of epidermal phospholipase A2. This increase was already apparent at 1 hr after treatment and reached a maximum by 12 hr; enzyme activity was still elevated at 72 hr. The magnitude of the increase and the kinetics of appearance are certainly very suggestive that the elevation in enzyme activity results in the production of the substrate for the enhanced prostaglandin levels observed in epidermis after TPA administration.

In our experiments, we determined the effects of the non-promoter, phorbol, of the moderately-active promoter, the didecanoate of phorbol ester, and of the non-promoter irritant, acetic acid. These results are presented in Table 5.

Table 5

Phospholipase A2 Activity in Mouse Epidermis

Treatment (no of Groups)	Phospholipase Activity (% increase)
Phorbol (concentration equivalent to TPA), 18-24 hr (3)	0
Phorbol ester-didecanoate (equivalent to TPA), 18-24 hr (3)	49
Acetic Acid (333 μmol), 12-15 hr	30
24 hr	0

Table 6

Epidermal Phospholipase A2 as Effected by
Topical 3MC

Conditions (no of Groups)	% Arachidonate released/μg DNA/hr
Control (6)	3.76
3MC, 6 hr (5)	5.65 (50%)
, 12 hr (3)	4.69 (25%)
, 24 hr (2)	3.62

The moderately-active, dedecanoyl phorbol ester, produced a 49% increase in epidermal phospholipase A2 specific activity, while phorbol itself was inactive. The non-
promoter irritant, acetic acid, however, also caused an
elevation in this activity although transient and not of
great magnitude, i.e., 30% as opposed to 500% for TPA.

Finally, we tested the efficacy of the complete carcinogen, 3MC, upon epidermal phospholipase A2 (Table 6).

Enzyme specific activity was elevated (50%) by 6 hr
after the topical administration of 25 μg of 3MC. At 12 hr,
a 25% increase was noted while enzyme activity returned to
normal values by 24 hr.

DISCUSSION

Although little is known of the mechanisms of action of
promoters, circumstantial evidence would tend to implicate
the plasma membrane as the target site. In this regard, the
existence of a high-affinity binding "receptor" would be
suggested. Indeed, largely through the work of Blumberg's
laboratory (reviewed in Blumberg 1981), such a substance has
been found.

Levine and his colleagues (Levine and Hassid, 1977;
Levine 1977; Ohuchi and Levine 1978) have presented evidence
obtained in a 3MC-transformed kidney cell culture that the
prostaglandins may be participants in or mediators of the
promotion phase. They have reported a marked stimulation in
prostaglandin synthesis in these cells after addition of TPA
to the medium. The implication of prostaglandins in promotion of mouse epidermis also draws from the results of
several laboratories (Verma et al 1977; Ashendel and Boutwell 1979; Furstenberger and Marks 1980) as well as our own
(Bresnick et al 1979). In these studies on TPA-treated
mouse epidermis, either an increase in PGE$_2$ was demonstrated
or the blockade of a TPA-mediated effect was observed after
administration of indomethacin, a potent inhibitor of the
cyclooxygenase component of the prostaglandin synthetase
system.

In view of the fact that the polyunsaturated fatty acid
substrate for prostaglandin synthesis, arachidonic acid,
must be generated in mammalian cells by the catabolism of

membrane, we decided to investigate an enzyme responsible for such an action, phospholipase A2. It should be mentioned that Levine and Hassid (1977) had previously reported using their already-transformed kidney cell line that this activity was elevated after TPA addition. Our own results confirm this report and extend the action of TPA to include the biological target for promoters, mouse epidermis. The elevated phospholipase A2 activity occurs as early as 1 hr and reaches a maximum by 12 hr after topical administration of TPA. This time frame is certainly in accord with the kinetics of appearance of PGE_2 in mouse epidermis after application of TPA, i.e., maximum by 24 hr. Thus, it appears to us that the binding of TPA to an epidermal plasma membrane causes an activation of the membranal phospholipase A2, with the subsequent release of intracellular arachidonic acid and the consequent elaboration of PGE_2 (or other pre-cursor). It is our belief that this action is a principal mediator of the promoter activity of TPA and other sub-stances, e.g., 3MC. Our data also suggest that the irritant properties of TPA contribute to a small extent to phospho-lipase A2 activation since the non-promoter irritant, acetic acid, caused a small elevation in this membranal enzyme. It would appear to us that the isolation of the phorbol ester receptor and a study of its properties particularly in relationship to activation of phospholipase A2 would be important research targets and should be pursued with vigor.

ACKNOWLEDGEMENTS

It is a pleasure to acknowledge the help of our colla-borators in the conduct of some of this research, Drs. R. Bonney and P. Wightman of the Merck Institute for Thera-peutic Research, Rahway, NJ. The support of the NIH in the form of CA20711 is also greatfully acknowledged.

REFERENCES

Ashendel CL, Boutwell RK (1979). Prostaglandin E and F levels in mouse epidermis are increased by tumor-proto-ting phorbol esters. Biochem Biophys Res Commun 90:623.

Blumberg PM (1981). In vitro studies on the mode of action of the phorbol esters potent tumor promoters. CRC Crit Rev in Tox 9:199.

Boutwell RK (1978). Biochemical mechanisms of tumor promotion. In Slaga TJ, Sirak A, Boutwell RK (Eds): "Carcinogenesis, A Comprehensive Survey", Vol 2, NY, Raven Press, p 49.

Bresnick E, Meunier P, Lamden M (1979). Epidermal prostaglandins after topical application of a tumor promoter. Cancer Lett 7:121.

Bresnick E, Bailey G, Bonney RJ, Wightman P (in press). Phospholipase activity in skin after application of phorbol esters and 3-methylcholanthrene. Carcinogenesis.

Brune K, Kalin H, Schmidt R, Hecker E (1978). Inflammatory, tumor initiating and promoting activities of polycyclic aromatic hydrocarbons and diterdione esters in mouse skin as compared with their prostaglandin potency in vitro. Cancer Lett 4:333.

Burton K (1956). A study of the conditions and mechanisms of the diphenylamine reaction for the colorimetric estimation of deoxyribonucleic acid. Biochem J 62:315.

Ferriera SH, Vane JR (1974). New aspects of the mode of action of non steroid anti-inflammatory drugs. Ann Rev Pharmacol 14:57.

Furstenberger G, Marks F (1980). Early prostaglandin E synthesis is an obligatory event in the induction of cell proliferation in mouse epidermis in vivo by phorbol ester TPA. Biochem Biophys Res Communs 92:749.

Jaffe BM, Behrman HR (1974). Prostaglandins and prostaglandin metabolites in "Methods of Hormone Radioimmunoassay" NY, Academic Press, p 19.

Karim SMM, Rao B (1976). Prostaglandins and Tumors in Karim SMM (ed). in "Prostaglandins:physiological and Pathological Aspects". Lancaster, MTP Press p 305.

Levine L (1977). Chemical carcinogens stimulate canine kidney (MDCK) cells to produce prostaglandins. Nature 268:447.

Levine L, Hassid A (1977). Effects of phorbol-12,13-diesters on prostaglandin production and phospholipase activity in canine kidney (MDCK) cells. Biochem Biophys Res Communs 79:477.

Lowry OH, Rosebrough NJ, Farr AL, Randall RJ (1951). Protein measurement with the folin phenol reagent. J Biol Chem 193:265.

Ohucki K, Levine L (1978). Stimulation of prostaglandin synthesis in tumor cells by tumor-promoting phorbol-12,13-diesters in canine kidney (MDCK) cells. J Biol Chem 253:4783.

Verma AK, Rice WM, Boutwell RK (1977). Prostaglandin and skin tumor promotion:inhibition of tumor promoter-induced ornithine decarboxylase activity in epidermis by inhibitors of prostaglandin synthesis. Biochem Biophys Res Communs 79:1160.

Van Duuren BL, Banerjee S, Witz G (1976). Fluorescence studies on the interaction of the tumor promoter phorbol myristate acetate and related compounds with rat liver plasma membranes. Chem-Biol Inter 15:233.

Zubroff J, Sarma DSR (1976) A nonradioactive method for measuring DNA damage and its repair in nonproliferating tissue. Anal Biochem 70:387.

Prostaglandins and Cancer: First
International Conference, pages 217-238
© 1982 Alan R. Liss, Inc., 150 Fifth Avenue, New York, NY 10011

RECEPTOR BINDING AND CELLULAR EFFECTS
OF TUMOR PROMOTERS

Ann D. Horowitz and I. Bernard Weinstein

Division of Environmental Science and
Cancer Center/Institute of Cancer Research,
Columbia University, New York, N.Y. 10032

INTRODUCTION

In contrast to chemicals which initiate carcinogenesis
by binding covalently to cellular DNA, tumor promoters appear to act primarily on the cell surface membrane (for reviews see Slaga et al. 1978; Weinstein et al. 1979a). Some
of the membrane effects which have been observed for
12-0-tetradecanoyl-phorbol-13-acetate (TPA) and related compounds are listed in Table 1. These include alterations in
phospholipid metabolism, cell-cell communication, membrane
transport, and interaction of hormones with their receptors.
The membrane-related activities of the phorbol esters which
we will be discussing in detail here are stimulation of choline release and arachidonic acid release from cellular
phospholipids and inhibition of binding of epidermal growth
factor (EGF) to its receptor.

Several indirect lines of evidence suggest that phorbol
esters may act by binding to and usurping the functions of a
cell surface receptor that is normally utilized by an endogenous growth factor (Weinstein et al. 1977; Lee and Weinstein, 1978a). The evidence in favor of this hypothesis includes the following points: (a) TPA and related compounds
act in a concentration range similar to that of several hormones and growth factors (i.e., 0.1-10nM), (b) these compounds display similar structure-function relationships in
cells from diverse species and tissues, and (c) like known
hormones, they induce highly pleiotropic effects which vary
considerably depending on the target cell.

Table 1
Effects of TPA on Cell Surfaces and Membranes in Cell Culture

Altered Na/K ATPase
Increased Uptake 2-deoxyglucose, ^{32}P, ^{86}Rb
Increased Membrane Lipid "Fluidity"
Increased Release Arachidonic Acid, Prostaglandins
Altered Morphology and Cell-Cell Orientation
Altered Erythroleukemia Cell Adhesion
Increased Pinocytosis
Altered Fucose-Glycopeptides
Decreased LETS Protein
"Uncoupling" of β-Adrenergic Receptors
Inhibition of Binding of EGF to Receptors
Inhibition of Binding of Thyrotropin-releasing hormone
  and somatostatin to receptors
Decrease in Acetylcholine Receptors
Synergistic Interaction with Growth Factors
Inhibition of Metabolic Cooperation
Increased release and incorporation of choline

  For specific references see Slaga et al (1978), Weinstein et al (1977), (1979a), (1979b), Weinstein (1980), Diamond et al (1978), and text.

Recently, membrane associated receptors which bind phorbol esters specifically and with high affinity have been demonstrated in a wide variety of cell types (Driedger and Blumberg, 1980; Fisher et al. 1981; Shoyab and Todaro, 1980; Horowitz et al. 1981a; Solanki et al. 1981; Solanki and Slaga, 1981). The binding affinities of various phorbol esters (Driedger and Blumberg, 1980; Shoyab and Todaro, 1981) and related tumor promoters (Umezawa et al. 1981) to the phorbol receptor correlate well with their relative biologic activities.

We wish to present here some of our studies of the phorboid receptor in relation to the cellular effects of phorbol esters.

CHARACTERISTICS OF PHORBOL ESTER BINDING

Initially, we attempted to study phorbol ester binding to monolayers of Hela and rat embryo cells using ^{3}H-TPA (Lee and Weinstein, 1978; Horowitz and Weinstein, unpublished studies). However, we were unable to demonstrate saturable binding. The specific binding of ^{3}H-TPA may have been masked by the extensive nonspecific partitioning of TPA into

Table 2

Characterization of Phorboid Receptors in Various Cell Types

	Cell Type	K_{D_1} (nM)	Number/ Cell	K_{D_2} (nM)	Number/ Cell
			Phorboid Receptors		
CREF N	Rat Embryo fibroblast[a]	7.6[b]	1.6×10^5	710[b]	2.8×10^6
CREF A	Rat Embryo fibroblast	7	3.8×10^5	1,700	4×10^6
CREF A2	Variant of CREF A	18	1×10^6	–[c]	–[c]
E-11	Adenovirus-transformed Rat Embryo fibroblast[a]	11	1.5×10^5	1,100	1.4×10^6
K-22	Rat liver epithelial[d]	26	2.5×10^5	1,450	9.4×10^6
TS 19-10	TPA-Sensitive Friend erythroleukemia cells[e]	8[f]	3×10^4	800[f]	3×10^6
TR 19-4	TPA-Resistant Friend erythroleukemia cells[e]	8[f]	3×10^4	800[f]	3×10^6
B-35	NEU-transformed rat neuronal cell[g]	25	4.1×10^5	–[c]	–[c]
B-103	NEU-transformed rat neuronal cell[g]	36	4.5×10^5	–[c]	–[c]
B-49	NEU-transformed rat cell with neuronal and glial characteristics[g]	8.7	1.6×10^5	330	5.4×10^6
B-15	NEU-transformed rat glial cell[g]	40	1.5×10^6	–[c]	–[c]
B-92	NEU-transformed rat glial cell[g]	37	1.4×10^6	–[c]	–[c]
SC-9	RSV-transformed rat cerebellar cells[h]	15	1.8×10^5	700	3.3×10^6
WC-5	RSV-transformed rat cerebellar astrocyte[h]	3	2×10^4	380	1.3×10^6

(We would like to thank Dr. Giotta of the Salk Institute for cell lines B-35 through WC-5. Lines B-35 through B-92 were isolated by Dr. D. Schubert of the Salk Institute.) (See following page for footnotes)

the lipid phases of the cell. Blumberg and his colleagues initiated the use of ^{3}H-phorbol-12-13-dibutyrate, (^{3}H PDBu) a less hydrophobic and somewhat less potent analog of TPA to demonstrate saturable binding of phorbol esters (Driedger and Blumberg, 1980). Using ^{3}H PDBu, specific binding of the phorbol esters has been demonstrated in almost every mammalian cell type tested, with the exception of mature erythrocytes (Driedger and Blumberg, 1980; Shoyab and Todaro, 1980; Dunphy et al. 1980; Solanki et al. 1981; Horowitz et al. 1981a; Solanki and Slaga, 1981; Fisher et al. 1981). In the course of our studies, we have determined the binding constants and receptor numbers in a wide variety of cell types (Table 2). In general, one or two classes of receptor are found in each cell type. In most cases, the high affinity site, with a K_D in the range of 3 to 17 nM is present at $0.2\text{-}4\text{X}10^5$ sites per cell. Where a second, lower affinity site is observed the K_D is 300 nM or greater, and the number of sites is greater than $1\text{X}10^6$ per cell. Some variation in receptor number occurs within a cell line depending on the growth state of the cells at the time of assay. When only one binding site is detected the affinity for PDBu appears to be lower (K_D of 12-41 nM), but the number of sites is, in general, higher. In the case of cell lines of glial origin (B-15 and B-92, Table 2) as many as $2\text{X}10^6$ high affinity sites per cell are present. This observation is in accord with the results of Nagle et al. (1981) showing that brain tissue contains a very large number of phorboid receptors. Our studies on brain tumor cell lines suggest that the glial rather than the neuronal cells contribute to the large number of receptors in brain.

We have studied binding to the phorboid receptor in greatest detail in CREF N cells, an established line derived from Fisher rat embryo cells by Dr. Paul Fisher (Fisher et al. 1980). CREF N cells have normal morphology and growth control. These cells contain two classes of binding sites, one with a K_D of 8nM at $1.6\text{X}10^5$ sites/cell and the other with a K_D of 710nM at $2\text{X}10^6$ sites/cell (Horowitz et al. 1981a).

Table 2, Abbreviations: NEU, N-ethylurea; RSV, Rous Sarcoma Virus. Footnotes: a) Fisher et al (1980) b) Horowitz et al (1981) c) Only a single class of binding sites observed d) Weinstein et al (1975) e) Fibach et al (1978) f) Fisher et al (1981) g) Schubert et al (1974), Stallcup et al (1976), Stallcup (1977) h) Giotta et al (1980).

The K_D of the high affinity binding site is in the same range as the concentration of PDBu required for biologic effects. The significance of the weaker binding site is not known. Binding of ^3H PDBu to the phorboid receptor is rapid and reversible in these cells. Binding is complete within 30 minutes at $37^\circ C$, and dissociation of pre-bound ^3H PDBu can be obtained within 60 min at $37^\circ C$ (Horowitz et al. 1981a). Binding and dissociation are slower at $4^\circ C$. The Scatchard plot of ^3H PDBu binding obtained after equilibrium is reached at $4^\circ C$ is identical to that obtained at $37^\circ C$. Specific receptor binding can also be demonstrated in a crude membrane fraction from CREF N cells in the same manner as originally described by Driedger and Blumberg (1980).

The biologic responses to phorbol esters show great specificity according to the stereochemistry of the ring system and to the ester functions attached to it (Hecker, 1978; Weinstein et al. 1977; Yamasaki et al. 1981). In CREF N cells, binding of ^3H PDBu shows similar specificity. It is not inhibited by the inactive compounds phorbol or $4-\alpha$-phorbol-didecanoate, but it is strongly inhibited by TPA, and more weakly by PDBu and mezerein (Table 3)(Horowitz et al. 1981a). Other laboratories have studied the binding of additional phorbol esters to the phorboid receptor and find a full correlation with biologic activity (Driedger and Blumberg, 1980; Shoyab and Todaro, 1980). Some tumor promoters and anti-leukemic compounds from other plant species, although of differing chemical structures, have similar effects on cultures of mammalian cells as do the phorbol esters (Weinstein et al. 1977; Wigler et al. 1978; Lee and Weinstein, 1978; Umezawa et al. 1981). We have measured the dose inhibiting ^3H PDBu binding by 50% (ID_{50}) of several of these compounds in CREF N cell monolayers. The results are shown in Table 3. In addition, we have listed the ED_{50} (50% effective dose) for inhibition of ^{125}I EGF binding for those compounds for which data are available. Some of these data were obtained using different cell types, but they are included for comparison. The indole alkaloid teleocidin B is derived from Streptomyces 2A 1563 (Fujiki et al. 1979). It is a potent tumor promoter (Fujiki et al. 1981), and is strongly inhibitory of ^{125}I EGF binding in C3H 10T1/2 cells (Umezawa et al. 1981). It also inhibits ^3H PDBu binding quite strongly (Umezawa et al. 1981, and Table 3). A structurally similar toxin, lyngbyatoxin A (Cardellina et al. 1970) is derived from a blue-green alga (Lyngbya majuscula Gomont). Lyngbyatoxin A is also a potent inhibi-

Table 3
Inhibition of PDBu and EGF Binding by Various Compounds

	PDBu Binding ID_{50} (ng/ml)	EGF Binding ID_{50} (ng/ml)		
Cell Type:	CREF N	CREF N	C3H 10T½	Hela
Compound				
TPA	4[a,d]	0.7[c]	0.5	2.5[b]
PDBu	12.5[c]	4[c]	-	-
Teleocidin B	2.7[a]	-	1.0[a]	-
Lyngbyatoxin A	3.3[c]	-	-	-
Mezerein	20[d]	-	-	4.7[b]
Gnidipalmin	>1000[c]	500	-	>100[b]
Gnilatimacrin	16[c]	1.2	-	4.5[b]
Gnidilatin	48[c]	5.7	-	21.5 [b]
Phorbol	N.I.[d]	-	-	N.I[b]
4-α-PDD	N.I.[d]	-	-	N.I[b]

Abbreviations: ID_{50}--concentration inhibiting binding by 50%; N.I.--not inhibitory
Teleocidin B and Lyngbyatoxin kindly provided by Dr. T. Sugimura.
Footnotes: a--Umezawa et al (1981); b--Lee and Weinstein (1978b); c--Horowitz, A.D. and Weinstein, I.B. (unpublished data); d--Horowitz et al (1981).

tor of ^{3}H PDBu binding to its receptor (Table 3). We have also studied some plant diterpenes with structures similar to the phorbol esters, which have been reported to have anti-leukemic activity (Kupchan and Baxter, 1975; Kupchan et al. 1976 a & b). Of these compounds, gnidilatin and gnilatimac-rin have been previously reported to stimulate induction of plasminogen activator (Wigler et al. 1978) and to inhibit binding of ^{125}I EGF to Hela cells (Lee and Weinstein, 1979), whereas gnidipalmin was much less active. In the ^{3}H PDBu binding assay, gnidilatin and gnilatimacrin were potent inhibitors, whereas gnidipalmin was inactive up to 250 ng/ml. It is striking that compounds of such divergent chemical structures can bind with high affinity to the same receptor. They are all somewhat amphipathic molecules with ring systems that have hydrophilic as well as hydrophobic residues.

CELLULAR EFFECTS OF TUMOR PROMOTERS

Inhibition of Epidermal Growth Factor Binding

An initial reason for investigating the effect of phorbol esters on ^{125}I EGF receptor binding was the similarity in effects shared by phorbol esters and EGF. Subsequent studies have shown that they do not, in fact, occupy the same receptor. Recently, phorbol esters have also been shown to inhibit binding of somatostatin and thyrotropin-releasing hormone to their receptors in GH_4C_1 pituitary cells (Osborne & Tashjian 1979; Jaken et al. 1981). However, for reasons that are not apparent the phorbol esters cause preferential inhibition of EGF-receptor binding (Lee and Weinstein, 1979; Shoyab et al. 1979).

In CREF N cells, the inhibition of ^{125}I EGF binding by PDBu occurs at a somewhat lower concentration of PDBu than does the inhibition of ^3H PDBu binding. This same phenomenon is observed with TPA, and is probably true for the other tumor promoters listed in Table 3. For PDBu, the ID_{50} for PDBu binding is 12.5 ng/ml, whereas that of EGF binding is 4ng/ml. This could be explained in two different ways: 1) if EGF binding is only sensitive to phorbol ester binding to the higher affinity binding site, or 2) if there are excess, "spare" phorboid receptors, and only a fraction of receptors need be occupied to produce a biologic response. A non-linear dependence of biologic response on receptor occupancy has been observed in many hormone receptor systems. It has been explained by postulating that the biologic response is mediated by an enzymatic reaction or second messenger, or by movement in the plane of the membrane (Strickland and Loeb, 1981; Ariens et al. 1979; Kahn, 1976; Jacobs and Cuatrecasas, 1976). Lee and Weinstein (1979b, 1980) showed that the inhibition of EGF binding by phorbol esters is indirect; it does not occur at $4°C$ or in isolated cellular membranes. We have suggested that the diverse cellular effects of the phorbol esters, such as inhibition of EGF binding, may be mediated by alterations in membrane structure, perhaps due to the activation of phospholipases (Mufson et al. 1981; Fisher et al. 1981; Weinstein et al. 1980, 1981; Lee and Weinstein, 1979, 1980).

We have also found that the amphipathic membrane-active polypeptides δ-hemolysin and melittin inhibit EGF binding to its receptor (Umezawa et al. 1981 Horowitz et al. 1980). Both polypeptides stimulate the activity of cellular phospholipase A_2, causing arachidonic acid release and subsequent prostaglandin synthesis (Durkin and Shier, 1981; Mollay et al. 1976; Umezawa et al. 1980; Mufson et al. 1979). However, exogenous phospholipase A_2 alone does not inhibit EGF binding (Lee and Weinstein, 1980; Shoyab and Todaro, 1981). Another membrane-perturbing agent, phospholipase C,

Table 4
Stimulation of Choline Release from
C3H 10T½ Cells by Various Agents

Additions	Maximum ^{3}H cpm Released	$\underline{ID}_{50}$
None	2,000	N.A.*
TPA	6,900	5.5ng/ml
PDBu	6,000	13 ng/ml
Human Serum	16,000	15 mg/ml
Human Serum Factor	2,800	N.A.*

*N.A.: not applicable

The assay was performed as described in Mufson et al (1981), except that DMEM, rather than DMEM plus 10% calf serum, was used during the assay. Choline release was measured after incubation for 60 minutes at 37°C. The C3H 10T½ cells were 10-15th passage. The maximum concentration of human serum factor tested was 140 μg/ml.

has recently been reported to inhibit EGF binding to its receptor (Shoyab & Todaro, 1981). Thus the binding of EGF to its receptor appears to be a sensitive measure of perturbation of membrane structure. As such, it has been a useful method to follow the membrane effects of the phorbol esters. It has been observed that certain polycyclic aromatic hydrocarbon carcinogens also induce inhibition of EGF receptor binding through indirect mechanisms (Ivanovic and Weinstein, 1981). This may relate to their capacity to exert tumor promoting-like activity. Glucocorticoids have the opposite effect, increasing the binding of EGF to its receptor (Ivanovic and Weinstein, 1981; Baker and Cunningham, 1978).

Stimulation of Choline Release

The stimulation of choline release from C3H 10T1/2 cells by TPA has been previously studied by this laboratory in the presence of 10% calf serum. The 50% effective dose (ED_{50}) was about 30 ng/ml of TPA (Mufson et al. 1981). In view of our recent studies on the effects of serum on PDBu binding (discussed below) we repeated the study in Dulbecco's modified Eagle's medium (DMEM), in the absence of serum. The concentration dependence was shifted to a lower concentration, in better agreement with the activity of TPA in other assay systems. In DMEM, the ED_{50} for choline release by TPA was 5.5 ng/ml and for PDBu 13ng/ml (20nM)

(Table 4). This effect is less sensitive to phorbol ester concentration than is EGF binding. This is consistent with the hypothesis that activation of phospholipases and perturbations in membrane structure are important in mediating the inhibition of EGF binding by phorbol esters.

The tumor-promoting phorbol esters have been shown to stimulate arachidonic acid release and subsequent prostaglandin synthesis in a wide range of cell types (Levine and Hassid, 1977; Yamasaki et al. 1979; Mufson et al. 1979; and papers by Levine, and Bresnick, and Furstenberger, this symposium).

We have found (Mufson et al. 1981) that the TPA-induced release of choline from cellular phospholipids probably precedes the release of arachidonic acid. Inhibitors of protein synthesis inhibit TPA-stimulated arachidonic acid release, but not choline release (Mufson et al. 1979; Mufson et al. 1981). The calcium ionophore A23187 enhances arachidonic acid and prostaglandin release, without stimulating choline release. A hypothetical scheme showing how TPA-induced choline release may be related to arachidonic acid release and to increased incorporation of choline into phospholipids has been presented by Mufson et al. (1981) (see also Weinstein et al. 1980). Briefly, binding of phorbol ester tumor promoters to their membrane receptors may activate a phospholipase C or D. The phospholipase, in conjunction with a phosphatase, would give rise to choline and diacylglycerol. The diacylglycerol could then be hydrolyzed by a diacylglycerol lipase to release arachidonic acid. The diacylglycerol could also be reincorporated into phosphatidylcholine. It is also possible that arachidonic acid is released directly from phospholipid by the action of phospholipase A_2. These metabolic events could produce membrane structural changes, signals, or second messengers that might mediate subsequent cytoplasmic and nuclear events in tumor promotion.

INHIBITION OF PDBu BINDING BY A SERUM FACTOR

As mentioned previously, we have postulated that the phorboid receptor may normally be utilized by an endogenous ligand. The search for an endogenous ligand of the phorboid receptor led us to test numerous growth factors and physiologic fluids for ability to inhibit PDBu binding. The results are summarized in Tables 5 and 6. In Table 5

Table 5
Substances That Did Not Inhibit ^{3}H-PDBu
Binding to CREF Cells

Substances	Concentration Tested (μg/ml)
Phorbol	1.0
4-α-phorbol didecanoate	1.0
Epidermal Growth Factor	0.05
Fibroblast Growth Factor	0.10
Platelet-Derived Growth Factor	0.10
T-Cell Growth Factor	C.M.[1]
Arginine Vasopressin	0.15
Lysine Vasopressin	0.30
Luteinizing Hormone Releasing Hormone	0.50
Thrombin	2.5 (units/ml)
Fetuin	1000
Transcortin	5.0
Human Chorionic Gonadotropin	100
Thymopoeitin	50
Ubiquitin	50
T3	0.33
Ganglioside GM_1	0.15
Total Brain Gangliosides	0.15
Neurotensin	25
Hepatic Proliferation Inhibitor	100
Cortisol	5.0
Fluocinolone Acetonide	45
Diazepam	30
Cytochalasin B	1.0
Concanavalin A	0.10
Wheat Germ Agglutinin	0.10
4-α-Methyl Glucoside	3×10^4

[1]C.M.:Conditioned medium from normal peripheral blood
lymphocytes stimilated with PHA was a gift from Dr. R.
Mertelsmann(M.S.-K.C.C.). It was tested at a dilution
of 1:4./Hepatic Proliferation Inhibitor: derived from rat
liver, McMahon, T. B. and Iype, P. T. (1980).

diverse growth factors corticosterioids, lectins and other
compounds are listed. None of these showed inhibitory activity at the concentrations tested. Epidermal growth factor, at a concentration sufficient to saturate its cellular
receptors, did not inhibit ^{3}H PDBu binding. Prostaglandins
E_1, E_2, and $F_{2\alpha}$ have been tested in other laboratories

Table 6
Inhibition of ^{3}H-PDBu Binding by Various Physiologic Fluids

Test Substance	Approximate ID_{50}*(mg/ml)
Calf Serum	11
Fetal Calf Serum	11
Pooled Human Serum	4
Pregnant Human Serum	2
Platelet Depleted Human Serum	4
Lipoprotein Depleted Human Serum	4
Rhesus Monkey Serum	8
Rat Serum	1
Human Amniotic Fluid	2
Rat Embryo Homogenate	0.3
Rat Liver Homogenate	1
Human Cerebrospinal Fluid	- **
Rhesus Monkey Cerebrospinal Fluid	-
Pregnant Human Urine (10x)	-
Human Milk	-
Human Serum Albumin	25

*ID_{50} is defined as the concentration of test substance required to produce 50% inhibition of specific H-PDBu binding to rat embryo cells./**Designated no activity detected when tested at a final concentration of 50% physiological fluid in the binding assay buffer. Cerebrospinal fluid was used as such. Urine was first dialyzed and then concentrated ten-fold by evaporation.

and been found to have no effect (Driedger and Blumberg, 1980; Shoyab and Todaro, 1980). The sera and other physiologic fluids which we have tested are listed in Table 6. We have found that sera from several species, including human, and human amniotic fluid were potent inhibitors of ^{3}H PDBu binding. Human serum albumin was slightly inhibitory, but much less so than the corresponding concentration of serum.

We have partially purified, by 2 chromatographic steps, an inhibitory factor from human serum. It is labile to heating at 70°C for 10 min, precipitable by 80% ethanol, is anionic at neutral pH, and has a molecular weight of about 60,000 (Horowitz et al. 1981a). We characterized its effect on PDBu binding in a variant of CREF cells (CREF A2) which has only a single binding site for ^{3}H PDBu (Table 1), since this facilitated binding studies. A double-reciprocal plot

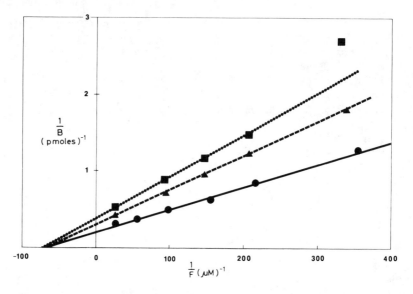

<u>Figure 1</u>. Double-Reciprocal plot of PDBu Binding in the presence of the serum factors. Specifically bound PDBu (B) is in pmoles. Free PDBu (F) is in µmoles/liter. Binding was determined in the presence of 0 (- ● -), 13 (- ▲ -), and 27 (.. ■ ..) µg/ml of serum factor. A tracer amount of 3nM ^{3}H PDBu was used. The assay was conducted in assay buffer (2 volumes of DMEM to one volume of phosphate buffered saline (PBS) plus 1mg/ml bovine serum albumen), as described by Horowitz et al (1981) on 5.6X10^6 CREF A2 cells per dish, at 37°C. Nonspecific binding was that observed in the presence of 50µM PDBu, and has been subtracted from all points.

of PDBu binding in the presence of 0,13 and 27 µg/ml of the partially purified serum factor is shown in Figure 1. The serum factor reduced the number of available phorboid receptors from 4.6X10^5 to 3.6X10^5 and 2.9X10^5 per cell respectively without altering their apparent affinity. This type of behavior is typical of non-competitive inhibition. In further experiments, the inhibition of PDBu binding by the serum factor was found to be rapid and reversible at 4°C (Horowitz et al. 1981b). The inhibition reached an equilibrium value rapidly, which makes it unlikely that it acts by enzymatically destroying the PDBu. Nor does the serum factor act by irreversible inactivation of the phorboid recep-

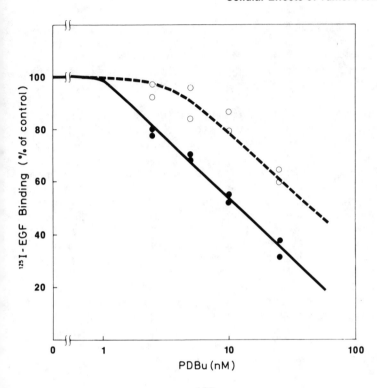

Figure 2. Inhibition of ^{125}I EGF Binding by PDBu in the presence of human serum factor. Binding of 0.7 ng/ml of ^{125}I EGF was measured in the presence (- O -) and absence (- ● -) of 150 µg/ml of serum factor. Results from two experiments are shown. Binding is given as percent of binding in the absence of serum factor and PDBu. All values are corrected for nonspecific binding. The assay was conducted in 24 well culture dishes at 5.5 X 10^5 cells/well. Assay was conducted as described by Lee and Weinstein (1978b).

tors, but probably by physically blocking access of PDBu to the receptor.

We were concerned that the serum factor might act by binding or trapping ^{3}H PDBu thereby preventing it from binding to the phorboid receptor. However, in a gel filtration assay, we were unable to detect any binding of ^{3}H PDBu by partially purified serum factor. Unfractionated serum did, however, bind ^{3}H PDBu (Horowitz, Greenebaum, Nicolaides, Woodward & Weinstein, manuscript in preparation). It appears, therefore, that the serum factor acts by interacting with phorboid receptors or with sites on the membrane that influence the activity of the phorboid receptors.

We have also investigated the influence of the serum factor on certain cellular responses to PDBu. By itself, the serum factor is inactive in stimulating arachidonic acid or choline release from C3H 10T 1/2 cells (Table 4, and unpublished observations, Horowitz, Okin and Weinstein), or in inhibiting ^{125}I EGF binding to CREF cells (Figure 2). In all 3 of these assays, however, whole human serum is quite effective. We also studied the effect of purified human serum factor on the inhibition of ^{125}I EGF binding by PDBu. As can be seen in Figure 2, the inhibition of ^{125}I EGF binding required a higher concentration of PDBu when the serum factor was present. Thus in the absence of serum factor 50% inhibition of EGF binding was obtained with 10nM PDBu; whereas in the presence of 150μg/ml serum factor 50nM of PDBu was required to produce the same inhibition. These results are consistent with what we calculate for the amount of PDBu receptor binding that occurs in the presence of this concentration of serum factor based on the data in Figure 1.

DOWN REGULATION OF THE PHORBOID RECEPTOR.

When CREF N cells are cultured in the continuous presence of PDBu and ^{3}H PDBu binding is measured after removal of all bound and free PDBu, a decrease in the binding of ^{3}H PDBu is observed (Figure 3). This decrease arises from a decrease in the number of available receptors as determined by Scatchard analysis, and therefore may be referred to as "down-regulation."

In Figure 4, the concentration dependence of the down regulation is displayed. The 50% effective dose for down-regulation is 8nM, which is the K_{D50} of the high affinity binding site in these cells (Horowitz et al. 1981). At a concentration of PDBu higher than that at which the high-affinity site is saturated, no further down-regulation of phorboid receptors is seen. The down regulation reaches only about 50% of the control binding in these cells. It is complete within 6 hours in the presence of 100nM PDBu. Down-regulation of phorboid receptors has also been reported

Time-Course of Down-Regulation of PDBu Receptors

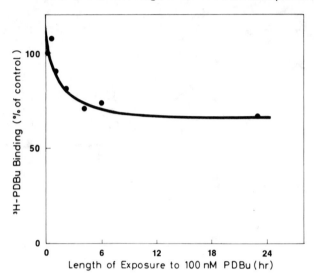

Figure 3. CREF N cells in 5 cm culture dishes were grown in DMEM plus 10% calf serum, plus or minus 100 nM PDBu. At the end of the incubation period, cell monolayers were washed with PBS and incubated in fresh assay buffer at 37°C for 30 minutes to allow all bound PDBu to dissociate. The monolayer was washed again in PBS and fresh assay buffer and ^{3}H PDBu were added. Specific binding of ^{3}H PDBu is given as % of control binding. The control plates were not pretreated with 100nM PDBu.

in other cell types (Solanki et al. 1981; Jaken et al. 1981). In its susceptibility to down-regulation, the phorboid receptor behaves like other known cellular receptors. However, following down regulation of the receptor, CREF N cells, unlike Hela cells (Lee & Weinstein, 1980), remain sensitive to the inhibition of EGF binding by PDBu (Horowitz and Weinstein, unpublished observations). This suggests that at least 40% of the phorboid receptors in CREF N cells are spare receptors, not required for the full biologic response to PDBu.

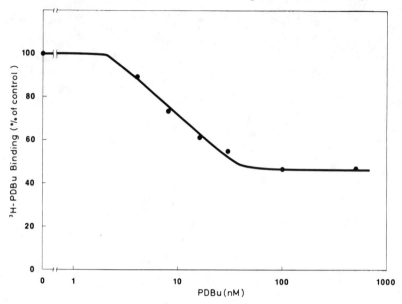

Figure 4. Concentration Dependence of Down-Regulation of Phorboid Receptors: Varying amounts of PDBu were added to monolayers of CREF N cells in DMEM plus 10% calf serum in 5 cm tissue culture dishes. Monolayers were incubated with the PDBu for 44 hours. At the end of the incubation period, free and bound PDBu were removed as described in Figure 3. Specific binding of 3nM ^{3}H PDBu was measured and is given as % of control binding. A parallel set of plates was treated and reserved for cell counts. All values are corrected for cell numbers.

CONCLUSION

The phorboid receptor behaves in a manner consistent with our knowledge of other cellular receptors: it shows high affinity (8-30nM K_D); the binding constants of various ligands correlate well with relative biologic activity; ligand binding is reversible; and partial down-regulation of the receptor occurs in the continued presence of ligand.

We have isolated a substance from human sera which

strongly inhibits phorbol ester binding in a non-competitive manner. However, the putative endogenous ligand for the phorboid receptor remains elusive. At the present time it is not clear whether or not the serum factor we have isolated plays a role in host susceptibility to carcinogenesis. If so, our findings suggest that it may have a protective rather than an enhancing role. On the other hand, very little is known about the normal biologic role of the phorboid receptor.

Some of the earliest cellular responses to phorbol esters involve changes in lipid metabolism. Evidence suggests that these changes, and changes in membrane structure may play an important role in cellular response to phorbol esters. Following partial down-regulation of phorboid receptors, cells continue to be responsive to phorbol esters. This suggests an excess of phorboid receptors. Continued studies may help elucidate the role of the phorboid receptor and the role of host and cellular factors in tumor promotion.

ACKNOWLEDGMENTS

We would like to thank Maria Nicolaides, Kim Woodward and Dr. Ellen Greenebaum for their valuable collaboration in various aspects of these studies, and Ester Okin for her assistance in the choline and arachidonic acid release assays. We would like to thank Drs. Paul Fisher and G. Giotta for providing certain cell lines, and Drs. Larry Witte, Dewitt Goodman, P. T. Iype, T. Sugimura, and R. Mertelsmann, among others, for samples used in these experiments.

This research was supported by National Cancer Institute Grant CA 26056 and CA 21111, and an award from the Dupont Company. The authors express their gratitude to Patricia Kelly for her valuable assistance in the preparation of this manuscript.

REFERENCES

Ariens EJ, Beld AJ, Rodrigues de Miranda JF, Simonis AM (1979). The Pharmacon-Receptor-Effector Concept: A Basis for Understanding the Transmission of Information in Biological Systems. In O'Brien RD (ed): "The Receptors: A Comprehensive Treatise," New York: Plenum Press, Vol 1, p 33.

Baker JB, Cunningham DD (1978). Glucocortocoid-mediated alteration in growth factor binding and action: analysis of the binding change. J Supramol Struc 9:69.

Cardellina JH, Marner FJ, Moore RE (1979). Seaweed Dermatitis: Structure of Lyngbyatoxin A. Science 204:193.

Diamond L, O'Brien TG, Rovera G (1978). Tumor Promoters: Effects on Proliferation and Differentiation of Cells in Culture. Life Sci 23:1979.

Driedger PE, Blumberg PM (1980). Specific Binding of phorbol ester tumor promoters. Proc Nat Acad Sci USA 77:567.

Dunphy WG, Delclos KB, Blumberg PM (1980). Characterization of specific binding of [^{3}H]phorbol 12,13-dibutyrate and [^{3}H]phorbol 12-myristate 13-acetate to mouse brain. Cancer Res 40:3635.

Durkin JP, Shier WT (1981). Staphylococcal delta toxin stimulates endogenous phospholipase A$_2$ activity and prostaglandin synthesis in fibroblasts. Biochem Biophys Acta 633:467.

Fibach E, Yamasaki H, Weinstein IB, Marks PA, Rifkind RA (1978). Heterogeneity of murine erythroleukemia cells with respect to tumor promoter-mediated inhibition of cell differentiation. Cancer Res 38:3685.

Fisher PB, Cogan U, Horowitz AD, Schachter D, Weinstein IB (1981). TPA Resistance in Friend Erythroleukemia Cells: Role of Membrane Lipid Fluidity. Biochem Biophys Res Commun 100:370.

Fisher PB, Dorsch-Hasler K, Weinstein IB, Ginsberg HS (1980). Interactions between initiating chemical carcinogens, tumor promoters, and adenovirus in cell transformation. J Teratogen Carcinogen Mutagen 1:245.

Fujiki H, Mori M, Nakayasu M, Terada M, Sugimura T (1979). A possible naturally occurring tumor promoter, teleocidin B from Streptomyces. Biochem Biophys Res Commun 90:976.

Fujiki H, Mori M. Nakayasu M, Terada M, Sugimura T, Moore RE (1981). Indole alkaloids; dihydroteleocidin B, teleocidin and lyngbyatoxin A, a new class of tumor promoters. Proc Nat Acad Sci 78:3872.

Giotta GJ, Heitzmann J, Cohn M (1980). Properties of two temperature sensitive Rous sarcoma virus transformed cerebellar cell lines. Brain Res 202:445.

Hecker E (1978). Structure-Activity Relationships in Diterpene Esters Irritant and Cocarcinogenic to Mouse Skin. In Slaga TJ, Sivak A, Boutwell RK (eds): "Mechanisms of Tumor Promotion and Cocarcinogenesis," New York: Raven Press Vol 2, p. 11.

Horowitz AD, Greenebaum E, Weinstein IB (1981). Identification of receptors for phorbol ester tumor promoters in intact mammalian cells and of an inhibitor of receptor binding in biologic fluids. Proc Nat Acad sci 78:2315.

Horowitz AD, Greenebaum E, Weinstein IB (1981b). A factor from human serum inhibits binding of ^{3}H-phorbol-12,13-dibutyrate (PDBu) to rat embryo cells. Proc 72nd Annual Mtng Am Assoc Cancer Res, abstract 538, p 136.

Ivanovic V, Weinstein IB (1981). Glucocorticoids and benzo[a]pyrene have opposing effects on epidermal growth factor-receptor binding. Nature (in press).

Jacobs S, Cuatrecasas P (1976). The Mobile Receptor Hypothesis and "Cooperativity" of Hormone Binding: Application to Insulin. Biochem Biophys Acta 433:482.

Jaken S, Tashjian AH, Blumberg PM (1981). Characterization of Phorbol Ester Receptors and Their Down Modulation in GH_4C_1 Rat Pituitary Cells. Cancer Res 41:2175.

Kahn CR (1976). Membrane Receptors for Hormones and Neurotransmitters. J Cell Biol 70:261.

Kupchan SM, Baxter RL (1975). Mezerein: Antileukemic Principle Isolated from Daphne Mezereum L. Science 187:652.

Kupchan SM, Shizuri Y, Sumner WC Jr, Haynes HR, Leighton AP, Sickles BR (1976a). Isolation and Structural Elucidation of New Potent Antileukemic Diterpenoid Esters from Gnidia Species. J Org Chem 41:3850.

Kupchan SM, Uchids I, Branfman AR, Daily RG, Fei BY (1976b). Antileukemic Principles Isolated from Euphorbiaceae Plants. Science 191:571.

Lee LS, Weinstein IB (1978a). Uptake of the Tumor Promoting Agent 12-0-tetradecanoyl-phorbol-13-acetate by Hela Cells. J Env Pathol Toxicol 1:627.

Lee LS, Weinstein IB (1978b). Tumor-Promoting Phorbol Esters Inhibit Binding of Epidermal Growth Factor to Cellular Receptors. Science 202:313.

Lee LS, Weinstein IB (1979). Mechanism of tumor promoter inhibition of cellular binding of epidermal growth factor. Proc Nat Acad Sci USA 76:5168.

Lee LS, Weinstein IB (1980). Studies on the mechanism by which a tumor promoter inhibits binding of epidermal growth factor to cellular receptors. Carcinogenesis 1:669.

Levine L, Hassid A (1977). Effects of phorbol-12,13-diesters on prostaglandin production and phospholipase activity in canine kidney (MDCK) cells. Biochem Biophys Res Commun 79:477.

McMahon TB, Iype PT (1980). Specific Inhibition of Proliferation of Non-Malignant Rat Hepatic Cells by a Factor from Rat Liver. Cancer Res 40:1249.

Mollay C, Kreil G, Berger H (1976). Action of phospholipases on the cytoplasmic membrane of Eschorichia Coli. Stimulation by Melittin. Biochem Biophys Acta 426:317.

Mufson RA, DeFeo D, Weinstein IB (1979). Effects of phorbol ester tumor promoters on arachidonic acid metabolism in chick embryo fibroblasts. Molec Pharmacol 16:569.

Mufson RA, Laskin JD, Fisher PB, Weinstein IB (1979). Melittin shares certain cellular effects with phorbol ester tumour promoters. Nature 280:72.

Mufson RA, Okin E, Weinstein IB (1981). Phorbol Esters Stimulate the Rapid Release of Choline from Cellular Phosphatidyl Choline. Carcinogenesis (in press).

Nagle DS, Jaken S, Castagna M, Blumberg PM (1981). Variation with embryonic development and regional localization of specific ^{3}-phorbol-12,13-dibutyrate binding to brain. Cancer Res 41:89.

Osborne R, Tashjian AH Jr (1979). Phorbol Diesters Modulate Peptide Hormone Binding to Pituitary Cells. In "Program and Abstracts of the 61st Meeting of the Endocrine Society," (Abstract 684) p 243.

Shoyab M, Todaro GJ (1980). Specific high affinity cell membrane receptors for biologically active phorbol and ingenol esters. Nature 288:451.

Shoyab M, Todaro GJ (1981). Perturbation of Membrane Phospholipids Alters the Interaction between Epidermal Growth Factor and Its Membrane Receptor. Arch Biochem Biophys 206:222.

Slaga T, Sivak A, Boutwell RK (1978). "Carcinogenesis, Mechanisms of Tumor Promotion and Cocarcinogenesis." New York: Raven Press, Vol 2.

Solanki V, Slaga TJ (1981). Specific binding of phorbol ester tumor promoters to intact primary epidermal cells from Sencar mice. Proc Nat Acad Sci USA 78:2549.

Solanki V, Slaga TJ, Callahan M, Huberman E (1981). Down-regulation of Specific Binding of [20-3H] phorbol 12,13-dibutyrate and phorbol-ester induced differentiation of human promyelocytic leukemia cells. Proc Nat Acad Sci USA 78:1722.

Stallcup WB (1977). Nerve and Glial Specific Antigens on Cloned Neural Cell Lines. Cellular Neurobiology 1977:165.

Stallcup WB, Cohn M (1978). Correlation of surface antigens and cell type in cloned cell lines from the rat central nervous system. Experimental Cell Research 98:285.

Strickland S, Loeb JN (1981). Obligatory Separation of Hormone binding and biological response curves in systems dependent upon secondary mediators of hormone action. Proc

Nat Acad Sci USA 78:1366.
Umezawa K, Weinstein IB, Shaw WV (1980). Staphylococcal delta-hemolysin inhibits cellular binding of epidermal growth factor and induces arachidonic acid release. Biochem Biophys Res Commun 92:625.
Umezawa K, Weinstein IB, Horowitz A, Fujiki H, Matsushima T, Sugimura T (1981). Similarity of teleocidin B and phorbol esters tumor promoters in effects on membrane receptors. Nature 290:411.
Weinstein IB (1981). Studies on the mechanism of action of tumor promoters and their relevance to mammary carcinogenesis. In McGrath CM, Brennan MJ, Rich MA (eds): "Cell Biology of Breast Cancer," New York: Academic Press, p 425.
Weinstein IB, Horowitz AD, Mufson RA, Fisher PB, Ivanovic V, Greenebaum E (1981). Results and Speculations Related to Recent Studies on Mechanisms of Tumor Promotion. In "Symposium on Cocarcinogenesis and Biological Effects of Tumor Promoters," Elmau, Germany: Raven Press (in press).
Weinstein IB, Lee LS, Fisher PB, Mufson RA, Yamasaki H (1979a). Action of Phorbol Ester in Cell Culture: Mimicry of Transformation, Altered Differentiation and Effects on Cell Membrane. J Supramol Struc 12:195.
Weinstein IB, Lee LS, Fisher PB, Mufson RA, Yamasaki H (1979b). The Mechanism of Action of Tumor Promoters and a Molecular Model of Two Stage Carcinogenesis. In Emmelot P, Kriek E (eds) "Environmental Carcinogenesis," Elsevier, Amsterdam: North Holland Biomedical Press, p 265.
Weinstein IB, Mufson RA, Lee LS, Fisher PB, Laskin J, Horowitz A, Ivanovic V (1980). Membrane and Other Biochemical Effects of the Phorbol Esters and Their Relevance to Tumor Promotion. In Pullman B, Ts'o POP, Gelboin H (eds) "Carcinogenesis: Fundamental Mechanisms and Environmental Effects," Amsterdam: R. Reidel Pub Co, p 543.
Weinstein IB, Wigler M, Pietropaolo C (1977). The action of tumor-promoting agents in cell culture. In Hiatt HH, Watson JO, Winston JA (eds) "Origins of Human Cancer," New York: Cold Spring Harbor, p 751.
Weinstein IB, Yamaguchi N, Gebert R, Kiaghn ME (1975). The use of epithelial cell cultures for studies on the mechanism of transformation by chemical carcinogens. In Vitro II:130.
Wigler M, Defeo D, Weinstein IB (1978). Induction of Plasminogen Activator in Cultured Cells by Macrocyclic Plant Diterpene Esters and Other Agents Related to Tumor Promotion. Cancer Res 38:1434.

Yamasaki H, Mufson RA, Weinstein IB (1979). Phorbol Ester Induced Prostaglandin Synthesis and ^{3}H-TPA Metabolism by TPA Sensitive and TPA Resistant Friend Erythroleukemia Cells. Biochem Biophys Res Commun 89:1018.

Yamasaki H, Weinstein IB, Van Duuren BL (1981). Induction of erythroleukemia cell adhesion by plant diterpene tumor promoters: A quantitative study and correlation with in vivo activities. Carcinogenesis 2:537.

**Prostaglandins and Cancer: First
International Conference, pages 239-254
© 1982 Alan R. Liss, Inc., 150 Fifth Avenue, New York, NY 10011**

ON THE ROLE OF PROSTAGLANDINS IN THE INDUCTION OF EPIDERMAL
PROLIFERATION, HYPERPLASIA AND TUMOR PROMOTION IN MOUSE SKIN

G. Fürstenberger, M. Gross and F. Marks

German Cancer Research Center, Institute of
Biochemistry
D - 6900 Heidelberg, F.R.G.

I. INTRODUCTION

Studies on the biochemical mechanisms underlying the induction of epidermal hyperproliferation and hyperplasia may
lead to a better understanding of epidermal wound healing,
of many proliferative skin diseases and even of events related to chemical carcinogenesis - especially of the process
of tumor promotion. One prerequisite is the establishment of
models which allow strict control of the first and subsequent stages of the proliferative processes. They should enable us to find a clue to key biochemical events in the
highly complex process of induction of epidermal hyperproliferation. Our model is mouse skin, stimulated to proliferate
by mechanical devices, chemical mitogens and tumor promoters.

II. PROTOTYPES OF EPIDERMAL HYPERPROLIFERATION IN MOUSE
SKIN

Based upon biochemical criteria, we distinguish at least
three types of hyperproliferation in adult mouse skin. Proliferation type 1 is evoked by non-damaging stimuli like skin
massage, type 2 by superficial wounding of the epidermis (removal of the horny layer by means of sandpaper rubbing) and
type 3 by full skin wounding (Table 1). Proliferation type 1
is characterized by an increase of the flow rate of epidermal
cells, while maintaining the normal steady state of tissue
homeostasis (Bertsch et al., 1976). Proliferation types 2 and
3 are characterized by an alteration of the homeostatic equilibrium of the epidermis. The increase of cell proliferation

Table 1: Types of epidermal proliferation induced by mechanical and chemical stimuli in mouse skin in vivo

stimulus mechanical	chemical	type of epidermal proliferation: biochemical criteria	ref.
skin massage	4-O-methylTPA	1: increase of flow rate maintaining the normal steady state equilibrium in epidermis; maintainance of G_1 chalone control	a) b)
epidermal wounding	Ti$_8$, RPA, mezerein, A 23187	2: alteration of the steady state equilibrium in epidermis, release from G_1 chalone control, epidermal hyperplasia	a)c) d)e) f)g) h)
full skin wounding	TPA	3: alteration of the steady state equilibrium in epidermis, release from G_1 chalone control, epidermal hyperplasia and tumor promoting potency	h) i) j) k)

a) Bertsch et al., 1976; b) Fürstenberger et al., 1981e;
c)d)e) Marks et al., 1978, 1979, 1981c; f)g) Fürstenberger
et al., 1972, 1981a; h) Slaga et al., 1980; i) Hennings et
al., 1970; j) Clark-Lewis et al., 1978; k) Argyris, 1981.

is consistently followed by a hyperplastic reaction (Marks
et al., 1978). Contrary to proliferation types 1 and 2, type
3 exerts a tumor promoting potency (Hennings and Boutwell,
1970; Clark-Lewis and Murray, 1978; Argyris, 1981). Moreover,
manipulations inducing proliferation types 2 and 3 have been
shown to release the epidermis from the inhibitory effect of
epidermal G_1 chalone, a tissue-specific endogenous inhibitor
of the G_1-S-transition, whereas in proliferation type 1 the
epidermis remains under G_1 chalone control (Table 1; Marks
et al., 1978).

The three proliferation types can also be induced by
chemical agents. Their chemical structures are depicted in
Figure 1. The phorbol ester 12-O-tetradecanoylphorbol-13-
acetate (or TPA) is a strong irritant skin mitogen and a potent tumor promoter (Slaga et al., 1978). Methylation of the

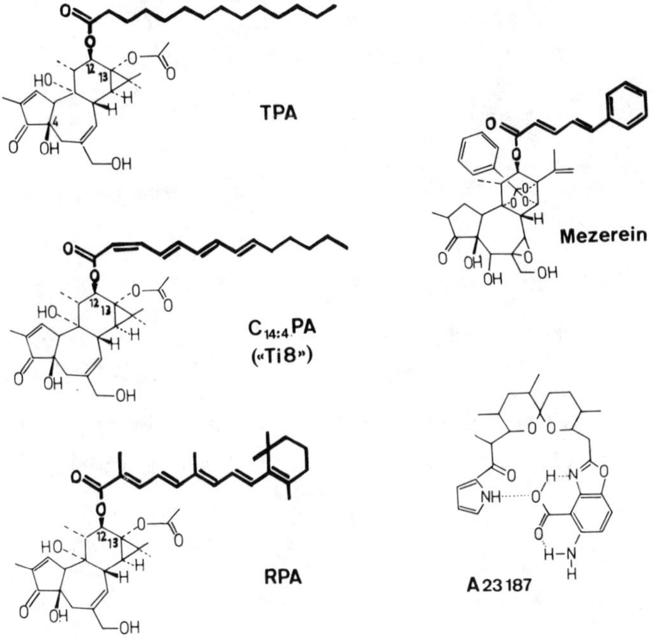

Fig. 1 Chemical structures of tumor promoter TPA and
non-promoting TPA analogues, of mezerein and
of the ionophore A 23187.

4-hydroxyl function of TPA results in an almost complete loss
of the irritant and tumor promoting activity (Hecker, 1978)
and a considerable weakening of the mitogenic potency (Fürstenberger et al., 1981e). The introduction of conjugated
double bonds into the long chain fatty acid residue of TPA,
as in 12-O-2cis,4trans,6,8-tetradecatetraenoylphorbol-13-ace-
tate (Ti$_8$; Marks et al., 1979), or its substitution by retinoic acid, as in 12-O-retinoylphorbol-13-acetate (RPA; Fürstenberger et al., 1981a,b), yield agents that provoke skin
inflammation and epidermal hyperproliferation as efficiently
as an equimolar dose of TPA, while possessing negligible tumor promoting activity. This also holds true for mezerein,
the unsaturated daphnane orthoester (Fürstenberger and Hecker,
1972; Mufson et al., 1979; Slaga et al., 1980) and for the
cation ionophore A 23187, a compound with a completely different chemical structure (Marks et al., 1981c).

Based upon the biochemical criteria listed in Table 1,
the non-irritant phorbol ester derivative 4-O-methyl TPA in-

duces proliferation type 1, the irritant mitogens Ti_8, RPA mezerein and ionophore A 23187 evoke proliferation type 2 and TPA-type tumor promoters bring about proliferation type 3.

III. ON THE ROLE OF PROSTAGLANDINS IN THE INDUCTION OF CELL PROLIFERATION AND HYPERPLASTIC TRANSFORMATION IN MOUSE EPIDERMIS

The increasing body of evidence in the literature indicating that prostaglandins might be involved in the control of growth and differentiation of skin (Kischer, 1969; Eaglestein and Weinstein, 1975; Hammarström et al., 1975, 1979; Lowe and Stoughton, 1977; Bentley-Philipps, 1977; Ziboh et al., 1977), as well as the hypothesis that phorbol esters might exert their biological effects via prostaglandin receptor interaction (Smythies et al., 1975, 1979), prompted us to investigate the role of prostaglandins in the induction by TPA of epidermal cell proliferation and hyperplasia.

However, TPA did not turn out to be a prostaglandin E agonist as measured by competition binding studies (Fürstenberger and Marks, 1979a), and the prostaglandins E and F themselves did not affect normal epidermal cell proliferation (Fürstenberger and Marks, 1978). On the other hand, it was demonstrated that TPA-stimulated induction of ornithine decarboxylase activity, as part of a biochemical cascade leading to epidermal hyperproliferation (O'Brien et al., 1975; Verma and Boutwell, 1977) and TPA-stimulated cell proliferation (Fürstenberger and Marks, 1978) both could be inhibited by the cyclooxygenase inhibitor indomethacin (Flower et al., 1972), indicating that prostaglandins might be involved in these processes.

Due to the lipophilic structure of TPA and based upon data on the subcellular localization of specific TPA binding sites in various tissues, including epidermis (Delclos et al., 1980; Ashendel and Boutwell, 1981; Dunphy et al., 1981), TPA probably interacts with cellular membranes. In mouse epidermis, the immediate response to such an interaction is the biosynthesis of prostaglandins. Using primary epidermal cells and a murine epidermal cell line we have shown that the TPA-induced prostaglandin release is preceded by liberation of arachidonic acid, released from membrane phospholipids (Fürstenberger et al., 1981c,d). In vivo, the prostaglandin E (PGE) content of mouse epidermis reaches a first maximum after only 10 minutes, followed by a second peak

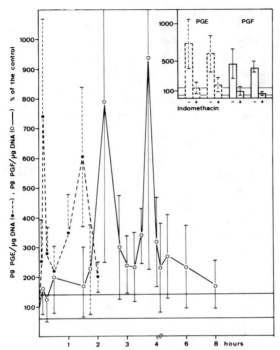

Fig. 2 Levels of prostaglandin E (●---) and F
(O——) in mouse epidermis in vivo after topical application of TPA. Mice were treated
with 0.1 ml acetone or 10 nmol TPA dissolved
in 0.1 ml acetone and killed at the times indicated. The prostaglandins were extracted
from frozen epidermis, isolated by thin-layer
chromatography and determined by radioimmunoassay. Each experimental point represents the
mean ± S.D. for 9-24 mice. The horizontal lines
represent the average S.D. of the control values (treatment with acetone) as obtained with
36 animals (7.1 ± 2.5 pg PGE/μg DNA = 100%;
4.3 ± 1.7 pg PGF/μg DNA). Inserts, results when
1.1 μmol indomethacin was applied topically
30 min prior to TPA. The PGE content was determined 10 to 90 min, the PGF content 150 and
210 min after TPA treatment. N = 6 ± S.D.

after 90 minutes (Fig. 2; Fürstenberger and Marks, 1980).
The increase of epidermal prostaglandin F (PGF) also occurs
biphasically, with a first peak at about 2 hours and a second maximum at 4 hours after treatment (Fig. 2). At later

time points, the levels of both PGE and PGF increase, as
also shown by others (Ashendel and Boutwell, 1979; Bresnick
et al., 1979). If the early prostaglandin response is inhibited by indomethacin (Fig. 2), the stimulation by TPA of
ornithine decarboxylase activity (Verma and Boutwell, 1977;
Verma et al., 1980), of epidermal DNA synthesis and of mitotic activity (Fürstenberger and Marks, 1978) is strongly
inhibited, whereas other responses to TPA such as skin inflammation (Marks et al., 1981c) and the increase of epidermal phosphodiesterase activity (Marks and Fürstenberger,
1980) remain unaffected. Interestingly, the proliferation
rate of the normal epidermis is not inhibited by indomethacin using a comparable dose (Fürstenberger and Marks, 1978).
The inhibition of epidermal hyperproliferation and hyperplasia by indomethacin can be specifically overcome by low
doses of PGE_1 or PGE_2 (but not by $PGF_{2\alpha}$) applied topically
and simultaneously with TPA. This strongly indicates that
E-prostaglandins selectively mediate the mitogenic stimulus
(Fürstenberger and Marks, 1978). Applied to the normal skin,
PGE_2 alone turns out to evoke negligible mitogenic activity.
This result shows that, besides its stimulatory activity on
PGE biosynthesis, TPA enhances the responsiveness of the
epidermis to PGE_2 immediately after treatment (Fürstenberger
and Marks 1978). Indomethacin administration 30 minutes after
TPA application does not interfere with epidermal hyperproliferation (Fig. 3; Fürstenberger and Marks, 1980). This
result excludes the indomethacin inhibition being due to
toxic effects of the drug and indicates that the very early
burst of PGE synthesis is the key event, whereas the second
peak of PGE synthesis and the subsequent synthesis of PGF
are obviously not obligatory for the mediation of the mitogenic effect of TPA (Fig. 3).

In epidermal cells in culture, TPA induces a similar
sequence of biochemical events, i.e., stimulation of prostaglandin synthesis, induction of ornithine decarboxylase activity and DNA synthesis (Fürstenberger et al., 1981c,d). In
contrast to the in vivo situation, the experiments with indomethacin do not reveal any relationship between prostaglandin synthesis and cellular proliferation using a murine
epidermal cell line. However, in primary guinea pig epidermal
cells, TPA-stimulated DNA synthesis turns out to be prostaglandin-dependent (Fürstenberger et al., 1981d).

Summarizing the data, we have established that: 1. TPA
is not able to induce epidermal hyperproliferation in the
absence of PGE, i.e. when its endogenous synthesis is inhibited by indomethacin; 2. PGE_2 is unable to induce epidermal

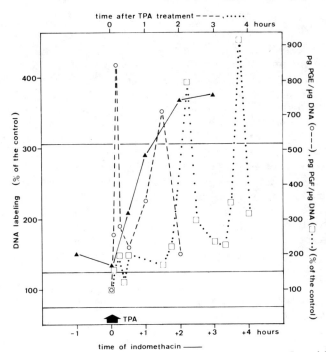

Fig. 3 Relationship between the kinetics of epidermal
PGE (O---) and PGF (□●●●) synthesis induced by
TPA and the effect on epidermal DNA labeling
of varying the time interval between indomethacin and TPA treatment (▲——). Mice were treated with 0.1 ml acetone or 10 nmol TPA dissolved
in 0.1 ml acetone and killed at the times indicated for determination of the epidermal PGE and
PGF contents (see Figure 1). To determine the
effect of indomethacin on DNA labeling, mice
were treated with 0.1 ml acetone or indomethacin
(1.1 μmol/0.1 ml acetone) or TPA (10 nmol/0.1 ml
acetone) and killed 18 hours after TPA treatment.
Labeled thymidine was injected i.p. one hour
prior to sacrifice. The horizontal lines indicate either control (acetone-treated) DNA labeling: 51 ± 13 cpm/μg DNA, or DNA labeling 18
hours after TPA treatment: 201 ± 49 cpm/μg DNA,
N = 10.

hyperproliferation in the absence of TPA; 3. PGE$_2$ applied
simultaneously with TPA enhances the mitogenic effect of the
latter;4. indomethacin does not significantly inhibit nor-

mal epidermal cell proliferation. Accordingly, we conclude that PGE_2 and TPA act synergistically and that the early synthesis of PGE_2 is a necessary but not sufficient event in the induction by TPA of epidermal hyperproliferation and hyperplasia. Thus, in mouse epidermis in vivo and in primary epidermal cells in culture, the stimulatory effect of TPA on prostaglandin biosynthesis which has been also observed in other systems (Brune et al., 1978; Humes et al., 1978; Levine et al., 1978; Tashijan et al., 1978; Mufson et al., 1979; Yamasaki et al., 1979; Crutchley et al., 1980) can be related to a distinct physiological reaction.

The role of prostaglandins in the biochemical cascade leading to the induction of the different types of hyperproliferation in mouse skin is summarized in Table 2. In an appropriate dose, the almost non-irritant and non-promoting phorbol ester derivative 4-O-methyl TPA induces epidermal hyperproliferation along a pathway which does not involve early prostaglandin E synthesis, induction of ornithine decarboxylase activity or release of G_1 chalone responsiveness. This hyperproliferation is not followed by a hyperplastic transformation of the epidermis. The same holds true for the mitogenic effect of skin massage, indicating that proliferation type 1 is prostaglandin-independent (Bertsch et al., 1976; Marks et al., 1979, 1981a; Fürstenberger et al., 1979, 1981e). The almost non-promoting irritant skin mitogens Ti_8, RPA, mezerein and ionophore A 23187 cause epidermal hyperproliferation, followed by a sustained hyperplasia via a prostaglandin-dependent pathway. This involves the induction of ornithine decarboxylase activity and release from G_1 chalone control. Epidermal wounding (removal of the horny layer) follows the same prostaglandin-dependent pathway, characterized as proliferation type 2 (Fürstenberger and Hecker, 1972; Bertsch et al., 1976; Marks et al., 1979, 1981a,c; Fürstenberger et al., 1979, 1981a,b). Since PGE_2 does not induce epidermal hyperproliferation but acts synergistically with a mitogen, the question arises as to whether the epidermal damage itself is a mitogenic trigger or whether growth factors are released upon injury, the activity of which is modified or amplified by PGE. Proliferation type 3, provoked by full skin wounding or by a tumor promoter such as TPA, is characterized by a similar sequence of biochemical events, i.e., prostaglandin synthesis, induction of ornithine decarboxylase activity and release from G_1 chalone responsiveness (Fürstenberger and Marks, 1978, 1980; Bertsch and Marks, 1981; Marks et al., 1981a). These results indicate that the prostaglan-

Table 2: Biochemical parameters of the induction of proliferation by mechanical and chemical stimuli in mouse skin in vivo. In the doses indicated the mitogenic effects of the chemical agents are of comparable degree.

prolif. type	mitogenic stimulus	dose (nmol/animal)	skin inflammation	hyperprolifera-tion	hyper-plasia	mediation by prosta-glandins	ODC induc-tion	G_1 chalone refracto-riness	tumor promo-tion
1	skin massage	–	no	yes	no	no	very weak	no	no
	4-O-Me-TPA	400	no	yes	weak	no	no	no	very weak
2	Ti_8	2-10	yes	yes	yes	partially	yes	yes	very weak
	RPA	2-10	yes [a,b]	yes [b]	yes [b]	yes	yes	yes	very weak [a,b]
	mezerein	2-10	yes	yes	yes	yes	yes	yes	very weak
	A 23187	100	yes	yes	yes	yes	yes	yes	no
	epidermal wounding	–	yes	yes	yes	yes	yes	yes	no
3	TPA	2-10	yes	yes	yes	yes	yes	yes	yes
	full skin wounding	–	yes	yes	yes	yes	yes [d]	yes	yes [c,d] yes [e]

a) Fürstenberger and Hecker 1972; b) Mufson et al., 1979; Slaga et al. 1980;
c) Hennings and Boutwell 1970; d) Clark-Lewis 1978; e) Argyris 1981.

din-dependent epidermal hyperproliferation and hyperplasia is not a sufficient but obviously a necessary condition of tumor promotion. Moreover, the prostaglandin-mediated hyperplasia - as the reaction of the epidermis to wounding - may be regarded as an essential part of a self-defense mechanism of the epidermis, with PGE immediately synthesized and released upon tissue damage as an SOS signal. This process would then be obligatory for the induction of the regenerative process.

IV. ON THE ROLE OF PROSTAGLANDINS IN TUMOR PROMOTION

Since tumor promoters induce a prostaglandin-mediated hyperplastic transformation of the epidermis which may be necessary for tumor promotion, indomethacin should inhibit the process of tumor promotion at least by influencing the proliferative aspect of the whole process. The results of tumor promotion experiments indicate a dose-dependent inhibitory effect of indomethacin, as measured as tumor rate or tumor yield (Table 3), confirming data obtained by others (Slaga et al., 1973; Viaje et al., 1977; Verma et al., 1980). However, no inhibitory effect of indomethacin on tumor promotion was observed using the Sencar mouse (Fischer et al., 1980a,b). To our surprise, inhibition of tumor promotion by indomethacin in our NMRI mice can be reversed by simultaneous treatment with $PGF_{2\alpha}$ but not with PGE_2 (Table 3). Contrary to PGE_2, $PGF_{2\alpha}$ is not able to release the indomethacin inhibition of the induction by TPA of cell proliferation. Whether this change in the epidermal responsiveness to prostaglandins reflects an alteration of the chronic hyperplastic epidermis or whether F-type prostaglandins are involved in a promotion-specific effect remains to be established.

A further investigation of the functions and the mechanism of action of prostaglandins in epidermal hyperproliferation and in skin tumor promotion promises to yield more information on the nature of endogenous regulatory mechanisms in epidermis and their disturbance by wounding, mitogenic stimuli and tumor promoting agents.

Table 3: Effect of indomethacin and prostaglandins on TPA-induced tumor promotion.

For each group , 16 female NMRI mice (7 weeks old) were initiated by topical application of 100 nmol dimethylbenz(a)anthracene (dissolved in 0.1 ml acetone) on the shaved back skin. One week later the treatments with either acetone (controls), prostaglandins, indomethacin, and TPA were started. Indomethacin was applied 30 min prior to and prostaglandins simultaneously with each TPA-application.

treatment	nmol/animal	Tumor formation					
		after 12 weeks		after 15 weeks		after 18 weeks	
		rate %	yield %	rate %	yield %	rate %	yield %
acetone		0	0	0	0	0	0
TPA	5	100	4.6	100	7.4	100	7.2
TPA + indomethacin	5+ 75	67	3.4	78	4.2	84	4.6
TPA + indomethacin	5+25	64	3.2	72	4.1	72	4.2
TPA + indomethacin	5+550	36	0.7	44	1.7	44	1.6
TPA + indomethacin+ PGE$_2$	5+550+15	36	0.9	56	1.6	50	1.6
TPA + indomethacin+ PGE$_2$	5+550+60	50	1.1	56	1.9	62	1.9
TPA + indomethacin+ PGF$_{2\alpha}$	5+550+15	44	1.9	78	3.0	86	3.2
TPA + indomethacin+ PGF$_{2\alpha}$	5+550+30	72	3.1	86	4.1	92	4.8
PGE$_2$	30	0	0	0	0	0	0
PGF$_{2\alpha}$	30	0	0	0	0	0	0

REFERENCES

Argyris TS (1981). The regulation of epidermal hyperplastic growth. CRC Critical Reviews in Toxicology 9:151.
Ashendel CL, Boutwell RK (1979). Prostaglandin E and F levels in mouse epidermis are increased by tumor-promoting phorbol esters. Biochem Biophys Res Commun 90:623.
Bentley-Philipps CB, Paulli-Jorgensen H, Marks R (1977). The effects of prostaglandins E_1 and $F_{2\alpha}$ on epidermal growth. Arch Derm Res 257:233.
Bertsch S, Csontos K, Schweizer J, Marks F (1976). Effect of mechanical stimulation on cell proliferation in mouse epidermis and on growth regulation by endogenous factors (chalones). Cell Tissue Kinet 9:207.
Bertsch S, Marks F (1981). A comparative study on wound healing in neonatal and adult mouse epidermis in vivo. Cell Tissue Kinet, in press.
Bresnick E, Meunier P, Lamden M (1979). Epidermal prostaglandins after topical application of a tumor promoter. Cancer Lett 7:121.
Brune K, Kalin H, Schmidt R, Hecker E (1978). Inflammatory, tumor initiating and promoting activities of polycyclic aromatic hydrocarbons and diterpene esters in mouse skin as compared with their prostaglandin releasing potency in vitro. Cancer Lett 4:333.
Clark-Lewis J, Murray AW (1978). Tumor promotion and the induction of epidermal ornithine decarboxylase activity in mechanically stimulated mouse skin. Cancer Res 38:494.
Crutchley DJ, Conanan LB, Maynard JB (1980). Induction of plasminogen activator and prostaglandin biosynthesis in HeLa Cells by 12-O-tetradecanoylphorbol-13-acetate. Cancer Res 40:849.
Delcos KG, Nagle DS, Blumberg PM (1980). Specific binding of phorbol ester tumor promoters to mouse skin. Cell 19:1025.
Dunphy WG, Kochenburger RJ, Castagna M, Blumberg PM (1981). Kinetics and subcellular localization of specific (H)phorbol-12,13-dibutyrate binding by mouse brain. Cancer Res 41: 2640.
Eaglestein WH, Weinstein GD (1975). Prostaglandin and DNA synthesis in human skin. Possible relationships to ultraviolet light effects. J Invest Dermatol 64:386.
Fischer SM, Gleason FL, Bohrman JS, Slaga TJ (1980). Prostaglandin modulation of phorbol ester skin tumor promotion. Carcinogenesis 1:245.
Fischer SM, Gleason, GL, Mills GD, Slaga TJ (1980). Indome-

thacin enhancement of TPA tumor promotion in mice. Cancer Lett 10:343

Flower RJ, Gryglewski R, Herbaczyuska-Cedro K, Vane JR (1972) The effects of antiinflammatory drugs on prostaglandin biosynthesis. Nature New Biol 238:104.

Fürstenberger G, Hecker E (1972). Zum Wirkungsmechanismus cocarcinogener Pflanzeninhaltsstoffe. Planta Med 22:241.

Fürstenberger G, Marks F (1978). Indomethacin inhibition of cell proliferation induced by the phorbol ester TPA is reversed by prostaglandin E_2 in mouse epidermis in vivo. Biochem Biophys Res Commun 84:1103.

Fürstenberger G, DeBravo M, Bertsch S, Marks F (1979). The effect of indomethacin on cell proliferation induced by chemical and mechanical means in mouse epidermis in vivo. Res Commun Chem Pathol Pharmacol 24:533.

Fürstenberger G, Marks F (1979). Tumor promoter 12-O-tetradecanoylphorbol-acetate is not a prostaglandin E type agonist. Cancer Lett 6:73.

Fürstenberger G, Marks F (1980). Early prostaglandin E synthesis is an obligatory event in the induction of cell proliferation in mouse epidermis in vivo by the phorbol ester TPA. Biochem Biophys Res Commun 92:749.

Fürstenberger G, Berry DL, Sorg B, Marks F (1981a). Skin tumor promotion by phorbol esters is a two-stage process. Proc Natl Acad Sci USA, in press.

Fürstenberger G, Berry DL, Sorg B, Marks F (1981b). The phorbol ester of vitamin A acid is an irritant mitogenic agent and an incomplete tumor promoter in mouse skin in vivo. J Cancer Res Clin Oncol 99:A26.

Fürstenberger G, Delescluse C, Fischer SM, Richter H, Marks F (1981c). Early induction of the arachidonic acid cascade and stimulation of DNA synthesis by TPA in murine and guinea pig epidermal cells in culture. In Hecker E, Fusenig NE, Kunz W, Marks F, Thielmann HW (eds): "Cocarcinogenesis and Biological Effects of Tumor Promoters", Carcinogenesis, a Comprehensive Survey, Vol , New York: Raven Press, in press.

Fürstenberger G, Richter H, Fusenig NE, Marks F (1981d). Arachidonic acid and prostaglandin E_2 release and enhanced cell proliferation induced by the phorbol ester TPA in a murine epidermal cell line. Cancer Lett 11:191.

Fürstenberger G, Richter H, Argyris RS, Marks F (1981e). 4-O-Methyl TPA is not an appropriate negative control compound for studies on the biological effects of phorbol ester tumor promoters. Submitted for publication.

Hammarström S, Hamberg M, Samuels B, Duell M, Stawiski M,

Vorhees JJ (1975). Increased concentrations of nonesterified arachidonic acid, 12L-hydroxy-5,8,10,14-eicosatetraenoic acid, prostaglandin E_2 and prostaglandin $F_{2\alpha}$ in epidermis of psoriasis. Proc Natl Acad Sci USA 72:5130.

Hammarström S, Lindgren JA, Marcelo C, Duell EA, Anderson Th F, Vorhees JJ (1979). Arachidonic acid transformation in normal and psoriatic skin. J Invest Dermatol 73:180.

Hecker E (1978). Structure-activity relationships in diterpene esters, irritant and cocarcinogenic to mouse skin. In Slaga TJ, Sivak A, Boutwell RK (eds): "Mechanisms of Tumor Promotion and Cocarcinogenesis" Carcinogenesis, a Comprehensive Survey, Vol. 2, New York: Raven Press, p 11.

Hennings H, Boutwell RK (1970). Studies on the mechanism of skin tumor promotion. Cancer Res 30:312.

Kischer CW (1969). Accelerated maturation of chick embryo skin treated with a prostaglandin (PGB_1): An electron microscopic study. Am J Anat 124:491.

Levine L, Hassid A (1977) Effects of phorbol-12,13-diesters on prostaglandin production and phospholipase activity in canine kidney (MDCK) cells. Biochem Biophys Res Commun 79: 477.

Lowe NJ, Stoughton RB (1977). Effects of topical prostaglandin E_2 analogue on normal hairless mouse epidermal DNA-synthesis. J Invest Dermatol 68:134.

Marks F, Bertsch S, Grimm W, Schweizer J (1978). Hyperplastic transformation and tumor promotion in mouse epidermis: possible consequences of disturbances of endogenous mechanisms controlling proliferation and differentiation. In Slaga TJ, Sivak A, Boutwell RK (eds): "Mechanisms of Tumor Promotion and Cocarcinogenesis", Carcinogenesis, a Comprehensive Survey, Vol 2, New York: Raven Press, p 97.

Marks F, Bertsch S, Fürstenberger G (1979). Ornithine decarboxylase activity, cell proliferation and tumor promotion in mouse epidermis in vivo. Cancer Res 39:4183.

Marks F, Fürstenberger G (1980). Effect of phorbol ester application and other mitogenic treatments on 3',5'-cyclic-nucleotide phosphodiesterase activity in mouse epidermis in vivo. Hoppe Seyler's Z Physiol Chem 361:1641.

Marks F, Berry DL, Bertsch S, Fürstenberger G, Richter H (1981a). On the relationship between epidermal hyperproliferation and skin tumor promotion. In Hecker E, Fusenig NE, Kunz W, Marks F, Thielmann HW (eds): "Cocarcinogenesis and Biological Effects of Tumor Promoters" Carcinogenesis, a Comprehensive Survey, Vol , New York: Raven Press, in press.

Marks F, Bertsch S, DeBravo M, Fürstenberger G (1981b). Studies on the trigger mechanism of epidermal hyperplasia. In Marks R, Christophers E (eds): "The Epidermis in Disease", Lancaster: MRP press, p 193.

Marks F, Fürstenberger G, Kownatzki, E (1981c). Prostaglandin E-mediated mitogenic stimulation of mouse epidermis in vivo by divalent cation ionophore A 23187 and by tumor promoter TPA. Cancer Res 41:696.

Mufson, RA, Defeo D, Weinstein IB (1979). Effects of phorbol ester tumor promoters on arachidonic acid metabolism in chick embryo fibroblasts. Mol Pharmacol 16:569.

Mufson RA, Fischer SM, Verma AK, Gleason GL, Slaga TJ, Boutwell RK (1979). Effects of 12-O-tetradecanoylphorbol-13-acetate and mezerein on epidermal ornithine decarboxylase activity, isoproterenol-stimulated levels of cyclic adenosine 3,5-monophosphate, and induction of mouse skin tumors. Cancer Res 39:4791.

O'Brien TG, Simsiman RC, Boutwell RK (1975). Induction of the polyamine synthetic enzymes in mouse epidermis and their specificity for tumor promotion. Cancer Res 35:2426.

Slaga TJ, Scribner JD (1973). Inhibition of tumor initiation and promotion by anti-inflammatory agents J Natl Cancer Inst 51:1723.

Slaga TJ, Sivak A, Boutwell RK (1978). "Mechanism of Tumor Promotion and Cocarcinogenesis, A Comprehensive Survey, Vol 2, New York: Raven Press.

Slaga TJ, Fischer SM, Nelson K, Gleason GL (1980). Studies on the mechanism of skin tumor promotion: evidence for several stages of promotion. Proc Natl Acad Sci USA 77:3659.

Smythies JR, Bennington F, Morin RD (1975). On the molecular structure of receptors for cocarcinogens and some anti-cancer drugs. Psychoneuroendocrinology 1:123.

Smythies JR (1979). On the molecular structure of some prostaglandin receptors. Prostaglandins and Medicine 2:393.

Tashjian AH, Ivey JL, Delclos B, Levine L (1978). Stimulation of prostaglandin production in bone by phorbol esters and melittin. Prostaglandins 16:221.

Verma AK, Rice HM, Boutwell RK (1977). Prostaglandins and skin tumor promotion: Inhibition of tumor promoter-induced ornithine decarboxylase activity in epidermis by inhibitors of prostaglandin synthesis. Biochem Biophys Res Commun 79:1160.

Verma AK, Ashendel CL, Boutwell RK (1980). Inhibition by prostaglandin synthesis inhibitors of the induction of epidermal ornithine decarboxylase activity, the accumulation of prostaglandins, and tumor promotion caused by 12-O-tetradecanoylphorbol-13-acetate. Cancer Res 40:308.

Viaje A, Slaga TJ, Wigler M, Weinstein IB (1977). The effects of antiinflammatory agents on mouse skin tumor promotion, epidermal DNA synthesis, phorbol ester-induced proliferation and production of plasminogen activator. Cancer Res 37:1530.

Yamasaki H, Mufson RA, Weinstein IB (1979). Phorbol ester induced prostaglandin synthesis and (^{3}H)-TPA metabolism by TPA-sensitive and TPA-resistant Friend erythroleukemia cells. Biochem Biophys Res Commun 89:1018.

Ziboh VA, Lord JT, Penney NS (1977). Alterations of prostaglandin E_2-9-ketoreductase activity in proliferating skin. J Lipid Res 18:37.

**Prostaglandins and Cancer: First
International Conference, pages 255-264
Published by Alan R. Liss, Inc., 150 Fifth Avenue, New York, NY 10011**

MODULATION OF PROSTAGLANDIN SYNTHESIS AND TUMOR PROMOTION

Susan M. Fischer and Thomas J. Slaga

Biology Division, Oak Ridge National Laboratory

Oak Ridge, Tennessee 37830

Investigations into the role of prostaglandins in tumor promotion began with the observation that 12-0-tetradecanoyl-phorbol-13-acetate (TPA) induces cytotoxicity, inflammation and vascular permeability changes (Janoff et al 1970). Although most promoters appear to be irritants that induce epidermal hyperplasia, not all irritants or inflammatory hyperplastic agents are promoters (Berenblum 1944 and Saffiotti & Shubik 1963). The essential nature of inflammation to tumor promotion was suggested by several studies (Belman & Troll 1972 and Scribner & Slaga 1973) which showed that the anti-inflammatory steroids dexamethasone and fluocinolone acetonide could completely suppress tumor promotion in mouse skin. Besides being strong inhibitors of TPA induced inflammation and epidermal DNA synthesis, they have also been shown to inhibit prostaglandin biosynthesis at the level of phospholipase A_2 (Flower 1978, Blackwell et al 1980).

The second series of observations implicating the prostaglandins in TPA induced inflammation are the stimulation of phospholipid metabolism in mouse skin (Rohrschneider & Boutwell 1973), the demonstration that some methyl esters of fatty acids, such as methyl 12-oxo-trans-10-octadecanoate, are weak tumor promoters (Arffman & Glavind 1971) and that these and several related oxidation products of fatty acids are also highly hyperplasiogenic in the epithelial newt skin test (Glavind & Arffman 1970).

There are numerous reports that TPA induces prostaglandin production in a variety of systems. Using dog kidney cells (MDCK) Levine and Ohuchi (1978) found that TPA, but not

the non-promoting 4α-phorbol 12,13-didecanoate stimulated
arachidonic acid release, prostaglandin biosynthesis and
morphological changes. Bresnick et al (1979) as well as
Verma et al (1980) reported that TPA induces a striking increase in the PGE levels in CD-1 mouse skin. Additionally,
Verma et al (1977) demonstrated that the inhibition of TPA
induced ornithine decarboxylase by indomethacin could be
overridden by the addition of PGE's but not PGF's.

The above studies suggested that tumor promotion could
be modified (or perhaps mimicked) through the application of
either exogenous prostaglandins or inhibitors of prostaglandin synthesis. We therefore began our studies on the
involvement of prostaglandins in promotion by looking at the
effect of topical application of the various prostaglandins
either alone or with TPA on initiated mouse skin. In most
of our studiés tumors were induced on SENCAR mice by the two
step procedure of initiation (one application of a subcar-
cinogenic dose of 7,12-methylbenz(a)anthracene) and promotion (repetitive applications of the noncarcinogenic promoter TPA). The results of this series of experiments (described in detail by Fischer et al 1980a) suggested that the
effects of the different prostaglandins on tumor production
depends both on the particular agent used as well as the time
of application. More specifically, $PGF_{2\alpha}$ enhances TPA promotion by 30 to 60% at doses of 1-10 ug. PGE_1, on the other
hand, inhibits TPA tumor production even at doses as low as
1 ug. Experiments with PGE_2 showed that time of application
with respect to TPA is important. When PGE_2 was applied 45
min or more before TPA, a slight enhancement in tumors was
seen but if PGE_2 was applied within 15 min of TPA, a 30-40%
inhibition occurred. Arachidonic acid had little effect at
lower doses but showed dramatic inhibition at doses over 100
ug. On the other hand, linoleic acid at the same doses had
no effect on TPA-induced tumors, suggesting that arachidonic
acid is active not because of its fatty acid characteristics
but because it is a direct precursor to the prostaglandins
and lipoxygenase products. It is important to note that
none of the PG's tested or arachidonic acid had tumor promoting ability when used alone on initiated mice.

While the results of the above studies suggested that the
prostaglandins are involved in promotion, this approach is
complicated by the fact that TPA induces PG synthesis on its
own in which the exogenously added prostaglandin may have an
effect on the endogenously generated prostaglandin. For this

reason, the next series of studies involved the use of inhibitors of various pathways of arachidonic acid metabolism.
As has been previously mentioned, the steroidal anti-
inflammatory agents, which have been reported to inhibit
phospholipase A_2, are very potent inhibitors of tumor promotion as is the phospholipase inhibitor dibromoacetophenone
(see Table 1). Based on this information it was felt that
the non-steroidal anti-inflammatory agents such as indomethacin should also inhibit promotion, particularly since
Verma et al (1977) had demonstrated that indomethacin suppresses TPA induced ornithine decarboxylase activity in the
CD-1 mouse skin. In later studies he reported (1980) that
indomethacin also inhibited promotion, as did Furstenberger
& Marks (1980) in the NMRI mouse. However, as has been previously reported by our laboratory (Fischer et al 1980b) in
the SENCAR mouse, indomethacin can both enhance and inhibit
promotion in a dose dependent and time dependent manner depending on the dose range used. Indomethacin is most effective in enhancing or inhibiting promotion when applied 2
hr prior to TPA. Enhancement of promotion occurs at doses
of 25 to 100 ug. Doses above 100 ug (i.e. 200 ug) are inhibitory and the skin sloughing that results at these doses
suggests this inhibition is due to toxicity. Results from
preliminary experiments currently underway in our laboratory
on CD-1 and SENCAR mice suggests that the difference between
the two stocks of mice may be one of differing sensitivities
to indomethacin and that with the low doses, indomethacin can
enhance tumor production in CD-1 mice and at high doses can
inhibit. The effectiveness of indomethacin in enhancing
tumor promotion is most striking using the multi-stage promotion protocol in which a limited number of TPA applications
(first stage) is followed by repetitive applications of
mezerein (second stage), a weak complete promoter (Slaga et al
1980 a & b). As shown in Fig. 1, when indomethacin is given
2 hr before TPA in the first stage of the two-stage promotion,
enhancement is dramatic (200%). Additional experiments (data
not shown) have given similar results (enhancement of up to
500% depending on the dose of indomethacin). Indomethacin
has only a mildly enhancing effect on the second stage of promotion. Preliminary studies (not shown) suggest that indomethacin can slightly induce dark cells alone as well as enhancing the induction by TPA. This corresponds well with the
fact that TPA (and other first stage promoters) induces "dark"
basal cells (Klein-Szanto et al 1980) to a much larger extent
than does mezerein.

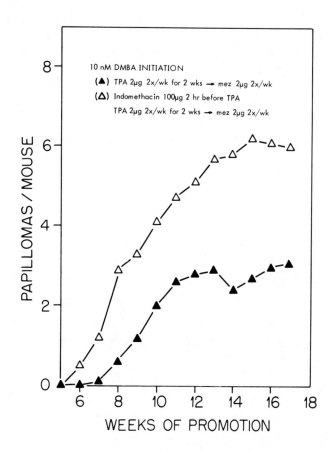

Figure 1. Indomethacin enhancement of stage one of multi-stage tumor promotion. Promotion was carried out by applying indomethacin (100 ug) 2 hr prior to TPA (1 ug) twice weekly for 2 weeks (stage one) followed by twice weekly applications of mezerein (2 ug) for the remainder of the experiment (stage two).

In additional tumor experiments, inhibitors were employed that were effective in blocking both the lipoxygenase and cyclo-oxygenase pathways or only thromboxane synthesis. As shown in Table 1, phenidone, an inhibitor of both lipoxygenase and prostaglandin synthetase, inhibits promotion by 45% when applied with TPA. Another dual inhibitor, 5,8,11,14 eico-satetraenoic acid (ETYA) reduced the tumor yield by 45% when given 2 hr before TPA. The thromboxane synthetase inhibitors

imidazolacetophenone and imidazol-phenol (RO22-3581 and -3582,
Hoffman-LaRoche) also significantly inhibited tumor promotion
suggesting that thromboxane may be integrally involved.
Measurement of thromboxane levels in skin after TPA treatment
are currently under study. The phospholipase inhibitor, dibromoacetophenone, has been shown in two different experiments to almost completely block promotion at the 500 ug dose
level.

Table 1

Group	Inhibitor	Amount (ug)	papillomas per mouse at 15 wks	% Inhibition
1	dibromoacetophenone	50	7.1	none
2	"	100	5.5	5
3	"	500	0.8	86
4	ETYA (2 h before TPA)	100	3.2	45
5	RO-22-358-2	100	1.5	75
6	RO-22-3581	100	3.9	34
7	phenidone	100	3.2	45
8	none	---	5.8	--

The effect of prostaglandin or thromboxane synthetase
inhibitors on TPA tumor promotion. Groups of 30 SENCAR mice,
7 to 9 weeks old, received a single topical application of
10 nmole 7,12 dimethylbenz[a]anthracene in 0.2 ml acetone.
After 1 week, twice weekly applications of 1 ug TPA were
given for 15 weeks. The inhibitors were applied simultaneously except where noted. The number and incidence of
papillomas were recorded weekly.

The results of the inhibitor studies suggested not only
that arachidonic acid metabolites are important, and perhaps
even essential in tumor promotion, but also that the most important metabolites may not be the prostaglandins themselves.
It has been shown in human platelets (Hamberg 1974), that inhibition of prostaglandin synthesis results in elevated
levels of the hydroperoxy- and hydroxy-eicosatetraenoic acid
(HPETE and HETE). Since these products may be important in
cell proliferation, as indicated by the high levels found in
the hyper-proliferative disease psoriasis (Hammarstrom 1979),
they may be responsible, at least in part, for the hyperplasia
and inflammation seen with TPA treatments. It was of interest,
therefore to determine whether indomethacin could cause an

elevation of HPETE's in TPA treated mouse skin. This was done by using primary cultures of adult mouse epidermal cells, prelabelled with ^{14}C-arachidonic acid, and exposing them to TPA with and without indomethacin for appropriate time periods. The acidified media was extracted twice with ethyl acetate, and small volumes of the dried extract applied to silica thin layer plates which were developed in an "A-9" solvent system (Hamberg et al 1966). Arachidonic acid, various prostaglandins and a mixture of HPETE's (kindly provided by L. Marnett) were used as reference compounds. After the standards were visualized by iodine vapors, the appropriate corresponding sample zones were scraped for scintillation counting. The results, shown in Fig. 2, indicate that indomethacin does shunt arachidonic acid into the lipoxygenase pathway. It is also striking that the major products of arachidonic acid metabolism in cultured adult epidermal cells appear to be the lipoxygenase products. This information further suggested that the HPETE's are intimately involved in promotion; tumor experiments using a mixture of HPETE's (supplied by L. Marnett) are currently underway.

The HPETE's are also interesting in light of the recent work by Slaga et al (1981) that shows that certain peroxides can act as tumor promoters. In particular, he has studied benzoyl peroxide, a widely used anti-acne agent which is also a free radical generating compound, and found that it has complete promoting ability. Other free radical generating peroxides such as lauryl peroxide and chloroperbenzoic acid also have promoting activity (T. J. Slaga, unpublished data). The involvement of free radicals in promotion has been previously suggested by Goldstein et al (1981), who showed that phorbol ester tumor promoters stimulate superoxide anion radical production by human polymorphonuclear leukocytes and that the tumor promoter-induced free radicals can be inhibited by such inhibitors of promotion as protease inhibitors, retinoids and anti-inflammatory steroids (Goldstein et al 1979). Recently Slaga et al (unpublished data) found that butylated hydroxyanisole and butylated hydroxytoluene are effective inhibitors of TPA and benzoyl peroxide promotion. The generation of free radicals during the promotion process may lead directly or indirectly to membrane lipid peroxidation and genome damage, in a manner similar to that found in radiation-induced carcinogenesis.

Of the many biochemical effects elicited by TPA, one of the more interesting changes is that of inhibition of

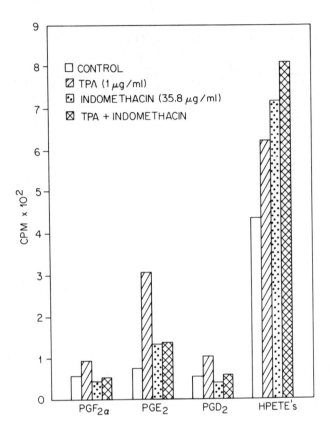

Figure 2. In vitro hydroperoxyeicosatetraenoic acid (HPETE's) production in adult murine epidermal cells in response to TPA and indomethacin. Primary cultures prelabeled with $[^{14}C]$arachidonic acid were treated for 4 hr with either acetone, 1 ug/ml TPA, 35.8 ug/ml indomethacin, or both. Prostaglandins and HPETE's were extracted from the media and separated by TLC.

metabolic cooperation as seen in the cell communication assay described by Yotti et al (1979) and Murray & Fitzgerald (1979). In this assay, wild-type Chinese hamster V79 cells (6-thioguanine-sensitive) reduce the number of colonies formed by 6-thioguanine resistant cells through a form of intracellular communication (Yotti et al 1979). TPA effectively inhibits this communication as does benzoyl peroxide, although to a lesser extent (Slaga et al 1981).

They suggested that the mechanism by which benzoyl peroxide promotes skin tumors may result from membrane changes caused by free radicals. This suggested the possibility that the HPETE's might also inhibit metabolic cooperation. As seen in Table 2, the ability of the HPETE's (a mixture supplied by L. Marnett) to inhibit cell communication indicates that they behave as would be expected of a weak tumor promoter.

Table 2

Dose ug/ml	Agent	Recovery (% ± S.E.)
0	---	12.7 ± 1.99
0.01	HPETE's	14.6 ± 1.97
0.1	HPETE's	20.0 ± 1.07*
0.01	TPA	73.4 ± 5.46

Effects of HPETE's (mixture supplied by L. Marnett) on the recovery of 6-thioguanine-resistant Chinese hamster V79 cells. The procedure has been described (Yotti 1979); S.E., standard error; the 0.1 ug HPETE is significantly different (p =.05) from the acetone control using the Student's t-test.

The above studies indicate that while the prostaglandins or other metabolites of arachidonic acid metabolism that have been tested to date are not tumor promoters themselves, they play an integral part in the underlying mechanism of tumor promotion. The thromboxanes, prostacyclin and leukotrienes have not yet been tested; information on the contribution of these to tumor promotion will be of value. Additional work is clearly needed to clarify the role(s) of the specific arachidonate metabolites in tumor promotion.

References

1 Arffmann E, Glavind J (1971). Tumor promoting activity of fatty acid methyl esters in mice. Experientia 27:1465.
2 Belman S, Troll W (1972). The inhibition of croton oil promoted mouse skin tumorigenesis by steroid hormones. Cancer Res 32: 450.
3 Berenblum I (1944). Irritation and carcinogenesis. Arch Pathol 38: 233.
4 Blackwell GJ, Cornuccio R, DiRosa M, Flower RJ, Parente L, Persico P (1980). Macrocortin: a polypeptide causing the anti-phospholipase effect of glucocorticoids. Nature 287: 147.

5   Bresnick E, Meunier P, Lamden M (1979). Epidermal
    prostaglandins after topical application of a tumor pro-
    moter. Cancer Letters 7: 121.
6   Fischer SM, Gleason GL, Bohrman JS, Slaga TJ (1980a).
    Prostaglandin modulation of phorbol ester skin tumor
    promotion. Carcinogenesis 1: 245.
7   Fischer SM, Gleason GL, Mills GD, Slaga TJ (1980b). Indo-
    methacin enhancement of TPA tumor promotion in mice.
    Cancer Letters 10: 343.
8   Flower RJ (1978). Steroidal anti-inflammatory drugs as
    inhibitors of phospholipase A_2. In Galli C et al (eds):
    "Adv in Prostaglandin and Thromboxane Research" Vol 3,
    New York: Raven Press, p 105.
9   Furstenberger G, Marks F (1980). Studies on the role of
    prostaglandins in the induction of cell proliferation
    and hyperplasia and in tumor promotion in mouse skin.
    In Hecker E et al (eds): "Symp. on Cocarcinogenesis and
    Biological Effects of Tumor Promoters" Raven Press (in
    press).
10 Glavind J, Arffmann E (1970). The possible carcinogenic
    properties of altered lipids. Acta path microbiol scand
    Sect A 78: 345.
11 Goldstein BD, Witz G, Amoruso M, Troll W (1979). Pro-
    tease inhibitors antagonize the activation of polymorpho-
    nuclear leukocyte oxygen consumption. Biochem Biophys
    Res Commun 88: 854.
12 Goldstein BD, Witz G, Amoruso M, Stone DS, Troll W (1981).
    Stimulation of human polymorphonuclear leukocyte super-
    oxide anion radical production by tumor promoters. Cancer
    Letters 11: 157.
13 Hamberg M, Samuelsson B (1966). Prostaglandins in human
    seminal plasma. J Biol Chem 241: 257.
14 Hamberg M, Svensson J, Samuelsson B (1974). Prosta-
    glandin endoperoxides: A new concept concerning the mode
    of action and release of prostaglandins. Proc Natl Acad
    Sci 7: 3824.
15 Hammarstrom S, Lindgren JA, Marcelo C, Duell EA,
    Anderson TF, Voorhees JJ (1979). Arachidonic acid trans-
    formations in normal and psoriatic skin. J Invest
    Dermatol 73: 180.
16 Janoff A, Klassen A, Troll W (1970). Local vascular
    changes induced by the cocarcinogen phorbol myristate
    acetate. Cancer Res 30: 2568.
17 Klein-Szanto AJP, Major SK, Slaga TJ (1980). Induction
    of dark keratinocytes by 12-0-tetradecanoyl-phorbol-13-
    acetate and mezerein as an indicator of tumor-promoting-
    efficiency. Carcinogenesis 1: 399.

18   Levine L, Okuchi K (1978). Stimulation by carcinogens
      and promoters of prostaglandin production by dog kidney
      (MDCK) cells in culture. Cancer Res 38: 4142.
19   Murray AW, Fitzgerald DJ (1979). Tumor promoters inhibit
      metabolic cooperation in cocultures of epidermal and 3T3
      cells. Biochem Biophys Res Commun 91: 395.
20   Rohrschneider LR, Boutwell RK (1973). The early stimu-
      lation of phospholipid metabolism by 12-0-tetradecanoyl-
      phorbol-13-acetate and its specificity for tumor promotion
      Cancer Res 33: 1945.
21   Saffiotti U, Shubik P(1963). Studies on promoting action
      of skin carcinogenesis. Natl Cancer Inst Monogr 10: 489.
22   Scribner JD, Slaga TJ (1973). Multiple effects of dexa-
      methasone on protein synthesis and hyperplasia caused by
      a tumor promoter. Cancer Res 33: 542.
23   Slaga TJ, Fischer SM, Nelson KG, Gleason GL (1980a).
      Studies on the mechanism of skin tumor promotion: Evi-
      dence for several stages in promotion. Proc Natl Acad
      Sci. 77: 3659.
24   Slaga TJ, Klein-Szanto AJP, Fischer SM, Weeks CE, Nelson
      K, Major S (1980b). Studies on the mechanism of action
      of anti-tumor promoting agents: Their specificity in two-
      stage promotion. Proc Natl Acad Sci 77: 2251.
25   Slaga TJ, Klein-Szanto AJP, Triplett LL, Yotti LP (1981).
      Skin tumor-promoting activity of benzoyl peroxide, a
      widely used free radical-generating compound. Science
      213: 1023.
26   Verma AK, Rice HM, Boutwell RK (1977). Prostaglandins
      and skin tumor promotion: Inhibition of tumor promoter-
      induced ornithine decarboxylase activity in epidermis by
      inhibitors of prostaglandin synthesis. Biochem Biophys
      Res Commun 79: 1160.
27   Verma AK, Ashendel CL, Boutwell RK (1980). Inhibition by
      prostaglandin synthesis inhibitors of the induction of
      epidermal ornithine decarboxylase activity, the accumu-
      lation of prostaglandins and tumor promotion caused by
      12-0-tetradecanoyl-13-acetate. Cancer Res 40: 308.
28   Yotti LP, Chang CC, Trosko JE (1979). Elimination of
      metabolic cooperation in Chinese Hamster cells by a tumor
      promoter. Science 206: 1089.

Prostaglandins and Cancer: First
International Conference, pages 265-271
© 1982 Alan R. Liss, Inc., 150 Fifth Avenue, New York, NY 10011

THE SOURCE OF ARACHIDONATE FOR PROSTAGLANDIN SYNTHESIS BY
MDCK CELLS

M. Waite, L. Daniel, G. Beaudry

Department of Biochemistry
Bowman Gray School of Medicine, Wake Forest Univ.
Winston-Salem, North Carolina 27103

Levine and co-workers demonstrated that the cocarcinogen
tetradecanoyl phorbol acetate (TPA) caused MDCK cells to
release arachidonate (C20:4) from cellular lipid and to
convert the C20:4 to prostaglandins through the action of
the cyclooxygenase system (Hong and Levine, 1976; Levine and
Moskowitz, 1979; Levine and Ohuchi, 1978; Ohuchi and Levine,
1978). This response is long acting, continuing over a
period of many hours. It was inferred that the deacylation
process was catalyzed by a phospholipase A_2 and that the
stimulation of the cyclooxygenase was dependent upon protein
synthesis (Ohuchi and Levine, 1978). At present there is
considerable controversy over the mechanism of deacylation.
On one hand the group of Smith and Silver concluded that a
phospholipase A_2 is responsible for deacylation in platelets
(Bills et al., 1977; McKean et al., 1981). Rittenhouse-
Simmons (1981), the groups of Majerus (Bell and Majerus,
1980) and of Cuatrecasas (Lapetina et al., 1980) have
proposed that the combined action of a phospholipase C and a
diglyceride lipase was involved. We have provided evidence
that a phospholipase A_2 is responsible for the deacylation
in human and rabbit neutrophils (Chilton et al., 1981; Walsh
et al., 1981a,b). These cells respond acutely to stimuli,
giving maximal deacylation and lipoxygenase or cyclooxygenase
response within minutes. The purpose of this study was to
contrast this acute response with a chronic one, that is,
one that continues to have activity over a period of hours.
In this way we should better understand the various
mechanisms by which cells respond to stimuli by producing
C20:4 metabolites.

For this study we labeled cells with [³H]C20:4 and [¹⁴C]C16:0 (palmitate) for 24 h. The [³H]C20:4 was incorporated into position 2 of phosphatidylethanolamine (PE) and plasmalogen, phosphatidylcholine (PC), and phosphatidylinositol (PI), in that order of percentage of incorporation. On the other hand [¹⁴C]C16:0 was incorporated into PC, PE, sphingomyelin, neutral lipids, and PI, in that order. About 30% of the [¹⁴C]C16:0 was converted to [¹⁴C]C18:1 (oleate); a total of 65% of the [¹⁴C] acids were incorporated into position 1 of the phospholipids. By quantitating the phospholipids, determining the fatty acid composition of each phospholipid, and knowing the [³H]C20:4 content of each phospholipid, we calculated the specific activity of [³H]C20:4 in each phospholipid.

When the labeled cells were challenged with TPA (10^{-10} to 10^{-6} M for 1 h) or the ionophore A23187 (10^{-8} to 10^{-5} M for up to 5 h) the phospholipids were deacylated (Table 1). TPA, unlike A23187, also activated the cyclooxygenase system and produced PGE₂ and PGF₂α that were released from the cells.

Table 1

Identification of products of [³H]20:4 release
from MDCK cells

Product	[³H]Arachidonate release by:			
	No treatment	A23187	TPA	TPA + A23187
Fatty acid	4,341	29,109	8,113	56,501
PGE₂	2,082	3,445	13,582	9,287
PGF₂α	219	387	1,069	1,014
TXB₂	522	1,045	2,585	2,185
Phospholipid	438	2,439	891	3,199
Other	703	1,976	3,302	5,075

MDCK cells were incubated for 18 h with [³H]20:4. The medium was then removed and the cells were washed with minimum essential medium (MEM) without serum. The cells were incubated in MEM without serum ± 10^{-8} M TPA and after 1 h the medium was removed and replaced with MEM ± 10^{-5} M A23187. After 5 h the medium was removed, extracted, and the extract was analyzed by TLC.

When the cellular phospholipids were examined 24 h after stimulation with TPA (10^{-8} M) we found the ethanolamine class of lipids to be the major donors of C20:4. Interestingly, the plasmalogen was the primary source.

Table 2

Origin of arachidonate; percentage derived from each phospholipid

Lipid	Percentage
PE	29.6
Plasmalogen PE	42.6
PS + PI	19.3
PC	8.5

^{32}P labeled cells were cultured 24 h post stimulation with TPA. The extracted lipids were separated by thin layer chromatography and the [^{32}P] content and acyl composition of each lipid was determined and compared with unstimulated cells. The percentages were calculated as the percentage of each lipid times the loss of arachidonate in that lipid.

Indomethacin at a concentration of 1 µg/ml completely blocked the cyclooxygenase system and reduced the deacylation by about 50%. It is possible that the observed reduction in deacylation is the result of product inhibition in which free fatty acid reduced the deacylation. On the other hand, it is possible that indomethacin has no effect on the deacylation but stimulates the incorporation of free fatty acid into phospholipids.

In order to determine if the deacylation process is specific for C20:4, we labeled the cells with various polyunsaturated fatty acids (Table 3). All of the acids used were released when the cells were stimulated. Direct comparison of the relative extent of deacylation of these acids cannot be made, however, since we did not determine the specific activities of each in the various phospholipids.

Table 3

Release of incorporated [^{14}C] fatty acids 12 hours
post stimulation with 10^{-8} M TPA

Fatty acid	Deacylation product		Total prostaglandin	
	+	–	+	–
	% of total label incorporated			
18:2^{9,12}	11.8	4.1	1.0	0.2
20:3^{5,8,11}	15.1	5.8	0.1	0.1
20:3^{8,11,14}	14.4	4.6	5.2	0.5
20:4^{5,8,11,14}	18.0	2.7	5.7	0.4

Cells were labeled with the appropriate [^{14}C] fatty
acid for 18 h. Stimulation with 10^{-8} M TPA was then for
1 h. After the stimulation cells were washed and 1 ml of
HMEM-10 was added. Samples were taken 12 h post stimulation.
The sample of C20:3^{5,8,11} was the generous gift of
Dr. Howard Sprecher.

The acyl composition of the phospholipids was determined
after incubation with or without TPA (Table 4). As was
found with the [^{3}H]C20:4 the ethanolamine lipids were the
primary donors of C20:4. The C20:4 was replaced by saturated
fatty acids primarily, C16:0 and C18:0. Interestingly, PC
contained very little C20:4.

In these studies we were unable to detect any other
products of the proposed deacylation pathways, namely
lysolipids, diglycerides, monoglycerides, or phosphatidic
acid. In order to better understand the process of the
deacylation, we studied the effect of TPA on the incorporation
of [^{32}P] into phospholipids and found TPA caused about a 20%
increase in the incorporation of [^{32}P] into the phospholipids.
This suggests that TPA stimulates the synthesis de novo of
phospholipid. On the other hand, TPA decreased the
incorporation of [^{3}H]C20:4 into phospholipids, primarily PE
and PI. This we interpreted to be a reflection of increased
turnover of the [^{3}H]C20:4 in the presence of TPA. It was

Table 4

Effect of TPA on the phospholipid acyl composition of MDCK cells

Phospholipid	TPA	Fatty acid[a]					
		16:0	16:1	18:0	18:1	20:3	20:4
Diacyl-PE	−	5.4	0.7	26.0	52.7	2.0	13.2
	+	7.4	1.1	28.7	55.8	1.1	5.9
Alk-1-enyl PE	−	8.7	1.6	6.7	65.5	—[b]	17.5
	+	14.1	5.4	14.9	62.6	—	2.9
PI + PS	−	4.0	—	43.7	35.2	7.4	9.8
	+	4.2	1.1	44.3	42.7	4.2	3.3
PC	−	22.1	4.8	13.2	55.5	1.7	2.6
	+	22.3	5.6	13.4	55.7	1.4	1.6

[a]Mass percent.
[b]Not detectable.

significant to note that over a 4 h period 12 h after TPA treatment free $[^3H]C20:4$ was not acted upon by the cyclooxygenase; only after the $[^3H]C20:4$ was incorporated into phospholipid and subsequently released did TPA cause increased prostaglandin synthesis. When we examined the effect of TPA on the loss of $[^3H]C20:4$ and $[^{32}P]$ from phospholipids in prelabeled cells, we found that the $[^3H]C20:4$ decreased more rapidly than $[^{32}P]$. These results, along with the results with $[^{14}C]C16:0$, suggest to us that a deacylation catalyzed by phospholipase A_2 followed by reacylation is the primary pathway stimulated by TPA (and probably ionophore). However, since the de novo synthesis of phospholipids is also stimulated somewhat, we cannot totally exclude at this time other pathways of deacylation being involved in deacylation.

ACKNOWLEDGMENTS

This work was supported by grant CA-12197 and National Research Service Award CA-06885 from the National Institutes of Health, grant R807770 from the Environmental Protection Agency, and a grant from the Forsyth Cancer Service.

REFERENCES

Bell RL, Majerus PW (1980). Thrombin-induced hydrolysis of phosphatidyl inositol in human platelets. J Biol Chem 255:1790.
Bills TK, Smith JB, Silver MJ (1977). Selective release of arachidonic acid from the phospholipids of human platelets in response to thrombin. J Clin Invest 60:1.
Chilton FH, O'Flaherty JT, Walsh CE, Thomas MJ, Wykle RL, DeChatelet LR, Waite M (1981). Platelet activating factor: stimulation of the lipoxygenase pathway in polymorphonuclear leukocytes by 1-0-alkyl-2-0-acetyl-sn-glycero-3-phospho-choline. J Biol Chem, submitted for publication.
Hong SCL, Levine L (1976). Stimulation of prostaglandin synthesis by Bradykinin and thrombin and their mechanisms of action on MC5-5 fibroblasts. J Biol Chem 251:5814.
Lapetina EG, Billah MM, Cuatrecasas P (1980). Rapid acylation and deacylation of arachidonic acid into phosphatidic acid of horse neutrophils. J Biol Chem 255:10966.

Levine L, Moskowitz MA (1979). α and β-adrenergic stimulation of arachidonic acid metabolism in cells in culture. Proc Natl Acad Sci USA 76:6632.

Levine L, Ohuchi K (1978). Retinoids as well as tumour promoters enhance deacylation of cellular lipids and prostaglandin production in MDCK cells. Nature 276:274.

McKean ML, Smith JB, Silver MJ (1981). Formation of lysophosphatidylcholine by human platelets in response to thrombin . Support for the phospholipase A_2 pathway for the liberation of arachidonic acid. J Biol Chem 256:1522.

Ohuchi K, Levine L (1978). Stimulation of prostaglandin synthesis by tumor-promoting phorbol-12,13-diesters in canine kidney (MDCK) cells. J Biol Chem 253:4783.

Rittenhouse-Simmons S (1981). Differential activation of platelet phospholipases by thrombin and ionophore A23187. J Biol Chem 256:4153.

Walsh CE, DeChatelet LR, Thomas MJ, O'Flaherty JT, Waite M (1981a). Effect of phagocytosis and ionophores on release and metabolism of arachidonic acid from human neutrophils. Lipids 16:120.

Walsh CE, Waite M, Thomas MJ, DeChatelet LR (1981b). Release and metabolism of arachidonic acid in human neutrophils. J Biol Chem 256:7228.

**Prostaglandins and Cancer: First
International Conference, pages 273–280
© 1982 Alan R. Liss, Inc., 150 Fifth Avenue, New York, NY 10011**

MODULATION BY INDOMETHACIN, PROSTAGLANDINS AND RETINYL-
ACETATE OF RAT LIVER ORNITHINE DECARBOXYLASE ACTIVITY
INDUCED BY TUMOR PROMOTORS *in vivo*

Dr.Arnold Bisschop and Lucio A.A.van Rooijen

Laboratory for Carcinogenesis and Mutagenesis,
National Institute of Public Health, P.O.Box 1,
3720 BA Bilthoven, The Netherlands

Epidermal tumors on mice can be induced by a two-stage
procedure. In the first stage, called initiation, normally
a single subthreshold dose of carcinogen is applied resulting
in the generation of initiated cells. During the second stage,
promotion, administration of tumor promotor finally leads to
the development of tumors from the previously initiated cells
(Slaga 1978). Although tumor promotion is a long-term process
depending on repeated treatments with promotor, it is generally believed that the responses seen after a single promotor
application are representative for the mechanism of promotion
(Marks 1981). Application of the most potent tumor promotor
12-0-tetradecanyolphorbol-13-acetate (TPA) leads to a multitude of metabolic changes in epidermal cells *in vivo* as well
as *in vitro* (Yuspa 1976; Fürstenberger 1980; Marks 1981). A
striking and perhaps the most extensively studied biochemical
response after tumor promotor treatment is the induction of
ornithine decarboxylase (ODC). Intracellular induction of
epidermal ODC, and presumably also of liver ODC (Weiner 1980;
Bisschop 1981; Kishore 1981), by phorbol esters including
TPA, is believed to be an essential although not sufficient
component of the tumor promotion process (O' Brien 1976;
Yuspa 1976; Verma 1980).

   Vitamin A and its analogs, collectively called retinoids,
inhibit the *in vitro* growth of several cell lines and prevent
the development of various epithelial tumors. Although the
mechanism of vitamin A action is not fully understood it has
been demonstrated in a number of cases that application of
retinoids prior to tumor promotors prevented the induction
of ODC (Verma 1979a; Verma 1979b; Haddox 1979; Bisschop 1981;

Lichti 1981).

Recently, considerable attention has been given to the role of prostaglandins (PGs) in tumor promotion, because of the hyperplasic and inflammatory features of the response on tumor promotors (Fürstenberger 1980; Marks 1981). Moreover, synthesis of PGs occurs in a number of malignant tumors including human breast tumors (Rolland 1980). Studies (Fischer 1980a; Fischer 1980b) indicate that TPA promotion of skin tumors in mice can be modified by PGs. The mechanism by which PGs act in tumor promotion is still unclear. However, the observations of Verma (1977; Verma 1980) that prostaglandin synthetase inhibitors depressed the induction of OCD activity by TPA, and that this effect was completely overcome by treatment with either PGE_1 or PGE_2 are of great importance for the further elucidation of the mechanism of TPA-mediated tumor promotion.

The purpose of this paper is to investigate the mechanism of ODC induction in rat liver by TPA and phenobarbital (PB). Especially the modulating effects of retinyl-acetate (RA), indomethacin, PGE_2, and $PGF_{2\alpha}$ are examined.

It appears from Fig. 1 that a transient increase of ODC activity is observed in the liver of rats which were given a single i.p. dose of 20 μg TPA/kg b.w. Increase of this enzymatic activity occurs after a lag period of two hours and maximal ODC activity is measured 4 hours after injection of the tumor promotor. The two hour lag period is probably not due to a possible low transport rate of TPA to the liver, since uptake studies with 3H-TPA reveal the presence of considerable amounts in the liver even a few minutes after i.p. injection of the tumor promotor (data not shown). The transient character of the TPA-dependent ODC activity change in rat liver is in agreement with previous observations in several systems, although in rat liver the increase is much less pronounced (5-6 fold) than in mouse epidermis (O' Brien 1976; Yuspa 1976; Mufson 1979; Weiner 1980). Induction of ODC activity in rat liver is also seen after injection of PB, a well known rat liver tumor promotor (Peraino 1980) (Fig. 1). Like in the case of TPA, maximal ODC activity is reached 4-5 hours after treatment, and also a lag-time of two hours is observed. The main difference between TPA- and PB-induced ODC activity is the rate at which ODC activity declines after the maximum. This difference might reflect a different effect of the tumor promotors on the cellular

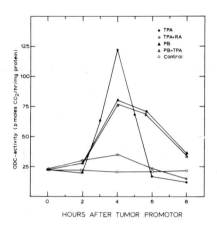

HOURS AFTER TUMOR PROMOTOR

Fig. 1. Induction of rat hepatic ODC activity by i.p. injection of TPA or PB, and the effect of pretreatment with RA.
Groups of 8 female Wistar rats, 3-4 weeks old received a
single i.p. injection of 20 μg TPA or 100 mg PB/kg body
weight. Some groups of rats received 2 μg RA/kg b.w. 1 hr
prior to injection of TPA or PB. At different times after
tumor promotor treatment rats were killed by abdominal
exsanguination under ether anaesthesia and the livers were
quickly removed and transferred in ice-cold 0.02 M KH_2PO_4-
buffer pH 7.2 containing 0.04 mM pyridoxalphosphate,
2 mM dithiothreitol, 0.1 mM EDTA, 5 mM NaF and 0.5 mM phenyl-
methylsulphonylfluoride. Homogenization in a Potter-Elvehjem
yielded homogenates which were centrifuged for 1 hr at
105.000 g in the cold. The supernatants were assayed in duplicate for ODC activity. (Van Wijk 1981; Bisschop 1981).

events leading to the inactivation of ODC. Another explanation might be found in the different times that the hepatocytes are exposed to effective concentrations of TPA and PB,
in consequence of differences in uptake rates, metabolism or
excretion of the promotors. With respect to the role of RA,
Fig. 1 demonstrates that a single dose of 20 mg RA/kg b.w.,
when applied 1 hour prior to TPA or PB has a differential
effect on the induction of ODC by the tumor promotors. Whereas the induction of ODC by TPA is almost completely inhibited
(85%), the same dose of RA has no effect on PB-dependent ODC
induction. For the interpretation of these observations it is
assumed that RA, as may be expected, functions always at the
same cellular site(s), independent of the tumor promotor used.

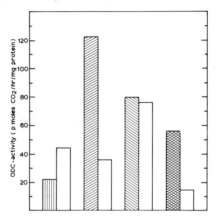

Fig. 2. Induction of rat hepatic ODC activity by either TPA and PB individually or simultaneously.
Groups of 5 or more rats received the following i.p. injections: 20 µg TPA/kg b.w. (▨); 100 mg PB/kg b.w. (▧); 20 µg TPA + 100 mg PB/kg b.w. (▓); control rats (▥) received solvent only. In each pair the open block demonstrates the effect of i.p. injection of 20 mg RA/kg b.w. 1 hr prior to treatment with tumor promotor(s). Rats were killed 4 hrs after tumor promotor injection. (For experimental details see Fig. 1).

TPA is thought to exert its intracellular effect *via* binding to specific membrane receptors (Driedger 1980), whose affinity for its ligand is supposed to be reduced or abolished by retinoids. Inhibition of binding of TPA thus should prevent the transmembrane signal which ultimately gives rise to ODC induction. Until now no specific membrane receptors for PB are described, so it is not known whether the insensitivity of PB-induced ODC activity to RA is based on the absence of specific membrane receptors whose affinity can be modulated by retinoids or that possible existing receptors are insensitive for RA.

Two other interesting phenomena are shown in Fig. 2. Firstly it appears that 20 mg RA/kg b.w. itself causes about a twofold increase of basal ODC activity. Possibly RA interacts at cellular sites *via* which ODC is normally induced. However, the actual mechanism underlying this phenomenon remains to be established. Secondly, Fig. 2 shows that when

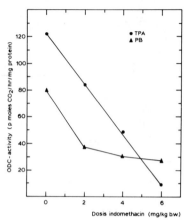

Fig. 3. Effect of indomethacin on tumor promotor-induced liver ODC activity.
Groups of 5 or more rats received increasing doses of indomethacin 1 hr prior to injection with either 20 µg TPA or 100 mg PB/kg b.w.. Rats were killed 4 hrs after treatment with tumor promotor. (For experimental details see Fig. 1).

doses of TPA and PB, which individually enhance ODC activity to 122 and 80 p moles CO_2/hr/mg protein, are administered simultaneously, it only results in an ODC activity of 56 p moles CO_2/hr/mg protein. Since the ODC activity obtained after simultaneous administration is not additive it possibly may be concluded that induction by TPA and PB does not occur in separate populations of liver cells which would be sensitive for either TPA or PB alone. The apparent mutual depression of the induction of ODC by the tumor promotors might be due to cytotoxicity, which also is suggested for the effects when higher than optimal inducing doses of TPA or PB alone are applied (Bisschop 1981). Possibly a more general principle underlies the observations. Lipophilic compounds like TPA and RA, interact at specific sites in the membrane, but cause also a more general "membrane perturbation" which may perhaps give rise to changes in the control of cellular processes such as the induction of ODC (Marks 1981; Fisher 1979).

Corresponding to the observations with indomethacin in mouse epidermal cells it appears that i.p. administration of indomethacin 1 hr prior to TPA blocks the induction of ODC activity in a dose-dependent manner (Fig. 3). At 6 mg

indomethacin/kg b.w. induction of ODC activity by TPA is completely blocked and even control level ODC has been decreased
to about 50% under these experimental conditions. In contrast
to the observations with TPA, PB-induced ODC activity in rat
liver seems to be only partly sensitive to the action of
indomethacin (Fig. 3). Administration of 2 mg indomethacin/
kg b.w. inhibits the induction of ODC activity with 70%,
whereas higher doses indomethacin upto 6 mg/kg b.w. almost do
not further decrease this level. Obviously, for the induction
of ODC activity by TPA in rat liver PGs synthesis is a necessary event. Similar observations were described for TPA-induced ODC in mouse epidermis (Verma 1977; Verma 1980; Marks
1981).

Table 1
Effect of PGE_2 and $PGF_{2\alpha}$ on rat hepatic ODC activity induced
by TPA or PB

PROMOTOR	ODC activity after PG treatment (p moles CO_2/hr/mg protein)		
	None	PGE_2	$PGF_{2\alpha}$
None	20	7	15
TPA	122	62	97
PB	80	26	39

Groups of 5 or more rats received 0.4 mg PGE_2 or PGF_2/kg b.w.
1 hr prior to injection of 20 µg TPA or 100 mg PB/kg b.w..
Rats were killed 4 hrs after tumor promotor treatment or
5 hrs after PG treatment when no tumor promotion was injected.

The suggestion that PGs are involved in the induction of
ODC activity was further tested by the application of 0.4 mg
PGE_2 or $PGF_{2\alpha}$/kg b.w. 1 hour prior to tumor promotor treatment.
However, in contrast to what was expected, both PGE_2 and $PGF_{2\alpha}$
are inhibitory on the induction of ODC by TPA and PB (Table 1)
Perhaps the PG effects are not due to the PGs themselves but
result from metabolism of the applied PGs *in vivo*. Another
explanation might be that extracellular PGs have effects different from intracellularly synthesized PGs.

From the observations described in this paper it is
concluded that the mechanism of intracellular induction of

rat hepatic ornithine decarboxylase by TPA closely resembles
that in mouse skin, according to its sensitivity to retinoids
and prostaglandin synthetase inhibitors. Further investigations are being carried out in order to establish the different modes of action of TPA and PB as inducers of ODC in
rat liver, especially in relation to the involvement of PGs.

Bisschop A, Rooijen van LAA, Derks HJGM, Wijk van R (1981).
Induction of rat hepatic ornithine decarboxylase by the
tumor promotors 12-0-tetradecanoylphorbol-13-acetate and
phenobarbital in vivo; effect of retinyl-acetate. Carcinogenesis: accepted for publication.
Driedger PE, Blumberg PM (1980). Specific binding of phorbol
ester tumor promotors. Proc Natl Acad Sci USA 77:567.
Fisher PB, Flamm M, Schachter D, Weinstein IB (1979). Tumor
promotors induce membrane changes detected by fluorescence
polarization. Biochem Biophys Res Commun 86:1063.
Fischer SM, Gleason GL, Hardin LG, Bohrman JS, Slaga TJ (1980a).
Prostaglandin modulation of phorbol ester skin tumor promotion. Carcinogenesis 1:245.
Fischer SM, Gleason GL, Bohrman JS, Slaga TJ (1980b). Prostaglandin enhancement of skin tumor initiation and promotion.
Advances in Prostaglandin and Thromboxane Research 6:517.
Fürstenberger G, Marks F (1980). Early prostaglandin E synthesis is an obligatory event in the induction of cell pro-
liferation in mouse epidermis in vivo by the phorbol ester
TPA. Biochem Biophys Res Commun 92:749.
Haddox HK, Scott KFF, Russels DH (1979). Retinol inhibition
of ornithine decarboxylase induction and G1 progression in
chinese hamster ovary cells. Cancer Res 39:4930.
Kishore GS, Boutwell RK (1981), Induction of mouse hepatic
ornithine decarboxylase by skin application of 12-0-tetra-
decanoylphorbol-13-acetate. Experientia 37:179. Birkhäuser
Verlag, Basel (Schweiz).
Lichti U, Patterson E, Hennings H, Yuspa SH (1981). Differential retinoic acid inhibition of ornithine decarboxylase
induction by 12-0-tetradecanoylphorbol-13-acetate and by
germicidal ultraviolet light. Cancer Res 41:49.
Marks F, Fürstenberger G, Kownatzki E (1981). Prostaglandin
E-mediated mitogenic stimulation of mouse epidermis in vivo
by divalent cation ionophore A23187 and by tumor promotor
12-0-teradecanoylphorbol-13-acetate. Cancer Res 41:696.
Mufson RA, Fischer SM, Verma AK, Gleason GL, Boutwell RK
(1979). Effects of 12-0-tetradecanoylphorbol-13-acetate and
mezerein on epidermal ornithinedecarboxylase activity,

isoproterenol-stimulated levels of cyclic adenosine 3':5'-monophosphate, and induction of mouse skin tumors in vivo. Cancer Res 39: 4791.

O' Brien TG (1976). The induction of ornithine decarboxylase as an early, possibly obligatory, event in mouse skin carcinogenesis. Cancer Res 36: 2644.

Peraino C, Staffeldt EF, Haugen DA, Lombard LS, Stevens FJ, Fry RJM (1980). Effects of varying the dietary concentration of phenobarbital on its enhancement of 2-acetylamino-fluorene-induced hepatic tumorigenesis. Cancer Res 40:3268.

Rolland PH, Martin PM, Jacquemier J, Rolland AM, Toga M (1980). Prostaglandin in human breast cancer: Evidence suggesting that an elevated prostaglandin synthesis is a marker of high metastatic potential for neoplastic cells. J Natl Cancer Inst 64:1061.

Slaga TJ, Sivak A, Boutwell RK (eds.) (1978). Carcinogenesis Vol.2. New York, Raven Press.

Verma AK, Rice HM, Boutwell RK (1977). Prostaglandins and skin tumor promotion: Inhibition of tumor promotor-induced ornithine decarboxylase activity in epidermis by inhibitors of prostaglandin synthesis. Biochem Biophys Res Commun 79:1166.

Verma AK, Boutwell RK (1979a). Vitamin A acid (retinoic acid) a potent inhibitor of 12-0-tetradecanoylphorbol-13-acetate induced ornithine decarboxylase activity in mouse epidermis. Cancer Res 37:2196.

Verma AK, Shapas BG, Rice HM, Boutwell RK (1979b). Correlation of the inhibition by retinoids of tumor promotor-induced mouse epidermal ornithine decarboxylase activity and of skin tumor promotion. Cancer Res 39:419.

Verma AK, Ashendel LS, Boutwell RK (1980). Inhibition by prostaglandin synthesis inhibitors of the induction of epidermal ornithine decarboxylase activity, the accumulation of prostaglandins, and tumor promotion caused by 12-0-tetradecanoylphorbol-13-acetate. Cancer Res 40:308.

Weiner RA, Byus CV (1980). Induction of ornithine decarboxylase by 12-0-tetradecanoylphorbol-13-acetate in rat tissues. Biochem Biophys Commun 97:1575.

Wijk van R, Louwers HAPM, Bisschop A (1981). The induction of ornithine decarboxylase and DNA synthesis in rat hepatocytes after a single administration of diethylnitrosamine. Carcinogenesis 2:34.

Yuspa SH, Lichti U, Ben T, Patterson E, Hennings H, Slaga TJ, Colburn NH, Kelsey W (1976). Phorbol esters stimulate DNA synthesis and ornithine decarboxylase activity in mouse epidermal cell cultures. Nature (Lond.) 262:402.

Prostaglandins and Cancer: First
International Conference, pages 281–287
© **1982 Alan R. Liss, Inc., 150 Fifth Avenue, New York, NY 10011**

ARACHIDONIC ACID METABOLISM AND INDUCTION OF PLASMINOGEN
ACTIVATOR IN HeLa CELLS BY TUMOR-PROMOTING PHORBOL ESTER

David J. Crutchley and James R. Maynard

Research Division, Miami Heart Institute

Miami Beach, Florida 33140

Transformed cells usually contain elevated levels of
plasminogen activator (PA) when compared to their normal
counterparts. PA is a serine protease which converts the
inactive serum zymogen plasminogen to the fibrinolytic
enzyme plasmin. In addition to their importance in hemostasis, PA and plasmin may facilitate tumor metastasis by
proteolytic digestion of extracellular matrix. In cultured
cells, PA can be induced by several structurally diverse
compounds, including tumor-promoting phorbol esters, retinoids, calcium ionophore, and epidermal growth factor (Chou,
et al., 1977; Lee and Weinstein, 1978; Wilson and Reich,
1978). All of these compounds also stimulate cellular deacylation and arachidonic acid (AA) release (Knapp, et al.,
1977; Levine and Hassid, 1977; Levine and Ohuchi, 1978;
Ohuchi and Levine, 1978). AA is further metabolized by at
least two pathways: via cyclooxygenase to prostaglandins
and thromboxanes or via lipoxygenase to leukotrienes and
other hydroxylated fatty acids. We have investigated whether
metabolites of AA mediate the induction of PA. HeLa cells
were chosen for study since they contain relatively high
levels of PA which increase further following incubation
with the tumor-promoting phorbol ester 12-O-tetradecanoyl-
phorbol-13-acetate (TPA) (Lee and Weinstein, 1978). Our
results show that prostaglandins and other cyclooxygenase metabolites of AA do not mediate the induction of PA, but suggest
that lipoxygenase metabolites may play a role in this process.

METHODS

HeLa cells (American Type Culture Collection) were

grown in Eagle's minimal essential medium supplemented with
10% heat-inactivated fetal calf serum, 5 mM L-glutamine, 50
µg/ml streptomycin, and 50 units/ml penicillin. Confluent
cells in 35 mm dishes were incubated for 6 hr with 2 ml serum-
free medium containing TPA and drugs. After incubation conditioned medium was removed and centrifuged, and E- and F-type
prostaglandins were measured by radioimmunoassay (Clinical
Assays). Cells were washed twice with ice-cold saline A
solution containing 20 mM Hepes, pH 7.4, scraped into the
same solution, and collected by centrifugation. Cells were
extracted with 1 ml Tris buffer (0.1 M, pH 8.1) containing
0.1% Triton X-100. PA in cell extracts was measured by using
a ^{125}I-fibrin dish assay (Unkeless, et al., 1973) with added
human plasminogen (Deutsch and Mertz, 1970). Omission of
plasminogen abolished fibrinolysis. Assays were carried out
at room temperature for up to 3 hr, and results are expressed
in terms of a urokinase internal standard.

RESULTS AND DISCUSSION

HeLa cells had readily measurable PA, which increased
when the cells were incubated with 0.5-50 nM TPA (Figure 1,
left panel). Conditioned medium from untreated cells contained small amounts of prostaglandins E_2 and $F_{2\alpha}$, which
increased significantly when the cells were incubated with
the same doses of TPA (Figure 1, right panel). Changes in
PA were detected after 6 hr, and reached a peak after 18-
24 hr; in contrast, increases in prostaglandins were detected
after 1 hr (data not shown). Hence, changes in AA metabolism
precede those in PA, a finding which is consistent with a
regulatory role of AA metabolites in the induction of the
protease.

The effects of three compounds known to inhibit AA
metabolism were then investigated. The compounds were indomethacin, which blocks cyclooxygenase (Vane, 1971), eicosatetraynoic acid (ETYA) which blocks both cyclooxygenase and
lipoxygenase (Hamberg and Samuelsson, 1974), and nordihydroguaiaretic acid, which readily blocks lipoxygenase but appears
to block cyclooxygenase only at high concentrations (Hamberg,
1976; Panganamala, et al., 1977). Figure 2 shows that indomethacin, 0.01-3 µM, had no effect on the induction of PA.
However, these doses of indomethacin were more than sufficient
to inhibit cyclooxygenase. For example, indomethacin at 0.03
µM reduced the levels of PGE_2 in media from TPA-treated cells

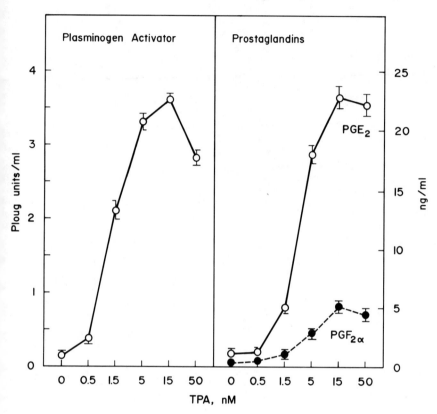

Figure 1. Stimulation of PA and prostaglandin biosynthesis by tumor-promoting phorbol ester TPA. HeLa cells were incubated for 18 hr with serum-free medium containing 0.5-50 nM TPA. PA in cell extracts (left panel) and prostaglandins E_2 and $F_{2\alpha}$ in conditioned medium (right panel) were then measured. Each point is mean±S.E. of quadruplicate dishes.

from 15.1±1.9 ng/ml to 0.9±0.1 ng/ml, while levels of $PGF_{2\alpha}$ fell from 4.5±0.8 ng/ml to 0.2±0.1 ng/ml (mean±S.E., quadruplicate dishes). At 0.1 μM and higher, indomethacin reduced the levels of both prostaglandins to below the limits of detection by the assay (0.1 ng/ml). Thus, in HeLa cells, metabolites of AA derived via cyclooxygenase do not appear to mediate the induction of PA by TPA. Similar results have

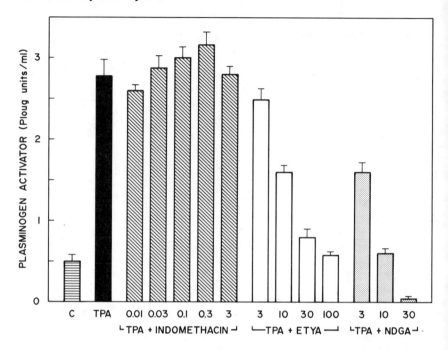

Figure 2. Effects of inhibitors of AA metabolism on the induction of PA in HeLa cells by TPA. Extracts from control cells (▨) showed PA activity. This increased following 6 hr exposure to 15 nM TPA (■). Indomethacin 0.01-3 µM (▨) had no effect on TPA-induced PA. In contrast, ETYA 3-100 µM (□) and nordihydroguaiaretic acid 3-30 µM (NDGA) (▨) produced dose-dependent suppression of TPA-induced PA. Each point is mean±S.E. of triplicate or quadruplicate dishes

been obtained in human foreskin fibroblasts and canine kidney (MDCK) cells (Crutchley, et al., 1980), chick embryo fibroblasts (Mufson, et al., 1979) and mouse macrophages (Hamilton, 1980).

In contrast to indomethacin, the lipoxygenase inhibitors ETYA and nordihydroguaiaretic acid both inhibited the induction of PA by TPA (Figure 2). The inhibition was dose-related; the approximate ID_{50} values were 10 µM for ETYA and 5 µM for nordihydroguaiaretic acid. In contrast to their effects on PA in cells treated with TPA, both inhibitors had relatively little effects on PA in untreated cells (data not shown). Moreover, neither inhibitor produced observable effects on cellular morphology or trypan blue exclusion. Measurement of the cytosolic enzyme lactate dehydrogenase in HeLa cell homogenates showed that incubation of the cells for 6 hr with 15 nM TPA had no effect on levels of the enzyme (control, 20.0 ± 1.1 U/mg; TPA, 22.8 ± 1.3 U/mg; mean$\pm$S.E., n=6). Similar results were obtained with cells incubated with TPA plus 30 μM ETYA (23.3 ± 0.9 U/mg, n=3) or TPA plus 10 μM nor-dihydroguaiaretic acid (19.7 ± 1.2 U/mg, n=3). It is therefore unlikely that the inhibitors exerted their effects on PA induction via non-specific cytotoxicity.

Several of the biological effects of the tumor-promoting phorbol esters have been attributed to their ability to increase cellular prostaglandin synthesis, including ornithine decarboxylase induction (Verma, et al., 1980), epidermal cell proliferation (Furstenberger and Marks, 1980), and bone resorption (Tashjian, et al., 1978). However, other effects appear to be independent of prostaglandins, including morphology changes in MDCK cells (Ohuchi and Levine, 1978). The increased choline phospholipid synthesis induced in bovine lymphocytes by TPA may be mediated via lipoxygenase metabolites of AA (Wertz and Mueller, 1980). Our results suggest that such metabolites may also mediate at least in part the induction of PA. Certainly, the possible contribution of lipoxygenase metabolites to the biological effects of TPA deserves further investigation.

ACKNOWLEDGMENTS

We wish to thank Dr. W. E. Scott of Hoffmann-LaRoche for a gift of ETYA. This study was supported in part by Grant HL-25864 from the National Heart, Lung and Blood Institute.

REFERENCES

Chou I-N, Roblin RO, Black PH (1977). Calcium stimulation of plasminogen activator secretion/production by Swiss 3T3 cells. J Biol Chem 252:6256.
Crutchley DJ, Conanan LB, Maynard JR (1980). Induction of plasminogen activator and prostaglandin biosynthesis in HeLa cells by 12-O-tetradecanoylphorbol-13-acetate. Cancer

Res 40:849.

Deutsch DG, Mertz ET (1970). Plasminogen: purification from human plasma by affinity chromatography. Science 170:1095.

Furstenberger G, Marks F (1980). Early prostaglandin E synthesis is an obligatory event in the induction of cell proliferation in mouse epidermis in vivo by the phorbol ester TPA. Biochem Biophys Res Commun 92:749.

Hamberg M (1976). On the formation of thromboxane B_2 and 12L-hydroxy-5,8,10,14-eicosatetraenoic acid (12ho-20:4) in tissues from the guinea pig. Biochim Biophys Acta 431:651.

Hamberg M, Samuelsson B (1974). Prostaglandin endoperoxides. Novel transformations of arachidonic acid in human platelets. Proc Natl Acad Sci USA 71:3400.

Hamilton JA (1980). Stimulation of macrophage prostaglandin and neutral protease production by phorbol esters as a model for the induction of vascular changes associated with tumor promotion. Cancer Res 40:2273.

Knapp HR, Oelz O, Roberts LJ, Sweetman BJ, Oates JA, Reed PW (1977). Ionophores stimulate prostaglandin and thromboxane biosynthesis. Proc Natl Acad Sci USA 74:4251.

Lee L-S, Weinstein IB (1978). Epidermal growth factor, like phorbol esters, induces plasminogen activator in HeLa cells. Nature (Lond) 274:696.

Levine L, Hassid A (1977). Epidermal growth factor stimulates prostaglandin biosynthesis by canine kidney (MDCK) cells. Biochem Biophys Res Commun 76:1181.

Levine L, Ohuchi K (1978). Retinoids as well as tumour promoters enhance deacylation of cellular lipids and prostaglandin production in MDCK cells. Nature (Lond) 276:274.

Mufson RA, DeFeo D, Weinstein IB (1979). Effects of phorbol ester tumor promoters on arachidonic acid metabolism in chick embryo fibroblasts. Mol Pharmacol 16:569.

Ohuchi K, Levine L (1978). Stimulation of prostaglandin synthesis by tumor-promoting phorbol-12,13-diesters in canine kidney (MDCK) cells. J Biol Chem 253:4783.

Panganamala RV, Miller JS, Gwebu ET, Sharma HM, Cornwell DG (1977). Differential inhibitory effects of vitamin E and other antioxidants on prostaglandin synthetase, platelet aggregation and lipoxidase. Prostaglandins 14:261.

Tashjian AHJr, Ivey JL, Delclos B, Levine L (1978). Stimulation of prostaglandin production in bone by phorbol diesters and melittin. Prostaglandins 16:221.

Unkeless JC, Tobia A, Ossowski L, Quigley JP, Rifkin DB, Reich E (1973). An enzymatic function associated with transformation of fibroblasts by oncogenic viruses. Chick embryo fibroblast cultures transformed by avian tumor

viruses. J Exp Med 137:85.
Vane JR (1971). Inhibition of prostaglandin synthesis as a mechanism of action for aspirin-like drugs. Nature (New Biol) 231:232.
Verma AK, Ashendel CL, Boutwell RK (1980). Inhibition by prostaglandin synthesis inhibitors of the induction of epidermal ornithine decarboxylase activity, the accumulation of prostaglandins, and tumor promotion caused by 12-O-tetradecanoylphorbol-13-acetate. Cancer Res 40:309.
Wertz PW, Mueller GC (1980). Inhibition of 12-O-tetradecanoylphorbol-13-acetate-accelerated phospholipid metabolism by 5,8,11,14-eicosatetraynoic acid. Cancer Res 40:776.
Wilson EL, Reich E (1978). Plasminogen activator in chick fibroblasts: induction of synthesis by retinoic acid; synergism with viral transformation and phorbol ester. Cell 15:385.

CELL REPLICATION/PROLIFERATION

**Prostaglandins and Cancer: First
International Conference, pages 291-296**
© **1982 Alan R. Liss, Inc., 150 Fifth Avenue, New York, NY 10011**

PLATELET DERIVED GROWTH FACTOR ACTION: A MOLECULAR ANALYSIS
OF BALB/C-3T3 AND TRANSFORMED BALB/C-3T3 CELLS

Charles D. Scher, Ronald L. Dick, Kathryn L.
Locatell, and Charles D. Stiles

Sidney Farber Cancer Institute and Harvard Medical
School, Boston, MA 02115

The replication of the BALB/c-3T3 mouse cells and its
transformed derivatives provides a useful model system for
analyzing cellular growth control. The growth of BALB/c-3T3
cells in tissue culture is regulated by recently characterized
polypeptide growth factors present in serum (Ross 1978; Scher
1979). These cells proliferate until they deplete the medium
of an essential serum growth factor. Under the usual tissue
culture conditions, the BALB/c-3T3 cells stop replicating
when they become confluent. The addition of serum, or
purified growth factors, stimulates a round of cell replication. Recent evidence suggests that transformed cells have
lost the requirement for one or more growth factors, and thus
grow to a higher cellular density (Scher 1978; Stiles 1979).
In this paper we review the activities of serum derived growth
factors in order to provide a perspective on cellular growth
control and transformation.

Recent evidence demonstrates that each growth factor
present in serum regulates a distinct cell cycle event in
BALB/c-3T3 cells. The platelet derived growth factor (PDGF),
which is present in serum but not in plasma, induces the first
event in the cell cycle by inducing density arrested BALB/c-3T3
to become "competent" to replicate (Pledger 1977). PDGF is
released from the alpha granules of platelets into serum
during the clotting process. PDGF-treated competent cells
(but not incompetent cells) respond to growth factors present
in plasma by synthesizing DNA. A brief treatment with PDGF
(as little as 0.5 hours) is sufficient to induce competence.
PDGF-treated cells remain competent for as long as thirteen
hours after PDGF is removed.

Unlike PDGF, the growth factors in plasma must be present continuously in order to initiate the mitogenic response (Pledger 1978). Furthermore, the sequence of growth factor addition is critical. PDGF-treated cells respond to plasma by initiating DNA synthesis. In contrast, plasma treated cells transferred to PDGF supplemented medium (lacking plasma) do not enter the S phase (Pledger 1978). Thus, PDGF primes cells to respond to the growth factors present in plasma

PDGF is a heat (100°C) stable polypeptide with a molecular weight of 32,000. It is a highly cationic molecule (isoelectric point 9.8 - 10.2), which appears to consist of two peptide chains held together by disulfide bonds. Like other polypeptide hormones, it is active at about 10^{-10}M (Antoniades 1979; Heldin 1979).

The growth factors present in plasma which stimulate PDGF-treated cells to synthesize DNA have also been characterized. One group of these growth factors is the somatomedins, polypeptides which have a marked amino acid sequence homology to proinsulin. The somatomedins appear to regulate cartilage growth and ultimately total body height and weight in mammals (Van Wyk 1978). Their plasma concentration is regulated by pituitary growth hormone. Animals lacking a pituitary gland have low levels of somatomedin and are of short stature. PDGF-treated BALB/c-3T3 cells synthesize DNA poorly if transferred to medium supplemented with plasma from a hypophysectomized rat. Supplementation of the plasma with a somatomedin (10^{-9}-10^{-11}M) allows the cells to synthesize DNA (Stiles 1979). Thus, the somatomedins have been characterized as being require for DNA synthesis. High concentrations of insulin (10^{-6}M) can replace somatomedin to permit S phase entry.

The epidermal growth factor (EGF) is another polypeptide hormone which is necessary for optimal cell replication. Mouse EGF was initially purified from the submaxillary gland of male mice; its human counterpart (urogastrone) is present in plasma. Mouse EGF is an acidic polypeptide with a molecular weight of 6045; it is active at 10^{-11}M in stimulating cell replication (Carpenter 1979). We have recently utilized serum-free medium to study the hormonal requirements for DNA synthesi (Scher 1981). We found that PDGF, EGF and somatomedin (or insulin) together induce density arrested BALB/c-3T3 cells to undergo a single round of DNA synthesis. A high concentration of either PDGF, EGF or somatomedin alone induced a weak growth response; however, in combination these agents act at

10^{-9}-10^{-11}M to stimulate the majority of cells to undertake a single round of DNA synthesis in serum-free medium.

Both EGF and somatomedin interact rapidly with their respective receptors. The binding of EGF to its receptor suffices to stimulate the receptor's kinase activity. However, prolonged treatment with these hormones is required for DNA synthesis (Carpenter 1979). PDGF also binds rapidly to specific membrane receptors (Heldin 1981) and like EGF and somatomedin serves to induce a pleotypic response (Abelson 1979). It appears to regulate cellular receptors for EGF (Wrann 1980) and somatomedin (Clemmons 1980). It appeared likely that PDGF had a different mechanism of action than the other growth factors because only a brief treatment is sufficient to induce a growth response. Furthermore, unlike EGF or insulin, it causes transient centriole deciliation in density-arrested BALB/c-3T3 cells (Tucker 1979).

The response to PDGF can be transferred from PDGF-treated BALB/c-3T3 cells to untreated cells using fusion techniques (Smith 1981). After treatment with PDGF, the cells are taken up with trypsin and fused with untreated cells using Sendai virus. The fused cells are plated in plasma supplemented medium lacking PDGF. Three types of heterokaryons (i.e. fused cells) are found after such treatment. In a typical experiment, 24% of PDGF treated cells that became fused to other PDGF-treated cells synthesized DNA, whereas, only 2% of untreated cells fused to other untreated cells entered the S phase. Approximately 14% of hybrids between PDGF-treated cells and untreated cells synthesized DNA. Both nuclei of these heterokaryons entered the S phase. The cytoplasts from enucleated PDGF-treated cells could also be used to transfer this second signal. The PDGF modulated second signal appears to be a gene product which arises within four hours of PDGF treatment. It appears to be a gene product because addition of actinomycin D, or other inhibitors of RNA synthesis, prevent the generation of the PDGF modulated mitogenic signal.

Because the PDGF modulated mitogenic signal can be transferred from cell to cell, we studied the synthesis of gene products in PDGF-treated cells. Density arrested BALB/c-3T3 cells were treated with PDGF or plasma in the presence of ^{35}S-methionine to label cellular proteins. The proteins were separated by one or two dimensional gel electrophoresis; they were characterized and their rate of synthesis quantified by fluorography. We found that the treatment of cells with

PDGF rapidly caused the cells to synthesize a family of cytoplasmic proteins (molecular weights, 29,000-70,000) (Pledger 1981; Scher 1981). One of these proteins (pI, 29,000) appeared within 40 minutes of PDGF addition, and another (pII, 35,000) appeared within an hour. These proteins were synthesized in response to pure PDGF but not in response to whole plasma, or to purified EGF or insulin. Their synthesis was prevented by inhibitors of RNA synthesis, such as actinomycin D, suggesting that their synthesis is regulated at the level of gene transcription. The rate of pI and pII synthesis was governed by the PDGF concentration; at optimal PDGF concentrations, the rate of pI synthesis increased ten-fold, and pII synthesis five-fold compared to plasma treated cultures.

To provide evidence that the synthesis of PDGF-modulated proteins regulates competence, we isolated and cloned a BALB/c-3T3 cell line which doesn't require PDGF for growth (Pledger 1981; Scher 1981). These variant cells (ST3T3) were recognized because they were spontaneously trans-formed, growing to a six-fold higher saturation density than BALB/c-3T3 cells. Unlike BALB/c-3T3 cells, suspensions of ST3T3 cells are tumorigenic in nude mice.

The ST3T3 cells become growth arrested, before S phase, at confluence. Insulin alone induces DNA synthesis with PDGF and/or EGF having little, if any, effect. The ST3T3 cell line synthesizes the PDGF-modulated proteins constitutively in the absence of PDGF. Although the function of these PDGF modulated proteins is not known, it appears likely that they are required for the PDGF-induced mitogenic response. Con-stitutive synthesis of these proteins may provide a mechanism for causing cellular transformation.

Abelson HT, Antoniades HN, Scher CD (1979). Uncoupling of RNA and DNA synthesis after plasma stimulation of G_0-arrested BALB/c-3T3 cells. Biochem Biophys Acta 561:269.

Antoniades HN, Scher CD, Stiles CD (1979). Purification of human platelet-derived growth factor. Proc Natl. Acad Sci USA 76:1809.

Carpenter G, Cohen S (1979). Epidermal growth factor. Ann Rev Biochem 48:193.

Clemmons DR, Van Wyk JJ, Pledger WJ (1980). Sequential addition of platelet factor and plasma to BALB/c-3T3 fibroblast cultures stimulates somatomedin-C binding early in cell cycle. Proc Natl Acad Sci USA 77:6644.

Heldin C-H, Westermark B, Wasteson A (1979). Platelet-derived growth factor: purification and partial characterization. Proc Natl Acad Sci USA 76:3722.

Heldin C-H, Westermark B, Wasteson A (1981). Specific receptors for platelet-derived growth factor on cells derived from connective tissue and glia. Proc Natl Acad Sci USA 78:3664.

Pledger WJ, Stiles CD, Antoniades HN, Scher CD (1977). Induction of DNA synthesis in BALB/c-3T3 cells by serum components: Reevaluation of the commitment process. Proc Natl Acad Sci USA 74:4481.

Pledger WJ, Stiles CD, Antoniades HN, Scher CD (1981). An ordered sequence of events is required before BALB/c-3T3 cells become committed to DNA synthesis. Proc Natl Acad Sci USA 75:2839.

Pledger WJ, Hart CA, Locatell KL, Scher CD (1981). Platelet-derived growth factor modulated proteins: constitutive synthesis by a transformed cell line. Proc Natl Acad Sci USA 78: 4358.

Ross R, Vogel A (1978). The platelet-derived growth factor. Cell 14:203.

Scher CD, Pledger WJ, Martin P, Antoniades H, Stiles CD (1978). Transforming viruses directly reduce the cellular growth requirement for a platelet derived growth factor. J Cell Physiol 97:371.

Scher CD, Shephard RC, Antoniades HN, Stiles CD (1979). Platelet-derived growth factor and the regulation of the mammalian fibroblast cell cycle. Biochim Biophys Acta 560:217.

Scher CD, Hendrickson SL, Whipple AP, Gottesman MM, Pledger WJ (1981). Constitutive synthesis of platelet-derived growth factor modulated proteins by a tumorigenic cell line. In Sirbasku D, Pardee AB (eds): "Ninth Cold Spring Harbor Conference on Cell Proliferation - Growth of Cells in Hormonally Defined Media", New York:Cold Spring Harbor Press, in press.

Smith JC, Stiles CD (1981). Cytoplasmic transfer of the mitogenic response to platelet-derived growth factor. Proc Natl Acad Sci USA 78:4363.

Stiles CD, Capone GT, Scher CD, Antoniades HN, Van Wyk JJ, Pledger WJ (1979). Dual control of cell growth by somatomedins and platelet-derived growth factor. Proc Natl Acad Sci USA 76:1279.

Tucker RW, Scher CD, Stiles CD (1979). Centriole deciliation associated with the early response to growth factors but not to SV40. Cell 18:1065.

Van Wyk JJ, Underwood LE (1978). The somatomedins and their

actions. In Litwach G (ed):"Biochemical Actions of Hormones",
New York:Academic Press, p101.
Wrann M, Fox CF, Ross R (1980). Modulation of epidermal growth
factor receptors on 3T3 cells by platelet-derived growth
factor. Science 210:1363.

Prostaglandins and Cancer: First
International Conference, pages 297-307
© 1982 Alan R. Liss, Inc., 150 Fifth Avenue, New York, NY 10011

ENDOGENOUS PROSTAGLANDIN PRODUCTION AND CELL
REPLICATION IN VITRO

Sven Hammarström

Department of Chemistry, Karolinska Institutet,

S-104 01 Stockholm, Sweden

Certain prostaglandins, notably PGE_1, PGE_2, PGD_2 and PGI_2, stimulate the formation of cyclic AMP in a number of tissues and cells (Samuelsson et al., 1979). The stimulation involves binding to specific receptors and activation of adenylate cyclase. Cyclic AMP seems to have a role in the regulation of cell growth: Exogenous cyclic AMP derivatives inhibit cell division, confluent, contact-inhibited cells have higher levels of cyclic AMP than growing cells and several transformed cells have lower levels of cyclic AMP than corresponding non-transformed cells (Pastan et al., 1975). Prostaglandins produced by tumor cells might thus inhibit proliferation of cells involved in host-defense mechanisms against cancer cells. These observations led us to investigate endogenous prostaglandin production by normal and transformed fibroblasts and to determine its effects on cyclic AMP formation and cell growth.

Effects of Polyoma Virus Transformation on Prostaglandin Formation

Baby hamster kidney fibroblasts transformed by poly-oma virus synthesized and released considerable amounts of prostaglandin E_2 into the growth media (up to 4.1 µg PGE_2/100 µg of cellular DNA in 72 hr, see Table 1). Significant amounts of prostaglandin $F_{2\alpha}$ (up to 0.11 µg/100 µg of cellular DNA) were also formed (Hammarström et al., 1973). On the other hand, regular baby hamster kidney fibroblasts, produced much smaller quantities of PGE_2 ($\leq$ 0.06 µg/100 µg of DNA) and $PGF_{2\alpha}$ (< 0.01 µg/100 µg of DNA (Table 1). Cells transformed by a temperature sensi-

Table 1. PGE_2 and $PGF_{2\alpha}$ levels in cells and growth media

Cell line	Growth temperature	Cell density	Cell density µg DNA/100 mm dish
BHK Cl 13	39°	High	74
BHK Cl 13	39°	Low	41.6
BHK Cl 13	37°	High	87.5
BHK Cl 13	37°	Low	41.8
BHK Cl 13	31°	High	99.6
BHK Cl 13	31°	Low	42.4
BHK ts-3 Cl 7C	39°	High	89.6
BHK ts-3 Cl 7C	39°	Low	40.8
BHK ts-3 Cl 7C	31°	High	158
BHK ts-3 Cl 7C	31°	Low	71.2
BHK Wt Cl 2A	39°	High	138.5
BHK Wt Cl 2A	39°	Low	33.2
BHK Wt Cl 2A	31°	High	154.4
BHK Wt Cl 2A	31°	Low	37.2

✶ Not analyzed.
From (Hammarström et al., 1973).

tive mutant of polyoma virus synthesized PGE_2 and $PGF_{2\alpha}$ in amounts intermediate to those mentioned above. The quantities produced were 2-3 fold higher at the permissive temperature (31°) than at the non-permissive temperature (39°) (PGE_2:≤0.51 at 31° and ≤ 0.16 µg/100 µg DNA at 39°; $PGF_{2\alpha}$ ≤ 0.016 at 31° and ≤ 0.007 µg/100 µg DNA at 39° (Table 1).

More detailed investigations were performed using Balb/c 3T3 fibroblasts transformed by polyoma virus (Goldyne et al., 1980; Hammarström, 1977; Roos et al., 1980). Figure 1A shows the concentrations of PGE_2 and $PGF_{2\alpha}$ in growth media from these cells at various times after initiation of the cultures. These concentrations increased with time throughout the experiment. Figure 1B shows corresponding values for media from regular Balb/c 3T3 fibroblasts. In this case, it is obvious that no net synthesis of PGE_2 occurred after 24 hr in culture whereas the concentrations of $PGF_{2\alpha}$ increased also after day 3. This suggested that polyoma virus transformation changes the regulation of prostaglandin E_2 and $F_{2\alpha}$ biosynthesis in fibroblasts. Other prostaglandins were also produced in

of normal and polyoma virus transformed BHK cultures

ng PGE$_2$/100 μg of cellular DNA			ng PGE$_1$/100 μg of cellular DNA		
Cells	Medium	Sum	Cells	Medium	Sum
2.6	22.8	25.4	1.4	5.1	6.5
2.8	12.6	15.4	6.4	8.1	14.5
3.0 *	31.9	34.9	1.5	5.8	7.3
-	22.2	-	1.2	8.7 *	9.9
4.2	20.1	24.3	1.2	- *	-
4.5	61.0	65.5	4.3	-	-
9.4	161.9	171.3	1.9	6.1	8.0
7.3 `	153.2	160.5	2.5	7.0	9.5
10.0	269.9	279.9	1.1	9.7	10.8
16.1	512.8	528.9	1.3	15.7	17.0
63.5	1,226	1,290	4.5	73.2	77.7
74.0	1,692	1,766	3.4	31.8	35.2
35.3	664.5	699.8	1.7	20.7	22.4
132.5	4,065	4,198	8.5	113.0	121.5

increased amounts by polyoma virus transformed 3T3 fibroblasts (Goldyne et al., 1980). Thus, the concentrations of PGE$_1$ and 6-keto PGF$_{1\alpha}$ (hydrolysis product of PGI$_2$) were circa 100 times higher in media from polyoma virus transformed compared to regular 3T3 fibroblasts. On the other hand, circa 10 times lower amounts of PGE$_1$ and PGI$_2$ were produced by both cell types in comparison to the amounts of PGE$_2$ formed by the same cells.

Mechanism of Altered Prostaglandin Biosynthesis in Polyoma Virus Transformed Fibroblasts (Roos et al., 1980)

As mentioned above, regular 3T3 fibroblasts produced prostaglandin E$_2$ for a period of less than 24 hr following a medium change. The time course of stimulation of PGE$_2$ synthesis by serum was therefore determined by analyzing the amounts of PGE$_2$ released into phosphate-buffered saline during 60 min at various times after the medium change (Fig. 2). Maximal synthesis (0.2 μg PGE$_2$/100 μg DNA) was observed 30 min after medium change. After 3 hr, less than 0.05 μg/100 μg DNA was produced. For compar-

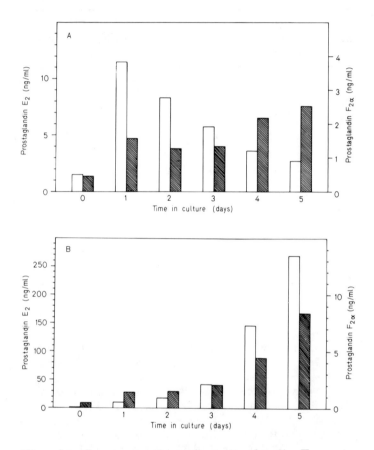

Fig. 1. Concentration of prostaglandin E_2 (open bars) and prostaglandin $F_{2\alpha}$ (hatched bars) in cell culture media from 3T3 fibroblasts (A), and polyoma-virus-transformed 3T3 (py 3T3)cells (B) (From Hammarström, 1977).

ison, corresponding analyses were also performed using polyoma virus transformed 3T3 fibroblasts. These cells produced circa 1 μg PGE_2/100 μg DNA · 60 min at all times following medium change, suggesting that synthesis was independent of serum stimulation. Therefore, polyoma virus transformation appears to alter mechanisms

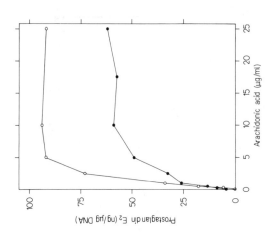

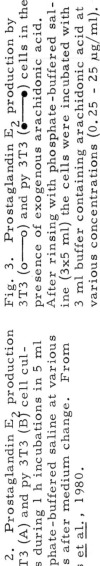

Fig. 3. Prostaglandin E_2 production by 3T3 (o——o) and py 3T3 (•——•) cells in the presence of exogenous arachidonic acid. After rinsing with phosphate-buffered saline (3x5 ml) the cells were incubated with 3 ml buffer containing arachidonic acid at various concentrations (0.25 - 25 $\mu g/ml$). Prostaglandin E_2 levels were determined after 20 min and corrected for DNA content. From Roos et al., 1980.

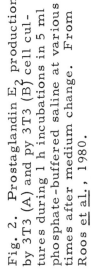

Fig. 2. Prostaglandin E_2 production by 3T3 (A) and py 3T3 (B) cell cultures during 1 h incubations in 5 ml phosphate-buffered saline at various times after medium change. From Roos et al., 1980.

which normally decrease prostaglandin E_2 synthesis following a stimulus (e.g. by serum).

Addition of arachidonic acid markedly stimulated prostaglandin E_2 synthesis in both 3T3 and polyoma virus transformed 3T3 cells (Fig. 3). This showed that the concentration of precursor fatty acid was rate-limiting in PGE_2 biosynthesis in these cells and suggested that polyoma virus transformation might alter the rate of release of arachidonic acid from cellular lipids. In fact it had been previously observed (Hammarström, 1977) that the levels of free arachidonic acid are higher in growth media from polyoma virus transformed compared to regular 3T3 fibroblasts (Fig. 4). This would be compatible with increased acyl hydrolase activity in the transformed cells with release of liberated acids into the medium.

To determine the hydrolytic release of arachidonic acid from regular and polyoma virus transformed 3T3 fibroblasts, the cells were labeled by growth in medium

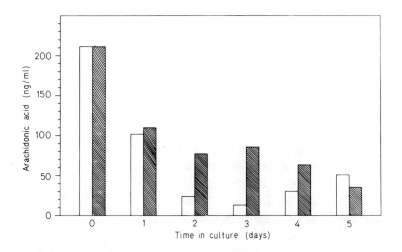

Fig. 4. Arachidonic acid concentrations in the growth media from 3T3 fibroblasts (open bars) and polyoma-virus-transformed 3T3 fibroblasts (hatched bars). The analyses were performed by quantitative mass spectrometry. From Hammarström, 1977.

containing $[1-^{14}C]$ arachidonic acid for 16 hr. After rinsing, the release of radioactivity from the cells into the
medium was determined (Fig. 5). Chromatographic analyses indicated that 90% of the radioactivity in the cells
was bound in the phospholipid fraction and 10% in the neutral ester lipid fraction. Both cell types released about
10% of the radioactivity during the first 60 min after the
medium change. During the next 71 hr, the transformed
cells released an additional 22% of the labeled arachidonic
acid from cellular lipids whereas the regular 3T3 cells
released less than 4% during the same period of time.

It has recently been demonstrated that corticosteroids
are effective inhibitors of arachidonic acid release (Hong
and Levine, 1976) in various cells and that the mechanism
of action is induction of a phospholipase A_2 inhibiting
protein (Blackwell et al., 1980; Hirata et al., 1980).
When added to polyoma virus transformed 3T3 fibroblasts,

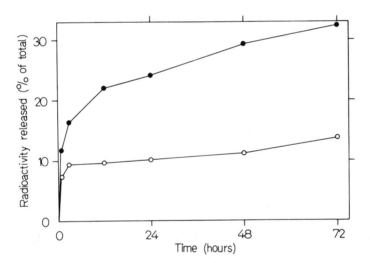

Fig. 5. Release of radioactivity from 3T3 (o——o)
and py 3T3 (●——●) cells prelabeled with $[1-^{14}C]$
arachidonic acid. Cultures were incubated for
16 h in media containing radio labeled arachidonic
acid (0.02 µCi/ml, 50-60 Ci/mol). After rinsing
the cells, fresh medium was added and samples
were taken at intervals for radioactivity determinations. From Roos et al., 1980.

hydrocortisone totally prevented further prostaglandin E_2 synthesis. No effect of the steroid on PGE_2 levels in media from corresponding 3T3 fibroblasts was observed.

These results strongly suggest that polyoma virus transformation of 3T3 fibroblasts increases the basal acyl hydrolase activity in the cells. This leads to release of arachidonic acid from cellular lipids and to increased synthesis of PGE_2, $PGF_{2\alpha}$ and PGI_2. In addition, dihomo-γ-linolenic acid is released since PGE_1 is synthesized by the transformed cells.

The effects of polyoma virus transformation on the activities of the enzymes which convert arachidonic acid to PGE_2 (prostaglandin endoperoxide synthase and prostaglandin endoperoxide-E isomerase) and which metabolize prostaglandin E_2 (probably 15-hydroxyprostaglandin dehydrogenase) in 3T3 cells were also determined. After addition of saturating concentrations of arachidonic acid, the initial rates of PGE_2 synthesis were greater (2.9-fold) in regular compared with transformed cells. The rate of degradation of PGE_2 (determined in the presence of 1 μM indomethacin to inhibit endogenous synthesis) was the same in regular and transformed cells ($t_{1/2}$ = 45 h). The decreased capacity to synthesize prostaglandin E_2 in the transformed compared to the regular cells confirms that the activities of these enzymes is not rate-limiting for PGE_2 synthesis in polyoma virus transformed 3T3 fibroblasts.

Stimulation of Cyclic AMP Synthesis and Inhibition of Cell Growth by Endogenous Prostaglandin E_2 Formation in Polyoma Virus Transformed 3T3 Fibroblasts

Prostaglandin E_2 stimulates or inhibits adenylate cyclase in various cells (Samuelsson et al., 1979). It seemed of interest, therefore, to determine if endogenous prostaglandin production in polyoma virus transformed 3T3 fibroblasts had effects on cyclic AMP synthesis and cell growth. Measurements of cyclic AMP showed that virus transformed fibroblasts had higher levels than regular 3T3 cells, particularly when the concentrations of PGE_2 were high in the growth medium (Claesson et al., 1977; Lindgren et al., 1979; see Fig. 6A and B, days 7-11, ▨ : PGE_2, o——o: cAMP). More frequent growth medium changes decreased the concentrations of PGE_2 and also the levels of

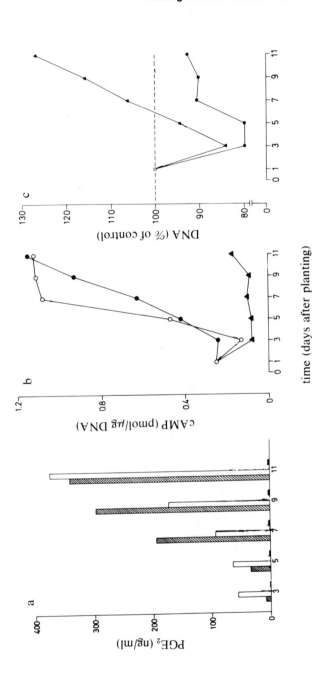

Fig. 6. Effects of indomethacin and indomethacin plus PGE₂ on PGE₂ concentrations in growth media (a), cyclic AMP levels in cells (b), and DNA contents/dish (c). Symbols: control without additions (▨, o——o), 1 μM indomethacin (▨, ▲-▲), and 1 μM indomethacin plus 10, 75, 75, 25, 120, 30, 180, 85, 300 and 250 ng/ml of PGE₂ on days 1-10, respectively (□, ●——●). From Lindgren et al., 1979.

cyclic AMP (Claesson et al., 1977). Conclusive
evidence that PGE_2 synthesis was involved in the regulation
of cyclic AMP concentrations was obtained using inhibitors
of prostaglandin biosynthesis (aspirin, indomethacin, and
5, 8, 11, 14-eicosatetraynoic acid) and exogenous additions
of PGE_2 (Claesson et al., 1977; Lindgren et al., 1979).
At minimal doses which inhibited PGE_2 synthesis completely the rise in cyclic AMP concentrations with time was abolished (results using 1 μM indomethacin are shown in Fig.
6A and B ▨ : PGE_2 ▲ : cAMP). At lower concentration of
indomethacin (10 nM) partial inhibition of PGE_2 synthesis
and partial lowering of cyclic AMP levels (not shown) were
observed (Fig. 6A and B). Daily additions of PGE_2 to cells
treated with 1 μM indomethacin (10, 75, 75, 25, 120, 30,
180, 85, 300 and 250 ng/ml on days 1-10, respectively)
gave similar values of PGE_2 in media (□) and cyclic AMP
in cells (●——●) as observed in the control cultures which
received neither indomethacin nor PGE_2 (▨ and o——o)
Fig. 6A and B). Cell growth was measured as amounts of
DNA/dish in the same experiments (Fig. 6C). The results
showed that 1 μM indomethacin significantly stimulated
growth (30%; ▲ - ▲). 10 nM indomethacin had no effect (not
shown) and 1 μM indomethacin plus the daily PGE_2 additions
mentioned above decreased growth by about 10% (●——●).
Moreover, 10-20% reductions in DNA contents were observed on day 3 in all experiments with indomethacin. This
initial inhibitory effect may be due to inhibition of $PGF_{2\alpha}$
synthesis since $PGF_{2\alpha}$ can stimulate cell proliferation
(Jimenez de Asua et al., 1975).

   In summary, the results presented indicate that virus
transformation of mammalian cells can alter the regulation
of phospholipase A_2, leading to enhanced formation of
prostaglandins. The endogenously produced prostaglandins
influence cyclic AMP levels and growth of the tumor cells
in vitro. It is possible that prostaglandins produced by
virus transformed cells in vivo will inhibit the proliferation
also of tumor killing cells, thereby facilitating the survival
of tumor cells in the host animal.

ACKNOWLEDGMENT

   Supported by a grant from the Swedish Cancer Society
(1503-03X).

REFERENCES

Blackwell GJ, Carnuccio R, DiRosa M, Flower RJ, Parente L, Persico P (1980). Macrocortin: A polypeptide causing the antiphospholipase effect of glucocorticoids. Nature 287:147.

Claesson HE, Lindgren JÅ, Hammarström S (1977). Prostaglandin E_2 production in 3T3 cells transformed by polyoma virus raises the intracellular adenosine 3´:5´monophosphate levels. Eur J Biochem 74:13.

Goldyne ME, Lindgren JÅ, Claesson HE, Hammarström S (1980). Endogenous synthesis of prostaglandins E_1 and I_2 in 3T3 fibroblasts transformed by polyoma virus. Prostaglandins 19:155.

Hammarström S, Samuelsson B, Bjursell G (1973). Prostaglandin levels in normal and transformed baby hamster kidney fibroblasts. Nature New Biol 243:50.

Hammarström S (1977). Prostaglandin production by normal and transformed 3T3 fibroblasts in cell culture. Eur J Biochem 74:7.

Hirata F, Schiffmann E, Venkatasubramanian K, Salomon D, Axelrod J (1980). A phospholipase A_2 inhibitory protein in rabbit neutrophils induced by glucocorticoids. Proc Natl Acad Sci USA 77:2533.

Hong SL, Levine L (1976). Inhibition of arachidonic acid release from cells as the biochemical action of anti-inflammatory corticosteroids. Proc Natl Acad Sci USA 73:1730.

Jimenez de Asua L, Clingan D, Rudland, PS (1975) Initiation of cell proliferation in cultured mouse fibroblast by prostaglandin $F_{2\alpha}$. Proc Natl Acad Sci USA 72:2724.

Lindgren JÅ, Claesson HE, Hammarström S (1979). Endogenous prostaglandin E_2 synthesis inhibits growth of polyoma virus transformed 3T3 fibroblasts. Exp Cell Res 124:1.

Pastan IH, Johnson GS, Anderson WB (1975). Role of cyclic nucleotides in growth control. Ann Rev Biochem 44:491.

Roos P, Lindgren JÅ, Hammarström S (1980). On the mechanism of elevated prostaglandin E_2 production in 3T3 fibroblasts transformed by polyoma virus. Eur J Biochem 108:279.

Samuelsson B, Goldyne M, Granström E, Hamberg M, Hammarström S, Malmsten C (1979). Prostaglandins and thromboxanes. Ann Rev Biochem 47:997.

**Prostaglandins and Cancer: First
International Conference, pages 309-331
© 1982 Alan R. Liss, Inc., 150 Fifth Avenue, New York, NY 10011**

THE REGULATION OF DNA REPLICATION IN ANIMAL CELLS BY
PROSTAGLANDIN $F_{2\alpha}$

Luis Jimenez de Asua[*], Angela M. Otto,
Marie-Odile Ulrich, Jorge Martin-Perez
and George Thomas

Friedrich Miescher-Institut, P.O.Box 273,
CH-4002 Basel, Switzerland

"Nature is a labyrinth in which the very haste you move
with will make you lose your way"
                                        Francis Bacon

     Proliferation of normal animal cells is regulated
through a reproducible program of signals and molecular
events which lead to chromosomal DNA replication and cell
division. In spite of numerous studies on the biochemistry
and molecular biology of resting and stimulated mammalian
cells, the regulation of cell proliferation is not yet understood. It has become evident that the isolation of growth
factors is an important prerequisite for elucidating the
cascade of molecular events which culminate in the initiation of DNA replication. Another prerequisite for the study
of molecular events involved in the regulation of DNA replication is the availability of cloned cell lines, which can
be grown under defined conditions, become arrested in the
G_o/G_1 phase, and can be stimulated to initiate DNA synthesis
by specific growth factors. Swiss 3T3 cells have provided a
useful model system, since they can be stimulated by different growth factors of which the structure is known:
epidermal growth factor (EGF) (Carpenter, Cohen 1979),
Prostaglandin $F_{2\alpha}$ ($PGF_{2\alpha}$)(Jimenez de Asua et al. 1975). and
vasopressin (Rozengurt et al. 1979).

---

[*] I dedicate this article to Luis F. Leloir on the
occasion of his 75th birthday.

Prostaglandins are a group of molecules with closely related structures eliciting different activities on a wide variety of target cells. Since the chemical structure of the different prostaglandins are known (Fig. 1), it has been possible to correlate the presence of certain molecular groups on the basic structure with their effects in certain cells.

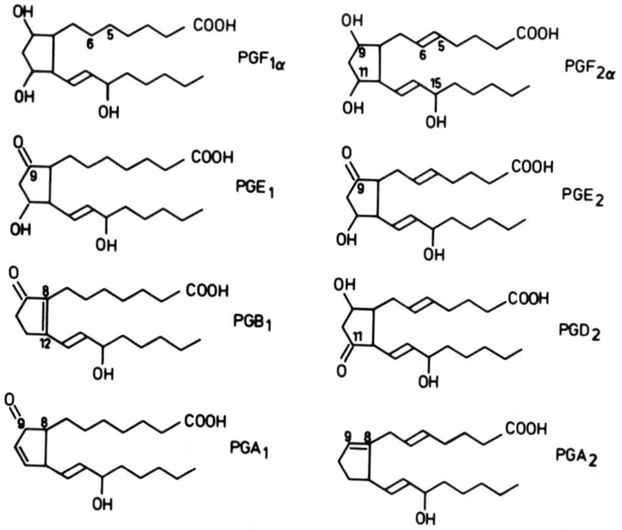

Fig. 1. Structure of different prostaglandins.

The mitogenic effect of $PGF_{2\alpha}$ on Swiss 3T3 cells was first observed by L. Jimenez de Asua and P.S. Rudland during their postdoctoral training in Dr. R. Dulbecco's laboratory in London. Two different clues led them to test the effect of $PGF_{2\alpha}$ on cell proliferation. First, it had been reported that transformed cells which produce and release growth promoting substances (Bürk 1973) were also releasing $PGF_{2\alpha}$ and PGE_2 (Sykes and Maddox 1972; Hammarström et al.1973). Second, it was observed that $PGF_{2\alpha}$ and insulin stimulated 2-deoxyglucose uptake with biphasic kinetics similar to those observed with serum (Jimenez de Asua and Rozengurt 1974) (Fig. 2). An increase in the cell number was observed when $PGF_{2\alpha}$ alone or with insulin was added to quiescent Swiss 3T3 cells (Jimenez de Asua et al. 1975).

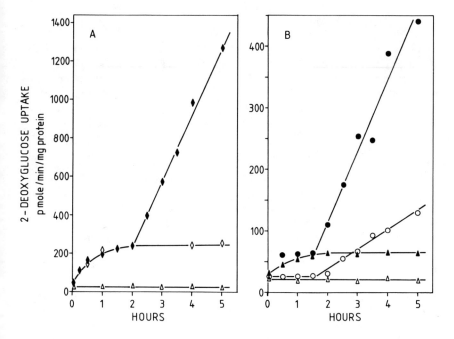

Fig. 2. Stimulation of 2-deoxyglucose uptake by fetal calf serum, PGF$_{2\alpha}$ and insulin in quiescent Swiss 3T3 cells. Concentrations used were for serum 15%, cycloheximide (10 μg/ml), PGF$_{2\alpha}$ (400 ng/ml), and insulin (1 μg/ml). (A) Δ, no addition; ◆, serum; ◊ serum + cycloheximide, (B) Δ, no addition; ▲, insulin; O, PGF$_{2\alpha}$; ●, PGF$_{2\alpha}$ + insulin. The uptake of ^{3}H-2-deoxyglucose was determined as described in Materials and Methods.

  In what follows, we shall discuss four different aspects of the effect of PGF$_{2\alpha}$ on the stimulation of cell proliferation:
1. The specificity of the effect of PGF$_{2\alpha}$ and the requirement of certain molecular groups for the mitogenic activity.
2. The biochemical events which occur prior to the initiation of DNA synthesis.
3. The regulation of DNA replication by PGF$_{2\alpha}$ and its interaction with insulin and hydrocortisone.
4. Comparison of PGF$_{2\alpha}$ with EGF in regulating the initiation of DNA replication.

MATERIALS AND METHODS

Cell Cultures. Swiss mouse 3T3 cells (Todaro and Green 1963)
were propagated in Dulbecco-Vogt's modified Eagle's medium
containing streptomycin (100 mg/ml), penicillin (100 units/
ml) and 10% fetal calf serum as previously described
(Jimenez de Asua et al 1977a).

Measurement of the initiation of DNA synthesis and determination of rate constant for entry into S phase. Cells were
plated at 1.6 x 10^5 per 35 mm dish in 2 ml of Dulbecco-
Vogt's modified Eagle's medium supplemented with 6% fetal
calf serum and low molecular weight nutrients. Three days
after seeding, the cells were given fresh medium supplemented as indicated (Jimenez de Asua et al.1977a) and then
allowed to become confluent and quiescent in 3-4 days. Such
3T3 cultures had a saturation density of 3.3 x 10^4 cells
per cm^2 and gave a very low labeling index (> 0.5%) after
28 hours. All additions were made directly to the conditioned medium. Cells were radioactively labeled for autoradiography by exposing them to 1 μM [methyl-^{3}H]thymidine
(3 μCi/ml) from the time of additions until the times
indicated in each experiment. Pairs of cultures were then
processed for autoradiography and the labeling index was
determined by counting 1800 cells. Determination of rate
constants for entry into S phase was as previously described
(Jimenez de Asua et al.1977a).

Polysome profiles and preparation of ribosomal proteins for
two-dimensional polyacrylamide gel electrophoresis. Cells
were plated at 5.0 x 10^5 per 100 mm dish in 10 ml of cultured medium supplemented as described for the assay of DNA
synthesis. Isolation and analysis of polysomes were performed as described (Thomas et al.1977). For analysis of
ribosomal proteins by two-dimensional electrophoresis,
cells were labeled with 1.5 μCi/ml of ^{35}S-methionine at
the time they received fresh medium as described for DNA
synthesis. Resting or stimulated cells were extracted and
processed for electrophoretic analysis (Thomas et al.1980).

Measurements of 2-deoxyglucose uptake. For determination
of the 2-deoxy-D[1-^{3}H]glucose, the cells were plated as for
DNA synthesis. Uptake was determined as previously
described (Jimenez de Asua et al.1977b).

<u>Materials</u>. Prostaglandins: A$_1$(PGA$_1$), A$_2$(PGA$_2$), B$_1$(PGB$_1$), D$_2$(PGD$_2$), E$_1$(PGE$_1$), E$_2$(PGE$_2$), F$_{1\alpha}$(PGF$_{1\alpha}$), F$_2$(PGF$_2$), 15-Keto-PGF$_{2\alpha}$, (15s) 15-methyl-PGF$_{2\alpha}$, (15s) 15-methyl-PGF$_2$ - methyl-ester, 15-methyl-ether-PGF$_{2\alpha}$, 15-epi-PGF$_{2\alpha}$, 16-diα methyl-PGF$_2$, and 13,14-dihydro-PGF$_{2\alpha}$, 6-keto-PGF$_{2\alpha}$ and prostacyclin (PGI$_2$) were generously supplied by Dr. John Pike, Upjohn Co.. Epidermal growth factor (EGF) was the generous gift of Dr. Stanley Cohen, Vanderbilt University. Crystalline insulin and thymidine were purchased from Sigma. [Methyl-^{3}H]thymidine (18 Ci/mmol) and 2-deoxy-D-[1-^{3}H]-glucose (22 Ci/mmol) were obtained from the Radiochemical Centre, Amersham, England. ^{35}S-methionine (670 Ci/mmol) was obtained from New England Nuclear. Prostaglandins were dissolved in absolute ethanol and diluted so that the final concentration of ethanol in the culture medium was 0.01%.

RESULTS AND DISCUSSION

Specificity of the Effect of PGF$_{2\alpha}$ on the Initiation of DNA Synthesis

The effect of PGF$_{2\alpha}$ on the initiation of DNA synthesis in quiescent Swiss 3T3 is specific compared to other prostaglandins with closely related structure.(Fig.3). Addition of PGF$_2$ in a concentration range of 2 ng/ml to 3 µg/ml stimulated DNA synthesis, the labeling index reached a plateau of 21% at 200 ng/ml within 28 hours (Fig.3A). The presence of physiological concentrations of insulin which alone has no stimulatory effect in these cells (Jimenez de Asua et al.1977a; Otto et al.1979), potentiates the effect of PGF$_2$ (Fig. 3B). It decreased the saturating concentration of PGF$_{2\alpha}$ to 30 ng/ml and produced its maximal effect by increasing the value of the labeling index to 55%. (Fig.3B).

In contrast, PGD$_2$, PGE$_2$, PGE$_1$ and PGF$_{1\alpha}$ had a stimulatory effect only at concentrations above 150 ng/ml (Fig.3A) but their maximal effect even in the presence of insulin never reached the same value observed at lower concentrations of PGF$_{2\alpha}$ (Fig. 3B). PGF$_{1\alpha}$, a close analogue of PGF$_{2\alpha}$ which lacks the C5-C6 double bond, alone or with insulin produced an increase of 10% and 40%, respectively, on the labeling index only at a concentration above 1 µg/ml (Fig.3A and B). PGE$_2$ as well as PGD$_2$, which have a keto group replacing the hydroxyl group in the C9 and C11, respectively, showed even less effect when added alone or with insulin (Fig.3A and B). PGE$_1$, which differs from PGE$_2$

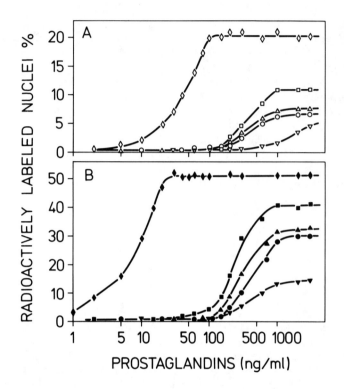

Fig. 3. Effect of increasing concentrations of prosta-
glandins D_2, E_2, E_1, $F_{1\alpha}$ and $F_{2\alpha}$, alone or with insulin,
on the initiation of DNA synthesis in Swiss 3T3 cells.
(A) O, PGD_2; △, PGE_2; ▽, PGE_1; ◻, $PGF_{1\alpha}$ and ◇, $PGF_{2\alpha}$.
(B) ●, PGD_2 + insulin; △, PGE_2 + insulin; ▼, PGE_1 + insulin;
■, $PGF_{1\alpha}$ + insulin and ◆, $PGF_{2\alpha}$ + insulin. Insulin was
added at 50 ng/ml. Determination of labeling index was as
described in Materials and Methods.

in that it lacks the C5-C6 double bond, was the least effective of these five prostaglandins. Furthermore, prostaglandins with no hydroxyl groups on C9 and C11, such as
PGA_1, PGA_2 and PGB_1 were incapable of stimulating DNA synthesis in resting Swiss 3T3 cells within 28 hours (Fig. 4).
Only in the presence of insulin (50 ng/ml) did PGA_1 and PGA_2
exhibit a marginal effect on the labeling index at concentrations between 0.1-1 µg/ml. Thus, both hydroxyl groups on

C9 and C11 as well as the C5–C6 double bond are essential to confer specificity to PGF$_{2\alpha}$ in stimulating the initiation of DNA synthesis in Swiss 3T3 cells.

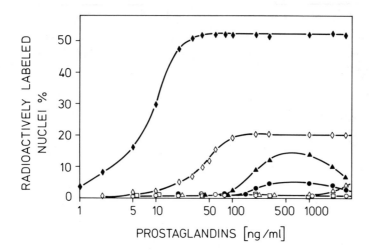

Fig. 4. Effect of increasing concentrations of prostaglandins A$_1$, A$_2$, and B$_1$, alone or with insulin, on the initiation of DNA synthesis in Swiss 3T3 cells. Open symbols: without insulin; closed symbols: with insulin. ○, ●, PGA$_1$; △, ▲, PGA$_2$; □, PGB$_1$; ◇, ◆, PGF$_{2\alpha}$. Insulin was added at 50 ng/ml. Determination of labeling index was described in Materials and Methods.

Is the double bond between C13 and C14 essential for the stimulatory activity of PGF$_{2\alpha}$? Reduction of the C13–C14 double bond by addition of two hydrogens results in a less active molecule at lower concentrations (Table 1). However, addition of a saturating amount of 13,14–dihydro-PGF$_{2\alpha}$ (200 ng/ml) to resting Swiss 3T3 cells results in the same labeling index of about 20% as observed with PGF$_{2\alpha}$. Likewise, only at higher concentrations of 13,14–dihydro-PGF$_{2\alpha}$ was the synergistic effect with insulin like that observed with PGF$_{2\alpha}$. This indicates that the C13–C14 double bond plays only a secondary role in the specificity of PGF$_{2\alpha}$ for the stimulation of DNA synthesis.

Table 1. Effect of $PGF_{2\alpha}$, 15-keto-$PGF_{2\alpha}$, 15-epi-$PGF_{2\alpha}$ and 13,14-dihydro-$PGF_{2\alpha}$, alone or with insulin, on the initiation of DNA synthesis in quiescent Swiss 3T3 cells.

Additions		Labeling Index (%)	
		without insulin	with insulin
None		0.4	0.7
$PGF_{2\alpha}$	30 ng/ml	6.8	51.6
	300 ng/ml	21.0	51.0
15-Keto-$PGF_{2\alpha}$	30 ng/ml	0.5	0.8
	300 ng/ml	0.7	0.9
15-Epi-$PGF_{2\alpha}$	30 ng/ml	0.5	14.3
	300 ng/ml	6.1	51.9
13,14-Dihydro-$PGF_{2\alpha}$	30 ng/ml	1.4	34.6
	300 ng/ml	20.0	51.0
Serum 10%		97.5	99.0

Labeling index was determined as indicated in Materials and Methods. Insulin was added at 50 ng/ml.

However, the presence of the hydroxyl group on the C15 as well as its stereospecificity on $PGF_{2\alpha}$ is important for the stimulation of the initiation of DNA replication and cell division. 15-Keto-$PGF_{2\alpha}$, the metabolic product of $PGF_{2\alpha}$, has no stimulatory activity even at high concentrations and in the presence of insulin (Table 1). Furthermore, epimerization of the C15 hydroxyl group of $PGF_{2\alpha}$ to 15-epi-$PGF_{2\alpha}$ dramatically reduced the stimulatory effect on the initiation of DNA synthesis (Table 1). At a saturating concentration of 15-epi-$PGF_{2\alpha}$ (300 ng/ml), the maximal value of the labeling index was only 6% in 28 hours. However, when 15-epi-$PGF_{2\alpha}$ was added with insulin, the stimulation was similar to that observed with $PGF_{2\alpha}$ plus insulin, except that for the maximal value 300 ng/ml of 15-epi-$PGF_{2\alpha}$ was required (Table 1).

When the C15 hydrogen on $PGF_{2\alpha}$ is substituted by a methyl or methyl-ether group, as in 15-methyl-$PGF_{2\alpha}$ and 15-methyl-ether-$PGF_{2\alpha}$, there is little change in the ability of the molecule to stimulate DNA synthesis (Table 2).

Table 2. Effect of different methyl-derivatives of $PGF_{2\alpha}$, alone or with insulin, on the initiation of DNA synthesis in quiescent Swiss 3T3 cells.

Additions	Labeling Index %	
	without insulin	with insulin
None	0.5	0.7
$PGF_{2\alpha}$		
30 ng/ml	6.8	51.6
300 ng/ml	21.0	51.0
(15s) 15-Methyl-$PGF_{2\alpha}$		
30 ng/ml	9.5	54.1
300 ng/ml	24.0	54.0
(15s) 15-Methyl-$PGF_{2\alpha}$-methyl-ester		
30 ng/ml	10.1	52.4
300 ng/ml	23.6	54.0
15-Methyl-ether-$PGF_{2\alpha}$		
30 ng/ml	5.8	51.1
300 ng/ml	21.6	50.9
16,16-Dimethyl-$PGF_{2\alpha}$		
30 ng/ml	7.1	51.8
300 ng/ml	22.0	52.0
Serum 10%	98.1	--

Labeling index was determined as indicated in Materials and Methods. Insulin was added at 50 ng/ml.

Likewise, two methyl groups on the neighbouring C16, as in 16,16-dimethyl-$PGF_{2\alpha}$, did not alter the stimulatory activity of the molecule. Also, with two methyl groups at different parts of the molecule, 15-methyl-PGF_2-methyl-ester was as active as PGF_2 (Table 2). It therefore seems that when the hydroxyl group on C15 is in its right position, methyl groups on C15 itself as well as on C16 and the carboxyl group have very little or no effect on the specificity of $PGF_{2\alpha}$ for the stimulation of DNA synthesis.

Fig. 5 shows more clearly the concentration of $PGF_{2\alpha}$ required for half maximal stimulation of DNA synthesis in Swiss 3T3 cells. In the presence of insulin the half-maximal concentration was reduced by a factor of almost 5 from 110 to 24 nM. Furthermore, this presentation of the data also shows that 15-methyl-ether-$PGF_{2\alpha}$ and 16,16-dimethyl-$PGF_{2\alpha}$ have very similar, and in the presence of insulin, even the same half-maximal concentrations as $PGF_{2\alpha}$.

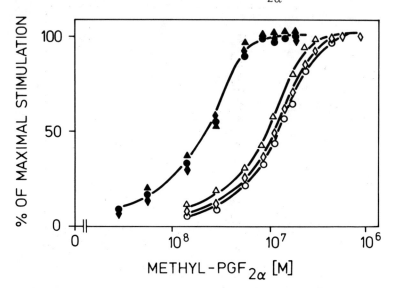

Fig. 5. Percentage of maximal stimulation as a function of the logarithmic concentration of $PGF_{2\alpha}$ and its methyl-derivatives, alone or with insulin. Open symbols : without insulin; closed symbols: with insulin; ◇, ◆, $PGF_{2\alpha}$, △, ▲, (15s) 15-methyl-$PGF_{2\alpha}$, ○, ●, 16,16-dimethyl-$PGF_{2\alpha}$. The percentage of stimulation at each concentration was calculated from the maximal value of the labeling index at the saturating concentration of each prostaglandin. Maximal values without or with insulin are given in Table 3.

Other compounds, such as PGI_2 or its metabolite 6-keto-$PGF_{1\alpha}$ did not have any stimulatory effect on DNA synthesis, even in the presence of insulin. This selective effect of $PGF_{2\alpha}$ suggests that Swiss 3T3 cells may have a specific receptor complex.

$PGF_{2\alpha}$ was also specific for other cells in stimulating the initiation of DNA synthesis. When added to confluent quiescent 3T6 cells in serum-free medium supplemented with vitamin B12 (O'Farrell et al.1979), PGF$_2$ at 1.0-300 ng/ml increased the fraction of labeled nuclei$^\alpha$to a plateau of 20% (Fig. 6). As in 3T3 cells, insulin also had a syner-

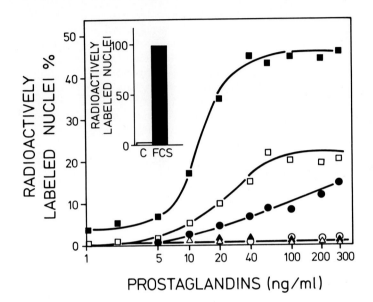

Fig. 6. Differences between PGE$_1$, PGE$_2$ and PGF$_{2\alpha}$ on the initiation of DNA synthesis in resting 3T6 cells alone or with insulin. 3T6 cells were plated in Dulbecco's-Vogt's modified Eagle's medium supplemented with 100 ng/ml of vitamin B12 as described by O'Farrell et al.1979. Additions were as follows: open symbols: without insulin; closed symbols: with insulin; O, ●, PGE$_2$; $\triangle$, ▲, PGE$_1$; $\square$, ■, PGF$_{2\alpha}$. Insert: White bar: control, dark bar: fetal calf serum 10%. Insulin was added at 50 ng/ml. Labeling index was determined as indicated in Materials and Methods. (Reprinted from O'Farrell et al.1979).

gistic effect in these cells by decreasing the saturating concentration of PGF$_{2\alpha}$ to 30 ng/ml and increasing the labeling index to 45%. The stimulatory effect of PGF$_2$ and insulin was less than that of serum (Fig.6,insert). When added in the same concentration range as PGF$_{2\alpha}$, PGE$_1$ and PGE$_2$ had no stimulatory effect (Fig. 6). Only in the

presence of insulin did PGE_2 increase the labeling index up
to about 15%. The stimulation of DNA synthesis by $PGF_{2\alpha}$ was
also observed in secondary mouse fibroblasts (O'Farrell et
al.1979) and in human lung fibroblasts (Taylor and Polgar
1977). In contrast to Swiss 3T3 cells, Balb/c 3T3 were not
stimulated to initiate DNA synthesis by $PGF_{2\alpha}$ alone. However,
when PGF_2 was added with a low concentration of serum, a synergistic effect on the labeling index was observed (O'Farrell
et al. 1979). These results indicate that the specificity
of PGF_2 to stimulate DNA synthesis depends on the cell type
and may be dependent on low concentrations of other growth
factors. It appears that the stimulatory effect of $PGF_{2\alpha}$ has
a restricted cell specificity, which has also been described
for platelet derived growth factor (Heldin et al.1981). In
contrast, EGF, which has the same stimulatory effect as
$PGF_{2\alpha}$ in Swiss 3T3 cells, is stimulatory for a wider spectrum of cell types (Heldin et al.1981).

Biochemical Events Stimulated by Prostaglandin $F_{2\alpha}$

    In Swiss 3T3 cells, $PGF_{2\alpha}$ (300 ng/ml) selectively
stimulates a number of different biochemical events which
occur during the prereplicative phase. Within minutes of
$PGF_{2\alpha}$ addition to quiescent cells, there is a rapid increase in $^{86}Rb^+$-uptake, a measurement of Na^+/K^+-ATPase
activity. PGE_1 and PGE_2 produced a similar effect only at
very high concentrations (40 ug/ml). At this concentration,
PGE_1 also increases cAMP levels. The stimulation of $^{86}Rb^+$-
uptake is not affected by cycloheximide, but is rapidly inhibited by ouabain (Lever et al.1976).

    $PGF_{2\alpha}$ also stimulates phosphate uptake, which follows
biphasic kinetics. The early phase is insensitive to
cycloheximide but can be partially inhibited by ouabain,
suggesting a coupling to $^{86}Rb^+$-uptake. The second phase,
occurring 1 1/2 hour after $PGF_{2\alpha}$ addition, is blocked by
cycloheximide, suggesting that this phase is protein synthesis dependent. Again, PGE_1 and PGE_2 were effective only
at 40 ug/ml (Lever et al.1976).

    The activation of glucose transport also follows bi-
phasic kinetics (Fig. 2), where the second phase is cycloheximide sensitive. $PGF_{2\alpha}$ stimulates only the second phase
of glucose transport occurring about 1 1/2 hours after the
addition and increasing up to 6 hours. Other prostaglandins,
which at the same concentration as $PGF_{2\alpha}$ did not initiate
DNA synthesis, such as PGB_1, PGE_1 and PGE_2, also did not

increase 2-deoxyglucose uptake (Table 3).

Table 3. Stimulation of 2-deoxyglucose uptake by different prostaglandins in confluent quiescent Swiss 3T3 cells.

Additions		% of Stimulation
None		100
PGF$_{2\alpha}$	300 ng/ml	750
PGE$_1$	300 ng/ml	166
PGE$_2$	300 ng/ml	231
PGB$_1$	300 ng/ml	198
Serum	10%	3950

Determinations of 2-deoxyglucose transport were done after 6 hours of additions as indicated in Materials and Methods. The control value without additions was 86 pmol/min/mg of protein.

Experiments with PGF$_2$ in combination with insulin and hydrocortisone, however, indicate that early ion fluxes can be dissociated from the stimulation of DNA synthesis (Lever et al.1980). Thus, while PGF$_2$ may be specific among the tested prostaglandins for stimulating these early bio-chemical events as it is specific for stimulating the ini-tiation of DNA synthesis, there appears to be no absolute requirement of these early events for DNA synthesis (Dul-becco 1975; Holley 1980b). The stimulation of the early ion fluxes may be related to other pathways triggered by PGF$_{2\alpha}$ unrelated to DNA replication but necessary for other metabolic events associated with cell growth.

It has been well established that protein synthesis is an essential requirement for DNA replication (Brooks 1977). Two events correlating with an increase in protein syn-thetic activity are multiple phosphorylation of 40s ribo-somal protein S6 and the shift of inactive 80s monosomes into translating polysomes. Recent evidence has suggested that phosphorylation of S6 is a prerequisite for this shift (Thomas et al.1980). In resting cells S6 is mainly in its unphosphorylated form (Fig.7A). Within two hours following PGF$_{2\alpha}$ addition S6 becomes increasingly phosphorylated (Fig.7C). The more phosphorylated S6 becomes the slower its migration in two-dimensional polyacrylamide gel electro-phoresis, resulting in five phosphorylated forms (Thomas et

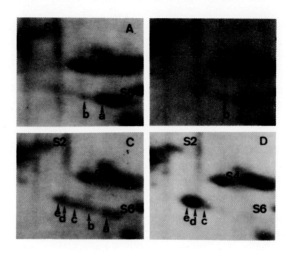

Fig. 7. Two-dimensional polyacrylamide gels of ^{35}S-methio-
nine labeled ribosomal proteins derived from (A) resting
cells, or cells treated for 2 hours with (B) 15-keto-PGF$_{2\alpha}$
(300 ng/ml), (C) PGF$_{2\alpha}$(300 ng/ml), or (D) 10% serum.
Preparation of ribosomal proteins and gel electrophoresis
was carried out as described in Material and Methods.

al.1979). PGF$_{2\alpha}$ also causes a partial shift of 80s monosomes into translating polysomes (Fig.8C). 15-keto-PGF$_{2\alpha}$,
which does not initiate DNA synthesis (Table 1), has no
effect on either S6 phosphorylation (Fig.7B) or polysome
formation (Fig.8a). During this time serum stimulates
maximally both biochemical events (Fig.7D,8D)(Thomas et al.
1980,1981). The extent to which these two processes are
stimulated by PGF$_{2\alpha}$ and serum correlates well with their
effects on the initiation of DNA synthesis (Table 1).
These results suggest that the extent of S6 phosphorylation
and the activation of protein synthesis are somehow involved in regulating the rate of initiation of DNA synthesis.

It has been shown in Swiss 3T3 cells that upon stimulation by PGF$_{2\alpha}$ and insulin there are changes in the metabolism of nonhistone nuclear proteins at the end of the lag
phase (Jimenez de Asua et al.1979). More recently, changes
in at least 18 cytoplasmic proteins have been observed
2 hours after serum stimulation; 8 of them appear to be
under transcriptional control (Thomas et al.1981b). It re-

mains to be investigated which of these changes are also produced by PGF$_{2\alpha}$ and how the addition of insulin will further affect these changes.

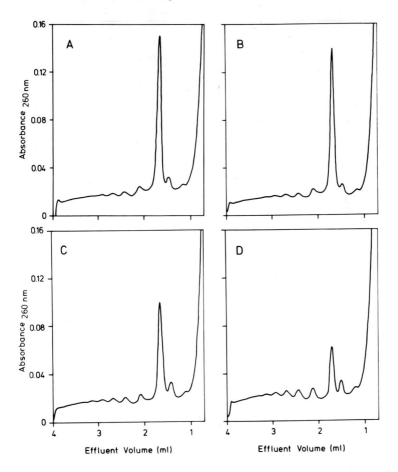

Fig. 8. Analytical sucrose gradients of total cytoplasmic polysomes derived from (A) resting cells, or cells treated for 2 hours with (B) 15-keto-PGF$_{2\alpha}$ (300 ng/ml), (C) PGF$_{2\alpha}$ (300 ng/ml), or (D) 10% serum. Samples were prepared and run on sucrose gradients as described in Materials and Methods.

$PGF_{2\alpha}$ and the Regulation of DNA Replication: Interactions with Hormones and Other Compounds

When $PGF_{2\alpha}$ stimulates the initiation of DNA replication, it induces two different phenomena: 1.) a prereplicative period (lag phase) of invariable length, and 2.) events regulating the rate at which the cells enter S phase. As shown in Table 4, $PGF_{2\alpha}$ at 60 ng/ml and at 300 ng/ml as well as 10% FCS induce the same length of the lag phase of 15 hours. Thus, the length of the lag phase is independent of the growth factor concentration above a minimal amount. On the other hand, upon completion of the lag phase the rate of entry into S phase is regulated by the growth factor concentration. The latter process appears to follow first order kinetics and is quantified by a rate constant. Table 4 shows the rate constants of two concentrations of $PGF_{2\alpha}$ as well as that of 10% FCS.

Table 4. Effect of the addition of two concentrations of $PGF_{2\alpha}$ on the length of the lag phase and the rate of initiation of DNA synthesis in Swiss 3T3 cells.

Additions		Lag Phase (hr)	Rate Constant $(x\ 10^{-2}/hr)$
None		--	0.04
$PGF_{2\alpha}$	60 ng/ml	15	1.10
	300 ng/ml	15	1.80
FCS 10%		15	25.90

Determination of the rate constants for entry into S phase is described in Materials and Methods. (Reprinted from Jimenez de Asua et al. 1977).

These two phenomena have been interpreted as requiring two different signals or sets of events to be triggered by a growth factor: signal 1.) is postulated to induce the events required for the temporally controlled progression through the lag phase, and signal 2.) regulates those events determining the rate of initiation of DNA synthesis.

Events regulating the final rate of entry into S phase are apparently occurring not only towards the end of the lag phase, but also at earlier times. Two different hormones, hydrocortisone and insulin, which by themselves do not initiate DNA synthesis, can modulate the rate constants

given by PGF$_{2\alpha}$. Hydrocortisone dramatically reduces the
rate constants of PGF$_2$ or PGF$_{2\alpha}$ plus insulin. However, this
effect is observed only when hydrocortisone is added within
the first 5 hours of the lag phase; thereafter it has no
effect (Jimenez de Asua et al.1977a). This indicates that
some event during the first five hours of the lag phase is
involved in determining the rate of initiation of DNA synthesis occurring at the end of the lag phase. In contrast,
insulin can increase the rate constant when added at 8 or
15 hours of the lag phase, indicating that it is affecting
some later event(s) involved in the initiation of DNA synthesis. Also, microtubule-disrupting agents, such as colchicine or colcemid, have a synergistic effect with PGF$_{2\alpha}$
and PGF$_{2\alpha}$ plus insulin, but the enhancement of the rate
constant is observed only when these agents are present during the first 8 hours of the lag phase (Otto et al.1979).
Thus, another event, sensitive to microtubule organization,
during the first part of the lag phase is involved in regulating the rate of entry into S phase. These modulating
interactions with other compounds indicate that PGF$_{2\alpha}$ induces a series of regulatory steps occurring at particular
times during the lag phase, which in concert determine the
final rate at which the cell population enters S phase
(Jimenez de Asua et al.1979).

PGF$_{2\alpha}$ and EGF Regulate Different Pathways of Events

A structurally unrelated growth factor is EGF, which
displays a similar pattern of interaction with hydrocortisone, insulin and microtubule-disrupting drugs to that
of PGF$_{2\alpha}$ in stimulating the initiation of DNA synthesis in
Swiss 3T3 cells (Otto et al.1981). Both PGF$_{2\alpha}$ and EGF are
present in tissue fluids as for example milk (Markelonis
et al.1975; Carpenter 1980; Reid et al.1980) which raises
a basic question: Do these two growth factors act through
a common sequence of events leading to DNA synthesis, or
does each growth factor trigger some different event?

When PGF$_{2\alpha}$ and EGF were added together to quiescent
Swiss 3T3 cells, a synergistic effect on the entry into
S phase is observed upon completion of the lag phase of
15 hours (Fig.9). Adding PGF$_{2\alpha}$ 6 hours after EGF (Fig.9A)
or vice versa (Fig.9B) also results in a synergistic enhancement of the rate constant though less than for
simultaneous additions. However, when PGF$_{2\alpha}$ is added 10 or
15 hours after EGF (or vice versa), then the synergistic

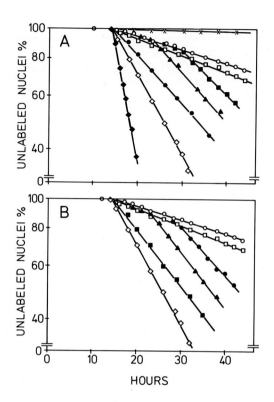

Fig. 9. Fraction of cells that remains unlabeled after syn-
chronous or nonsynchronous addition of EGF, PGF$_{2\alpha}$ or serum.
(A) x, no addition; o, EGF; □, PGF$_{2\alpha}$; ♦, serum; EGF with
PGF$_{2\alpha}$ added at: ◇, 0 hr; ●, 6 hr; ▲, 10 hr; ■, 15 hr;
(B) □, PGF$_{2\alpha}$; O, EGF. PGF$_{2\alpha}$ with EGF added at: ◇, 0 hr;
■, 6 hr; ▲, 10 hr; O, 15 hr. Additions were as follows:
PGF$_2$ 300 ng/ml, EGF 20 ng/ml, and serum 10%. (Reprinted
from Jimenez de Asua et al.1981).

effect is delayed until 10 or 15 hr after the end of the lag
phase, i.e. 15 hr after the second addition. These results
indicate that PGF$_{2\alpha}$ and EGF, while probably having those
events in common which are modulated by hydrocortisone,
insulin and microtubule-disrupting drugs, nevertheless differ in some other events which can cooperate to produce a
synergistic effect. Furthermore, EGF and PGF$_{2\alpha}$ can interact

optimally only when both are added at the beginning of the lag phase; the delay in the synergistic effect suggests that the events can no longer be integrated later during the lag phase. But apparently the events of the second growth factor can still interact with the previously added growth factor, resulting in a synergistic effect when the second one has completed its sequence.

In the presence of insulin the rate constants of EGF and PGF$_{2\alpha}$ alone or together are enhanced and the pattern of interaction between EGF and PGF$_{2\alpha}$ is conserved (Fig.10).

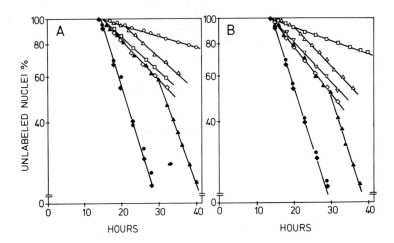

Fig. 10. Fraction of cells that remains unlabeled after synchronous or nonsynchronous addition of EGF, PGF$_{2\alpha}$ and insulin. (A) ○, EGF. EGF with insulin added at: ◇, 0 hr; □, 6 hr; △, 15 hr. EGF plus insulin with PGF$_2$ added at: ◆, 0 hr; ●, 6 hr; ▲, 15 hr. (B) □, PGF$_{2\alpha}$. PGF$_{2\alpha}$ with insulin added at: ◇, 0 hr; ▽, 6 hr; △, 15 hr. PGF$_2$ plus insulin with EGF added at: ◆, 0 hr; ●, 6 hr; ▲, 15 hr. PGF$_{2\alpha}$ and EGF were added as in Fig. 9. Insulin was added at 50 ng/ml.(Reprinted from Jimenez de Asua et al.1981).

The difference is that when PGF$_{2\alpha}$ is added 6 hours after EGF plus insulin, the synergistic effect is the same as if it had been added at the beginning. This figure shows also the basic difference in the interaction of another growth factor

and of insulin with a growth factor which has set the lag
phase. When insulin is added at 8 hours of the lag phase,
there is no delay in the synergistic effect, and when insulin is added at 15 hours, only 4-5 hours are required to
produce the enhancement of the rate constant. This phenomenon is observed also with $PGF_{2\alpha}$ and EGF together (Jimenez
de Asua et al.1981).

The interaction between $PGF_{2\alpha}$ and EGF for regulating
the initiation of DNA replication suggests that these two
growth factors act through different sequences of events
that can be integrated through some common event(s) during
the lag phase. It can be postulated that $PGF_{2\alpha}$ and EGF differ in signal 2 (regulating the rate constant). Whether signal 1, which induces the lag phase, is also different, cannot be conclusively deducted from these results. Interaction
between other growth factors may reveal other regulatory
steps during the lag phase. It is becoming evident with the
acknowledgement of the increasing complexity of the regulation of DNA replication that none of the cell cycle models
proposed suffice to account for the different types of
interactions of growth factors and hormones (Holley 1980a,b).
Furthermore, as suggested earlier, different growth factors may act through separate pathways of molecular events
(Jimenez de Asua 1980).

While the results discussed above have been restricted
only to the role of $PGF_{2\alpha}$ on the initiation of DNA replication in Swiss 3T3 cells, other results show that modifications of endogenous synthesis of prostaglandins are reflected in changes in the rate of proliferation of transformed and cancer cells (Thomas et al.1974; Lindren et al.
1979). Certainly, a few more years will be required to
understand exactly how prostaglandins regulate the signals
and molecular events leading to DNA replication and cell
division.

ACKNOWLEDGEMENTS

We thank Debora Mackenzie, Gary Thomas and Dr. Denis
Monard for constructive criticisms and corrections of the
manuscript. While part of this research was being carried
out at the Imperial Cancer Research Fund Laboratories,
L.J.de A. was a Special Fellow of the Leukemia Society of
America, Inc.

REFERENCES

Brooks RF (1977). Continuous protein synthesis is required to maintain the probability of entry into S phase. Cell 12:311.

Brooks RF, Bennett D, Smith JD (1980). Mammalian cell cycles need two random transitions. Cell 19:493.

Bürk RR (1973). A factor from a transformed cell line that affects cell migration. Proc Natl Acad Sci USA 70:369.

Carpenter G (1980). Epidermal growth factor is a major growth promoting agent in human milk. Science 210:198.

Carpenter G, Cohen S (1979). Epidermal growth factor. Ann Rev Biochem 48:193.

Dulbecco R (1975). The control of cell growth. Regulation by tumor-inducing viruses: A challenging problem. Proc Roy Soc London B 189:1.

Hammarström S, Samuelson B, Bjursell G (1973). Prostaglandin levels in normal and transformed baby hamster-kidney fibroblasts. Nature New Biol 243:50.

Heldin C-H, Westermark B, Wasteson A (1981). Specific receptors for platelet-derived growth factor on cells derived from connective tissue and glia. Proc Natl Acad Sci USA 78:3664.

Holley RW (1980). Control of animal cell proliferation. J Sup Mol Struct 13:191.

Holley RW (1980). Control of growth of kidney epithelial cells. In Jimenez de Asua L, Levi-Montalcini R, Shields R, Iacobelli S (eds): "Control Mechanisms in Animal Cells", New York: Raven Press, p 15.

Jimenez de Asua L (1980). An ordered sequence of temporal steps regulates the rate of initiation of DNA synthesis in cultured mouse cells. In Jimenez de Asua L, Levi-Montalcini R, Shields R, Iacobelli S (eds):"Control Mechanisms in Animal Cells", New York: Raven Press, p 173.

Jimenez de Asua L, Rozengurt E (1974). Multiple control mechanisms underlie initiation of growth in animal cells. Nature 251:624.

Jimenez de Asua L, Clingan D, Rudland PS (1975). Initiation of cell proliferation in cultured mouse fibroblasts by prostaglandin F$_{2\alpha}$. Proc Natl Acad Sci USA 72:2724.

Jimenez de Asua L, O'Farrell MK, Clingan D, Rudland PS (1977a). Temporal sequence of hormonal interactions during the prereplicative phase of quiescent cultured fibroblasts. Proc Natl Acad Sci USA 74:3845.

Jimenez de Asua L, O'Farrell MK, Bennett D, Clingan D, Rudland PS (1977b). Interaction of two hormones and their effect on observed rate of initiation of DNA synthesis in 3T3 cells. Nature 265:151.

Jimenez de Asua L, Richmond KMV, Otto AM, Kubler AM, O'Farrell MK, Rudland PS (1979). Growth factors and hormones interact in a series of temporal steps to regulate the rate of initiation of DNA synthesis in mouse fibroblasts. In Ross R, Sato GH (eds): "Hormones and Cell Culture". Cold Spring Harbor Conferences on Cell Proliferation, Cold Spring Harbor Laboratory 6:403.

Jimenez de Asua L, Richmond KMV, Otto AM (1981). Two growth factors and two hormones regulate initiation of DNA synthesis in cultured mouse cells through different pathways of events. Proc Natl Acad Sci USA 78:1004.

Lever J, Clingan D, Jimenez de Asua L (1976). Prostaglandin $F_{2\alpha}$ and insulin stimulate phosphate uptake and (Na^+, K^+) ATPase activity in resting fibroblast cultures. Biochem Biophys Res Comm 271:136.

Lever J, Richmond KMV, Otto AM, Jimenez de Asua L (1980). Dissociation of uridine and $(^{86}Rb^+)$ uptake from stimulation of DNA synthesis in Swiss 3T3 cells. Cell Biol Intern Rep 4:907.

Lindgren JA, Claesson HE, Hammarström S (1979). Endogenous prostaglandin E_2 synthesis inhibits growth of polyoma virus-transformed 3T3 fibroblasts. Exp Cell Res 118:311.

Markelonis G, Garbus J (1975). Alterations of intracellular oxidative metabolism as stimuli evoking prostaglandin biosynthesis. Prostag 10:1087.

O'Farrell MK, Clingan D, Rudland PS, Jimenez de Asua L (1979). Stimulation of the initiation of DNA synthesis and cell division in several cultured mouse cell types. Exp Cell Res 118:311.

Otto AM, Natoli C, Richmond KMV, Iacobelli S, Jimenez de Asua L (1981a). Glucocorticoids inhibit the stimulatory effect of epidermal growth factor on the initiation of DNA synthesis. J Cell Physiol 107:155.

Otto AM, Ulrich MO, Jimenez de Asua L (1981b). Epidermal growth factor initiates DNA synthesis after a time-dependent sequence of regulatory events in Swiss 3T3 cells. Interaction with hormones and growth factor. J Cell Physiol 108:145.

Otto AM, Zumbé A, Gibson L, Kubler AM, Jimenez de Asua L (1979). Cytoskeleton-disrupting drugs enhance effect of growth factors and hormones on initiation of DNA synthesis. Proc Natl Acad Sci USA 76:6435.

Reid B, Smith H, Friedman Z (1980). Prostaglandins in human milk. Pediatrics 66:870.

Rozengurt E, Legg A, Pettican P (1979). Vasopressin stimulation of mouse 3T3 cell growth. Proc Natl Acad Sci USA 76:1284.

Sykes JAC, Maddox IS (1972). Prostaglandin production by experimental tumors and effects of anti-inflammatory compounds. Nature New Biol 237:59.

Taylor L, Polgar P (1977). Self-regulation of growth by human diploid fibroblasts via prostaglandin production. FEBS Lett 79:69.

Thomas DR, Philpott GW, Jaffe BM (1974). The relationship between concentration of prostaglandin E and rates of cell replication. Exp Cell Res 84:40.

Thomas G, Siegmann M, Bowman PD, Gordon J (1977). The isolation and analysis of polysomes and ribosomal RNA from cells growing in monolayer culture. Exp Cell Res 108:253.

Thomas G, Siegmann M, Gordon J (1979). Multiple phosphorylation of ribosomal protein S6 during the transition of quiescent 3T3 cells into early G$_1$ and cellular compartmentalization of the phosphate donor. Proc Natl Acad Sci USA 76:3952.

Thomas G, Siegmann M, Kubler AM, Gordon J, Jimenez de Asua L (1980). Regulation of 40S ribosomal protein S6 phosphorylation in Swiss 3T3 cells. Cell 19:1015.

Thomas G, Siegmann M, Gordon J, Jimenez de Asua L, Martin-Perez J, Nielsen P (1981a). Serum-stimulation of quiescent 3T3 mouse cells to proliferate leads to increased phosphorylation of 40S ribosomal protein S6. In Rosen O, Krebs E (eds): "Protein Phosphorylation". Cold Spring Harbor Conference on Cell Proliferation. Cold Spring Harbor Laboratory 8:783.

Thomas G, Thomas G, Luther H (1981b). Transcriptional and translational control of cytoplasmic proteins following serum stimulation of quiescent Swiss 3T3 cells. Proc Natl Acad Sci USA (in press).

**Prostaglandins and Cancer: First
International Conference, pages 333–343**
© **1982 Alan R. Liss, Inc., 150 Fifth Avenue, New York, NY 10011**

HOST DEFENSE: TRILATERAL RELATIONSHIPS AMONG VIRUS
INFECTION, INTERFERON INDUCTION AND CELLULAR PROSTAGLANDIN
BIOSYNTHESIS

F. A. Fitzpatrick and D. A. Stringfellow

Pharmaceutical Research and Development
The Upjohn Company
Kalamazoo, Michigan

INTRODUCTION

Viruses, interferons, and prostaglandins, or other
arachidonic acid metabolites have all been linked, separately,
with the development and progression, or the arrest and
reversal of neoplastic disease (Stewart, 1979; Honn *et al.*
1981). However, the trilateral relationships between these
three factors are unclear. To study these relationships
we examined the influence of virus infection, *in vitro*,
on cellular prostaglandin biosynthesis. This model system
is simple and physiologically relevant. Furthermore, it
permits correlations of two biochemical parameters,
prostaglandin biosynthesis and interferon induction, with
two biological parameters, virus replication and virus cytotoxicity. Our results with several viruses infecting host
cells from different species indicated that the biological
parameters, cytotoxicity and virus replication, did not
correlate with altered cellular prostaglandin biosynthesis.
In contrast, there was a uniform increase in cellular
prostaglandin biosynthesis that correlated with interferon
induction. These results are discussed in terms of the
antineoplastic effects of prostaglandins and interferons.

EXPERIMENTAL

WI-38 and MRC-5 human lung fibroblasts, L_{929} murine L-
cell fibroblasts, VERO African green monkey kidney cells,
primary hamster embryo (HEC), primary chicken kidney (CK),
primary rabbit kidney (RK), and human foreskin fibroblast

(HFF) cells were cultured in 35 mm Petri dishes (Falcon Plastics, Oxnard, California) with 2 ml of modified Eagle's Medium (MEM) (Microbiological Associates, Rockville, Maryland), containing 10% v/v fetal calf serum (Sterile Systems Inc., Logan, Utah), 100 units of penicillin per ml, and 50 μg of streptomycin per ml.

Type I herpes simplex virus (HSV-I), strain 42-D and type II herpes simplex virus (HSV-II), strain 35-D were obtained from H. E. Renis, The Upjohn Company. Vesicular stomatitis virus (VSV), Indiana strain and vaccinia virus (VACC) were obtained from the American Type Culture Collection, Rockville, Maryland. Chikungunya virus (CV) was obtained from P. Russell, Walter Reed Medical Center. The Herts strain of Newcastle disease virus (NDV) was obtained from S. Baron (National Institutes of Health). All viruses were propogated and titered as previously described (Stringfellow and Glasgow, 1974).

Confluent monolayers (10^6 cells per plate) of the different cell types were infected with each virus. After a one hour absorption period, cell monolayers were rinsed twice with 2 ml of pH 7.4 phosphate buffered saline (0.9% w/v NaCl), and then 1 ml of fresh MEM was added to each plate. Medium was collected from duplicate plates at 0, 3, 6, 9, 24 and 48 hours, or at other times indicated, and each sample was assayed separately for interferon, prostaglandins, and virus as a function of time after infection. Prostaglandin E_2 and $F_{2\alpha}$ and thromboxane B_2 were determined by radioimmunoassay (Fitzpatrick and Gorman, 1978). Interferon was measured by VSV plaque reduction assays on appropriate, homologous cells. Viruses were titered for all experiments using a modified Dulbecco plaque assay (Dulbecco and Vogt, 1954). NDV and CV were assayed on monolayers of chicken kidney cells. HSV I, HSV II, VACC, and VSV were assayed on monolayers of rabbit kidney cells. The virus cytopathic effect (CPE) was determined microscopically.

RESULTS

Effects of Virus Infection

Figure 1 shows typical results for murine L929 cells infected with three DNA and three RNA viruses. The upper panel depicts the virus yields as a function of time after

Figure 1

Effect of Virus Infections on Prostaglandin Biosynthesis
and Interferon Induction

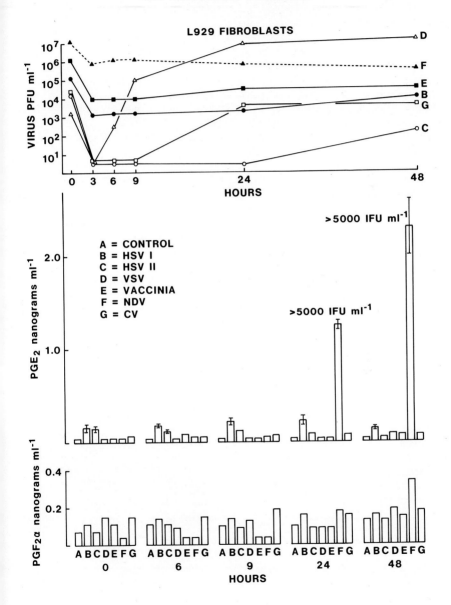

infection. The lower and middle panels depict the concentration of prostaglandin E_2 and prostaglandin $F_{2\alpha}$ in the culture media as a function of time after infection. Interferon titers, also, are noted in the middle panel. From 0 to 48 hours the only evident alteration in cellular prostaglandin biosynthesis coincided with interferon induction by Newcastle disease virus (NDV). When interferon titers were > 5000 units/mL, prostaglandin E_2 levels increased correspondingly. For all other virus host combinations, from 0 to 48 hours after infection, interferon levels were below 10 units/mL and cellular prostaglandin biosynthesis was unaltered by infectious viruses regardless of their replication and cytotoxic capabilities. These results suggest that interferon, but not viruses, stimulated prostaglandin formation. It is notable that NDV, itself, did not stimulate prostaglandin biosynthesis at any time prior to the appearance of interferon; consequently, the unique effect of NDV was dissociated temporally from direct virus-cell activation. Furthermore, the delayed effect of NDV was dissociated from viral uptake, maturation, and/or assembly since NDV is a non-productive infection in L_{929} cells, as shown in the top panel of Figure 1.

Detailed results for other host-virus combinations have been disclosed previously (Fitzpatrick and Stringfellow, 1979). Figure 2 summarizes the effect of several DNA and RNA viruses on prostaglandins and interferon production by

Figure 2

	L_{929}		HAMSTER EMBRYO		CHICK KIDNEY		HUMAN FORESKIN		HUMAN WI-38		HUMAN MRC-5		VERO MONKEY KIDNEY	
	PG	IF	PG	IF	PG	IF	PG	IF	PG	IF	PG	IF	PG	IF
HERPES I	↔	−	↔	−	↔	−	↔	−	↔	−	↔	−	↔	−
HERPES II	↔	−	↔	−	↔	−	↔	−	↔	−	↔	−	↔	−
VACCINIA	↔	−	↔	−	↔	−	↔	−	↔	−	↔	−	↔	−
NEWCASTLE DISEASE	↑	+	↑	+	↑	+	↑	+	↑	+	↑	+	↔	−
VESICULAR STOMATITIS	↔	−	↑	−	↔	−	↑	−	↔	−	↑	−	↔	−
CHIKUNGUNYA	↔	−	↔	−	↔	−	↑	+	↔	−	↑	+	↔	−

CODE: + = Interferon present
↑ = PG increased
− = Interferon absent
↔ = PG unaltered

8/8 Cases correlate ↑ +
31/35 Cases correlate ↔ −
3/35 Cases correlate ↑ −
Uniform correlation in 39/42 cases [90.4%]

host cells from five species. Increased cellular prostaglandin biosynthesis was uniformly related to the appearance
of interferon. Inducing viruses, such as Newcastle disease,
chikungunya or Sendai did not stimulate prostaglandin biosynthesis prior to the appearance of interferon; and they
had no effect that could be conclusively linked with their
replication cycle or cytopathic effect. The inability of
cells to modify their prostaglandin biosynthesis during
infection with severely cytopathic viruses was particularly
notable. For example, Table 1 shows that HSV I and HSV II
never stimulated prostaglandin formation although their
cytopathic effect ranged from 0% to 50%. Vaccinia and
vesicular stomatitis were even more destructive, with cytopathic effects ranging from 65% to 100%. Nevertheless, in
the majority of cases, they did not stimulate prostaglandin
biosynthesis. Vesicular stomatitis was an exception to
this generalization; however, this exception was confined
to certain, but not all host cells. For the inducing viruses,
Newcastle disease, chikungunya, and Sendai there was, likewise, no correlation between the cytopathic effect and
enhanced prostaglandin biosynthesis. The inability of
viruses to modify cellular prostaglandin biosynthesis during
such severe cell destruction is remarkable since cells are
exquisitely sensitive to scores of hormonal, neuronal,
mechanical, immunological, traumatic, or cytopathic stimuli,
all of which ordinarily enhance oxidative metabolism of
arachidonic acid. Consolidated results from Figure 2 and
Table 1 show 10/10 cases where interferon induction correlated with increased prostaglandin biosynthesis. In
32/35 cases, without interferon induction, cellular prostaglandin biosynthesis was unaltered suggesting that virus-
cell interactions do not necessarily activate the
phospholipase-cyclooxygenase enzyme complex responsible for
prostaglandin formation. Only 3/35 cases were exceptions
to these generalizations. These exceptions were peculiar
to vesicular stomatitis, and the exceptions themselves were
unique to some but not every host cell.

Effect of Transcription/Translation Inhibitors

When the experiments were repeated with cycloheximide
or actinomycin D added to the culture media one hour after
the virus infection, the results showed that the blockade
of interferon induction eliminated the stimulation of
prostaglandin biosynthesis [Table 2]. This result is

Table 1

Cell Type:	L929	CK	HFF	MRC-5	WI-38	WISH
Virus	Cytopathic Effect [% Monolayer Destruction]					
HSV I	0	25	50	50	50	—
HSV II	0	30	50	—	—	—
VSV	70	100	75+	80	—	—
VACC	65	75	90	80	—	—
NDV	75*	100*	80*	80*	100*	30*
CV	30	20	50*	30	—	—
Sendai	5*	—	—	50*	—	0*

*Increased prostaglandin biosynthesis was temporally related to interferon induction in these cases. The increase was not linked to the virus cytopathic effect.

+Increased prostaglandin biosynthesis occurred with VSV independent of interferon induction. VSV was the only exception; the effect of VSV was not evident in every host cell.

consistent with interferon mediated stimulation of cellular prostaglandin biosynthesis.

Table 2

EFFECT OF ACTINOMYCIN D AND CYCLOHEXIMIDE ON INTERFERON INDUCTION AND PROSTAGLANDIN BIOSYNTHESIS BY HUMAN CELL LINES DURING NDV INFECTION

Cell Type	Hours After Infection	Experimental Protocol	Interferon [Units · ml^{-1}]	Prostaglandin E$_2$ [Nanograms -ml^{-1}]
HFF	24	MEM + Actinomycin D*	<10	190 ± 14
HFF	24	MEM + NDV	490	248 ± 5
HFF	24	MEM + NDV + Actinomycin D	<10	180 ± 5
HFF	48	MEM + Actinomycin D	<10	251 ± 5
HFF	48	MEM + NDV	500	430 ± 16
HFF	48	MEM + NDV + Actinomycin D	<10	238 ± 12
MRC-5	24	MEM + Cycloheximide‡	<10	61 ± 15
MRC-5	24	MEM + NDV	500	529 ± 62
MRC-5	24	MEM + NDV + Cycloheximide	<10	84 ± 7
MRC-5	48	MEM + Cycloheximide	<10	60 ± 10
MRC-5	48	MEM + NDV	250	272 ± 16
MRC-5	48	MEM + NDV + Cycloheximide	<10	67 ± 14

*Actinomycin concentration = 1μg-ml^{-1}
‡Cycloheximide concentration = 50μg-ml^{-1}

Effect of Fibroblast Interferon Antibodies

Table 3 shows the effect of fibroblast interferon antibodies on cellular prostaglandin biosynthesis during infection with NDV. Prostaglandin E$_2$ levels increased coincident with interferon induction in human foreskin fibroblasts or L$_{929}$ cells infected with NDV. When sufficient IFN-β antibody was added to neutralize the interferon, prostaglandin E$_2$ biosynthesis was reduced nearly to its control level. The effect of the antibodies was species specific in accord with the known behavior of vertebrate interferons.

Table 3

HFF Cells

	PGE$_2$ [ng/mL]	IFN [units/mL]
Media Control	26 ± 2	<10
Media + NDV	365 ± 55	1200
Media + NDV + Human IFN-β Antibody	30 ± 6	<10

L929 Cells

	PGE$_2$ [ng/mL]	IFN [units/mL]
Media Control	<0.10	<10
Media + NDV	0.62 ± 0.02	4800
Media + NDV + Mouse IFN-β Antibody	0.25 ± 0.02	45
Media + NDV + Human IFN-β Antibody	0.75 ± 0.01	5000

Infection of Vero Cells

Vero cells lack the capacity to produce interferon (Wagner and Huang, 1965). Consequently, they are useful cells to distinguish effects caused by interferon from effects caused by other factors. Control experiments showed that Vero cells did not secrete interferon during infection with otherwise active inducing viruses, Newcastle disease and chikungunya; and they did not show increased cellular prostaglandin biosynthesis. The results imply that the ability of these viruses to stimulate prostaglandin formation in other host cells is linked to their ability to induce interferon in these cells.

Effect of Exogenous Interferon

Exogenous interferon can stimulate cellular prostaglandin biosynthesis (Yaron *et al.*, 1977). We confirmed this report. Human fibroblast interferon (10 units/mL) stimulated prostaglandin E$_2$ biosynthesis by MRC-5, HFF, WISH, and WI-38 cells. Mouse and rabbit interferons (40

units/mL) did not stimulate human cells; only species
homologous interferons were active in accord with the
typical behavior of interferons.

DISCUSSION

Why does interferon stimulate prostaglandin biosynthesis? The answer is uncertain, but it may relate to the
ability of prostaglandins to augment or regulate host
defense capabilities. For instance, vertebrates progressively lost their ability to produce interferons as a consequence of repeated exposure to viral infections or
neoplastic processes (Stringfellow, 1976). Prostaglandins,
in vivo, will restore the interferon response to afflicted
animals (Stringfellow, 1979). The cellular capacity for
sustained interferon production may depend on interferon
activation of prostaglandin biosynthesis. Prostaglandins
also decrease the cytotoxic effects of interferon *in vitro*
without reducing its antiviral effects (Wallach and Revel,
1979), consequently they ameliorate the viability and
function of cells that are producing interferon. A more
speculative but plausible link between interferon activity
and interferon activation of cellular prostaglandin biosynthesis may involve their antiproliferative effects.
Interferon may derive a portion of its antiproliferative
activity from its stimulation of biosynthesis of antiproliferative prostaglandins (Santoro *et al.*, 1976; Honn
et al., 1981)

The antineoplastic activity of interferon is not
exclusively related to its direct influence on cells.
Partly, interferon derives its effects from the activation
of a subset of cytotoxic lymphocytes called natural killer
(NK) cells. Both E and A type prostaglandin inhibit murine
NK activity, *in vitro*; and prostaglandin synthesis inhibitors potentiate NK activity, *in vitro* (Brunda *et al.*, 1980;
Tracey and Adkinson, 1980). These results have led to the
proposal that prostaglandins may regulate NK cell activity
in vivo. Prostaglandin dependent deactivation of NK cells
may counter interferon dependent activation. Evidence
suggests that prostaglandin E_2, especially, modulates many
biological response modifiers and their accompanying host
defense activities in a similar vein (Schultz *et al.*, 1978).
Regulation of lymphocyte and macrophage cytotoxicity by
prostaglandin E_2 may explain the unusual cellular tolerance

of viral insults without the activation of cellular prostaglandin biosynthesis: cells that relied on leukocyte
mediated anti-viral defense would create an advantage for
infectious viruses by synthesizing certain prostaglandins
that suppressed leukocyte activity. It is notable that
prostaglandin biosynthesis in cells transformed by oncogenic
viruses is abnormally high (Honn *et al.*, 1981), in contrast
to prostaglandin biosynthesis in cells exposed to infectious
virus (Fitzpatrick and Stringfellow, 1980). The influence
of prostaglandins on the immune system has been used to
explain the failure of the host defense system in the former
example (Plescia *et al.*, 1975); the absence of cellular
prostaglandin biosynthesis may contribute to the success of
the host defense system in the latter circumstance. Recent
results from other groups independently suggest that the
link between prostaglandins and interferon may explain the
pleiotypic effects of interferon (Pottathil *et al.*, 1980;
Chandrabose *et al.*, 1981).

References

Brunda M, Herberman R, Holden H (1980). Inhibition of
natural killer cell activity by prostaglandins. J Immunol
124:2682.
Chandrabose K, Cuatrecasas P, Pottathil R, Lang D (1981).
Interferon resistant cell line lacks fatty acid cyclooxygenase activity. Science 212:329.
Dulbecco R, Vogt M (1954). One step growth curve of Western
equine encephalitis in chicken embryo cells grown *in vitro*
and analysis of virus yields from single cells. J Exp Med
99:183.
Fitzpatrick F, Gorman R (1978). A comparison of imidazole
and 9,11-azoprosta-5,13-dienoic acid: two selective
thromboxane synthetase inhibitors. Biochim Biophys Acta
539:162.
Fitzpatrick F, Stringfellow D (1980). Virus and interferon
effects on cellular prostaglandin biosynthesis. J Immunol
125:431.
Honn KV, Bockman RS, Marnett LJ (1981). Prostaglandins and
cancer: a review of tumor initiation through tumor metastasis.
Prostaglandins 21:833.

Plescia O, Smith A, Grinwich K (1975). Subversion of the immune system by tumor cells and the role of prostaglandins. Proc Natl Acad Sci USA 72:1848.
Pottathil R, Chandrabose K, Cuatrecasas P, Lang D (1980). Establishment of the interferon mediated antiviral state: role of fatty acid cyclooxygenase. Proc Natl Acad Sci USA 77:5437.
Santoro M, Philpott G, Jaffe B (1976). Inhibition of tumor growth *in vivo* and *in vitro* by prostaglandin E. Nature 263:777.
Schultz R, Pavlidis N, Stylos W, Chirigos M (1978). Regulation of macrophage tumorocidal function: a role for prostaglandins of the E series. Science 202:320.
Stewart WE (1979). "The Interferon System." New York: Springer Verlag.
Stringfellow D, Glasgow L (1974). Hyporeactivity due to infection: recognition of a transferable hyporeactive factor in the serum of encephalomyocarditis virus infected mice. Infect Immun 10:1337.
Stringfellow D (1976). Murine leukemia: depressed response to interferon induction correlated with a serum hyporesponsive factor. Infect Immun 13:392.
Stringfellow D (1979). Prostaglandin restoration of the interferon response of hyporeactive animals. Science 201:376.
Tracey D, Adkinson F (1980). Prostaglandin synthesis inhibitors potentiate the BCG induced augmentation of natural killer cell activity. J Immunol 125:136.
Wallach D, Revel M (1979). Hormonal protection of interferon treated cells against double stranded RNA induced cytolysis. FEBS Letters 101:364.
Wagner P, Huang A (1965). Reversible inhibition of interferon synthesis by puromycin: evidence for an interferon specific messenger RNA. Proc Natl Acad Sci USA 54:1112.
Yaron M, Yaron D, Gurari-Rotman M, Revel M, Linder H, Zor U (1977). Stimulation of prostaglandin E production in cultured human fibroblasts by poly (I)·poly (C) and human interferon. Nature 267:457.

Acknowledgements

We thank W. E. Stewart II for providing antibodies against fibroblast interferons, and L. M. Missias for typing this manuscript.

Prostaglandins and Cancer: First
International Conference, pages 345–364
© 1982 Alan R. Liss, Inc., 150 Fifth Avenue, New York, NY 10011

THE POSSIBLE ROLES OF PROSTAGLANDIN SYNTHETASE AND CYTO-
PLASMIC SUPEROXIDE DISMUTASE IN INTERFERON ACTION IN
HOMOLOGOUS CELLS

K.A. Chandrabose[*]$_\pi$, Raveendran Pottathil[†],
Ernest C. Borden[π], Rebecca Fox[π], and Pedro
Cuatrecasas[*]

[*]Department of Molecular Biology, Wellcome
Research Laboratories, Research Triangle Park,
NC 27709
[†]Department of Pediatrics, University of Maryland,
School of Medicine, Baltimore, MD 21201
[π]Departments of Human Oncology and Medicine,
University of Wisconsin Clinical Cancer Center,
Madison, WI 53792

Interferon was originally described as an antiviral
substance produced by the host animal cells in reponse to
virus infection (Isaac and Lindenmann, 1957). Recent
evidence from various laboratories suggests that this
group of glycoproteins can also exert profound pleotropic
effects on homologous cells. Interferons have been implicated as modulators of phagocytosis (Donahoe and Huang,
1976), lymphocyte cytotoxicity (Gisler et al., 1975),
cell multiplication (Gresser et al., 1970) and neoplastic
proliferation ((Gresser and Tovey, 1978). It is now well
established that all these diverse properties can be
attributed to a single class of glycoproteins with antiviral activity (DeMaeyer-Guignard J and DeMaeyer-Guignard E,
1980). Much less is known however whether the biochemical
mechanism involved in the antiviral properties of IFN are
the same as those involved in the multitude of other
biological effects. In this chapter, we summarize data
which suggest that (1) IFN induces discrete and specific
changes in the composition of cell membrane lipids.
(2) The catalytic functions of cellular prostaglandin
synthetase (E.C.1.14.99.1) and cytoplasmic superoxide
dismutase (E.C.1.15.1.1.) appear to be required for such
changes (3). The membrane changes may be necessary
cellular events for IFN-mediated programming of homologous
cells to antiviral and possibly non-antiviral properties.

MATERIALS AND METHODS

Cells and IFN

Mouse sarcoma, S-180 (CCL.8) and human leukemic lymphoblast IM-9 (CCL.159) were purchased from American Type Culture Collection. L-cells were from Dr. Sam Baron, Department of Microbiology, University of Texas at Galveston. Human leukocyte IFN (α.IFN) (specific activity 2 x 10^6 units/mg protein) was prepared and purified at Wellcome Research Laboratories, Beckenham, England. L1210 S_6, mouse lymphocytic leukemia, the IFN resistant subline L1210 R_3, produced by growth of S_6 cells in presence of large concentrations of IFN ((Gresser et al., 1974) and mouse fibroblast IFN (β-IFN), specific activity, 2 x 10^7 units/mg protein were generous gifts from Dr. Ion Gresser, Institute De Recherches Scinetifiques Sur Le Cancer, Villejuif, France. Lipid extraction, fractionation, virus assays enzymatic analysis etc. were done according to previously published methods (Pottathil et al., 1980, 1981, Chandrabose et al, 1981a and 1981b).

NK cell cytotoxicity. Natural killing (NK) cell cytotoxicity was measured, as previously described (Zarling et al., 1979), in a 6-hour chromium release assay in which K562 cells were used as targets. K562 cells were labeled by incubating 5 x 10^6 cells in 1 ml of medium with 100 μCi/ml $Na_2{}^{51}CrO_4$, respectively, for 40 to 90 minutes. Labeled cells were then resuspended in medium, underlayered with 2 ml fetal bovine serum, and centrifuged at 400 x g, 3 minutes, 24°C to remove unincorporated isotope. After two such washes, target cells were diluted and added to microtiter wells at 2 x 10^3 cells per well for the chromium release assay. Lymphocytes were then added to the wells at cell concentrations in quadruplicate of 50:1, 25:1 and 12.5:1 are tested. After 6 hours incubation at 37°C in a 5% CO_2, humidified atmosphere, supernatants were collected utilizing a Titertek supernatant collection system based upon exponential fit model (Pross et al., 1981). 1 LU equals the number of cells required to produce 30% specific ^{51}Cr release. Specific release was calculated as

$$\frac{\text{cpm test wells - cpm spontaneous}}{\text{cpm maximum - cpm spontaneous}} \times 100$$

RESULTS

Formation of Less Polar Phospholipid Species as a Result
of IFN Action

The membranes of animal cells are composed of phospholipid molecules in a bipolar orientation forming a fluid
mosaic in which membrane proteins are dispersed with
specific orientations of their polar and apolar terminals
(Singer and Nicolson, 1972). The degree of unsaturation
in the hydrocarbon chains of fatty acids in phospholipid
molecules and the cholesterol content are the principal
structural components which regulate and maintain the
fluidity of membranes required for appropriate membrane
functions. When cells were treated with moderate concentrations of IFN (200-500 units/ml) a selective loss of
unsaturated fatty acids was observed in all of the major
phospholipids. The loss of unsaturated fatty acids
caused the formation of less polar species within each
class of phospholipids as detected by reverse phase thin
layer chromatography (Fig. 1a). The specific loss of
unsaturated fatty acids was seen without any increase in
lysolipids. The reaction elicited by IFN which results
in the loss of unsaturated fatty acids in phospholipids
has a broad specificity towards unsaturated fatty acids
in general rather than a given fatty acid of particular
chain length. Thus, when fatty acid methyl esters derived
from phosphatidyl ethanol amine from control and IFN
treated cells were separated by gas-liquid chromatography,
substantial losses of all unsaturated fatty acids, i.e.,
oleate (18:1), linoleate (18:2), linolenate (18:3), and
arachidonate (20:4) were obvious compared to the saturated
fatty acids, i.e., palmitate (16:0) and stearate (18:0)
(Fig. 1b).

The free cholesterol content of the IFN treated
cells was not different from that of the controls.
Therefore, the rigidity of membranes detected by E.S.R
spectroscopy after IFN treatment (Pfegger et al, 1981)
probably results from the selective loss of unsaturated
fatty acids observed from membrane lipids. The gas-liquid
chromatograms of fatty acid methyl esters from phosphatidyl
choline and phosphatidyl inositiol show profiles similar
to those of phosphatidyl ethanolamine (Chandrabose
et al., 1981a).

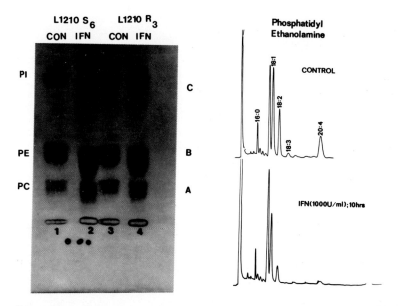

Fig. 1A. Formation of less polar phospholipid species as detected by thin layer chromatography as a result of IFN action on sensitive cells.

L1210 mouse leukemia cells were labelled with 1-^{14}C arachidonate (0.1 μCi/ml) and incubated with 1000 U/ml of mouse β-IFN where indicated. Total lipids were extracted and chromatographed on Whatman KC_{18} reverse phase TLC plates developed in methanol: water: chloroform (7/2/1)v/v, and autoradiographed on Kodak x-ray films.

Lane 1, IFN sensitive S_6 clone, control; Lane 2, IFN sensitive S_6 + IFN, 8 hrs; Lane 3, IFN resistant R_3 clone; Lane 4, IFN resistant R_3 + IFN, 8 hrs

Band A, Phosphatidylcholine; Band B, Phosphatidylethanolamine; Band C, Phosphatidylinositol

Radioactivity at the origin is associated with neutral lipid species.

Fig. 1B. Fatty acid methyl esters from phosphatidylethanolamine. typical gas-chromatographic tracing showing reduction of unsaturated fatty acids after IFN treatment.

The reverse-phase TLC of phospholipids of IFN sensitive L1210 S_6 and IFN resistant clones of L1210 R_3 mouse lymphocytic leukemia cells shows that (Fig. 1a) the resistant sub-line does not respond to IFN as would be expected, with lipid changes characteristic of the sensitive cells. A trend towards lower R_f values exhibited by phosphatidyl ethanolamine in these cells (Fig. 1a, line 4) may be explained by the observations a) that even the resistant R_3 cell population does contain a finite percentage of sensitive cells, and b) that the IFN induced changes are seen more dramatically in phosphatidyl ethanol amine because of the high unsaturated fatty acid content in this phospholipid, and consequently its high sensitivity towards the IFN induced change.

The species specificity of IFN action is apparently also manifested in these lipid changes. Thus, the changes were seen with mouse β IFN in mouse L, L929, S-180, and L1210 cells but are not observed in mouse cells with human IFN even at concentrations higher than 5000 U/ml. Furthermore the changes were seen in human lymphoma IM-9 with human IFN but not with mouse IFN. In both cases the IFN incubated with appropriate IFN antibodies prevented the IFN induced changes in the lipid in homologous cells as well as the development of antiviral state by IFN.

Time Course of the IFN Induced Lipid Changes

The lipid changes described take place relatively fast, and may be one of earliest IFN specific reactions seen in the sensitive cells. Changes are maximal at about 20-30 min depending upon the concentration of IFN and sensitivity of the cell to IFN. IFN induced synthesis of specific proteins is not translated until about 2 hrs after addition of IFN (Revel et al., 1980) (as shown by the cycloheximide sensitivity of IFN-induced enzymes and development of antiviral state). It is, therefore, reasonable to conclude that the composition changes of membranes induced by IFN involve only cellular enzymes.

The Possible Role of Prostaglandin Synthetase and Cytoplasmic Superoxide Dismutase in Membrane Lipid Changes
and in Development of Antiviral State

Prostaglandins have been implicated by Yaron et al.
to play a role in IFN action ((Yaron et al, 1977). These
investigators demonstrated increased prostaglandin synthesis with IFN and attributed this to one of the biological
effects of IFN in the treated cell. A different effect of
prostaglandins was reported by Stringfellow on the IFN-
system (Stringfellow et al., 1978). Recently, Fitzpatrick
and Stringfellow have investigated in detail the relationship of virus infection, interferon induction and prostaglandin production using various viruses and cell lines.
These studies show a close correlation between prostaglandin production and IFN titres in the virus infected
cells (Fitzpatrick and Strigfellow, 1980).

We have reported that a catalytically active prostaglandin synthetase is a required enzymatic function of the
cell for the complete development of antiviral state
induced by IFN (Pottathil et al., 1980). Inhibitors of
prostaglandin synthetase incubated with IFN, inhibited the
development of IFN-induced antiviral state. The extent of
suppression of the antiviral state by the inhibitors
correlated reasonably well with the potency and the stability of the inhibitor remaining in contact with the
cells. Thus, aspirin, despite being a potent inhibitor of
the enzyme, was much less effective than oxyphenyl butazone (Fig. 2). Aspirin is unstable in aqueous solutions
and is consequently ineffective against the newly synthesized enzyme which appears in the cells within approximately 4 hrs. The inhibitory activity of oxyphenyl butazone can be easily seen in the medium even after this
compound was incubated for 24 hrs with the cells.

An important observation is that none of the known
prostaglandins formed via the cyclo-oxygenase pathway was
found to substitute for the inhibited enzyme. In many
instances the products of cellular arachidonate metabolism
either by cyclo-oxygenase or lipoxygenase pathways were
found inhibitory to the IFN action (Fig. 2).

The hypothesis that the prostaglandin synthetase is a
necessary enzyme for IFN action was supported by the

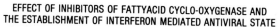

EFFECT OF INHIBITORS OF FATTYACID CYCLO-OXYGENASE AND
THE ESTABLISHMENT OF INTERFERON MEDIATED ANTIVIRAL STATE

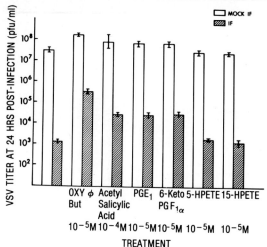

Fig. 2. Experiments were done in L-cell monolayers.
Additional experimental details may be found in Pottathil
et al. (1980). Inhibitor was added together with mouse
β-IFN (100 U/ml) and incubated for 24 hrs, before virus
challenge (multiplicity of infection, 1.0). Prostaglandins of E type, (PGE), 6 Keto prostaglandin $F_1\alpha$
(6 Keto PG $F_1\alpha$), 5 hydroperoxyeicosatetraenoic acid
(5HPETE) and 15 hydroperoxyeicosatetraenoic acid
(15·HPETE) are the most common oxygenation products of
cellular metabolism through cylo-oxygenase and lipoxygenase pathways.

observation that in IFN resistant, L1210 R_3 cells, the
specific activity of this enzyme was only less than 10% of
the sensitive S_6 clones (Fig. 3) (Chandrabose et al.,
1980). Fatty acid lipoxygenase, the only other enzyme
which metabolizes arachidonic acid though oxygenation
pathways, remains unaffected in R_3 cells. Thus a selective impairment of arachidonate metabolism involving only
the fatty acid cyclo-oxygenase was observed in these cells
as a result of selective growth in the presence of large
concentrations of IFN (Gresser et al., 1974). A related

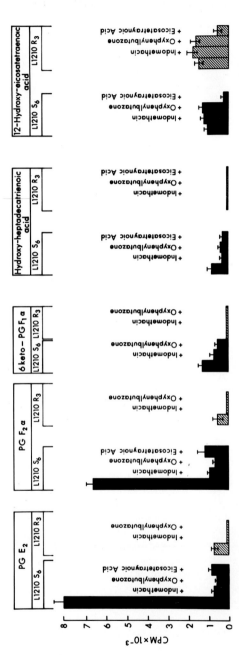

Fig. 3. Prostaglandin synthetase and lipoxygenase activities of L1210 S₆ and R₃ cells.
Suspension cultures of L1210 cells were grown in RPMI-1640 medium, with 10 percent
FCS. Cells were washed in phosphate-buffered saline (PBS) three times and resuspended in 0.1M
tris and 0.15M saline, pH 7.5, containing 1 μCi of [1-¹⁴C]arachidonate at a cell density of
20 x 10⁶ cells per milliliter. The cells were incubated at 37°C for 30 minutes. Formic acid
(100 μl) was then added, and after centrifugation the cell pellet and supernatant were extracted separately with a mixture of chloroform and methanol (2:1 by volume), Folch-partitioned,
and the lower chloroform layer was evaporated to dryness and chromatographed on silica gel G
plates. The solvent system used was the upper layer of a mixture of ethyl acetate isooctane,
acetic acid, and water (90:50:100, by volume). The radioactive bands were located by
autoradiography, scraped, and quantitated by scintillation spectrometry. I, indomethacin; O,
oxyphenylbutazone: and E, eicosatetraynoic acid. 12 Hydroxy icosatetraenoic acid, (the last
set in the figure) is the predominant lipoxygenase product in these cells.

observation regarding the requirement of prostaglandin synthetase for IFN sensitivity is the very low activity of this enzyme in primary cultures of mouse embryos. The specific activity of the enzyme increased progressively with passage. Activities comparable to those reported in mouse L cells or L1210 S_6 cells were obtained only after the 10th serial passage starting from a primary culture (unpublished observations). Other investigators have reported that IFN sensitivity of primary cultures is low, and that the ability of cells to respond to IFN increases with culture-age (Lindahl-Magnusson et al., 1971).

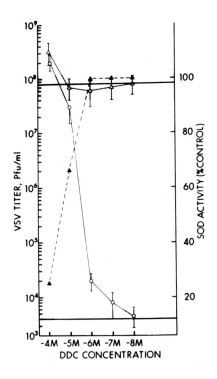

Fig. 4. Effect of diethyldithiocarbamate (DDC) concentration on the activity of superoxide dismutase and on virus yields of mouse β-IFN treated L-cells.

The upper shaded area represents the variation in virus yield with mock IFN. Lower shaded area represents the variation in virus yield after 200 U/ml of IFN for 8 hrs. ---, SOD activity; Δ---Δ, virus yield with mock IFN and DDC. 0--0--0, virus yield with 200 U/ml IFN + DDC; additional details in Pottathil et al. (1981).

The enzyme superoxide dismutase is coded by chromosome 21 in humans and chromosome 16 in mice. In these species, these chromosomes are also required for the IFN sensitivity. Superoxide dismutase has been shown to be syntenic with IFN sensitivity in somatic hybrids (Tan et al., 1973, Chang et al., 1975, Tan, 1977, Epstein et al., 1980, Cox et al., 1980). Because of some similarities in the reaction mechanisms in these two enzymes, we have investigated whether this enzyme is involved functionally in IFN sensitivity. We have shown recently (Pottathil et al., 1980) that an inhibitor of this enzyme blocked completely the development of antiviral activity by 200 U/ml of IFN (Fig. 4). The inhibitor diethyl dithiocarbamate (DDC) acts by chelating the metal ion copper present in the active site of the enzyme. After 2 hrs incubation of cells with 10^{-5}M DDC, if the medium is removed and replaced with fresh medium without DDC, there is no loss of the inhibitory effect on IFN action (Pottathil et al., 1981). However, if the cells are allowed to remain in the fresh medium with IFN, development of the antiviral state may be observed after 12-16 hrs. A parallel recovery of superoxide dismutase may be noticed during this period (Fig. 5).

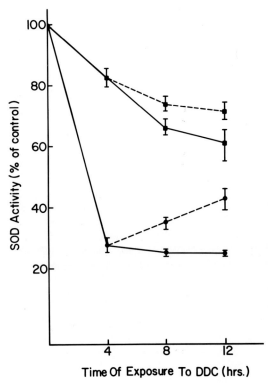

Fig. 5. Dose and time dependent inhibition by DDC and recovery of SOD. L cell monolayers were treated with DDC at final concentrations of 10^{-4} M, (A) or 10^{-5} M (B). The cultures were incubated at 37°C in CO_2 (5%). Medium from some cultures was removed after 4 hrs, replaced with fresh medium and further incubated for up to 12 hrs. Cells were harvested at different time intervals and SOD was quantitated (Pottathil et al., 1981). Dashed lines indicate where DDC-containing medium was replaced with fresh medium.

This Effect of Enzyme Inhibitors on the Lipid Changes
Induced by IFN

The data described so far has implicated the catalytic
function of two oxygen metabolizing cellular enzymes, and a
specific IFN induced membrane composition change to be required for sensitive cells to respond to appropriate IFN programming leading to the antiviral state. If the requirement of
these enzyme activities precedes the membrane changes, or if
they are required for these changes, during the programmed
sequence of IFN action, then the inhibition of enzyme activity should also prevent the membrane lipid changes, as well
as the development of a productive antiviral state. The
data described here and previously reported by us (Pottathil
et al., 1980) show that the development of the antiviral
state is indeed inhibited by these compounds. The membrane
lipid changes are also totally blocked if either oxyphenylbutazone or DDC is incubated with IFN (Fig. 6).

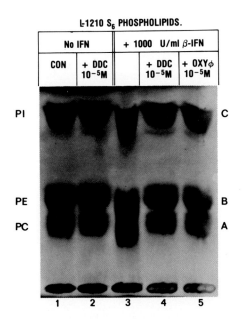

L-1210 S$_6$ PHOSPHOLIPIDS.

No IFN		+ 1000 U/ml β-IFN	
CON	+ DDC 10^{-5}M	+ DDC 10^{-5}M	+ OXYφ 10^{-5}M

PI   C

PE   B
PC   A

1   2   3   4   5

Fig. 6. Autoradiograph
of a thin layer chroma-
togram showing the ef-
fect of inhibitors of
IFN action on the IFN-
induced changes in phos-
pholipids.

Experimental details and
identification of lipid
bands are identical to
those in Fig. 1,A. Inhi-
bitors, when present,
were added together with
LFN and incubated for
8 hrs, before the lipids
were extracted and pro-
cessed.

Lane 1, L1210 S$_6$, IFN
sensitive cells control;
Lane 2, L1210 S$_6$ + 10^{5}M
diethyldithiocarbamate;
Lane 3, L1210 S$_6$ + 1000
U/ml β IFN; Lane 4,
L1210 S$_6$ + 10^{5}M diethyldithiocarbamate + 1000 U/ml IFN;
Lane 5, L1210 S$_6$ + 10^{5}M oxyphenylbutazone + 1000 U/ml IFN.

An interesting feature of such an inhibitory effect is that these compounds are effective only when added together with IFN or preincubated. The compounds have no effect on the development of the antiviral state once IFN has been in contact with the cell for more than 2 hrs. Thus, their effect appears to be on the initiation rather than the maintenance of antiviral activity.

Effect of Inhibition of Cyclooxygenase on IFN Enhanced Macrophage Phagocytosis

It is well documented that IFN enhances mononuclear cell functions like phagocytosis and macrophage tumorocidal activity (Huang et al., 1971, Schultz et al., 1978). We have extended our studies to the IFN mediated enhancement of phagocytosis by unstimulated peritoneal exudate macrophages. IFN at 100 U/ml caused nearly 6-fold increase in phagocytic activity in these cells. Preincubation, or addition of oxyphenylbutazone together with IFN resulted in 50% inhibition of the IFN induced enhancement in phagocytosis (Fig. 7). Thus, at least one non-antiviral property

EFFECT OF OXYPHENYLBUTAZONE ON THE INTERFERON MEDIATED
ENHANCEMENT OF Fc-MEDIATED PARTICLE UPTAKE BY
MACROPHAGES.

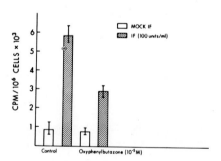

Fig. 7. Unstimulated peritoneal exudate cells were freshly harvested and plastic adherent cells were treated with 100 units of mouse β IFN/ml. Control and IFN treated macrophages were incubated for 4 hours at 37°C, washed repeatedly with fresh medium and incubated with ^{125}I-IgG coated sheep red blood cells (SRBC) at a ratio of 1000 SRBC/1 macrophage for 2 hours. SRBC has a specific radioactivity approximately equal to 0.0425 cts/cell.

of IFN is apparently affected in the same manner as the antiviral property suggesting that these diverse cellular functions activated by IFN should have had at least one common pathway influenced by the enzymatic function of prostaglandin synthetase.

Inhibition of IFN Induced NK Cell Activation by DDC

IFNs and IFN inducers are potent stimulants of natural killer (NK) cell activity (Einhorn et al., 1978, Trinchieri et al., 1978). NK cells, a population of Fc receptor bearing lymphocytes without markers of mature T or B cells, can initiate tumor cell lysis without prior antigenic sensitization and are not restricted by antigenic specificity. IFNs may serve a fundamental role in regulation of NK cell activity. Anti-IFN antisera inhibited not only stimulation of NK cell activity by IFN and poly I:poly C but also blocked basal NK cell activity (Djeu et al., 1979, Herberman et al., 1979).

It was thus our hypothesis that, if superoxide dismutase was a critical enzyme in mediation of the cellular effects of IFN, DDC should be a potent inhibitor of both basal and IFN stimulated NK cell activity. In specific, ^{51}Cr release assays using human lymphocytes and K562 target cells (described in Materials and Methods) a dose dependent inhibition by DDC was observed (Table 1).

Table 1

Effect of Diethyldithiocarbamate (DDC)

| | NK cell activity | |
| | Lytic units$_{30}$ x 10^7 cells) | |
DDC [M]	No IFN	IFN (800 units)
0	57	242
10^{-5}	32	158
10^{-4}	0	0

Ficoll-hypaque separated mononuclear cells were incubated with media or DDC for on hour. They were then incubated with αIFN (800 units/ml) for an additional hour. Specific ^{51}Cr release from K562 target cells was determined at effector: target cell ratios of 50:1, 25:1 and 12.5:1 after 6 hours incubation.

Both basal and interferon-stimulated NK cell cytotoxicity were inhibited by DDC (Table 1). DDC at 10^{-4}M
for 60 min was consistently effective. Under these
conditions, DDC did not result in any change in cell
viability, which was greater than 98% when assessed by
Eosin exclusion. Human basal NK cell activity was completely abrogated. A similar potent inhibition of
enhancement of NK cell activity by IFN was also observed.

DISCUSSION

One of the puzzling aspects of the data presented in
this chapter is that the common stable products of the
enzyme cannot substitute for the inhibited enzyme. PGE_2
is the most common and abundant prostaglandin product
synthesized and excreted by cultured fibroblasts. Not
only PGE_2, but also most other stable prostaglandins
tested were found to be inhibitory to development of
antiviral state by IFN to varying degrees. PGH_2, the
unstable endoperoxide which should conceivably supply all
the prostaglandins by appropriate metabolic conversions
was also ineffective in restoration of the antiviral
state in presence of the inhibitors of cyclo-oxygenase
(Pottathil et al., 1980). An interesting possibility is
that the PG-synthetase dependent co-oxidation reaction
(discussed elsewhere in this volume) might participate in
some early event in IFN action. If this is indeed happen-
ing, then the information available from data presented
would allows us to conclude that PG-synthetase should act
either before the lipid changes, or more likely the lipid
changes may be actually driven by this reaction. Such
conclusions should however await the complete elucidation
of the stochiometry of this reaction involving the phospholipids.

There are parallel observations in the literature
showing that pretreatment of cells with E_2 type prostaglandins are indeed inhibitory to various IFN mediated
biological activities. Trofatter and Daniels (1979)
reported inhibition of IF antiviral protection in human
fibroblasts by PGE_2. Inhibition of macrophage tumoricidal
function (Schultz and Chirgos, 1978a, Schultz et al.,
1978b) and suppression of the IFN-enhanced NK cell activity by E_2 type prostaglandins (Brunda et al., 1980) are
analogous observations. Data summarized in this chapter

show that the antiviral property and at least one non-antiviral property - the enhancement of phagocytosis by IFN - are both sensitive to inhibitors of cyclo-oxygenase function. It seems likely that this apparent paradox--that the function of cyclo-oxygenase is required for the development of an IFN mediated cellular event and that the same event is being inhibited by the product of the enzyme--may indeed be found applicable to various IFN mediated reactions. A partial explanation for such inhibitory properties of stable prostaglandins may be found in their ability to modulate cell membrane properties. Preliminary observations in our laboratory show that PGE$_2$ incubated with IFN does interfere with the specific membrane modification induced by IFN. This property of PGE$_2$ is probably independent of its ability to activate adenylate cyclase since a stable analogue of prostacyclin (carbon prostacyclin), at least equipotent in increasing cAMP concentrations, was not inhibitory to development of antiviral state by IFN (Pottathil et al., 1980).

What is the possible significance of the change in fluidity of cell membranes induced by IFN? The importance of specific growth factors (e.g., sarcoma growth factor and other tumor secreted growth factors) in maintaining the malignantly transformed phenotypes in vitro is discussed elsewhere in this volume. The productive interaction of a growth factor with its receptor, and the subsequent programmed processing of the hormone receptor complex are among the earliest events, before the complex array of transformation properties are manifested. The rigidity of membranes resulting from even 200-600 U/ml of IFN (a concentration that may be easily achieved in culture with inducers in vitro and therefore probably in vivo) is sufficient to prevent redistribution of specific receptors (Pfeffer et al., 1980). Ligand induced receptor redistribution is gaining increased acceptance as an important part of the mechanism of peptide hormone action. The question therefore arises whether the rigidity of the membrane necessary for the action of IFN would abort the receptor-ligand interaction or (appropriate redistribution of receptor-ligand complex) of a tumor specific growth factor required for the clonal proliferation of specific neoplasm (e.g., SGF and receptor). Decreased availability of serotonin receptors to serotonin binding after rigidifying the membranes artifically with lipids containing saturated fatty acids has been reported (Heron et al., 1980). We have found that IFN treatment inhibits specific

insulin binding to insulin receptors by about 50%. If
confirmed and extended, this might explain at least in
part the anti-neoplastic action of IFN, and why this
action may not be so universal.

There is inadequate information at present to answer
the question, "why such changes in cell membranes are
necessary, if at all, for IFN action." Although any model
based on incomplete information has to be necessarily
speculative, the kinetics of the reported changes allow
one to assign a limited sequence of events in which the
lipid changes might play a role. The time course of
phospholipid changes of IFN on homologous cells is very
rapid. It occurs before the minimum time required for
IFN-induced transcriptional or translational events can
possibly take place (Revel et al., 1980). Nevertheless, a
role for cellular enzymes is shown by the prevention of
these changes by various inhibitors described here which
have no effect on DNA, RNA or protein synthesis (unpublished
data). These compounds are profoundly inhibitory on the
development of the IFN-mediated antiviral state only if
applied before or during the time of incubation with IFN.
It is, therefore, tempting to postulate that the specific
modifications of cell membranes we observe are necessary
for the appropriate binding and processing of IFN in the
plane of the membrane, as is the case for many other
polypeptide hormones, before exerting its ultimate biological effects.

Scheme 1 summarizes the time course of what is known
about IFN action. The possible sequence in which the
membrane changes take place are indicated. This scheme in
general is taken from Revel et al. (1980) in which "rapid
membrane changes" was already labelled by the authors.

SUMMARY

Interferon induces specific compositional changes in
cell membrane lipids. The changes are maximal within
30 min after addition of interferon to homologous cells.
Therefore the membrane changes are not mediated by interferon induced enzymes which take considerably longer
times to be expressed. Compounds which inhibit fatty
acid cyclo-oxygenase and cytoplasmic superoxide dismutase
effectively block the interferon induced membrane composi-

tion changes. These compounds are also profoundly inhibitory to the development of the antiviral state, enhancement of phagocytosis and activation of natural killer cells by interferon. The membrane changes induced by interferon therefore appear to be a necessary cellular event required for productive programming of homologous cells for the characteristic manifestation of the pleotropic properties of interferon.

RECEPTOR-MEDIATED INTERNALIZATION HYPOTHESIS
AS APPLIED TO IFN ACTION

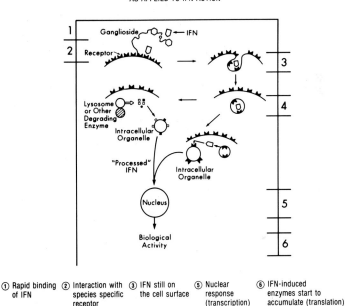

① Rapid binding of IFN	② Interaction with species specific receptor	③ IFN still on the cell surface	⑤ Nuclear response (transcription)	⑥ IFN-induced enzymes start to accumulate (translation)
	rapid membrane changes	④ Internalization of IFN and receptor (?)		Delayed biochemical response

TIME: 0 hr...1 hr....................2 hr..................3 hr..................12 hr

| binding to gangliosides (even in the cold) | binding to surface component coded by chr 21 | Inhibition by antibodies to or receptor | Antiviral state and enzyme induction becomes Act D resistant | Superinduction of antiviral state and enzyme by Act D |

Scheme 1

REFERENCES

Brunda MJ, Herberman RB, Holden HT (1980). Inhibition of
murine natural killer cell activity by prostaglandins.
J Immunol 124:2682.
Chandrabose KA, Cuatrecasas P, Pottathil R (1981a).
Changes in fatty acyl chains of phospholipids induced
by interferon in mouse sarcoma S-180 cells. Biochem
Biophys Res Commun 98:661.
Chandrabose KA, Cuatrecasas P, Pottathil R, Lang DJ
(1981b). Interferon resistant cell line lacks fatty
acid cyclo-oxygenase. Science 212:329.
Chang C, viginal M, Couillin P, Cong NV, Boue J, Boue A
(1975). Chromosomal localization of human genes govern-
ing the interferon induced antiviral sate. Proc Natl
Acad Sci USA 72:3129.
Cox DR, Epstein LB, Epstein CJ (1980). Genes coding for
sensitivity to interferon and soluble superoxide dimutase
are linked in mouse and man and map to chromosome 16.
Proc Natl Acad Sci 77:2168.
DeMaeyer-Guignard J, DeMaeyerGuignard E (1980). Electrophoretically pure interferon exerts multiple biological
effects. Ann NY Acad Sci 350:347.
Djeu TY, Heinbaugh JA, Holden HT, Herberman RB (1979).
Augmentation of mouse natural killer cell activity by
interferon and interferon inducers. J. Immunol 122:175.
Donahoe R, Huang KY (1976). Interferon preparations
enhance phagocytosis in vivo. Infect Immun 13:1250.
Einhorn S, Blomgren H, Strander H (1978). Enhancement of
spontaneous cytotoxicity of peripheral lymphocytes by
human leukocyte interferon. Int J Cancr 22:405.
Epstein LB, Cox DR, Epstein CJ (1980). Assignment of
genes for sensitivity to interferon and soluble superoxide dimutase to mouse chromosome 16. Ann NY Acad Sci
350:171.
Fitzpatrick FA, Stringfellow DA (1980). Virus and interferon effects on cellular prostaglandin biosynthesis.
J. Immunol 125:431.
Gisler R, Lindahl P, Gresser I (1975). Effects of interferon on antibody synthesis in vivo. J Immunol 113:438.
Gresser I, Bronty-Boye D, Thomas H, Macierra-Coelho
(1970). Interferon and cell division I. Inhibition of
the multiplication of the mouse leukemia L1219 cells in
vitro by interferon preparations. Proc Natl Acad Sci
USA 66:1052.

Gresser I, Bandu MT, Brouty-Boyé D (1974). Interferon and cell division IX. Interferon resistant L1210 cells - characteristics and origin. J Natl Cancer Inst 52:553.

Gresser I, Tovey MG (1978). Antitumor effects of interferon. Biochim Biophys Acta 516:231.

Herberman RB, Ortaldo JR, Bonnard GD (1979). Augmentation by interferon of human natural and antibody dependent cell mediated cytotoxicity. Nature 277:221.

Heron DS, Shinitzky M, Hershkowitz M, Samuel D (1980). Lipid fluidity markedly modulates the binding of seretonin to mouse brain membranes. Proc Natl Acad Sci USA 77:7463.

Huang KY, Donahoe RM, Gordon FB, Dressler HR (1971). Enhancement of phagocytosis by interferon containing preparations. Infect Immun 4:518.

Isaac A, Lindenmann J (1957). Virus interference I. The interferon. Proc Royal Soc B 147:258.

Lindahl-Magnusson P, Leary P, Gresser I (1971). Interferon and cell division VI. Inhibitory effect of interferon on the multiplication of mouse embryo and mouse kidney cells in primary cultures. Proc Soc Exp Biol Med 138:1044.

Pfeffer LM, Wang E, Tamm I (1980). Interferon inhibits the redistribution of cell surface components. J Exp Med 152:469.

Pfeffer LM, Wang E, Landsberger FR, Tamm E (1981). Assays to measure plasma membrane and cytoskeletal changes in interferon-treated cells. In Methods in enzymology, Interferons, ed. S. Pestka, Academic Press NY (in press).

Pottathil R, Chandrabose KA, Cuatrecasas P, Lang DJ (1980). Establishment of the interferon mediated antiviral state: Role of fatty acid cyclo-oxygenase. Proc Natl Acad Sci USA 77:5437.

Pottathil R, Chandrabose KA, Cuatrecasas P, Lang DJ (1981). Establishment of interferon mediated antiviral state: Possible role of superoxide dismutase. Proc Natl Acad Sci USA 78:3343.

Pross HF, Baines MG, Rubin P, Shragge P, Patterson MS (1981). Spontaneous human lymphocyte-mediated cytotoxicity against tumor target cells. IX The quantification of natural killer cell activity. J Clin Immunol 1:51.

Revel M, Kimchi A, Shulman L, Fradin A, Schuster E, Yakobson Y, Chernajovsky A, Schimidt AS, Bendori R (1980). Role of interferon induced enzymes in the antiviral and antimitogenic effects of interferon. Ann NY Acad Sci 350:459.

Schults RM and Chirgos MA (1978a). Similarities among factors that render macrophages tumorocidal in lymphokine and interferon preparations. Cancer Res 38:1003.

Schultz RM, Pavalidis NA, Stylos WA, Chirgos MA (1978b). Regulation of Macrophage tumorocidal function: A role for prostaglandin E series. Science 202:320.

Singer SJ, Nicolson GL (1972). The fluid mosaic model of the structure of cell membranes. Science 175:720.

Stringfellow DA (1978). Prostaglandin restoration of the interferon response of hyporeactive animals. Science 201:376.

Tan YH, Tischfield JA, Ruddle FH (1973). Linkage of the genes for human interferon induced antiviral protein and indophenol oxidase B traits to chromosome G-21. J Exp Med 137:317.

Tan YH (1979). Genetics of the human interferon system. In Stewert II (ed): "Interferons and their actions": CRC Press, p 73.

Trinchieri G, Santoli D, Koprowski H (1978). Spontaneous cell mediated cytotoxicity in humans: Role of inter- ferons and immunoglobulins. J Immunol 120:1849.

Trofatter KF, Daniels CA (1979). Possible role of prosta- glandins in exacerbation of Herpes Simplex virus infection. Inhibition of human cell's response to interferon production and of interferon's ability to mediate antibody dependent cell mediated cytotoxicity. Lab Invest 40:288.

Yaron M, Yaron I, Gurari Rotman D, Revel M, Lindner HR, Zor U (1977). Stimulation of prostaglandin E production in cultured human fibroblasts by poly (I) poly (C) and human interferon. Nature 267:457.

Zarling JM, Eskra L, Borden EC, Horoszewics J, Carter WA (1979). Activation of human natural killer cells cytotoxic for human leukemia cells by purified interferon. J Immunol 123:63.

**Prostaglandins and Cancer: First
International Conference, pages 365-368
© 1982 Alan R. Liss, Inc., 150 Fifth Avenue, New York, NY 10011**

STRUCTURAL ACTIVITY REQUIREMENT FOR PGA EFFECTS
ON TUMOR CELL GROWTH AND DIFFERENTIATION

W.A. Turner, D.R. Bennett, K.C. Thompson,
J.D. Taylor and K.V. Honn
Wayne State University, Detroit, MI 48202

INTRODUCTION

Prostaglandins of the "A" series (PGAs) have been
shown to inhibit tumor cell proliferation and induce
differentiation although the exact mechanism has been
unclear (Adolphe et al., 1973; Stein-Werblowsky, 1974;
Karmali et al., 1979; Honn et al., 1979; Santoro et al.,
1979). We propose that the structural requirement for
these effects is related to the presence of a reactive α,
β-unsaturated carbonyl group at the 10-11 position of the
cyclopentane ring (Fig. 1). For some time, citral, acro-

PGA$_2$ PGB$_2$

lein, and crotonaldehyde have been shown to be effective
anticancer agents (Boyland, 1940; Dittmar, 1940). The
toxic and carcinostatic activity of these compounds has
been attributed to the α, β-unsaturated aldehyde grouping
(Osato et al., 1953). These studies were initiated to
determine the structural requirement of the 10-11 α, β -
unsaturated double bond in PGA antitumor activity.

METHODS

To determine the effects on DNA synthesis, monodispersed B16 amelanotic melanoma cells (B16a) were collected
from whole tumors, incubated at intervals with various

prostaglandin treatments, and the resultant incorporation of ^{3}H-thymidine into DNA was measured (Honn et al., 1981). For these studies PGA$_1$ & PGA$_2$, 15 Epi PGA$_2$ (containing the 15R hydroxy group), and PGB$_1$ & PGB$_2$ (which possess a less reactive α, β-unsaturated carbonyl) were used for 4 hr at concentrations of 1-25 μg ml^{-1}. In addition PGA$_1$ and PGA$_2$ conjugated with reduced glutathione (GSH) at 5, 25, 50, & 100 μM (to reduce the 10-11 double bond) were also used in incubations for 4 hr at a concentration of 5 μg ml^{-1}.

For differentiation studies mouse neuroblastoma (ATCC, Rockville, Md) were grown as a monolayer (Prasad and Vernadakis, 1972). Prostaglandins were added to the cultures 24 h after plating. Differentiation was determined recording the % of cells exhibiting axon formation and morphology for 3 days. PGA$_1$, PGA$_2$, 15 Epi PGA$_2$, PGB$_1$, PGB$_2$ and PGE$_1$ were evaluated for inducing differentiation at concentrations of 5.0 or 10 μg ml^{-1}.

RESULTS

In B16a cell suspensions PGA$_1$ and PGA$_2$ produced a dose dependent inhibition of DNA synthesis (Table I). 15 Epi PGA$_2$ was equally as effective as PGA$_2$ in the inhibition of ^{3}H-thymidine incorporation. PGAs (5 μg ml^{-1}) conjugated with 25, 50, and 100 μM GSH failed to inhibit ^{3}H-thymidine incorporation. In addition PGB$_1$ and PGB$_2$ were also noninhibitory.

Table 1. ^{3}H Thymidine Incorporation   4 hr

Dose (μg/ml)		% Control	Dose (μg/ml)		% Control
PGA$_1$	1.0	79.1 ± 8.2	PGA$_2$* + GSH (25 M)		98.2 ± 3.8
PGA$_1$	10	88.4 ± 2.4	PGA$_2$* + GSH (50 M)		104.2 ± 2.6
PGA$_1$	25	56.0 ± 3.2	PGA$_2$* + GSH(100 M)		103.0 ± 1.8
PGA$_2$	1.0	78.6 ± 5.5	PGB$_1$	1.0	90.8 ± 0.1
PGA$_2$	5.0	71.6 ± 1.6	PGB$_1$	5.0	84.5 ± 1.2
PGA$_2$	10	60.1 ± 4.5	PGB$_1$	10	84.5 ± 2.9
PGA$_2$	25	31.2 ± 1.6	PGB$_2$	1.0	95.1 ± 1.8
Epi-PGA$_2$	1.0	61.5 ± 2.1	PGB$_2$	5.0	92.0 ± 2.0
Epi-PGA$_2$	5.0	48.3 ± 2.8	PGB$_2$	10	83.0 ± 0.9
Epi-PGA$_2$	10	30.3 ± 1.1			

*(5 μg/ml PGA$_2$)

In mouse neuroblastoma PGA_1, PGA_2, Epi PGA_2 (5.0 μg/ml) and PGE_1 (10 μg/ml), were effective in inducing differentiation above the level seen in untreated controls. PGB_1 and PGB_2 failed to induce differentiation above that seen in untreated controls.

DISCUSSION

PGA_1 and PGA_2 which possess the cyclopentenone moiety (α,β-unsaturated carbonyl) were effective inhibitors of DNA synthesis in B16 amelanotic melanoma and positive inducers of differentiation in mouse neuroblastoma cells. PGB_1 and PGB_2 which possess a less reactive (stericly hindered)α,β-unsaturated carbonyl did not cause an inhibition in DNA synthesis or induce differentiation. The importance of the α, β-unsaturated ketone group in PGA_2 is also shown with the glutathione treatments. Conjugation of the mercaptan to PGA_1 (at C_{11}) has been shown to occur at the site of the cyclopentenone moiety (Cagen et al., 1975; Cagen et al., 1976; Chandhari, 1978). In this study the reduction of the α, β unsaturated carbonyl in PGA_2 by GSH abolished the inhibition of ^3H thymidine incorporation. It was also shown that both the 15-OH epimers of PGA_2 (R or S) were equally effective in inhibiting DNA synthesis and inducing differentiation. The nature and stereospecificity of the substituents at position 15 of the prostaglandin molecule has been shown to be a critical determinant for platelet stimulating activity (MacIntyre et al., 1978). These modifications are apparently not important to the effects on DNA synthesis and differentiation as shown in these studies. The results here suggest that the reactiveα,β-unsaturated ketone group may be required for the antitumor effect exhibited by PGAs in vitro.

REFERENCES

Adolphe M, Giroud JP, Timsit J, Lechat P (1973) Etude comparative des effets des PGE_1, E_2 A_2, F_1 , F_2 sur la division des cellules Hela en culture. Compt Rend 277:537.
Boyland E (1940) Further experiments with aldehydes and their derivatives. Biochem J 34:1196.

Cagen LM, Fales HM, Pisano JJ (1976) Formation of glutathione conjugates of prostaglandin A_1 in human red blood cells. J Biol Chem 251:6550.

Cagen LM, Pisano JJ, Ketley JN, Habig WH, Jakoby WB (1975) The conjunction of prostaglandin A_1 and glutathione catalyzed by homogenous glutathione S-transferases from human and rat liver. Biochim et Biophys Acta 398:205.

Chardhari A, Anderson MW, Eling TE (1978) Conjugation of 15-keto-prostaglandins by glutathione s-transferases. Biochim et Biophys Acta 531:56.

Dittmar C (1940) Uber einige chemotherapeutisch bei wisksame vesbindungen. Z Krebsforsch 49:515.

Honn KV, Dunn JR, Morgan LR, Bienkowski M, Marnett LJ (1979) Inhibition of DNA synthesis in Harding-Passey melanoma cells by prostaglandins A_1 and A_2: comparison with chemotherapeutic agents. Biochem Biophy Res Comm 87:795.

Honn KV, Romine M, Skoff A (1981) Prostaglandin analogs as inhibitors of tumor cell DNA synthesis. Proc Soc Exp Biol Med 166:562.

Karmali RA, Horrobin DF, Menezes J, Patel P (1979) The relationship between concentrations of prostaglandins A_1, E_1, E_2 and F_2 and rates of cell proliferation. Phar Res Comm 11:69.

Osato s, Hanno H (1953) On chemotherapy of carcinoma. Gann 44:348.

Prasad KN, Vernadkis A (1972) Morphological and biochemical study in x-ray and dibutyryl cyclic-AMP-induced differentiated neuroblastoma cells. Exp Cell Res 70:27.

Santoro MG, Arrigo B, Jaffe BM (1979) Prostaglandin A_1 induces differentiation in Friend erythroleukemia cells. Prostaglandins 17:719.

Stein-Werblowsky R (1974) The effect of prostaglandin on tumor implantation. Experientia 30:957.

Prostaglandins and Cancer: First
International Conference, pages 369-373
© 1982 Alan R. Liss, Inc., 150 Fifth Avenue, New York, NY 10011

EFFECTS OF PROSTAGLANDIN "A" SERIES ON TUMOR CELLS IN VITRO

W.A. Turner, J.D. Taylor and K.V. Honn

Departments of Biological Sciences, Radiology
and Radiation Oncology
Wayne State University, Detroit, MI 48202

INTRODUCTION

Although a large amount of research has been conducted on the role of prostaglandins (PG) and cancer (for review see Karmali, 1980; Honn, et al., 1981) early reports of prostaglandin A (PGA) toxicity (Kagen et al., 1977) have limited their evaluation. Unlike the conflicting data concerning prostaglandin E's (PGEs) (Santoro et al., 1976; Santoro et al., 1977; Owen et al., 1980; Tutton and Barkla, 1980, Lupulescu, 1980), PGAs have been shown to inhibit tumor cell implantation (Stein-Werblowsky, 1974), growth in vivo (Favalli et al., 1980), and in vitro (Adolphe, et al., 1973; Eisenbarth et al., 1974; Honn et al., 1979; Karmali et al., 1979). In addition, PGAs have been shown to induce differentiation in Friend erythroleukemia cells (Santoro, 1979). This study investigates the effects of PGAs and their more stable 16-16 dimethyl analogues on proliferation and DNA synthesis in B16 amelanotic melanoma and Lewis lung carcinoma and on differentiation of 3T3-L1 mouse fibroblasts in vitro.

METHODS

B16 amelanotic melanoma (B16a) and Lewis lung carcinoma (3LL) (DCT Animal and Human Tumor Bank) tumors were disaggregated into monodispersed cell suspensions (Sloane, et al., 1981) for precursor incorporation and proliferation studies. PGA_1, PGA_2, di-me-PGA, and di-me-PGA_2 (Gift from Dr. John Pike, Upjohn) were used at concentrations of 1, 5,

10, or 25 µg ml^{-1} in all studies. Incorporation of ^{3}H-thymidine into DNA was measured at 4 and 20 hour inter- vals using B16a and 3LL cell suspensions. Proliferation studies in Eagle's MEM measured the growth rates of 3 x 10^4 PGA- treated B16a cells for 7 days. Recovery studies were conducted on B16a cells exposed to PGAs for only 4, 24, 48, or 72 hrs. Cell viabilities were monitored with trypan blue and LDH assays (Yochim and Clark, 1971). PGA induced conversion of 3T3-L1 mouse fibroblasts to adipocytes was evaluated with oil red O staining of triglycerides.

RESULTS

PGA$_1$ and PGA$_2$ and their dimethyl analogues were effective inhibitors of ^{3}H-thymidine incorporation in both tumor cell types. The inhibition was dose dependent and overall PGA$_2$ was the most effective inhibitor (Table 1).

Table 1. ^{3}H Thymidine Incorporation   % Control

Treatment	B16a	3LL
	20 h	20 h
PGA$_1$ 1µg/ml	100 ± 8.2	92.4 ± 6.8
PGA$_1$ 10µg/ml	52 ± 3.1	60.5 ± 2.6
PGA$_1$ 25µg/ml	42 ± 1.6	29.1 ± 1.0
PGA$_2$ 1µg/ml	94.4 ± 1.4	106.8 ± 4.0
PGA$_2$ 10µg/ml	32.9 ± 2.7	42.6 ± 1.1
PGA$_2$ 25µg/ml	12.9 ± 1.2	8.1 ± 0.4
dime-PGA$_1$ 1µg/ml	99.5 ± 6.6	90.9 ± 3.6
dime-PGA$_1$ 10µg/ml	43.3 ± 1.0	40.3 ± 1.9
dime-PGA$_1$ 25 µg/ml	22.4 ± 3.5	10.6 ± 0.7
dimePGA$_2$ 1µg/ml	85.0 ± 5.1	114 ± 1.6
dimePGA$_2$ 10µg/ml	40.9 ± 4.4	63.5 ± 13.9
dimePGA$_2$ 25µg/ml	22.6 ± 2.5	57.9 ± 9.4

Proliferation of B16a cells was significantly inhibited after 5 days of treatment with all PGAs at doses of 10 or 25 µg ml^{-1} (Table 2). PGA$_1$ and PGA$_2$ were more effective

Table 2. Proliferation B16a 5 Days

Treatment	Avg. # Cells	% Growth Inhibition
PGA$_1$ 1μg/ml	513,600	45
PGA$_1$ 10μg/ml	67,200	92.9
PGA$_1$ 25μg/ml	36,000	96.2
PGA$_2$ 1μg/ml	458,400	51
PGA$_2$ 10μg/ml	63,120	93.3
PGA$_2$ 25μg/ml	52,800	94.4
dime-PGA$_1$ 1μg/ml	943,200	0
dime-PGA$_1$ 10μg/ml	124,800	86.8
dime-PGA$_1$ 25μg/ml	60,000	93.7
dime-PGA$_2$ 1μg/ml	1,044,000	-11
dime-PGA$_2$ 10μg/ml	664,800	29.2
dime-PGA$_2$ 25μg/ml	442,400	52.9

than their dimethyl analogues. Analysis of growth media showed no difference in LDH levels between PGA treated and control cultures and no loss of viability was determined with trypan blue dye exclusion testing. B16a cells treated with PGA$_2$ for more than 48 hr did not show normal growth rates even if PGA treatment was stopped. If treatment was suspended within 48 hr, a normal growth rate was reacquired within 3 days. Light microscopy of PGA treated B16a cells showed a complete cessation of mitosis within 4 hr but it resumed to an above normal rate following removal of PGA. PGA$_2$ (5 μg ml^{-1}) effectively induced the differentiation of 3T3-L1 mouse fibroblasts into adipocytes in 3 weeks. Oil red O staining of triglycerides in PGA treated cultures was greater than in insulin treated controls.

DISCUSSION

This study has shown that PGAs effectively inhibit DNA synthesis and proliferation in B16a and 3LL cells in vitro. Others have shown that PGE$_2$ analogues were effective inhibitors of tumor cell proliferation in vivo (Santoro et al., 1977; Tutton and Barkla, 1980). The use of analogues of

PGAs does not appear to provide any advantage from these in vitro studies. Despite previous reports of PGA toxicity (Kagen et al., 1977) our LDH and trypan blue dye testing showed no toxic effects at doses as high as 10 μg ml^{-1}. The loss of cell numbers in proliferation studies is due to detachment of cells from the substratum and not a result of cell death. PGA has been shown to induce cell detachment in other cell types (Santoro et al., 1980). Light microscopy of PGA_2 treated cells reveals that the cells are arrested and do not undergo mitosis. PGA_2 inhibition of proliferation was reversible if treatment was withdrawal within 48 hr and the B16a cells were able to reacquire a normal growth rate within 3 days.

PGA_2 is a potent inducer of differentiation of 3T3-L1 mouse fibroblasts. PGA_1 has also been shown to induce differentiation in Friend erythroleukemia cells (Santoro et al., 1979). These effects on differentiation and tumor cell growth (inhibition) suggest that PGA compounds may prove beneficial in the treatment and control of neoplastic cell growth.

REFERENCES

Adolphe M, Giroud JP, Timsit J, Lechat P (1973). Etude comparative des effets des PGE_1, E_2, A_2, F_1, F_2 sur la division des cellules Hela en culture. Compt Rend 277:537.

Eisenbarth GS, Wellman DK, Lebovitz HE (1974). Prostaglandin A_1 inhibition of chondrosarcoma growth. Biochem Biophys Res Comm 60:1302.

Favalli C, Garaci E, Santoro MG, Santucci L, Jaffe BM (1980). The effects of PGA_1 on the immune response in B16 melanoma-bearing mice. Prostaglandins 19:587.

Honn KV, Bockman RS, Marnett LJ (1981) Prostaglandins and cancer: a review of tumor initiation through tumor metastasis. Prostaglandins 21:833.

Honn KV, Dunn JR, Morgan LR, Bienkowski M, Marnett LJ (1979). Inhibition of DNA synthesis in Harding-Passey melanoma cells by prostaglandins A_1 and A_2: Comparison with chemotherapeutic agents. Biochem Biophys Res Comm 87:795.

Kagen LJ, Neigel DT, Collins K, Robinson HJ (1977). Toxicity of prostaglandins A_1 and A_2 for cells in culture. In vitro 13:18.

Karmali RA (1980). Prostaglandins and cancer. Prostaglandins and Medicine 5:11.

Karmali RA, Horrobin DF, Menezes J, Patel P (1979). The relationship between concentrations of prostaglandins A_1, E_1, E_2 and F_2 and rates of cell proliferation. Phar Res Comm 11:69.

Lupulescu A (1980). Effects of prostaglandins on tumor transplantation. Oncology 37:418.

Owen K, Gomolka D, Droller MJ (1980). Production of PGE_2 by tumor cells in vitro. Canc Res 40:3167.

Santoro MG, Philipott GW, Jaffe BM (1976). Inhibition of tumor growth in vivo and in vitro by prostaglandin E. Nature 263:777.

Santoro MG, Philipott GW, Jaffe BM (1977). Inhibition of B16 melanoma growth in vivo by a synthetic analog of prostaglandin E_2. Canc Res 37:3774.

Santoro MG, Arrigo B, Jaffe BM (1979). Prostaglandin A_1 induces differentiation in Friend erythroleukemia cells. Prostaglandins 17:719.

Santoro MG, Benedetto A, Carruba G, Garaci E, Jaffe BM (1980). Prostaglandin A compounds as antiviral agents. Science 209:1032.

Sloane BF, Dunn JR, Honn KV (1981) Lysosomal cathepsin B: correlation with metastatic potential. Science 212:1151.

Stein-Werblowsky R (1974). The effect of prostaglandin on tumor implantation. Experientia 30:957.

Tutton PJM, Barkla DH (1980). Influence of prostaglandin analogues on epithelial cell proliferation and xenograft growth. Br J Cancer 41:47.

Yochim JM, Clark FW (1971). Lactate dehydrogenase activity in the uterus of the rat during the estrous cycle and its relation to intrauterine oxygen tension. Biol Reproduction 5:146.

Prostaglandins and Cancer: First
International Conference, pages 375-379
© 1982 Alan R. Liss, Inc., 150 Fifth Avenue, New York, NY 10011

THROMBOXANES AND PROSTACYCLIN: POSITIVE AND NEGATIVE
MODULATORS OF TUMOR CELL PROLIFERATION

Kenneth V. Honn, John R. Dunn and Jay Meyer
Departments of Radiation Oncology, Radiology and
Biological Sciences
Wayne State University, Detroit, MI 48202

INTRODUCTION: Thromboxane A_2 (TXA_2) and prostacyclin (PGI_2) exert antagonistic effects on platelet aggregation mediated by opposing effects on platelet cAMP. The rapid synthesis and short half-lives of these compounds make them ideal bioregulators. Recent evidence indicates that TXA_2 and PGI_2 are produced by a wide variety of tissues (Gorman et al., 1979), therefore we examined their effect on tumor cell proliferation and their relation to tumor cell cAMP production.

MATERIALS AND METHODS: B16 amelanotic melanoma (B16a) tumors were disaggregated and elutriated as described (Sloane et al., 1981). [^{3}H]-thymidine incorporation into acid-insoluble DNA was determined as previously described (Honn et al., 1981). Intracellular cAMP and cAMP released into culture media were determined by RIA. TXB_2; the TXA_2 mimicking agent, (15S)-hydroxy-11α, 9α-(epoxymethano) prosta-5Z, 13E-dienoic acid (U46619; Smith, 1980); thromboxane synthetase inhibitors, 9,11-diazo-prosta-5,13-dienoic acid (U51605) and 9,11-imminoepoxy-prosta-5,13-dienoic acid (U54701) (Fitzpatrick et al., 1978); a TXA_2 receptor antagonist, 9,11-epoxyimmino-prosta-5,13-dienoic acid (U54874; (Fitzpatrick et al., 1979); and PGI_2 were generously provided by Dr. John Pike, Upjohn Co.

RESULTS: B16a cells were cultured (7 da) in the presence of either TXB_2, the stable metabolite of TXA_2, or the TXA_2 mimicking agent (U46619). Both compounds produced a dose dependent significant stimulation of tumor cell proliferation with the TXA_2 mimicking agent effective at a dose of 1 µg ml^{-1} (Table 1). At 25 µg ml^{-1} TXB_2 increased proliferation 300%.

TABLE 1.

Effects of the TXA_2 mimicking agent, (15S)-hydroxy-11α, 9α-(epoxymethano) prosta-5Z, 13E-dienoic acid, on proliferation of B16a cells.

Treatment	Cell number X 10^5/plate
Control[a]	1.5 ± 0.2[b]
1.0 µg ml^{-1a}	2.3 ± 0.3
5.0 µg ml^{-1}	2.4 ± 0.2
15.0 µg ml $^{-1}$	2.8 ± 0.3

[a] Media and test compound were changed daily for 4 days.
[b] Mean ± SEM; n = 5

The mechanism of action of thromboxanes in the stimulation of tumor cell proliferation is unknown. Production of TXA_2 by tumor cells could prevent a rise in cAMP levels in response to normal external and/or internal growth regulators (e.g., hormones, growth factors, etc.). Incubation of B16a cells (48 hrs) with TXB_2 (25 µg ml^{-1}) decreased the basal level of intracellular cAMP and cAMP released into the media (Table 2). Cyclic GMP levels were unaffected by TXB_2. PGE_1 (1 µg ml^{-1}) increased B16a intracellular and release of cAMP over a time frame of 15-60 min (Table 2). Preincubation of B16a cells with TXB_2 (48 hr; 25 µg ml^{-1}) inhibited the cAMP response of B16a cells to PGE_1 (Table 2).

The endoperoxide analogues, U51605, U54701 and U54874, significantly reduced DNA synthesis by B16a tumor cells at non-cytotoxic doses (Table 3). The order of effectiveness was: U51605=U54874 > U54701.

Treatment of B16a melanoma cells in culture (7 da) with either PGI_2 or the thromboxane synthetase inhibitors (U51605, U54701) produced a significant dose-related inhibition of proliferation.

TABLE 2.

The Effects of Thromboxane B_2 and PGE_1 on cAMP Levels in B16a Cells.

	Media	Intracellular
Control	0.3300 ± 0.02[a]	0.09 ± 0.06
TXB_2[b]	0.0023 ± 0.002	0.03 ± 0.01
PGE_1 (15 min)[c]	0.4800 ± 0.030	0.34 ± 0.06
PGE_1 (30 min)	13.4000 ± 3.700	0.34 ± 0.05
PGE_1 (60 min)	19.0000 ± 5.000	0.21 ± 0.02
$TXB_2 + PGE_1$ (15 min)[d]	0.1100 ± 0.010	0.21 ± 0.03
$TXB_2 + PGE_1$ (30 min)	1.7000 ± 0.020	0.16 ± 0.08
$TXB_2 + PGE_1$ (60 min)	7.1000 ± 2.600	0.12 ± 0.03

(a) cAMP pmoles μg DNA^{-1}: Mean $\pm$ SEM; n=4; (b) Cells in log phase were pretreated with TXB_2 for 48 hrs prior to assay of cells and media for cAMP. Media were changed and fresh TXB_2 (25 μg ml^{-1}) was added at t_0 and at t_0 + 24 hrs.; (c) PGE_1 was added at a dose of 1 μg ml^{-1}. Media and cells were collected at 15, 30 and 60 min.; (d)Log phase growing cells were pretreated with TXB_2 as in (b) and challenged with PGE_1 (1 μg ml^{-1})

TABLE 3.

Inhibition of B16a melanoma cell DNA synthesis with thromboxane synthetase inhibitors and a thromboxane A_2 receptor antagonist.

Test Compound	Dose (μg ml^{-1})	B16a	
		4 hr	18 hr
U51605	1	73.2 ± 3.8[a]	67.0 ± 6.9
	10	33.7 ± 0.6	37.2 ± 1.5
	25	13.1 ± 1.0	3.5 ± 0.9
U54701	1	86.7 ± 8.6	115.2 ± 9.6
	10	50.0 ± 0.8	76.9 ± 2.6
	25	23.3 ± 1.0	23.6 ± 1.8
U54874	1	108.0 ± 7.0	115.4 ± 8.9
	10	70.9 ± 4.0	56.2 ± 1.4
	25	27.3 ± 1.3	4.3 ± 0.3

[a] % control; Mean $\pm$ SEM; n=4

DISCUSSION: Our results suggest the possibility of bidirectional control of tumor cell proliferation by the balance between endogenous and/or exogenous PGI_2/TXA_2. If this hypothesis is correct, then the following criteria should be substantiated by experimental fact: 1) thromboxane synthetase inhibitors should decrease tumor cell replication; 2) TXA_2 or its stable metabolite TXB_2 should enhance tumor cell proliferation; 3) the TXA_2 mimicking agent, (15S)-Hydroxy-11α, 9α-(epoxymethano) prosta-5Z,13E-dienoic acid, should enhance tumor cell proliferation; 4) exogenous TXB_2 should decrease basal tumor cell cAMP levels; 5) exogenous TXB_2 should blunt the rise in tumor cell cAMP response to external stimuli (e.g., PGE_1, PGE_2, growth factors, etc.); and 6) exogenous PGI_2 should decrease tumor cell proliferation. We have satisfied all of the above criteria by the results presented in this paper. In addition we have demonstrated that an agent (Nafazatrom, Bay g 6575) believed to stimulate PGI_2 production by vascular endothelium inhibits the growth of subcutaneous B16a tumors (Honn et al., in press). Collectively these results strongly suggest that modulation of PGI_2/TXA_2 ratios may be an important therapeutic locus in the control of tumor growth.

REFERENCES:

Fitzpatrick FA, Gorman RR (1978). A comparison of imidazole and 9,11-azo-prosta-5,13-dienoic acid. Two selective thromboxane synthetase inhibitors. Biochim Biophys Acta 539:162.

Fitzpatrick F, Gorman R, Bundy G, Honohan T, McGuire J, Sun F (1979). 9,11-imino-epoxyprosta-5,13-dienoic acid is a selective thromboxane A_2 synthetase inhibitor. Biochim Biophys Acta 573:238.

Gorman RR, Hamilton RD, Hopkins NK (1979). Prostacyclin and thromboxane A_2 biosynthesis and regulation of adenylate cyclase in human diploid cell lines. In Vane JR, Bergstrom S (eds.) "Prostacylin" New York:Raven Press, p. 85.

Honn KV, Romine M, Skoff A (1981). Prostaglandin analogs as inhibitors of tumor cell DNA synthesis. Proc. Soc. Exptl. Biol. Med. 166:562.

Honn KV, Meyer J, Neagos G, Henderson T, Westley C, Ratanatharathrom V. Control of tumor growth and metastasis with prostacyclin and thromboxane synthetase inhibitors: Evidence for a new antitumor and antimetastatic agent (Bay g 6575) In Jamieson GA (eds) "Interaction of Platelets and Tumor Cells. New York: Alan Liss Inc. (in press).
Sloane BF, Dunn JR, Honn KV (1981). Lysosomal cathepsin B: Correlation with metastatic potential. Science 212:1151.
Smith JB (1980). The prostanoids in hemostasis and thrombosis. Amer. J. Pathol. 99:743.

ACKNOWLEDGEMENTS: This work was supported by the National Institutes of Health grants CA29405, CA2997, The Milheim Foundation for Cancer Research and the Comprehensive Cancer Center of Metropolitan Detroit.

**Prostaglandins and Cancer: First
International Conference, pages 381–384**
© **1982 Alan R. Liss, Inc., 150 Fifth Avenue, New York, NY 10011**

THE EFFECT OF GAMMA RADIATION ON PROSTACYCLIN PRODUCTION IN
CULTURED PULMONARY ARTERY ENDOTHELIUM

G.L. Hahn, M. Menconi and P. Polgar

Department of Biochemistry, Boston University
School of Medicine, 80 East Concord Street
Boston, MA   02118

INTRODUCTION AND METHODS

     Endothelial cells comprise the inner lining of the mam-
malian circulatory system. These cells occupy a central position in vascular physiology. Recently, results from a number of laboratories have indicated that the prostaglandins
(PGs) may serve as critical messengers in the regulation of
physiological events in the circulatory system. Cultured
endothelial cells from the calf pulmonary artery exist as
homogeneous populations of cells. They have a finite life
span and present normal karyotypes even after long periods
in culture (Menconi and Polgar, 1981). As such they provide
excellent models for examination of the role of PGs in the
vasculature.

     The major product of arachidonate metabolism in endothel-
ial cells is prostacyclin (PGI_2). This appears to be true
under basal or stimulated conditions. However, the rate of
PGI_2 production is dependent to a large degree on the growth
state of the cell culture. We have previously demonstrated
that in fibroblasts, induced into a non-divisional "quiescent" state by lowered serum concentration, the synthesis of
PGs is significantly enhanced (Taylor, et al., 1981; Taylor
and Polgar, 1981). These observations indicate a correlation
between the ability to initiate cell division and the level
of PGs produced by the culture.

     To further evaluate this premise, we chose to examine
cells which had been rendered non-divisional by gamma irradiation. These cells remain viable for extended periods of

time but cannot be induced into mitosis. This report presents
the results of our examination of gamma irradiation induced
quiescence on PGI_2 production in cultured endothelial cells.

Endothelial cells were isolated from the intima of the
calf pulmonary artery by treatment with collagenase (Polgar
et al., 1980). Cells were maintained in McCoy's medium
plus 20% newborn or fetal bovine serum and fed every other
day. Cells to be used for experimental purposes were inoculated into 35mm petri dishes at densities of 30,000-60,000
cells per plate and used when confluent. Cultures were generally between 5 and 50 population doublings and contained
$1-2 \times 10^6$ cells per plate when used.

Confluent cultures, to be used for analysis, were last
fed 2 days prior to the experiment. Irradiated cultures were
exposed to 1000-3000 rads of gamma radiation in a dual[137] Cs
small animal irradiator. After a 30-60 min. recovery period
cells were preincubated for 3-5 hrs. in fresh medium containing 1%, 5% or 20% serum. Following preincubation, twice washed
cultures were incubated for 30 or 60 min. plus or minus any
additions. Unless otherwise indicated incubations were always
conducted in serum free McCoy's medium. Incubation medium was
assayed for PGs by radioimmunoassay (RIA) as previously reported (Polgar and Taylor, 1980).

RESULTS AND CONCLUSIONS

Homogeneous cultures of endothelial cells are capable of
producing PGI_2 (assayed as 6-keto $PGF_{1\alpha}$), TXA_2 (assayed as
TXB_2), PGE_2 and $PGF_{2\alpha}$. The PG profile of these cells is
presented in Table I. As indicated the major PG product of
these cells is PGI_2. This appears to be the case whether the
cells remain unstimulated or are presented with agents such
as bradykinin (BK) or the PG precursor arachidonic acid (ARA).
This finding is in keeping with much of what is known or suspected regarding the role of PGI_2 in vascular physiology.
Additionally the production of PGI_2 may be relevant to the
interaction between platelets and the endothelial lining of
the circulatory system.

The relationship between serum concentration, radiation
treatment and the rate of cell growth is presented in Table
II. Incubation of cells in medium containing 20% serum, the
normal culture medium, resulted in an approximate tripling of

cell density over a 48 hour period. If the serum concentration

TABLE I

PROSTAGLANDIN PRODUCTION BY ENDOTHELIAL CELLS IN CULTURE

NG/ML

PG TREATMENT	PGE_2	6-K $PGF_{1\alpha}$	TXB_2	$PGF_{2\alpha}$
CONTROL	0.4 ± 0.1	19.1 ± 3.7	$1.4 \pm .33$	1.8 ± 0.4
5.0 µG/ML BK	1.13 ± 0.4	54.2 ± 16.0	3.3 ± 1.2	3.5 ± 0.9
10uM ARA	3.8 ± 0	132.1 ± 11.5	9.2 ± 0.1	6.5 ± 0.6

ENDOTHELIAL CELLS WERE ISOLATED, MAINTAINED AND PREINCU-
BATED IN MEDIUM CONTAINING 5% SERUM AS DESCRIBED IN TEXT.
CULTURES WERE THEN INCUBATED FOR 30 MIN. WITH BRADYKININ
(BK) OR ARACHIDONIC ACID (ARA) IN SERUM FREE MCCOY'S MEDIUM.
FOLLOWING INCUBATION THE MEDIUM WAS REMOVED AND PG'S ASSAY-
ED BY RIA. EACH VALUE REPRESENTS THE MEAN ± S.E.M OF
AT LEAST 3 SEPARATE MEASUREMENTS.

is reduced to 1%, cell growth is severely inhibited showing
only a minimal increase over the 48 hour period. Treatment
of cultures with as few as 1000 rads of radiation completely
eliminates any further cell division, yet the cells remain
viable and can even be replated.

TABLE II

CELL GROWTH FOLLOWING GAMMA IRRADIATION

TOTAL CELLS

TREATMENT	20% SERUM	1% SERUM
CONTROL	$1.66 \times 10^6 \pm 6.8 \times 10^4$	$8.16 \times 10^5 \pm 4.6 \times 10^4$
1000 RADS	$5.13 \times 10^5 \pm 1.1 \times 10^4$	$4.49 \times 10^5 \pm 1.4 \times 10^4$

THE INITIAL CELL CONCENTRATION WAS $5.3 \times 10^5 \pm 4.0 \times 10^3$. CON-
FLUENT ENDOTHELIAL CULTURES WERE IRRADIATED AT 1000 RADS.
CULTURES WERE THEN FED WITH MEDIUM CONTAINING EITHER 1% OR
20% NEWBORN CALF SERUM. FORTY-EIGHT HOURS AFTER ADDITION OF
FRESH MEDIUM, CULTURES WERE TRYPSINIZED AND CELL NUMBER
DETERMINED ON A COULTER COUNTER. EACH COUNT IS THE MEAN ±
S.E.M. OF 3 SEPARATE CELL COUNTS ON EACH OF 3 PLATES.

The effect of cell growth and irradiation on PGI_2 production is demonstrated in Table III. Under all conditions examined irradiated cells were capacitated to produce more PGI_2
than their non-irradiated counterparts. This situation was
also true for cells induced into quiescence by lowered serum
concentration. Additionally the effect of these two treatments was cumulative, the highest levels resulting from cultures which had been both irradiated and preincubated in 1%
serum.

TABLE III

THE EFFECT OF GAMMA RADIATION AND SERUM
CONCENTRATION ON PGI_2 PRODUCTION

	6-KETO $PGF_{1\alpha}$ (NG/ML)	
TREATMENT	20% SERUM	1% SERUM
CONTROL	4.6 ± 0.2	26.3 ± 5.7
2400 RADS	8.5 ± 0.8	34.2 ± 4.7
5.0 µG/ML BK	22.6 ± 5.1	47.9 ± 5.2
2400 RADS & 5.0 µG/ML BK	39.0 ± 2.0	59.4 ± 0.9

ENDOTHELIAL CELLS WERE MAINTAINED, IRRADIATED AND
PREINCUBATED AS DESCRIBED IN TEXT. THEY WERE THEN
INCUBATED FOR 1 HOUR IN THE PRESENCE OR ABSENCE OF
BRADYKININ (BK) AS INDICATED. AT THE END OF THE
INCUBATION PERIOD MEDIA WAS REMOVED AND ASSAYED FOR
PGI_2 AS 6-KETO $PGF_{1\alpha}$ BY RIA. VALUES EXPRESSED ARE
THE MEAN ± S.E.M. OF MEASUREMENTS ON 3 PLATES.

The results of this study indicate that cells pretreated in such a fashion as to inhibit cell growth (e.g. decreased serum or γ irradiation) are capacitated for enhanced PGI_2 production. Therefore the state of cell growth appears to have profound effects on PG synthesis. This observation supports the previous reports that PGI_2 inhibits cell growth and promotes differentiation (Hopkins and Gorman, 1981). The role of PGI_2 levels may also be of clinical importance. A recent study indicates that PGI_2 may inhibit circulating, metastasized tumor cells from attaching to the endothelial lining (Honn, et al., 1981).

Honn KV, Cicone B, Skoff A (1981). Prostacyclin: A potent antimetastatic agent. Science 212:1270.

Hopkins NK, Gorman RR (1981). Regulation of 3T3-L1 fibroblast differentiation by prostacyclin. Biochem Biophys Acta 663:457.

Menconi M, Polgar P (1981). Aging and prostaglandin production by endothelial cells. Manuscript in preparation.

Polgar P, Taylor L (1980). Stimulation of PG synthesis by ascorbic acid. Prostaglandins 19:693.

Polgar P, Douglas W, Terracio L, Taylor L (1980). Release of arachidonic acid and its conversion to prostaglandins. Adv Prostaglandins and Thromboxane Res 6:225.

Taylor L, Polgar P (1981). Cell growth and PG synthesis. Submitted for publication, Prostaglandins.

Taylor L, Schneider E, Smith J, Polgar P (1981). Prostaglandin production and cellular aging. Mech Aging Dev 16:311.

This work was supported by N.I.H. HL 25776

**Prostaglandins and Cancer: First
International Conference, pages 385–389
© 1982 Alan R. Liss, Inc., 150 Fifth Avenue, New York, NY 10011**

INHIBITION OF GROWTH OF HAMSTER PANCREATIC DUCTAL ADENO-
CARCINOMA CELLS IN VITRO BY PGE_2 AND 16,16-DIMETHYL PGE_2 -
A PRELIMINARY REPORT

David T. Mayschak, M.D., M.A., Elena Glass, B.S.,
Scott Kacy, M.D., William Boerwinkle, M.S. Sam
Barranco, Ph.D., M. Wayne Flye, M.D.,Ph.D., Courtney
M. Townsend, Jr., M.D.
Departments of Surgery and Human Biological Chemistry
and Genetics, The University of Texas Medical Branch,
Galveston, Texas 77550

The relationship between prostaglandins (PG's) and the
growth of neoplasms remains unclear. PG's have been shown to
have both enhancing and an inhibitory effects on neoplastic
growth. Honn et al (1979) reported that PGA_1 and PGA_2 can
depress DNA synthesis and cell proliferation in Harding-Passey
melanoma cells. PG's of the E series inhibit incorporation
of thymidine, uridine and leucine by leukemic lymphoblasts
(Yang et al, 1976). Santoro and associates (1977) reported
a dose-dependent inhibition of B-16 melanoma growth in vivo
by a synthetic analog of PGE_2, 16,16-dimethyl PGE_2 (16,16-
$diMPGE_2$). Hofer and colleagues (1980) further found that
16,16-$diMPGE_2$ augments inhibitory effects of chemotherapeutic
agents on the mouse B-16 melanoma. Although the mechanism
was not determined, they speculated that either enhancement
of immunoresponsiveness or a direct antimitotic effect of
PG's was responsible for the increased inhibition produced by
this combination of PG's and chemotherapeutic agents.

There have been no reports of the effects of PG's on cell
cycle kinetics. Furthermore, PG's have not been previously
evaluated in a pancreatic cancer cell line.

The effects of the natural PGE_2 and synthetic 16,16-
$diMPGE_2$ on the growth characteristics and cell cycle kinetics
of the hamster H2T pancreatic ductal adenocarcinoma cell line
(Townsend et al, 1980) were examined in vitro. The effects
of PG's on the tumor cell doubling time were correlated with
the effects on survival fraction of treated cells and the
perturbations of cell cycle kinetics.

MATERIALS AND METHODS

Doubling Time. Known numbers of H2T cells in exponential growth were plated in 60 mm petri dishes. After 24 hours, different doses of either PGE_2 or 16,16-diMPGE_2 were added for the entire culture period. Twice daily for 120 hours the plates were examined microscopically and the total cell numbers in both treated cultures and untreated control cultures were determined by counting in a coulter counter (Model ZF).

Survival Fraction (SF). To determine the survival fraction, H2T cells were treated for only six hours with varying doses of PGE_2 and 16,16-diMPGE_2. Known numbers of washed cells were then plated and allowed to grow, undisturbed, for ten days. Plates were stained with methylene blue and colonies of 50 or more cells were counted. The ratio of colonies to numbers of cells initially plated yielded the plating efficiency (PE). The ratio of the PE of treated cells to that of untreated controls determined the survival fraction.

Flow Microfluorometry (FMF). Exponentially growing cells were plated and treated for six hours with different concentrations of PGE_2. At hourly intervals during and after treatment, cells were harvested and stained with ethidium bromide mithramycin. The stained nuclei were then analysed by flow microfluorometry to determine absolute numbers of cells in the G_1, S and G_2/M phases of the cell cycle. The percentage of treated cells in each phase was compared with untreated controls (Zante and co-workers, 1978).

Prostaglandins. PGE_2 and 16,16-diMPGE_2 were generously supplied by Dr. John E. Pike of the Upjohn Company (Kalamazoo, Michigan).

RESULTS

There was a dose dependent inhibitory effect of both PGE_2 and 16,16-diMPGE_2 on cell growth as expressed by prolongation of doubling time (T_d). T_d was increased by 50% compared to controls with high doses of 16,16-diMPGE_2 (75-100 µg/ml) and by 65% with equimolar doses of PGE_2 (Figure 1 A & B).

A six-hour treatment with 50 µg/ml PGE_2 killed 20% of the cells and 100 µg/ml 30%, as demonstrated by the survival fraction (SF). Equivalent doses of 16,16-diMPGE_2 produced

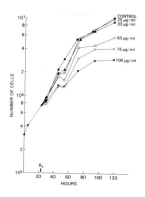 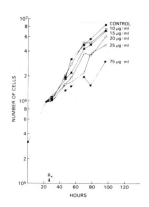

Figure 1A   Figure 1B

Figure 1A: Effect of various doses of PGE$_2$ on the doubling time of H2T cells.

Figure 1B: Effect of various doses of 16,16-dimethyl PGE$_2$ on the doubling time of H2T cells.

a more profound effect as judged by SF. It was found that at these doses of PGE$_2$ the H2T cells were caused to round up and come off the plate. However, doses of the PGE$_2$ below 50 µg/ml, which affected both T$_d$ and SF, brought about a change in cell morphology without affecting cell adhesion to the plate.

A 6-hour treatment with 50 µg/ml PGE$_2$ produced an increase of 160% in numbers of cells in the G$_2$/M phase of the cell cycle (expressed as percent of control), with corresponding changes in the S and G$_1$ phases (Figure 2). This blocking effect was seen as early as 3 hours after the addition of PG and was reversible; that is, the FMF histograms of treated cells reverted to control characteristics by 18 to 24 hours after treatment ended.

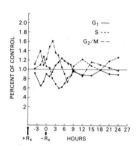

Figure 2

Figure 2: Effects of 6-hour treatment with 50 µg/ml of PGE$_2$ on the distribution of cells in the cell cycle as compared with control.

CONCLUSION

PGE$_2$ and 16,16-diMPGE$_2$ have a dose-dependent inhibitory effect on the doubling time and survival fraction of H2T cells in vitro.

At doses producing no more than 20% kill, PGE$_2$ has a reversible blocking effect on H2T cells in vitro, such that there is a transient build-up of cells in the G$_2$/M phase of the cell cycle.

Hofer D, Dubitsky AM, Jaffe BM (1980). Prostaglandin potentiation of the effect of chemotherapy on B-16 melanoma. Surgical Forum 31:417-419.

Honn K, Dunn J III, Morgan LR, Bienkowski M, Marnett LJ (1979). Inhibition of DNA synthesis in Harding-Passey melanoma cells by prostaglandins A$_1$ and A$_2$: Comparison with chemotherapeutic agents. Biochemical and Biophysical Research Communications 87:795-801.

Santoro JG, Philpott GW, Jaffee BM (1977). Inhibition of B-16 melanoma growth in vivo by a synthetic analog of Prostaglandin E$_2$. Cancer Research 37:3774-3779.

Townsend CM Jr, Franklin RB, Suddith RL, Thompson JC (1980).
Pancreatic ductal adenocarcinoma in continuous culture.
Surgical Forum XXXI:431-432.
Yang TJ, Dale JB, Machanoff R (1976). Effects of prostaglandins E_1, E_2 and $F_{2\alpha}$ on the growth of leukaemia cells in culture. Journal of Cell Science 20:199-206.
Zante J, Schumann J, Barlogie T (1978). New preparation and staining procedure for specific and rapid analysis of DNA distributions. In Göhde W, Schumann J, Büchner T (eds): "Pulse Cytometry." Ghent, Belgium: European Press, p 97ff.

**Prostaglandins and Cancer: First
International Conference, pages 391-396
© 1982 Alan R. Liss, Inc., 150 Fifth Avenue, New York, NY 10011**

CHANGES IN MICROTUBULE-ORGANIZATION AFFECT DIFFERENT EVENTS
REGULATING THE INITIATION OF DNA SYNTHESIS STIMULATED BY
PROSTAGLANDIN $F_{2\alpha}$ IN 3T3 CELLS

Angela M. Otto

Friedrich Miescher-Institut
P.O.Box 273
CH-4002 Basel. Switzerland

INTRODUCTION

Prostaglandin $F_{2\alpha}$ ($PGF_{2\alpha}$) has been shown to stimulate
the initiation of DNA replication in quiescent Swiss 3T3
cells (Jimenez de Asua et al.1977). Two different phenomena
are induced:
1. progression through a prereplicative period (lag phase)
   of about 15 hr, and
2. a rate of entry into S phase depending on the concentration of $PGF_{2\alpha}$ added.
Since the latter process appears to follow first order
kinetics, it is quantified by a rate constant (Jimenez de
Asua et al.1977). The stimulatory effect of $PGF_{2\alpha}$ can be
modulated by different hormones. such as insulin and hydrocortisone. at certain times of the lag phase. suggesting
that there is a time-dependent sequence of different regulatory events during the lag phase (Jimenez de Asua 1980).

Experiments with microtubule-disrupting drugs are indicating that the cytoskeleton. in particular the array of
microtubules. somehow plays a regulatory role in the initiation of DNA synthesis (Friedkin et al.1979; McClain et
al.1977; Otto et al 1979; Teng et al 1977).

This presentation will show that disassembly and re-
assembly of microtubules affects at least two different
events regulating the initiation of DNA replication stimulated by $PGF_{2\alpha}$.

MATERIALS AND METHODS

Swiss mouse 3T3 cells were propagated as described previously (Jimenez de Asua et al 1977). For determination of the labelling index and the rate constant, cells were grown in Dulbecco-Vogt's modified Eagle's medium supplemented with 6% fetal calf serum and low molecular weight components (O'Farrell et al 1979). Cultures were used when they had become confluent and quiescent 4 days after an intermediate medium change. Cells were labelled for autoradiography by exposing cultures to 3 µCi/ml. 1 µM [methyl-^{3}H]-thymidine from the time of addition of $PGF_{2\alpha}$. The rate constant for the kinetics of entry into S phase was determined as described before (Otto et al 1980).

$PGF_{2\alpha}$ was a generous gift of John Pike. Upjohn Company. Kalamazoo. USA. Crystalline insulin. colchicine and demecolcine (colcemid) were obtained from Sigma. [Methyl-^{3}H]-thymidine was from the Radiochemical Centre. Amersham. England.

RESULTS AND DISCUSSION

The rate of entry into S phase stimulated by $PGF_{2\alpha}$. alone or with a low concentration of insulin is enhanced by the simultaneous addition of colchicine (Table 1). Colchicine added alone to quiescent 3T3 cells does not stimulate DNA synthesis nor change the cell number in the monolayer. Lumicolchicine, an inactive analog of colchicine. has no effect on the stimulatory effect of $PGF_{2\alpha}$ or $PGF_{2\alpha}$ plus insulin (Otto et al 1979). Furthermore. when colchicine is aded at 8 hr or 15 hr after $PGF_{2\alpha}$, alone or with insulin, the kinetics are no longer enhanced. even though microtubules are disrupted. On the other hand, removal of colchicine at 5 hr of the lag phase resulted in the same synergistic effect as if it had remained present. The removal of colchicine allowed cell division (Otto et al 1979).

Colcemid also enhanced the stimulatory effect when added together with $PGF_{2\alpha}$ alone or plus insulin. Fig. 1 shows how the synergy is gradually reduced with later additions of colcemid. Similar results were obtained with colchicine (not shown). However. colcemid differs from colchicine in that removal of colcemid from the culture medium allows microtubules to reassemble within 2 hr. while

Table 1. Effect of colchicine on the rate of entry into S phase stimulated by PGF$_{2\alpha}$ alone or with insulin

Additions	rate constant (x 10^{-2}/ hr)
None	0.05
Insulin	0.10
Colchicine	0.08
PGF$_{2\alpha}$	1.80
PGF$_{2\alpha}$ + insulin	5.60
PGF$_{2\alpha}$ + colchicine	5.50
PGF$_{2\alpha}$ + insulin + colchicine	11.20
PGF$_{2\alpha}$ + (colchicine at 8 hr)	1.90
PGF$_{2\alpha}$ + insulin + (colchicine at 8 hr)	5.50
PGF$_{2\alpha}$ + insulin + (colchicine at 15 hr)	5.50
PGF$_{2\alpha}$ + (colchicine 0-5 hr)	5.40
PGF$_{2\alpha}$ + insulin + (colchicine 0-5 hr)	11.1

Additions were made to the culture medium in which cells became quiescent. Concentrations used were for PGF$_{2\alpha}$ 300 ng/ml. insulin 50 ng/ml and colchicine 2 μM. Colchicine was removed by aspirating the medium and washing the cells. Conditioned medium from quiescent parallel cultures was added with PGF$_{2\alpha}$ or PGF$_{2\alpha}$ + insulin. Rate constants were determined as previously described. The length of the lag phase was 15 hr in all cases. (Revised from Otto et al.1979).

after removal of colchicine many hours are required for repolymerization. As shown in Fig. 1, removal of colcemid during the first part of the lag phase results in loss of the synergistic effect. It appears that microtubules need to be disrupted up to 10 hr for the full synergistic effect.

When quiescent 3T3 cells are incubated for 8 hr with either colchicine or colcemid there is no change in the cell number of the monolayer. Adding PGF$_{2\alpha}$ and insulin to these preincubated cells results in a shortening of the lag phase

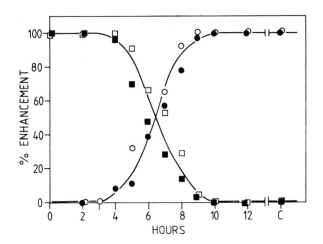

Fig. 1. Effect of later additions and early removals of colcemid on the stimulatory effect of $PGF_{2\alpha}$ or $PGF_{2\alpha}$ + insulin.
Additions of colcemid after $PGF_{2\alpha}$ (□) or $PGF_{2\alpha}$ + insulin (■),
at C: no addition of colcemid; removals of colcemid after
addition together with $PGF_{2\alpha}$ (o) or $PGF_{2\alpha}$ + insulin (●), at
C: no removal.

by about 2 hr without affecting the rate of entry into S
phase (Fig. 2). Even when colchicine or colcemid is removed
prior to the stimulation by $PGF_{2\alpha}$ and insulin the lag phase
is shortened irrespective of the resulting rate constant.
A 1 hr preincubation with colcemid prior to addition of
$PGF_{2\alpha}$ and insulin does not affect the length of the lag
phase (Fig. 2B).

These results indicate that at least two. independently
regulated events involved in the initiation of DNA synthesis
are sensitive to the organisation of microtubules. One event
involved in determining the length of the lag phase is altered by long term disruption of microtubules before $PGF_{2\alpha}$
induces progression through the lag phase. Another event
occurring in the early part of the lag phase. yet regulating the final rate of initiation of DNA synthesis upon
completion of the lag phase. is enhanced only by early disruption of microtubules; for the maximal accomplishment of

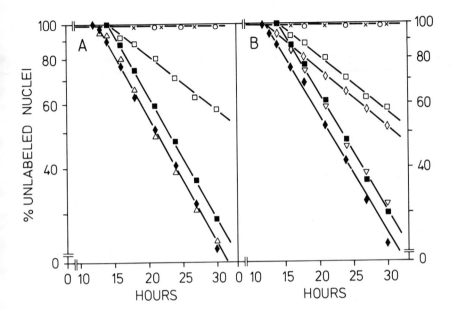

Fig. 2. Effect of preincubating quiescent Swiss 3T3 cells for 8 hr with colchicine or colcemid prior to stimulation by PGF$_{2\alpha}$ and insulin. Experimental procedures were as in Table 1. Concentrations used were for PGF$_{2\alpha}$ 300 ng/ml, insulin 50 ng/ml, colchicine 1 μM and colcemid 1 μM. A: (x) no addition, (o) colchicine alone, (□) PGF$_{2\alpha}$ and insulin, (■) PGF$_{2\alpha}$ + insulin + colchicine, (◆) colchicine added 8 hr before PGF$_{2\alpha}$ + insulin, (△) colchicine added for 8 hr and removed before adding PGF$_{2\alpha}$ + insulin. B: (x) no addition, (o) colcemid alone, (□) PGF$_{2\alpha}$ + insulin, (■) PGF$_{2\alpha}$ + insulin + colcemid, (▽) colcemid added 1 hr before PGF$_{2\alpha}$ + insulin, (◆) colcemid added 8 hr before PGF$_{2\alpha}$ + insulin, (◇) colcemid added for 8 hr and removed before adding PGF$_{2\alpha}$ + insulin.

this is putative event microtubules need to be disrupted for up to 10 hr of the lag phase. Which are the biochemical events sensitive to the organisation of microtubules and involved in regulating the initiation of DNA synthesis stimulated by PGF$_{2\alpha}$? This question will require intensive investigation.

ACKNOWLEDGEMENTS

I thank Drs. R.R. Bürk, L. Jimenez de Asua and D. Monard for corrective reading of the manuscript and M.-O. Ulrich for technical assistance.

REFERENCES

Friedkin ML, Legg A, Rozengurt E (1979). Anti-tubulin agents enhance the stimulation of DNA synthesis by polypeptide growth factors in 3T3 mouse fibroblasts. Proc Natl Acad Sci USA 76:3903

Jimenez de Asua L (1980). An ordered sequence of temporal steps regulates the rate of initiation of DNA synthesis in cultured mouse cells. In Jimenez de Asua L, Levi-Montalcini R, Shields S, Iacobelli S (eds): "Control Mechanisms in Animal Cells. Specific Growth Factors". New York: Raven Press. p. 173

Jimenez de Asua L, O'Farrell MK, Clingan D, Rudland PS (1977). Temporal sequence of hormonal interactions during the prereplicative phase of quiescent cultured fibroblasts. Proc Natl Acad Sci USA 74:3845

McClain D, D'Eustachio P, Edelman GM (1977). Role of surface-modulating assemblies in growth control of normal and transformed fibroblasts. Proc Natl Acad Sci USA 74:666

O'Farrell MK, Clingan D, Rudland PS, Jimenez de Asua L (1979). Stimulation of the initiation of DNA synthesis and cell division in several cultured mouse cell types. Exp Cell Res 118:311

Otto AM, Ulrich M-O, Jimenez de Asua L (1980). Does the cytoskeleton play a role in the initiation of DNA synthesis stimulated by growth factors? In Jimenez de Asua L, Levi-Montalcini R, Shields S, Iacobelli S (eds): "Control Mechanisms in Animal Cells. Specific Growth Factors". New York: Raven Press. p.209

Otto AM, Zumbé A, Gibson LJ, Kubler AM, Jimenez de Asua L (1979). Cytoskeleton-disrupting drugs enhance effect of growth factors and hormones. Proc Natl Acad Sci USA 76:6435

Teng M-K, Bartholomew JC, Bissell MJ (1977). Synergism between antimicrotubule agents and growth stimulants in enhancement of cell cycle traverse. Nature 268:739

CELL DIFFERENTIATION/MATURATION

**Prostaglandins and Cancer: First
International Conference, pages 399–413
© 1982 Alan R. Liss, Inc., 150 Fifth Avenue, New York, NY 10011**

ANTIGENIC AND HUMORAL CONTROL OF NORMAL AND LEUKEMIC HUMAN
MYELOPOIESIS

Louis M. Pelus

Sloan Kettering Institute for Cancer Research

1250 First Avenue, New York, N.Y. 10021

The development of techniques for the *in vitro* culture
and quantitation of specific types of hematopoietic stem and
progenitor cells in both man and mice has permitted the
investigation of mechanisms which control normal and abnormal
blood cell production. Homeostatic control of the production of these cells is a dynamic process of continuing cellular differentiation and proliferation under the influences
of specific positive and negative controls, which function
to maintain mature cell numbers within the tightly controlled limits noted *in vivo*. Within the myeloid cell lineage, it
is now well established that mature blood elements derive
from specific lineage restricted unipotent or bipotentially
committed progenitor cells. These cells are characterized by
extensive proliferative capacity within only a given cell
lineage, limited self renewal capacity, and dependence upon
specific stimulatory compounds for growth *in vitro*. In turn,
the committed progenitor cell compartment is maintained by
multipotential and pluripotential stem cells which have the
capacity for both self-renewal and the ability to give rise
to progenitor cells of several or all cell lineages (Till &
McCulloch, 1961; Fauser & Messner, 1978,1979; Johnson &
Metcalf, 1978).

Marrow culture studies have documented that the regulation of granulocyte-macrophage production entails interactions between specific bipotent progenitor cells, CFU-GM,
committed solely to granulocyte-macrophage differentiation,
and stimulatory and inhibitory substances derived from mature cells of these lineages. *In vitro*, CFU-GM proliferate

and differentiate in soft agar (Bradley & Metcalf, 1966;
Pluznik & Sach, 1966) forming colonies of granulocytes and/
or macrophages under the influence of specific growth stimulatory factors, GM-CSF (Chervenick & Boggs, 1970; Metcalf,
1973; Quesenberry & Levitt, 1979; Burgess & Metcalf, 1980).
Under normal circumstances, murine and human CFU-GM proliferation is limited by at least three naturally occuring
feedback regulators: polymorphonuclear neutrophil derived
lactoferrin (Broxmeyer et al.,1978) and monocyte-macrophage
derived acidic isoferritins (Broxmeyer et al.,1981) and
prostaglandin E (Pelus et al.,1979; Pelus et al.,1981).

EFFECTS OF PROSTAGLANDIN E ON CFU-GM PROLIFERATION

Studies on the regulation of human CFU-GM proliferation
indicate that prostaglandins of the E series inhibit the
clonal expansion of normal CFU-GM (colonies plus clusters)
in a dose dependent fashion over a concentration range of
10^{-5}M through 10^{-12}M (Figure 1).

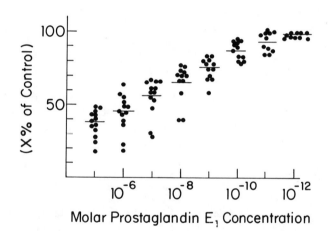

Molar Prostaglandin E_1 Concentration

FIGURE 1. The effects of PGE_1 on day 7 CFU-GM
(colonies plus clusters) proliferation by
10^5 nonadherent low-density (<1.074g/ml)
normal human bone marrow cells. Each point
represents the mean of quadruplicate cultures
for each normal donor tested.

Morphological analysis of proliferating clones demonstrates that the observed effect of prostaglandin E on total colony and cluster formation results from the selective inhibition of monocyte-macrophage clone-forming cells (Pelus et al., 1981). Mixed monocytoid-neutrophil clone formation was markedly less sensitive, and neutrophil and eosinophil clone formation essentially insensitive to the inhibitory effects of prostaglandin E. The molar concentrations of prostaglandin required for fifty percent inhibition of pure monycyte-macrophage, mixed monocytoid-neutrophil, neutrophil and eosinophil colony formation were found to be 5×10^{-9}M, 6×10^{-6}M, $>10^{-5}$M and $>10^{-5}$M, respectively. These dose titrations place the in vitro sensitivity of monocyte-macrophage but not granulocyte progenitor cells within physiologically demonstrable prostaglandin E limits and suggests that prostaglandin E could serve as a physiological regulator.

Specificity analysis, by comparison to a number of primary prostaglandins, endoperoxides, thromboxane, prostacyclin and 6-keto-$PGF_{1\alpha}$, indicates that the E series prostaglandins (PGE_1 and PGE_2) are at least 10 times more potent in inhibiting human CFU-GM proliferation than any other member of the prostaglandin family tested (Table 1).

PROSTAGLANDIN INSENSITIVITY OF CFU-GM FROM PATIENTS WITH CHRONIC MYELOID LEUKEMIA.

The ability to maintain and quantitate all types of hematopoietic progenitor cells has permitted the most detailed comparison of normal versus malignant cell populations available in any cell system. Analysis of prostaglandin sensitivity of CFU-GM populations from patients with leukemia has indicated that abnormal growth regulatory response characterizes many forms of leukemia and may play a role in leukemogenesis. Granulocyte-macrophage colony formation by CFU-GM from patients with chronic myeloid leukemia (CML) are virtually insensitive to inhibition by prostaglandin E, even by concentrations which maximally inhibit normal CFU-GM (Figure 2).

This defect occurs in spite of the presence of adequate numbers of proliferating monocytic clones, and is consistently observed at all stages of the disease. Furthermore, CFU-GM insensitivity persisted in three patients treated with aggressive chemotherapy which resulted in complete or partial Philadelphia chromosome (Ph[1]) conversion (Pelus

TABLE 1

THE EFFECTS OF VARIOUS PROSTAGLANDINS ON DAY 7 CFU-GM PRO-LIFERATION.

PROSTAGLANDIN	MOLAR CONCENTRATION for 50% INHIBITION OF *IN VITRO* CLONING[1]
PGH_2 (U-44069)	$5.8 \times 10^{-6}M$
PGH_2 (U-46619)	$4.8 \times 10^{-6}M$
Thromboxane B_2	$>10^{-5}M$
6-keto-$PGF_{1\alpha}$	$>10^{-5}M$
PGD_1	$8.5 \times 10^{-7}M$
PGD_2	$3 \times 10^{-8}M$
PGE_1	$4 \times 10^{-9}M$
PGE_2	$7 \times 10^{-9}M$
PGA_1	$5.6 \times 10^{-7}M$
PGA_2	$3.5 \times 10^{-7}M$
$PGI_2{}^{2}$	$>10^{-5}M$
$PGF_{1\alpha}$	$10^{-5}M$
$PGF_{2\alpha}$	$10^{-5}M$

1. *Determined by dose titration analysis on CFU-GM per 10^5 low density human bone marrow cells.*
2. *Stabalized in Tris buffer pH 9.5 prior to addition to agar culture.*

et al.,1980).

ASSOCIATION OF HLA-Dr(Ia) ANTIGENS WITH CFU-GM SENSITIVITY TO PROSTAGLANDIN E.

Investigation into the mechanism of action of prosta-glandin E on the proliferative capacity of human CFU-GM populations demonstrates that the effects of exogenously added prostaglandin E are selective for CFU-GM expressing HLA-Dr(Ia) antibodies. (Table 2). In four experiments, treatment of low density (<1.074g/ml) bone marrow cells with purified monoclonal mouse anti-human Ia antibody (NEI-011) plus complement (C') prior to agar culture, resulted in the cytolytic reduction of total CFU-GM (46-50%), with

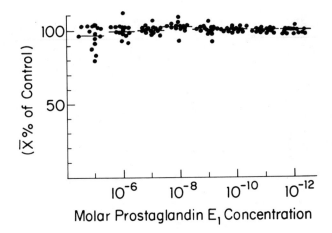

FIGURE 2. The effects of PGE_1 on day 7 CFU-GM
proliferation by 10^5 nonadherent low density
bone marrow cells from patients with CML.
Each point represents the mean of quadruplicate
cultures for each patient.

the resulting CFU-GM population being unresponsive to inhibition by prostaglandin E. Treatment with C' or αIa
alone did not alter or block the inhibitory effect of
prostaglandin E. Lack of responsiveness of CFU-GM was
observed following cytolytic treatment using concentrations
of 1/50 through 1/3000. Throughout this dilution range,
inhibition of CFU-GM proliferation of between 40% and 50%
is routinely observed (X 48 ± 4%, n = 38). Likewise, at all
antibody concentrations CFU-GM surviving cytolytic reduction
with αIa + C', were insensitive to prostaglandin E_1
throughout a dose response curve of 10^{-6}M through 10^{-12}M.

The ability to detect a subpopulation of regulatory
responsive CFU-GM can be demonstrated with three highly
purified mouse anti-human HLA-Dr monoclonal antibodies
(Table 3).

Based upon reported evidence that the expression of

TABLE 2

EFFECTS OF ANTI HLA-Dr ANTIBODIES ON CFU-GM SENSITIVITY TO INHIBITION BY PROSTAGLANDIN E_1.

ADDITION[2]	$\overline{X}$ CFU-GM AVERAGE, 4 EXPERIMENTS[1]·			
	MEDIA[3]	C'[3]	αIa^3	$\alpha Ia + C'^3$
Media	224±18	216±18	214±19	114±11(47 1%)[4]
10^{-7}M PGE$_1$	115±11	118±11	136±19	113±12

1. Total CFU-GM (colonies plus clusters) per 10^5 low density ($<$1.074g/ml) human bone marrow cells. Data represents the average of four separate experiments using four different bone marrow doners. Within each separate experiment, CFU-GM were determined from quadruplicate cultures.
2. Added to agar cultures upon initiation.
3. Treatment of bone marrow cells prior to soft agar culture. Monoclonal mouse anti-human HLA-Dr(Ia) antibody was used at a final dilution of 1/100.
4. $\overline{X}$ percentage Ia positive CFU-GM.

Ia-antigens on mature cells is transient and lost rapidly in culture (Beller & Unanue,1981; Steeg et al.,1980; Steinman et al.,1980), the expression of Ia-antigens and the regulatory response of CFU-GM was investigated as a function of time in culture. When incubated at 37^0C, a small decline in the number of Ia-positive CFU-GM and coincident reduction in prostaglandin responsiveness occured within 3 hours. After 6 hours, no significant presence of Ia-antigens could be detected by cytotoxicity, and correlated with the loss of prostaglandin E mediated inhibition (Table 4). Maintenance of CFU-GM at 4^0 or 23^0C for up to 24 hours, was without effect on the ability to detect Ia-antigens or upon sensitivity to inhibition by prostaglandin E (not shown), suggesting active shedding of Ia-antigens.

These studies provide evidence for the close association

TABLE 3

EFFECTS OF VARIOUS MONOCLONAL ANTI-HUMAN HLA-Dr(Ia) ANTI-BODIES.

MONOCLONAL ANTIBODY[1] (DILUTION)[2]	$\overline{X}$ CFU-GM[3]	
	MEDIA	$+10^{-7}M$ PGE$_1$
Media	459±13	267±14
C'	452±10	280±10
Anti-human HLA-Dr + C'		
NEI-011 (1:200)	290±5	264±16
OKIa$_1$ (1:200)	247±18	252±15
BD(L243) (1:200)	270±2	268±6

1. *Bone marrow cells were treated in a complement mediated cytotoxic assay prior to culture in semisolid agar.*
2. *Final antibody concentration used. Maximal activity was determined from prior dose response analysis.*
3. *CFU-GM per 10^5 low density human bone marrow cells. Data is expressed as $\overline{X}$ ± S.E. of quadruplicate cultures.*

between expression of CFU-GM Ia-antigens and the regulatory control of CFU-GM proliferation by prostaglandin E.

ASSOCIATION OF Ia-ANTIGENS AND PROSTAGLANDIN RESPONSIVENESS WITH S-PHASE OF THE CELL CYCLE.

Recent human and murine studies demonstrate the differential expression of Ia-antigens relative to changes in the DNA synthetic cycle (Lanier & Warner,1981; Sarkar et al., 1980). This suggested that perhaps the regulatory responsiveness and expression of Ia-antigens by CFU-GM might be related to the proportion of cells in S-phase of the cell cycle. Treatment of bone marrow cells with αIa + C' or high specific activity ^{3}H-Tdr resulted in essentially identical reduction of CFU-GM proliferation (Table 5). Furthermore, treatment of bone marrow cells sequentially

TABLE 4

LOSS OF SENSITIVITY TO CYTOTOXIC REDUCTION BY αIa ANTIBODY AND TO INHIBITION BY PROSTAGLANDIN E IN LIQUID CULTURE.

TIME	ADDITION[1]	$\overline{X}$ CFU-GM[2]	
		C'	αIa + C'[3]
3 hours	Media	282±6	146±5
	10^{-6}M PGE	154±7	147±4
6 hours	Media	244±14	228±3
	10^{-6}M PGE	220±15	233±4
24 hours	Media	289±12	268±24
	10^{-6}M PGE	280±7	284±16

1. *Prostaglandin E was added at the initiation of agar culture.*
2. *CFU-GM per 10^5 low density bone marrow cells placed into suspension culture.*
3. *Final αIa concentration of 1/100 (NEI-011) was used.*

with ^{3}H-Tdr followed by αIa + C' resulted in no further reduction of CFU-GM numbers than with either ^{3}H-Tdr or αIa + C' alone. Responsiveness of CFU-GM to inhibition by prostaglandin E was lost following either ^{3}H-Tdr or αIa + C' treatment (or both). These studies establish prostaglandin E as an S-phase inhibitor of CFU-GM and suggest that CFU-GM express Ia-antigenic determinants (or at least epitopic regions) only during S-phase, and coincident with the capacity to respond to regulation by prostaglandin E.

The detection of CFU-GM Ia-antigens only during S-phase of the cell cycle could be demonstrated using three different monoclonal anti-human HLA-Dr antibodies. (Figure 3).

ALTERED EXPRESSION OF Ia-ANTIGENS ON CFU-GM FROM PATIENTS WITH CML.

Granulocyte-macrophage colony forming cells from patients with CML are hyporesponsive to inhibition by

TABLE 5

SELECTIVE EFFECTS OF PROSTAGLANDIN E ON CFU-GM IN S-PHASE
AND EXPRESSING Ia-ANTIGENIC DETERMINANTS.

TREATMENT[1]	ADDITION	$\bar{X}$ CFU-GM[2]
None	Media	248±2
	10^{-7}M PGE$_1$	135±6 (46)
^{3}H-Tdr	Media	147±4
	10^{-7}M PGE$_1$	141±3 (4)
Tdr+^{3}H-Tdr	Media	250±3
	10^{-7}M PGE$_1$	144±3 (42)
αIa+C'	Media	134±16
	10^{-7}M PGE$_1$	133±7 (1)
^{3}H-Tdr+	Media	143±6
αIa+C'	10^{-7}M PGE$_1$	138±5 (3)

1. *Treatment of bone marrow cells prior to culture in soft*
   agar.
2. *Colonies plus clusters per 10^5 low density (<1.074g/ml)*
   human bone marrow cells.
3. *Percent inhibition of CFU-GM proliferation.*

prostaglandin E (Pelus *et al.*,1980). The relationship between expression of Ia-antigens on CML-CFU-GM and their
responsiveness to prostaglandin E was therefore investigated.
Throughout the anti-antibody dilution range of 1/100 to
1/1000 a consistent percentage (46-52%) of normal CFU-GM
were sensitive to αIa + C' dependent lysis. (Table 6).

In contrast, at all antibody dilutions, CFU-GM from
patients with CML were significantly less sensitive to
cytolytic reduction, although considerable heterogeneity
was observed. At the highest αIa antibody concentration
(1/100), little or no reduction in CFU-GM proliferation was
observed in 8 of 13 patients, while the percentage of Ia +

TABLE 6

QUANTITATION OF Ia-ANTIGEN POSITIVE CFU-GM FROM PATIENTS
WITH CML.

Ia-ANTIBODY DILUTION	$\overline{X}$ % Ia-POSITIVE CFU-GM[1]	
	NORMAL (n=14)	CML (n=13)
1:100	52±2	18±5* (0–46)[2]
1:250	46±3	10±5* (0–46)
1:500	49±3	18±4* (0–39)
1:1000	47±2	4±2* (0–16)

1. CFU-GM per 10^5 low density (<1.074g/ml) human bone marrow cells.
2. Range.
* Significantly lower than normal, P<.0005.

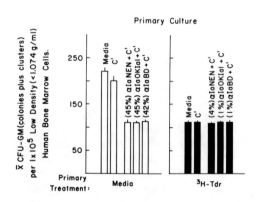

FIGURE 3. Detection of Ia-antigens on
CFU-GM before and after treatment
with high specific activity ^{3}H-Tdr.

TABLE 7

PROSTAGLANDIN RESPONSIVENESS AND Ia-EXPRESSION IN PATIENTS WITH CML.

MOLAR PROSTAGLANDIN E CONCENTRATION	CFU-GM[1] (% OF CONTROL)					
	CML, n=11		K.P.[2]		C.R.[3]	
	C'	αIa[4]+C'	C'	αIa+C'	C'	αIa+C'
10^{-5}M	84±4	88±4(14±5%)	46±5	100(46%)	38±6	85±2(36±2%)
10^{-6}M	97±2	99±2	66±1	–	46±3	100±3
10^{-7}M	100±3	100±1	84±6	–	68±2	–
10^{-8}M	–	–	90±4	–	88±1	–
10^{-9}M	–	–	98±3	–	98±2	–
10^{-10}M	–	–	100±1	–	100±1	–

1. CFU-GM per 1 x 10^5 low density bone marrow cells.
2. The prostaglandin responsiveness of this patient was analyzed on three separate occasions over an 18 month period. Quantitation of the number of Ia-antigen positive CFU-GM was performed only once.
3. The presence of Ia-antigens and prostaglandin responsiveness in this patient on two separate occasions during a 6 month period.
4. Monoclonal anti-human-HLA-Dr antibody was used at a final dilution of 1/100 (10μgm/ml).
5. Percentage of Ia-antigen positive CFU-GM detected.

CFU-GM in 5 patients were within the lower range of normal. However as antibody concentration was reduced, the number of Ia$^+$ CFU-GM in these patients decreased rapidly. Absent or reduced expression of Ia-antigens on CML CFU-GM coincident with insensitivity to prostaglandin E may therefore consti- ture the abnormal leukemic phenotype.

In two patients with CML (KP,CR) the ability to reduce CFU-GM proliferation by αIa + C' fell within normal range, and was still evident at an antibody dilution of 1/500. Considerable prostaglandin sensitivity could also be obser- ved in these patients, albeit still abnormal in comparison to normal. (Table 7). These results strongly contrast with the observed insensitivity to prostaglandin E inhibition displayed by CML CFU-GM in 11 of 13 patients with no or few detectable Ia$^+$ CFU-GM (Table 7).

SUMMARY

The lack of Ia-antigen expression on probable human pluripotent stem cells (Moore *et al.*, 1980), their occurrence on granulocyte-macrophage progenitor cells (Janossy *et al.*, 1978; Winchester *et al.*,1977), and their subsequent dis- appearance during differentiation (Moore *et al.*,1980; Janossy *et al.*,1978; Winchester *et al.*,1977) has suggested a role for Ia-antigens in the regulation of normal human myelopoiesis. These results extend this concept and indicate that a subpopulation of CFU-GM expresses Ia-antigens or at least epitopic determinants, relative to changes in the DNA synthetic cycle, which appears to be a cellular marker associated with responsiveness to growth regulation by prostaglandin E *in vitro*. The acquired loss of CFU-GM sensitivity to inhibition by prostaglandin E coincident with Ia-antigen shedding or metabolism supports this hypothesis. The *in vitro* studies described appear to define a normal regulatory phenotype for CFU-GM, characterized by respon- siveness to growth promotion by GM-CSF, expression of Ia- antigenic determinants and responsiveness to molecular (humoral) growth regulation by prostaglandin E.

Studies of growth regulation and differentiation of leukemic cells *in vitro*, has revealed a spectrum of speci- fic abnormalities in regulatory control which may play a role in leukemogenesis. While the demonstration that abnormal regulation contributes to the understanding of the patho- physiology of leukemia, it does not answer the question of why normal feedback regulators do not act against cells from patients with leukemia. A possible explanation is now apparent with the demonstration of regulatory responsiveness associated with expression of Ia-antigens. In patients with CML, an absence or decreased expression of Ia-antigens on CFU-GM can be demonstrated, and coincides with the abnormal regulatory response to prostaglandin E. These studies suggest that altered expression of Ia-antigens in CML correlates with hyporesponsiveness to prostaglandin mediated inhibition. Although the mechanism by which Ia-antigen expression and regulation by prostaglandin E are linked is unclear, the evidence supporting this association in normals is that the expression of CFU-GM Ia-antigens is coincident with, if not required for, the inhibitory effects of prostaglandin E. It it tempting to conclude, therefore, that the constitutive absence or diminution of Ia-antigen expression on CML CFU-GM is an important factor related to the abnormal response of CML. Of approximately 30 patients with CML studied thus far, only two have shown a residual, though subnormal, response to prostaglandin E. The striking observation is that these are the two patients with levels of CFU-GM Ia-antigens clearly higher than the other leukemic patients tested.

No single phenotypic change can be used unequivocally to determine or explain neoplastic transformation of hematopoietic cells. Collectively, the regulatory data described define an abnormal CFU-GM phenotype characterized by lack or altered expression of Ia-antigens and loss of normal regulatory responsiveness to prostaglandin E.

ACKNOWLEDGEMENTS

This work was supported by grant CA-28512 from the National Cancer Institute, DHEW. LMP is a Special Fellow of the Leukemia Society of America, Inc.

REFERENCES

Beller DI, Unanue ER (1981). Regulation of macrophage populations. II. Synthesis and expression of Ia-antigens by peritoneal exudate macrophages is a transient event. J

Immunol 126;263.

Bradley TR and Metcalf D (1966). The growth of mouse bone marrow cells *in vitro*. Aust J Exp Biol Med 44;287.

Broxmeyer HE, Smithyman A, Eger RR, Meyers PA and deSousa M (1978). Identification of lactoferrin as the granulocyte derived inhibitor of colony stimulating activity production. J Exp Med 148:1052.

Broxmeyer HE, Bognacki J, Dorner MH and deSousa M (1981). Identification of leukemia-associated inhibitory activity as acidic isoferritins. J Exp Med 153:1426.

Burgess AW and Metcalf D (1980). The nature and action of granulocyte-macrophage colony stimulating factors. Blood 56:947.

Chervenick PA and Boggs DR (1970). Bone marrow colonies: stimulation *in vitro* by supernatant from incubated blood cells. Science (Wash DC) 169:691.

Fauser AA and Messner HA (1978). Granuloerythopoietic colonies in human bone marrow, peripheral blood, and cord blood . Blood 52:1243.

Fausser AA and Messner HA (1979). Identification of mega-karyocytes, macrophages, and eosinophils in colonies of human bone marrow containing granulocytes and erythoblasts. Blood 53:1023.

Janossy G, Francis GE, Capellaro D, Goldstone AH and Greaves MF (1978). Cell sorter analysis of leukemia-associated antigens on human myeloid precursors. Nature 276:176.

Johnson GR and Metcalf D(1978). Nature of cells forming erythroid colonies in agar after stimulation by spleen conditioned medium. J Cell Physiol 94:243.

Lanier LL and Warner NL (1981). Cell cycle related hetero-geneity of Ia-expression on a murine B lymphoma cell line: Analysis by flow cytometry. J Immunol 126:626.

Metcalf D (1973). Regulation of granulocyte and monocyte-macrophage proliferation by colony stimulating factor (CSF): A review. Exp Hematol 1:185.

Moore MAS, Broxmeyer HE, Sheridan APC, Meyers PA, Jacobsen N and Winchester RJ (1980). Continuous human bone marrow culture: Ia-antigen characterization of probable pluripo-tent stem cells. Blood 55:682.

Pelus LM, Broxmeyer HE and Moore MAS (1981). Regulation of human myelopoiesis by prostaglandin E and lactoferrin. Cell Tissue Kinet 14: *in press*.

Pelus LM, Broxmeyer HE, Clarkson BD and Moore MAS (1980). Abnormal responsiveness of granulocyte-macrophage com-mitted colony forming cells from patients with chronic myeloid leukemia to inhibition by prostaglandin E.

Cancer Res 40:2512.

Pluznik DH and Sachs L (1965). The cloning of normal mast cells in tissue culture. J Cell Comp Physiol 66:319.

Quesenberry P and Levitt L (1979). Hematopoietic stem cells. N Eng J Med 301:819.

Sarkar S, Glassy MC, Ferrone S and Jones OW (1980). Cell cycle and the differential expression of HLA-A,B and HLA-Dr antigens on human B lymphoid cells. Proc Nat'l Acad Sci, USA 77:7297.

Steeg PS, Moore RN and Oppenheim JJ (1980). Regulation of murine macrophage Ia-antigen expression by products of activated spleen cells. J Exp Med 152:1734.

Steinman RM, Nogueira N, Witmer MD, Tydings JD and Mellman IS (1980). Lymphokine enhances the expression of Ia-antigens on cultured mouse peritoneal macrophages. J Exp Med 152:1248.

Till JE and McCulloch EA (1961). A direct measurement of the radiation sensitivity of normal mouse bone marrow cells. Radiat Res 14:213.

Winchester RJ, Ross GD, Jarowski CI, Wang CY, Halper J and Broxmeyer HE (1977). Expression of Ia-like antigen molecules on human granulocytes during early phases of differentiation. Proc Nat'l Acad Sci, USA 74:4012.

Prostaglandins and Cancer: First
International Conference, pages 415–423
© 1982 Alan R. Liss, Inc., 150 Fifth Avenue, New York, NY 10011

PROSTAGLANDINS, T-LYMPHOCYTE PRECURSORS AND CANCER

R.S. Bockman

Memorial Sloan-Kettering Cancer Center

]275 York Avenue, New York, New York   10021

1. INTRODUCTION

     With the development of newer in vitro techniques it
has been possible to maintain and support the growth of
human hematopoietic precursor cells. Using such systems the
roles of hormones and factors on stem cell proliferation and
differentiation has been examined. Initial pharmacological
experiments showed that prostaglandins (PG) could inhibit
the plating efficiency of one class of committed hematopoietic cell precursor (CFU-C) (Kurland & Moore, 1977). These
cells gave rise to mature granulocytes and macrophages. In
subsequent experiments endogenously synthesized PG could be
shown to have a physiologically relevant role in causing
feedback inhibition of factor initiated myelopoiesis (Kurland
et al., 1978a, 1978b, 1979; Miller et al., 1978). The
central modulating role of the monocyte/macrophage on stem
cell proliferation and differentiation was established when
these cells were identified as the prime producers of PG
(Kurland & Bockman, 1978; Bockman, 1981). Recent experiments
have demonstrated that only the monocyte descendents of the
CFU-C are inhibited by PG and that the activity rests within
the E class of PG (Pelus et al., 1979; Pelus et al., in press).
More recently we have examined a circulating T lymphocyte
which undergoes clonal expansion to form colonies of mature
T lymphocytes in soft agar (Bockman & Rothschild, 1979).
Previous studies had presented evidence that monocytes and
macrophages released a variety of factors some of which were
inhibitory, others that facilitated clonal T lymphocyte
expansion in soft agar (Claesson et al., 1977; Zeevi et al.,
1977). Suspecting that there might be a parallelism between

the CFU-C and CFU-Tl cell systems, the effect of prostaglandins and monocytes on T colony formation was examined (Bockman & Rotnschild, 1979). Our studies on PG regulation of CFU-Tl expansion in normal subjects and in select cancer patients will now be discussed.

2. Methods:

a. Isolation of mononuclear cells: Heparinized blood, marrow aspirate or lymph nodes which were mechanically disrupted to release cells were obtained from patients and normal subjects. The blood was diluted with phosphate-buffered saline (PBS), layered over a 2.3/1.0 gradient of Ficoll (9%, W/V) and hypaque, sodium diatrizoate (34%, W/V) and subjected to differential centrifugation. The mononuclear cells were harvested with a sterile pipette at the Ficoll/hypaque interface and washed thoroughly with McCoy's media. As pointed out in the original papers and as our own experience confirms in the Ficoll method of isolated mononuclear cells, about 80% of the cells are histologically identified as lymphocytes; the remainder are predominantly monocytes (Bockman & Rotnschild, 1979). Lymph node cells were washed with media and the number of phagocytic cells determined by particle ingestion. Enumeration of T and B cell percentages was carried out as part of immune parameter testing.

b. Prostaglandin E radioimmunoassay: To freshly obtained sera, culture media or tissue, a trace amount (10^{-12} g) of ^{3}H-PGE was added to permit calculation of percent recovery. Tissue samples were acidified with 0.3 M citric acid and then homogenized in the extracting solvents. Samples were initially extracted with petroluem ether to remove neutral fats. PG in samples were then extracted with acidified-ethylacetate- isopropanol or by the method of Folch. The organic phase was dried, solubilized in benzene-ethylacetate-methanol and applied to silicic acid columns. The columns were sequentially eluted using benzene-ethylacetate-methanol with increasing concentrations of methanol. The column effluents were dried and resolubilized in a gelatin-Tris buffer. Competitive binding between ^{3}H-PGE, and standard PGE or sample unknown to specific anti-PGE antibody was measured using a double -antibody RIA. Linearity of the standard curve plotted as the logit plot (ln B/BO vs log PG concentration) was an essential condition for data validity.

Since the silicic acid column clearly separates PGA, PGB and
$PGF_{2\alpha}$ from PGE we feel the assay was specific for the E
series. Occasional samples were subjected to thin-layer
chromatography (Bockman, 1981) to check extraction and fractionation procedures.

c. T Colony Assay: Human peripheral blood leukocytes
were isolated on Ficoll hypaque gradients as previously
described. Isolated cells were resuspended at a concentration of one million cells per ml and cultured with PHA or
other proliferative stimuli for 24 hours in McCoy's media.
Following the initial cultured period 0.3% Bacto-Agar was
added to the cell cultures. One ml aliquots of cells were
layered over a 0.5% agar under-layer containing 16ug of
PHA-P in 1 ml McCoy's 5A and 10% FCS and antibiotics in 35
mm petri dishes. The petri dishes were allowed to gel for
1/2 hour at room temperature and subsequently incubated for
4-8 days at $37^{\circ}C$ in a humidified atmosphere of 10% CO_2 in
air. At the end of the incubation period the plates were
scored for the number of colonies containing >50 cells at
40x magnification (Bockman & Rotnschild, 1979).

3. Results

a. Prostaglandin and T colony formation: In a soft agar
system, T colonies were shown to arise from a small subset
of phytonemagglutinin responsive T lymphocyte in peripheral
blood marrow aspirates and lymph nodes (Bockman & Rotnschild, 1979). Pooled cells from many colonies could be
shown to have specific functional activities. The addition
of PGE demonstrated a dose dependent inhibition of T colony
formation with a 50% point of inhibition occurring at 0.18
µM PGE_2, Table 1.

Table 1

Prostaglandin effect on T colony formation*
==

Prostaglandin	0.1	1.0	10	100	1000 nM
PGE_2	94	75	68	43	---
$PGF_{2\alpha}$	---	116	123	160	162
PGD	93	114	95	100	104

* Expressed as % of control

Prostaglandin E_1 was as potent as PGE_2 whereas PGD_2 was without effect at up to 10.0 μM concentration. These latter findings would suggest that the stereospecificity of the constituents on the pentane ring portion of the molecule, i.e. at positions C10 and C11 was critical for biologic effect. Low concentrations of $PGF_{2\alpha}$ (< 10μM) appeared to augment colony numbers whereas at concentrations of 10μM or greater $PGF_{2\alpha}$ was inhibitory. The addition of small numbers of normal monocytes or monocyte conditioned media to the soft agar underlayers mimicked the effect seen with PGE_2. The addition of prostaglandin synthetase inhibitors with low cell numbers of monocytes abrogated the inhibition caused by the monocytes. Finally, a highly significant correlation between endogenous levels of PGE measured by radioimmunoassay and T colony numbers was demonstrated (r=0.71, n=40, p<0.001). These data suggested that monocytes through their synthesis of PGE_2 could regulate the clonal expansion of circulating T cell precursors. In the previously quoted studies the implication was that PGE could serve as a physiologically relevant regulator of stem cell proliferation, but it clearly is not meant to imply that it is the only inhibitory agent. Indeed, other macrophage derived factors have been postulated to be key regulators (Claesson et al., 1977; Zeevi et al., 1977). Furthermore, our own studies demonstrated the, inability of prostaglandin inhibitors to block the inhibitory activity seen when large numbers of monocytes were added to the test system.

b. Prostaglandins, CFU-Tl and Hodgkin's Disease: In the previous section the inhibitory role of PGE on CFU-Tl was presented. It is now appropriate to continue that discussion and to ask to what extent monocyte derived PGE may contribute to the inhibition of the precursor T cell compartment in patients with Hodgkin's disease. We selected Hodgkin's disease for study since marked elevations of PGE had been noted in the media from mononuclear cell cultures of such patients (Goodwin et al., 1977). Profound immune cell deficits affecting several functional classes of T cells (Aisenberg, 1965; Levy & Kaplan, 1974; Twomey et al., 1975; Case et al., 1976; Hillinger & Herzig, 1978) suggested to us that impaired stem cell proliferation and differentiation might explain the immunosuppression seen in these patients. T colony formation by the peripheral blood and spleen mononuclear cells from 36 previously untreated patients with Hodgkin's disease was examined (Bockman, 1980). Progressive reduction in colony number was evident with advancing stage of disease whether peripheral blood or spleen cells were examined, Table 2.

Table 2

T Colony Formation in Hodgkin's Disease

===

	Stage II	Stage III
Patients	609 (209)*	416 (158)
with indometnacin+	1358 (355)	659 (165)
	n=14	n=14
Normal subjects	2274 (360)	
with indometnacin	2666 (378)	
	n=13	

* Mean colony counts/1 million cells plated +/- (sem)
+ Indometnacin 2 uM final concentration

Tne addition of indometnacin (2μM) caused a significant increase in T colony formation wnicn distinguisnes tne Hodgkin's disease patients from normal subjects in wnom no significant augmentation in colony formation was seen. A significant negative correlation of colony number witn stage of disease was noted. Wnile colony number was increased by tne addition of a prostaglandin-syntnetase innibitor to tne cultures, colony numbers could not be restored to normal levels in tne patients witn advanced stages of disease. Tnese data suggest tnat a progressive immunodepletion occurs at tne stem cell level with advancing stage of disease. Measurement of immune cell syntnesis of prostaglandins showed there to be augmented PGE levels, Table 3, and these levels increased witn advancing stage of disease. Cell separation experiments gave evidence tnat adnerent monocyte and macropnage syntnesis of PGE could account entirely for tne augmented levels measured. Wnen examined by tne tecnnique of tritiated aracnidonic acid conversion (Bockman, 1980) and tnin layer cnromatograpny it was evident tnat PGE_2 was tne major prostaglandin class syntnesized. A significant correlation coefficient ($r=-0.43$, $p<0.01$) was demonstrated by linear regression analyses of 40 paired samples

Table 3

PGE in Leukocyte Conditioned Media*
=====================================
ng PGE

Hodgkin's Disease	1.98 (0.36)	n=11
Breast Cancer	0.30 (0.07)	n=22
Normals	0.42 (0.08)	n=11

* One million cells cultured in McCoy's Media supplemented with 10% fetal calf serum.

comparing T colony number and PGE levels in patients with Hodgkin's disease. While there appeared to be a strong correlation between monocyte synthesis of PGE and depressed T colony counts this does not mean that depressed T colony formation was caused by the increased PGE production. Nevertheless, there appears to be sufficient evidence to conclude that excessive host production of PGE can suppress CFU-Tl colony formation. As an extrapolation of this latter conclusion, it seems worthwhile to test the premise that persistently elevated PGE levels may result in the progressive attrition of CFU-Tl to a point sufficient to result in depressed immunocompetence. Patients with newly diagnosed Hodgkin's disease are currently under long-term follow-up protocols in order to explore this premise.

4. Conclusion

Immune cell dysfunction and depressed immunocompetence are frequently associated with cancer and may contribute significantly to several of the morbidities which occur with cancer. The mechanisms which are responsible for these phenomena are poorly understood. In certain malignant conditions of which Hodgkin's disease serves as a prime example, immunodepletion and multifunctional immune cell disorders are found to progress with advancing stage of disease. In such patients excessive monocyte synthesis of prostaglandin E, a potent modulator of immune cell function, has been shown to occur. Since prostaglandins can exert their immunomodulatory effects at both the stem and mature T cell levels; it seems reasonable to speculate that augmented synthesis of prostaglandins may account for the disorders of T cell ontogeny and mature cell function seen in patients with Hodgkin's disease. Indeed, when it was looked for, the progressive loss of committed T stem cells could be shown to be significantly correlated with the increased levels of endogenous prostaglandins that occurs with advancing stage of disease. Such a correlation does not necessarily elucidate the actual mechanisms which lead to the depressed immune status seen in such patients but it is conceivable that disordered regulation of prostaglandin synthesis could result in specific alterations in T cell subpopulation frequency perhaps through the attrition of specifically committed T stem cells or the suppression of selected mature T cell classes.

Recent experiments have shown that mature T cell subpopulations can vary significantly in their responsiveness to exogenous prostaglandin. T cells which carry and express a receptor for the Fc portion of IgG (Tγ cells) could be shown to respond to PGE_2 with a 30 fold increase in cyclic adenosine monophosphate (cAMP) levels, whereas Tμ cells showed little or no response (Goodwin et al., 1979). Mature T cells separated on discontinuous albumin gradients were also shown to vary in their response to prostaglandin. T cells sedimenting with a high density (> 29% albumin fraction) showed a 60% reduction in their blastogenic response to PHA in the presence of 0.1 mM PGE. T cells of low density (< 26% albumin) had enhanced (20% increase over controls) PHA initiated blastogenesis when PGE was added to the cultures (Stobo et al., 1979). Clearly such data suggests that there is heterogeneity amongst physically separable subpopulations of mature T cells with regard to PGE responsiveness. Furthermore, the latter experiments would imply that PGE is a true modulator of cell function and not merely an inhibitor. It is intriguing to consider that such heterogeneity of PGE responsiveness may occur at the level of the CFU-T1 and that there may be differential susceptibility of the CFU-T1 committed to specific functional pathways.

5. References

Aisenberg, A.C. 1965. Quantitative estimation of the reactivity of normal and Hodgkin's disease lymphocytes with Thymidine-2^{14}C. Nature (Lond.) 205 :1233-1235.

Bockman, R.S. and M. Rothschild. 1979. Prostaglandin E inhibition of T lymphocyte colony formation. J. Clin. Invest. 64 :812-819.

Bockman, R.S.   1980.   Stage dependent reduction in T colony formation in Hodgkin's disease. J. Clin. Invest. 66 :523-31.

Bockman, R.S. 1981. Prostaglandin production by human blood monocytes and mouse peritoneal macrophages: synthesis dependent on in vitro culture conditions. Prostaglandins (21)1 :9-31.

Case, D.C., J.A. Hansen, E. Corrales, C.W. Young, B. Dupont, C.M. Pinsky and R.A. Good. 1976. Comparison of multiple in vivo and in vitro parameters in untreated patients with Hodgkin's disease. Cancer (Phila.) 38 :1807-1815.

Claesson, M.H., M.B. Rodger, G.R. Johnson, S. Whittingham and D. Metcalf. 1977. Colony formation by human T lymphocytes in agar medium. Clin. Exp. Immunol. 28 :526-534.

Goodwin, J.S., R.P. Messner, A.D. Banknurst, G.T. Peake, J.H. Saiki and R.C. Williams, Jr. 1977. Prostaglandin producing suppressor cells in Hodgkin's disease. N. Engl. J. Med. 297 :963-968.

Goodwin, J.S., P.A. Kaszubowski and R.C. Williams. 1979. Cyclic adenosine monophosphate response to prostaglandin E_2 on subpopulations of human lymphocytes. J. Exp. Med. 150 :1260-64.

Hillinger, S.M. and G.P. Herzig. 1978. Impaired cell-mediated immunity in Hodgkin's disease mediated by suppressor lymphocytes and monocytes. J. Clin. Invest. 61 :1620-1627.

Kurland, J. and M.A.S. Moore. 1977. Modulation of hemopoiesis by prostaglandins. Exp. Hematol. (Copenhag) 5 :357-73.

Kurland, J., R.S. Bockman, H. Broxmeyer and M.A.S. Moore. 1978. Limitation of excessive myelopoiesis by the extrinsic modulation of macrophage derived prostaglandin E. Science 199 :552-55.

Kurland, J., H. Broxmeyer, R.S. Bockman, L. Pelus and M.A.S. Moore. 1978. Role for monocyte-macrophage derived colony stimulating factor and prostaglandin E in positive and negative feedback control of myeloid

stem cell proliferation.
Blood 52 :388-407.

Kurland, J.I. and R.S. Bockman. 1978. Prostaglandin E production by human blood monocytes and mouse peritoneal macrophages. J. Exp. Med. 147 :952-957.

Kurland, J.I., L. Pelus, P. Ralph, R.S. Bockman and M.A.S. Moore. 1979. Induction of prostaglandin E synthesis in normal and neoplastic macrophages: a new role for colony stimulating factor(s). Proc. Natl. Acad. Sci. (U.S.A.) 76 :2326-30.

Levy, R. and H.S. Kaplan. 1974. Impaired lymphocyte function in untreated Hodgkin's disease. N. Engl. J. Med. 290 :181-186.

Miller, A.M., T.R. Russell, M.A. Gross and A.A. Yunis. 1978. Modulation of granulopoiesis: opposing roles of prostaglandin F and E. J. Lab. Clin. Med. 92 :983-990.

Pelus, L.M., H.E. Broxmeyer, J.I. Kurland and M.A.S. Moore. 1979. Regulation of macrophage and granulocyte proliferation. J. Exp. Med. 150 :277-92.

Pelus, L.M., H.E. Broxmeyer and M.A.S. Moore. 1981. Regulation of human myelopoiesis by prostaglandin E and lactoferrin. Cell Tissue Kinet. , in press.

Stobo, J.D., M.S. Kennedy and M.E. Goldyne. 1979. Prostaglandin E modulation of the mitogenic response of human T cells. J. Clin. Invest. 64 :1185-95.

Twomey, J.J., A.H. Laughter, S. Farrow and C.C. Douglass. 1975. Hodgkin's disease: An immunodepleting and immunosuppressive disorder. J. Clin. Invest. 56 :467-475.

Zeevi, A., I. Goldman and L.A. Rozenszajn. 1977. Stimulation and inhibition of human T lymphocyte colony cell proliferation by hemopoietic cell factors. Cell Immunol. 28 :235-247.

**Prostaglandins and Cancer: First
International Conference, pages 425-436
© 1982 Alan R. Liss, Inc., 150 Fifth Avenue, New York, NY 10011**

ROLE OF PROSTAGLANDINS ON THE GROWTH AND DIFFERENTIATION OF
FRIEND ERYTHROLEUKEMIA CELLS

M.G. Santoro and B.M. Jaffe

Center of Virology, C.N.R., O.O.R.R., Rome, Italy
and Department of Surgery, S.U.N.Y. Downstate
Medical Center, Brooklyn, New York

Murine erythroleukemic cells infected with the Friend
virus (FLC) provide an excellent model for the study of the
regulation of erythroleukemic differentiation. FLC grow in
suspension culture and can be induced in vitro to form morphologically and functionally mature cells of the erythroid
lineage upon stimulation with a wide variety of compounds
including dimethylsulfoxide (Friend et al., 1971) and other
planar polar compounds (Preisler and Lyman, 1975), butyric
acid and other short-chain fatty acids (Leder and Leder,
1975), hemin (Ross and Sautner, 1976), ouabain (Bernstein et
al., 1976), polymethylene bisacetamides (Reuben et al.,
1976), low doses of actinomycin D (Terada et al., 1978).
When induced to differentiate, FLC produce hemoglobin (Friend
et al., 1971) that presents an electophoretic pattern similar
to that of hemolysates of adult DBA/2j mice (Scher et al.,
1971), the strain from which the cells originated. Hemoglobin production is accompanied by morphological changes, increase in iron uptake and heme synthesis (Friend et al, 1971),
the appearance of erythrocyte membrane antigens (Ikawa et al.,
1973) and accumulation of mRNA for globin synthesis (Ross et
al., 1974).

Prostaglandins (PGs), and in particular prostaglandins
of the E series, are known to be implicated in the regulation
of cell proliferation and differentiation in several systems.
Stimulation of endogenous prostaglandins (mainly PGE) during
differentiation has been demonstrated in mouse myeloid leukemia cells (Honma et al., 1980), while administration of
exogenous PGEs promoted differentiation in neuroblastoma
(Prasad, 1972), mouse fibroblasts (Johnson and Pastan, 1971),

mouse myeloid leukemia cells (Honma et al., 1979), MDCK
cells (Lever, 1979), chick myoblasts (Zalin, 1979) and other
systems.

In addition, prostaglandins have been shown to play a
role in erythropoiesis. Arachidonic acid and PGs of the A
and E series stimulated erythropoiesis, measured by ^{59}Fe incorporation into newly formed red cells, as well as erythropoietin synthesis in exhypoxic polycytemic mice and isolated
perfused kidney (Dukes et al., 1973; Foley et al., 1978;
Paulo et al., 1973; Schooley and Mahlmann, 1971). Prostaglandins also stimulated in vitro erythropoiesis as measured
both by ^{59}Fe incorporation into heme of rat marrow cultures
(Dukes et al., 1975) and by an increase of mRNA synthesis
in liver cells of 12-day mouse embryos (Djaletti et al.,
1978). Our studies have determined the pattern of endogenous
PGE synthesis as well as the effect of exogenous PG administration during the growth and the differentiation process
of Friend Erythroleukemic cells.

The cell line used, GM-86 (clone 745) was provided by
the Institute for Medical Research, Camden, N.J. Cells were
maintained at 37^0C in Dulbecco's modified Eagle's medium
supplemented with 15% fetal calf serum and antibiotics, in a
5% CO_2, 95% air humidified atmosphere. Stationary-phase
cultures were defined as containing cells cultured for 120-
144 hr without media changes and which, although viable for
at least 96 more hours, did not replicate further.

The prostaglandins tested PGA_1, PGA_2, PGE_1, PGE_2, PGB_2,
PGD_2, $PGF_{2\alpha}$, TxB_2, 6-keto $PGF_{1\alpha}$ and the synthetic analogs,
16,16 dimethyl-PGA_2 methyl ester (di-M-PGA_2) were generously
provided by Dr. John Pike, Upjohn Company, Kalamazoo, Michigan. They were maintained as stock solutions in absolute
ethanol at -20^0C and diluted in tissue culture medium immediately before using. Control media contained identical
concentrations of ethanol (0.005%). Cellular DNA and protein
synthesis were measured by ^{3}H-thymidine and^{35}S-methionine
incorporation respectively. For hemoglobin determination,
samples of cells ($2x10^6$) were washed twice and lysed by
repeated freeze-thawings (3x). Hemoglobin was measured from
cell lysates using the technique of Crosby and Furth (1956).

PGE concentrations in media and supernatants were measured by radioimmunoassay after organic solvent extraction
and silicic acid chromatography as described previously

(Jaffe et al.,1973).Since more than 90% of the endogenous
prostaglandins are extruded,immediately after synthesis,
from the cells into the medium,media concentrations were
measured as a mean of quantitation of the amount of PGs syn-
thesized.PG determinations were corrected for appropiate
blanks;none of the compounds added to the medium,including
the PGE_2 analog,cross-reacted with the anti-PGE antibody
utilized.

Synthesis of Endogenous PGE During Growth and Differentiation
of FLC.

    In order to determine whether FLC synthesize prosta-
glandins during growth in vitro, aliquots of the supernatants of FLC cultures were collected and assayed for PGE
every 24 hours. Under control conditions,a peak of PGE
biosynthesis was reached at 24 hours after plating,and PGE
production decreased to the initial rate after 96 hours (Figure 1).Normal and Simian virus 40-transformed 3T3 fibroblasts had been reported to have a similar pattern of PGE
production (Hammarström,1977).

    In our system the growth of the cells at the time of
plating was important in determining both the growth pattern
and the amount of endogenous prostaglandins synthesized,as
well as the sensitivity of FLC to exogenous PGs.Figure 1
shows the pattern of growth and PGE synthesis of FLC derived
from logarithmically growing (fig.1A) and stationary (Fig.1B)
cultures plated at the same density (1×10^5 cells/ml) under
the same conditions.At 24 hours,the amount of PGE produced
by cells derived from stationary phase cultures was twice as
great as that produced by cells derived from log-phase cul-
tures.This difference in PGE production was associated with
a significant difference in the rate of proliferation (log
phase: $4.4 \pm 0.7 \times 10^5$ cells/ml;stationary phase: 2.2 ± 0.2
$\times 10^5$ cells/ml;at 24 hours).

    The levels of endogenous PGE were measured during DMSO-
induced differentiation in FLC derived from stationary phase
cultures.Figure 2 shows the cumulative PGE levels in cultures
treated with DMSO (1.5%),di-M-PGE_2 (1 µg/ml),and DMSO + di-
M-PGE_2. Both DMSO and di-M-PGE_2 alone significantly stimulated PGE production with a peak of 200% increase at 72 hours.
However,by 96 hours PGE synthesis returned to control levels.
Treatment with the combination of DMSO and di-M-PGE_2 produced a significant synergistic effect on the stimulation of
PGE synthesis which increased several fold at each data point
and did not decrease toward the end of the experimental period.

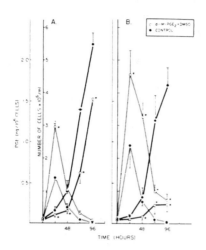

Fig.1.
PGE production
and growth pat-
tern of FL C de-
rived from log
(A) and statio-
nary (B) phase
cultures in the
presence and the
absence of D MSO
+ di-M-PGE$_2$.
* = p< 0.05.

In addition to the stimulation of PGE synthesis,treatment
with D MSO + di-M-PGE$_2$ produced a significant inhibition of
growth during the 96 hour period;this inverse correlation
between PGE synthesis and rate of cell replication was more
dramatic in cells derived from a resting population,in which
the marked stimulation of PGE biosynthesis was associated
with 90% inhibition of FL C replication at 96 hours.These two
parameters were significantly correlated (p<0.01),with a
correlation coefficient of 0.48 (n=69). An inverse relationship between prostaglandin biosynthesis and proliferation
rate has been previously reported in other tumor cell lines
(Thomas et al.,1974).

The stimulation of PGE synthesis as well as the inhibitory effect caused by DMSO and di-M-PGE$_2$ as inhibited by
more than 90% at 48 and 96 hours upon treatment with 10 $^\circ$ M
indomethacin;the mechanism by which D MSO and di-M-PGE$_2$ stimulate the PG synthetase system in FL C is unknown.

Effect of Exogenous Prostaglandins on the Growth and Differentiation of FL C .

The effect of a series of prostaglandins and prosta-

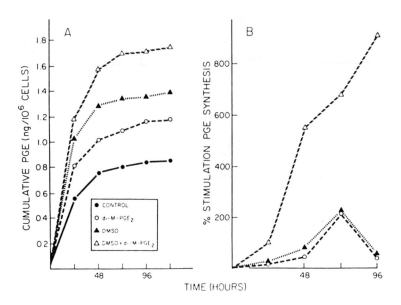

Figure 2. Cumulative production of PGE during the growth of FL C untreated or in the presence of DMSO,di-M-PGE$_2$ or DMSO + di-M-PGE$_2$. A = Cumulative PGE synthesis. B = Percent stimulation of PGE synthesis.

glandin-related compounds,on the growth of and hemoglobin production by FL C was tested.Figure 3 shows the effect of a wide variety of compounds on the growth of FL C cells. Cells derived from a stationary culture were plated at a density of 1 x 10^5 cells/ml and after four days of growth,cell numbers,cell viability and hemoglobin production were determined. Di-M-PGE$_2$ and PGD$_2$ were found to be slightly toxic to the cells (92% and 94% viability as compared to 98-100% viability in the normal range).Prostaglandins of the A and E series were found to inhibit FL C replication,the "2" series being more active than the "1" series. PGB$_2$,PGF$_{2\alpha}$,TxB$_2$ and 6-Keto PGF$_{1\alpha}$ had no significant effect on cell growth. Analogous results were obtained in the presence of 1.5% DMSO;in this case,however,the inhibition by PGA s and PGEs was even more pronounced. As anticipated in the previous section, cells derived from logarithmically

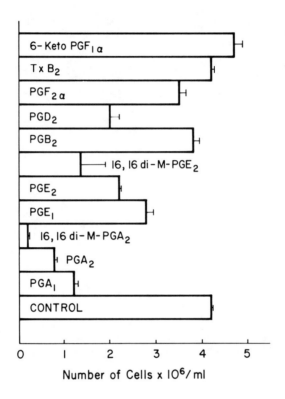

Figure 3. Effect of different prostaglandins and prostaglandin—related compounds on the replication of FLC. All compounds were tested at the concentration of 2 µg/ml.

growing populations were much less sensitive to the growth
inhibitory effect of these prostaglandins.Table 1 shows the
effect of PGA_1 (1 µg/ml) on DNA synthesis,measured as ^{3}H-thy-
midine incorporation,in FLC derived from stationary and log
phase cultures after 24 and 48 hours of treatment.
The reason for the different sensitivity to PGs of cells in
the stationary or log phase of growth is not clear. Hypothe-
tically,there might be a change in the prostaglandin receptors during the cell cycle or the cell might be able to respond to PG action only in some phases of the cell cycle.

Table 1. Effect of PGA_1 on DNA synthesis of FLC.

^{3}H-thymidine incorporation
(cpm x 10^3)

		24 hr	48 hr
Stationary	Control	454.9±10.3	518.4±12.7
	PGA_1	194.5±14.1*	139.6±43.9*
Log	Control	311.1± 8.3	352.8±16.4
	PGA_1	353.7±28.3	357.2±36.8

* = $p < 0.05$

This latter possibility has in fact being demonstrated in chick myoblasts (Zalin,1979) where only cells in the G_1 phase of the cell cycle were able to respond to PGE_1 with a transient rise in the intracellular levels of cyclic AMP and with precocious cell fusion to form syncytia.

In the absence of inducers,only a minimal portion of the FLC population undergoes spontaneous differentiation producing hemoglobin (0.2 to 0.4 µg Hb/10^6 cells).Addition of 1.5% DMSO to the medium induced hemoglobin production and more than 90% of the cells became benzidine-positive 5 days after DMSO administration. PGE_1,PGE_2,di-M-PGE_2,PGB_2,PGD_2,$PGF_{2\alpha}$,TxB_2 and 6-Keto $PGF_{1\alpha}$ did not induce hemoglobin production at the doses tested. Di-M-PGE_2 was,however,found to stimulate DMSO-induced differentiation,significantly increasing hemoglobin levels from 3.76±0.44 µg/10^6 cells to 6.85±0.30 µg/10^6 cells (Santoro et al.,1979a).

This stimulatory effect of di-M-PGE_2 was completely suppressed (as well as the growth inhibitory action) by treatment with 10^{-8} M indomethacin (4.35±0.87 µg/10^6 cells),suggesting that prostaglandins (not necessarely PGE) endogenously synthesized in response to DMSO + di-M-PGE_2 are responsible for this stimulatory effect.
Arachidonic acid was also shown to augment DMSO-induced differentiation. PGs of the A series were the only exogenous prostaglandins able to induce hemoglobin production in the absence of DMSO (Santoro et al.,1979b). Table 2 shows the effect

Table 2. Effect of PGA_1 on FLC differentiation.

Hemoglobin ($\mu g/10^6$ cells)

Cells derived from:

	stationary culture	log culture
Control	0.46±0.06	0.42±0.06
	(n=14)	(n=3)
PGA_1 (1 μg/ml)	1.29±0.13*	1.27±0.10*
	(n=12)	(n=3)
DMSO (1.5%)	4.02±0.26*	3.94±0.35*
	(n=17)	(n=4)

* = p < 0.05

of PGA_1 (2 μg/ml) on hemoglobin production in FLC derived from log and stationary cultures. In contrast to the inhibitory action on growth, that is selective for populations in stationary phase, PGA_1 induced differentiation in both stationary and log cultures, suggesting that the inhibition of proliferation was not a prerequisite for differentiation in this system.

The mechanism by which PGA_1 induces hemoglobin (Hb) synthesis in these cells is not known. PGA_1, at this dose, does not seem to affect the pattern of protein synthesis in FLC, measured by ^{35}S-methionine labeling and autoradiography after PAGE analysis (unpublished data). Although exogenous cyclic AMP and its derivatives do not influence differentiation in FLC, mediation by a stimulatory effect on the adenylate and guanylate cyclase cannot be excluded as a possible mechanism. The possibility of an action on heme synthesis should also be examined, since it has been reported that PGs and thromboxane A_2 play an important role in porphyrin biosynthesis and mitochondria ferrochetalase activity in liver cell culture (Morgan et al., 1979).

We have examined the effect on Hb production of simultaneous administration of erythropoietin (0.2 U/ml) and either PGA_1, PGA_2 or di-M-PGA_2, since it has been suggested that PGAs can bind actively to erythropoietin via glucuronide and sulphate ester bonds (Welch et al., 1979) and this binding may be necessary for its action (Dukes et al., 1975). In these studies erythropoietin did not stimulate hemoglobin synthesis either alone or in the presence of prostaglandins.

Effect of Inhibitors of Prostaglandin Synthesis.

While indomethacin,at the dose tested, had no effect on DMSO-induced differentiation in FLC,hydrocortisone (HC) was found to be a potent inhibitor of DMSO-induced hemoglobin production (Santoro et al.,1978).Hydrocortisone (10^{-7} -10^{-6} M) alone had no effect on FLC replication or differentiation, while simultaneous administration of HC and DMSO resulted in total inhibition of hemoglobin synthesis (Figure 4).

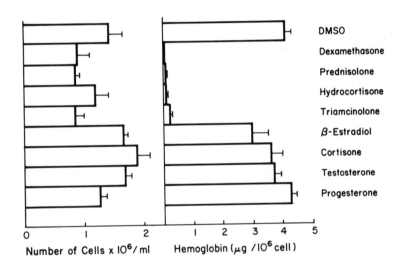

Figure 4. Effect of steroid hormones on DMSO-induced differentiation of FLC. Ethanolic solutions of different hormones were dissolved in medium containing 1.5% DMSO.Control and DMSO-containing media contained the same amount of ethanol (0.005%).The Hb content of the cells is expressed as $\mu g/10^6$ cells minus the control value (untreated cells contained 0.43±0.04 μg Hb/10^6 cells).

This effect was accomplished without any change in either the rate of cell proliferation or total protein synthesis. The effect was dose-related,with a maximal activity at concentrations of 10^{-6}-10^{-7} M.The inhibitory effect of hydrocortisone was also noted in DMF-(N,N,dimethylformamide) and PGA$_1$-induced Hb production (97 and 98% inhibition,respectively). Fig.4 shows the effect of several steroid hormones on DMSO-induced differentiation of FLC.Interestingly,at the concentrations tested (10^{-6} M),only the 11,17,dihydroxycorticosteroids were potent inhibitors of FLC differentiation.

In order to determine whether the hydrocortisone-mediated inhibitory action was due to the inhibition of endogenous PG biosynthesis,the effect of HC on PGE production was studied;we also examined the possibility of reversing this HC action by the addition of arachidonic acid and exogenous PGs.Hydrocortisone (10^{-6} M) lowered medium PGE concentrations by 48% in DMSO-treated FLC.However,the addition to DMSO + HC-containing medium of either arachidonic acid (1 μg/ml),PGE$_1$ (1 ng/ml),or di-M-PGE$_2$ (10 ng and 1 μg/ml) did not reverse HC action.

In summary,we have studied the pattern of PGE synthesis during the growth of both undifferentiated and differentiating FLC. Endogenously synthesized PGs were shown to be involved in regulating cell proliferation and stimulating DMSO-induced differentiation.Exogenous PGA$_1$ was able to induce hemoglobin production and,conversely,glucocorticosteroids were found to be potent inhibitors of FLC differentiation. The mechanism of these actions is not understood,and a detailed study of the effects of all prostaglandins and PG metabolites, including compounds produced by the lipoxygenase pathway,is necessary since more than one prostaglandin could be involved in modulating these actions.

This work was in part supported by grant 79.02385.65 from the CNR,in conjunction with the C.N.R.-National Science Foundation U.S.A.-Italy Cooperative Program,by grant 79.00370. 84 Progetto Finalizzato Virus,C.N.R.,and by grants CH 103 and CH 103A from the American Cancer Society.

References.

Bernstein A,Hunt DM,Crickley V and Mak TW (1976).Induction by ouabain of hemoglobin synthesis in cultured Friend erythroleukemic cells.Cell 9:375.
Crosby MH and Furth FW (1956).A modification of the benzidine method for measurement of hemoglobin in plasma and urine.Blood 11:380.
Djaletti M,Bessler H and Levi J (1978).Effect of PGA$_2$ on RNA synthesis in embryonic mouse erythroid cells.Nephron 21:345.

Dukes P,Shore N,Hammond D,Ortega J and Datta M (1973).Enhancement of erythropoiesis by prostaglandins.J Lab Clin Med 82:704.

Dukes P,Shore N, Hammond G and Ortega J (1975). Prostaglandins and erythropoietin action.In Nakao K et al.(eds):"Erythropoiesis", Tokyo: Tokyo University Press, p 3.

Foley J,Gross D,Nelson P and Fisher J (1978).The effects of arachidonic acid on erythropoietin production in exhypoxic polycythemic mice and the isolated perfused canine kidney. J Pharmac Exp Therapeutics 207:402.

Friend C,Scher W,Holland JG and Sato T (1971).Hemoglobin synthesis in murine virus induced leukemic cells in vitro: stimulation of erythroid differentiation by dimethylsulfoxide.Proc Nat Acad Sci (Wash) 68:378.

Hammarström S (1977).Prostaglandin production by normal and transformed 3T3 fibroblasts in cell culture.Eur J Biochem 74:7.

Honma Y,Kasukabe T and Hozumi M (1979).Inhibition of differentiation of cultured mouse myeloid leukemia cells by nonsteroidal antiinflammatory agents and counteraction of the inhibition by PGE.Cancer Res 39:2190.

Honma Y,Kasukabe T,Hozumi M and Koshihara Y (1980).Regulation of prostaglandin synthesis during differentiation of cultured mouse myeloid leukemia cells.J Cell Phys 104:349.

Ikawa Y,Furusawa M and Sugano H (1973).Erythrocyte membrane-specific antigens in Friend virus-induced leukemia cells. Bibl Hematol 39:955.

Jaffe BM,Behrman HR and Parker CW (1973).Radioimmunoassay measurement of prostaglandin E,A and F in human plasma. J Clin Invest 52:398.

Johnson GS and Pastan I (1971).Changes in growth and morphology of fibroblasts by prostaglandins.J Nat Cancer Inst 47:1357.

Leder A and Leder P (1975).Buryric acid,a potent inducer of erythroid differentiation in cultured erythroleukemia cells.Cell 5:319.

Lever J (1979).Inducers of mammalian cell differentiation stimulate dome formation in a differentiated kidney epithelial cell line.Proc Nat Acad Sci (Wash) 76:1323.

Morgan R,Horrobin D,Mankin M and Ally A (1979).Regulation of porphyrin-haeme biosynthesis by prostaglandins and thromboxane A_2 in liver cell culture.IV Intern. Prostaglandin Conference Abstracts,Wash DC,p 82.

Paulo L,Wilkerson R,Roh B,George W and Fisher J (1973).The effects of PGE_1 on erythropoietin production.Proc Soc Exp Biol Med 142:771.

Prasad K (1972).Morphological differentiation induced by prostaglandins in mouse neuroblastoma cell culture.Nature New Biol 236:49.

Preisler HP and Lyman G (1975).Differentiation of erythroleukemia cells in vitro:properties of chemical inducers.Cell Differen 4:179.

Reuben RC,Wife RL,Breslow R,Rifkind RA and Marks PA (1976).A new group of potent inducers of differentiation in murine erythroleukemic cells.Proc Nat Acad Sci (Wash) 73:862.

Ross J,Gielen J,Packman S,Ikawa Y and Leder P (1974).Globin gene expression in cultured erythroleukemic cells.J Mol Biol 87:697.

Ross J and Sautner D (1976).Induction of globin mRNA accumulation by hemin in cultured erythroleukemic cells.Cell 8: 513.

Santoro MG,Benedetto A and Jaffe BM (1978).Hydrocortisone inhibits DMSO-induced differentiation of Friend erythroleukemia cells.Biochem Biophys Res Comm 85:1510.

Santoro MG,Benedetto A and Jaffe BM (1979a).Effect of endogenous and exogenous prostaglandin E on Friend erythroleukemia cell growth and differentiation.Br J Cancer 39:259.

Santoro MG,Benedetto A and Jaffe BM (1979b).Prostaglandin A_1 induces differentiation in Friend erythroleukemia cells. Prostaglandins 17:719.

Sher W,Holland G and Friend C (1971).Hemoglobin synthesis in murine virus-induced leukemic cells in vitro.Blood 37:428.

Schooley J and Mahlmann L (1971).Stimulation of erythropoiesis in plethoric mice by prostaglandins and its inhibition by antierythropoietin.Proc Soc Exp Biol Med 138:523.

Terada M,Epner E,Nudel U,Salmon J,Fibach E,Rifkind RA and Marks PA (1978).Induction of murine erythroleukemia differentiation by actinomycin D.Proc Nat Acad Sci (Wash) 75: 2795.

Thomas D, Philpott GW and Jaffe BM (1974). The relationship between concentration of PGE and rates of cell replication. Exp Cell Res 84:40.

Welch E,Neal W,Lewis J,Lutcher C and Gardner E (1979).Prostaglandins associated with erythropoiesis regulatory factors (ERFs).IV Intern.Prostaglandin Conference Abstracts Wash DC,p 123.

Zalin R (1979).The cell cycle,myoblast differentiation and prostaglandins as a developmental signal.Develop Biol 71: 274.

Prostaglandins and Cancer: First
International Conference, pages 437-451
© 1982 Alan R. Liss, Inc., 150 Fifth Avenue, New York, NY 10011

ROLE OF PROSTAGLANDINS IN DIFFERENTIATION OF NEUROBLASTOMA
CELLS IN CULTURE

Kedar N. Prasad

University of Colorado Health Sciences Center
School of Medicine, 4200 East Nineth Avenue
Denver, Colorado 80262 USA

INTRODUCTION

It is now established that prostaglandins (PG's) are
produced in varying amounts by every tissue in the body,
except mature red blood cells. In addition, animal and
human tumors also produce prostaglandins (Karmali, 1980).
Recent studies suggest that PG's could induce cell
differentiation and growth inhibition in a variety of tumor
cells in culture. The extent and the type of effect of PG's
depends upon the type of tumor and the type of prostaglandin. For example, PG's induce differentiation and growth
inhibition in neuroblastoma (Prasad, 1972) and Friend
erythroleukemic cells (Santoro et $al.$, 1979); whereas, they
inhibit the growth of several mammalian cell lines
in $vitro$, including plasmocytoma (Naseem and Hollander,
1973), L-5178-Y-R mouse leukemia (Yang et $al.$, 1976), Hela
HEP-29 (Hamprecht et $al.$, 1973; Thomas et $al.$, 1974), B-16
melanoma (Santoro et $al.$, 1976; 1977), and fibroblasts
(Johnson and Pastan, 1971). These studies show that PG's
exhibit anticancer properties in $vitro$ by inducing
differentiation and by inhibiting growth. However, the
PGE series may promote the growth of certain tumors by
inhibiting the host's immune system (Goodwin et $al.$, 1980).
The purpose of this review is to discuss the role of PG's
in the differentiation of neuroblastoma cells in culture,
and to suggest a biological rationale for using PG's in
the management of tumors. All earlier studies (Prasad,
1975; 1980a) on the effects of PG's on NB cells have been
performed in the presence of serum; however, the success
of growing NB cells in hormone-supplemented serum free

medium (Bottenstein and Sato, 1979) has allowed the examination of the role of PG's on cell differentiation in the absence of complex serum factors. Therefore, the expression of PG-induced differentiated functions in NB cells cultured in serum free medium will also be discussed.

EFFECT OF PG-INDUCED MORPHOLOGICAL DIFFERENTIATION IN NB CELLS CULTURED IN SERUM-SUPPLEMENTED MEDIUM

Earlier studies (Prasad, 1972; Prasad and Sinha, 1978) have shown that PGE_1 and PGE_2 induce the morphological differentiation of mouse NB (NBP_2 and $NBA_{2(1)}$) cells in culture. This is evidenced by the formation of long neurites and an increase in the size of soma and nucleus. The formation of neurites occurs in dividing NB cells; however, the cell division eventually stops in PG-treated cultures. These differentiated NB cells also have increased levels of biochemically differentiated functions (Prasad, 1975). In clones NBP_2 and $NBA_{2(1)}$, most of the cells in PGE_1-treated cultures do not retract their neurites when PGE_1 is removed after 3 days of treatment and the cells are examined 1 day after removal (Prasad, 1975). However, PGE_1-resistant cells and partially affected cells exist in PGE_1-treated cultures; and these cells continue to divide and eventually reach confluency. The terminally differentiated cells die in culture (Prasad, 1980a). When PGE_1-treated NB cells are removed from the dishes (after 3 days of treatment) by incubating them in the presence of 0.25% pancreatin solution, the cells appear round without any neurites. When these cells are replated in dishes, the neurites are extended within an hour even though no prostaglandin has been added (Prasad and Kumar, 1974). This finding further suggests that PGE_1-induced morphological differentiation is irreversible, and this differentiated phenotype can reexpress in the absence of PGE_1.

The effect of various types of prostaglandins has been summarized in Table 1. The PGA series was more effective than the PGE series in causing morphological differentiation in the NBP_2 clone. PGA_2 also induced morphological differentiation and growth inhibition in a clone (NBE^-) which was relatively insensitive to PGE_1 for these criteria. These data show that PGE_1 and PGA_2 may have separate receptors. This possibility is supported by

Table 1

Effect of Prostaglandins (PG's) on the
Morphological Differentiation of Neuroblastoma
Cells Cultured in the Presence of Serum

NB Clone	Treatment	Morphological Differentiation (% of Total Cells)
NBP_2	Control with or without ethanol (0.5%)	< 1
NBP_2	PGE_1 (10 μg/ml)	43 ± 6*
NBP_2	PGE_2 (10 μg/ml)	46 ± 5
NBP_2	PGA_1 (2.5 μg/ml)	77 ± 6
NBP_2	PGA_2 (10 μg/ml)	91 ± 3
NBP_2	$PGF_{2\alpha}$ (10 μg/ml)	3 ± 1
NBE^-	Control with or without ethanol (0.5%)	4 ± 1
NBE^-	PGE_1 (10 μg/ml)	24 ± 3
NBE^-	PGA_2 (10 μg/ml)	93 ± 4

*Standard deviation

Cells (50,000) were plated in Lux tissue culture dishes
(60 mm), and prostaglandins were added 24 hrs later. The
medium and drug were changed after 2 days of treatment,
and the number of morphologically differentiated cells were
determined after 3 days of treatment. Cells having
neurites greater than 50 μm in length were considered
morphologically differentiated. Each value represents an
average of 6 samples.

another experiment using mouse melanoma cells in culture
(unpublished observation). PGE_1 did not cause morphological changes; however, PGA_2 markedly inhibited the growth
and induced morphological differentiation in melanoma
cells. Both PGA_2 and PGE_1 enhance the intracellular level
of cAMP in NB cells in culture (Table 2). These data show

Table 2

Effect of Prostaglandins on the Level
of cAMP in Neuroblastoma (NBP$_2$) Cells
Cultured in the Presence of Serum

Treatment	cAMP Level pmole/mg protein
Control	25 ± 4*
Ethanol (0.5%)	27 ± 5
PGE$_1$ (10 µg/ml)	64 ± 6
PGE$_2$ (10 µg/ml)	60 ± 7
PGA$_1$ (5 µg/ml)	89 ± 6
PGA$_2$ (10 µg/ml)	95 ± 7
PGF$_{2\alpha}$ (10 µg/ml)	24 ± 6

*Standard deviation

Cells (50,000) were plated in Lux tissue culture dishes
(60 mm). Fresh growth medium was changed 3 days after
plating. At 4 days after plating fresh growth medium was
added 15 min before the addition of prostaglandins (PG's).
Cells were incubated at 37° in the presence of a PG for 10
min, and then the level of cAMP was determined. Each
value represents an average of 6 samples.

that the receptors of both PGE$_1$ and PGA$_2$ are linked with
adenylate cyclase. It has been reported that the effect
of PGE$_1$ on morphological differentiation (NBP$_2$) was
dependent upon the type of serum (Prasad et $al.$, 1979),
being least in fetal calf serum (Table 3); however, PGA$_2$
was equally effective in fetal calf and in agammaglobulin
newborn calf serum. PGF$_{2\alpha}$ up to a concentration of
10 µg/ml did not affect the growth or morphological
differentiation of NB cells; however, at a higher
concentration (20 µg/ml), it inhibited the growth without
causing morphological differentiation (unpublished
observation).

Table 3

Effect of Serum Type on PG-induced
Morphological Differentiation of
Neuroblastoma (NBP$_2$) cells in Culture

Type of Serum	Treatment	Morphologically Differentiated Cells (% of Total Cells)
Fetal calf	Control	11 ± 2*
Fetal calf	PGE$_1$ (5 µg/ml)	14 ± 2
Fetal calf	PGA$_2$ (5 µg/ml)	88 ± 4
Agammaglobulin newborn calf	Control	2 ± 0
Agammaglobulin newborn calf	PGE$_1$ (10 µg/ml)	41 ± 3
Agammaglobulin newborn calf	PGA$_2$ (10 µg/ml)	91 ± 3

*Standard deviation

PG concentrations higher than those listed were toxic.
Cells (50,000) were plated in Lux tissue culture dishes
(60 mm); and drugs were added 24 hrs after plating. The
medium and drug were changed after 2 days of treatment,
and the number of morphologically differentiated cells
were determined after 3 days of treatment. Cells having
neurites greater than 50 µm in length were considered
morphologically differentiated. Each value represents an
average of 6 samples. A portion of data was obtained from
a previous publication (Prasad et $al.$, 1979).

EFFECT OF PG-INDUCED MORPHOLOGICAL DIFFERENTIATION IN NB
CELLS CULTURED IN HORMONE-SUPPLEMENTED SERUM FREE MEDIUM

It is known that serum contains complex factors, the
quantities of which vary dramatically from one batch of
serum to another, due to the differences in donor age, sex,
nutrition and physiological state (Waymouth, 1977).
Therefore, it is likely that serum factors may modify the
effect of PG's on NB cells. Indeed, the effect of PGE$_1$ on

morphological differentiation was dependent upon the type of serum used in the culture medium (Prasad *et al.*, 1979). Recent advances in tissue culture technology make it possible to grow neural tumor cells in the absence of serum. Bottenstein and Sato (1979) have reported that NB cells proliferate in hormone-supplemented serum free medium (F12 containing 5 μg/ml insulin, 100 μg/ml transferrin, 20 nM progesterone, 30 nM selenium and 100 μM putrescine). We have found that mouse NB cells (NBP$_2$), 4 days after plating, achieved a cell density which represents 70-75% of that found in 10% agammaglobulin newborn calf serum (Prasad, 1981). There was no significant increase in spontaneous morphological differentiation under the above growth conditions. PGE$_1$, PGE$_2$, PGA$_1$ and PGA$_2$ induced morphological differentiation (Table 4) and inhibited growth in NB cells cultured in serum free medium; however, the concentration requirement in serum free medium was 5-10 times less than that needed in serum-supplemented medium. These data show that serum factors modify the effect of PGE$_1$, PGE$_2$, PGA$_1$ and PGA$_2$ on NB cells in a quantitative sense. This was not an unexpected observation (Prasad, 1981). However, the effect of PGF$_{2\alpha}$ on NB cells was unexpected. For example, PGF$_{2\alpha}$, which does not affect the growth or morphology of NB cells cultured in serum-supplemented medium (Prasad, 1972), induced morphological differentiation and inhibited growth in NB cells cultured in serum free medium (Table 4). This suggests that the serum factors could mask the effect of a drug on NB cells. The mechanism of the modification of the effect of PGF$_{2\alpha}$ by serum factors is unknown; however, the following possibilities can be mentioned: (a) serum factors rapidly degrade PGF$_{2\alpha}$; and (b) serum factors prevent the binding of PGF$_{2\alpha}$ with its receptors, probably by forming a complex with it. When PG's were removed after 3 days of treatment, and the morphological differentiation was determined 1 and 2 days after removal; the percent of morphologically differentiated cells did not change at 1 day after removal, but it decreased at 2 days after removal. This is due to the fact that the fully differentiated cells die in culture, and PG-resistant cells and partially affected cells continue to divide and eventually reach confluency.

PROSTAGLANDINS AND BIOCHEMICAL DIFFERENTIATION

Table 4

Effect of Prostaglandins on Morphological
Differentiation of Mouse Neuroblastoma
(NBP2) Cells Cultured in the Presence
of Serum and Serum Free Medium

Treatment	Morphological Differentiation (% of Total Cells)	
	Serum Free	Serum
Control, untreated or treated with ethanol (0.5%)	3 ± 1*	< 1
PGE$_1$ (1 µg/ml)	82 ± 5	7 ± 2
PGE$_2$ (1 µg/ml)	65 ± 6	2 ± 1
PGA$_1$ (0.5 µg/ml)	62 ± 4	2 ± 1
PGA$_2$ (1 µg/ml)	75 ± 6	2 ± 1
PGF$_{2\alpha}$ (10 µg/ml)	51 ± 4	2 ± 1

*Standard deviation

Cells (50,000) were plated in Lux tissue culture dishes
containing medium with serum, and drugs were added 24 hrs
later. For the serum free medium (SFM) group, cells were
washed twice with SFM, and then SFM was added prior to
addition of drugs. The medium and drugs were changed after
2 days of treatment, and the number of morphologically
differentiated cells was determined after 3 days of
treatment. Cells having neurites greater than 50 µm in
length were considered morphologically differentiated.
Each value represents an average of 6 samples.

The effect of PG's on the level of biochemical
differentiation has been studied only in NB cells cultured
in medium with serum (Prasad, 1975; 1980a; 1980b; Prasad and
Sinha, 1978; Prasad and Kumar, 1974; Prasad et al., 1979).
PGE$_1$ increases the activities of tyrosine hydroxylase
(converts tyrosine to dopa), choline acetyltransferase
(converts choline to acetylcholine) and acetylcholinesterase
(degrades acetylcholine) in neuroblastoma cells in culture.

PROSTAGLANDINS AND CYCLIC NUCLEOTIDES

PGE_1 and PGE_2 increase the intracellular level of cAMP in NB cells (NBP$_2$) cultured in serum-supplemented medium (Prasad, 1975; Gilman and Nirenberg, 1971). PGA_1 and PGA_2 also increase the cAMP level in NB cells (Table 2). Thus, the effect of both the PGE series and the PGA series on differentiation is mediated by cAMP. $PGF_{2\alpha}$ does not increase the cAMP level in NB cells (Prasad, 1975). The effect of $PGF_{2\alpha}$ on the cAMP level in NB cells cultured in serum free medium has not been measured; therefore, it remains to be ascertained whether the effect of $PGF_{2\alpha}$ on morphological differentiation is mediated by cAMP. PGE_1-resistant cells exist even in a clonal line. There are some clones (NBE$^-$) which are less sensitive to PGE_1 (Sahu and Prasad, 1975); however, in the presence of an inhibitor of cyclic nucleotide phosphodiesterase (R020-1724), PGE_1 increases the intracellular level of cAMP to the same level, irrespective of their original sensitivity. This suggests that the activity of cAMP phosphodiesterase may be a limiting factor in the accumulation of cAMP after treatment of cells with PGE_1, rather than the alteration in the sensitivity of PGE_1 receptors. It has been reported (Matsuzawa and Nirenberg, 1975) that in a NB x glioma hybrid there are two distinct receptors for PGE_1, one of which is linked with adenylate cyclase, and the other of which is linked with guanylate cyclase. This was shown by the fact that a PGE_1-induced increase in the cGMP level is observed within a minute, and this response returned to a basal level soon after that. However, a PGE_1-induced increase in the cAMP level is also observed within a few minutes, but the response is maintained for a prolonged period of time. The significance of a PGE_1-induced rise in the cGMP level in mediating the expression of morphological differentiation is uncertain, but other cGMP-stimulating agents such as dibutyryl cGMP, or acetylcholine have no effect on morphological differentiation (Prasad, 1975).

An increase in the intracellular level of cAMP in neuroblastoma cells leads to the following changes in the cyclic nucleotide system: (a) increase in sensitivity of adenylate cyclase to dopamine and norepinephrine (Prasad and Gilmer, 1974); (b) increase in cAMP phosphodiesterase activity (Prasad and Kumar, 1973); (c) increase in cAMP binding proteins (Prasad *et al.*, 1976); and (d) increases

and decreases in cAMP-dependent and -independent phosphorylation of cellular proteins (Ehrlich *et al.*, 1977).

SOME OTHER BIOCHEMICAL CHANGES INDUCED BY PG'S

The synthesis of histones and the phosphorylation of
the H_1-histone are considered important biological events
for the proliferation of mammalian cells (Gurley *et al.*,
1972; 1974; Krause and Inasi, 1974). An elevation of the
intracellular level of cyclic AMP in neuroblastoma cells
markedly reduced the synthesis of histones and phosphorylation of the H_1-histone (Lazo *et al.*, 1976). Since the
above changes occur at the time of inhibition of cell
division and DNA synthesis (Prasad and Kumar, 1974), they
may be important biological signals for the dividing
neuroblasts to "turn off" cell division. The occurrences
of histone synthesis and the phosphorylation of the H_1-
histone may be necessary biological events for the
proliferating system (differentiated or embryonic); but
for the embryonic nerve cells, which must eventually stop
cell division, a continuation of these events after a
specified time during development may be indicative of
malignant change.

We have reported that there was no prominent change
in the synthesis or phosphorylation of nonhistone
chromosomal proteins in cyclic AMP-induced "differentiated"
cells (Lazo *et al.*, 1976). Other investigators (Burdman,
1972) have been unable to demonstrate any significant
changes in nonhistone chromosomal proteins during
development of the rat brain. However, we have observed
a small decrease in the synthesis and a small increase in
the phosphorylation of 40,000 dalton peptides in cyclic
AMP-induced "differentiated" cells. The significance of
this change in nonhistone protein is unknown. It has
been suggested (Elgin *et al.*, 1973) that a nonhistone
protein of the 40,000-50,000 dalton range may be involved
in DNA replication in mammalian cells. If this is true,
the changes in the synthesis and phosphorylation of
40,000 dalton peptides in the "differentiated" cells may
be a reflection of the inhibition of DNA synthesis that
occurs in these cells (Prasad and Kumar, 1974).

ACTIVITY OF LACTIC ACID DEHYDROGENASE AND PYRUVATE KINASE

PGE$_1$ also causes a three-fold increase in the activity
of lactic acid dehydrogenase (LDH), a rate limiting enzyme
in anaerobic glycolysis, in mouse neuroblastoma cells in
culture. It is well known that a shift from anaerobic
glycolysis to aerobic glycolysis occurs during differentiation of normal nervous tissue; however, the above
study shows this phenomenon did not occur in cAMP-induced
differentiated NB cells in culture (Prasad, 1980b). The
treatment of NB cells with 1% ethanol depresses pyruvate
kinase (converts phosphophenol pyruvate to pyruvate) by
about 2-fold; however, this decrease in PK activity was
prevented in the presence of PGE$_1$. This suggests that an
elevation of cAMP prevents ethanol-induced depression of
pyruvate kinase activity (Prasad, 1980b).

TUMORIGENICITY OF PGE$_1$-INDUCED DIFFERENTIATED CELLS

The tumorigenicity of differentiated cells is markedly
reduced or completely abolished, depending on the
experimental conditions. For example, in an uncloned cell
line, RO20-1724 (cyclic nucleotide phosphodiesterase
inhibitor), and PGE$_1$ only partially reduced the tumorigenicity of differentiated cells, whereas the combination
of PGE$_1$ with an inhibitor of cyclic nucleotide phosphodiesterase activity completely abolished the tumorigenicity
of "differentiated" cells (Table 5). This is consistent
with the observation that the tumor contains variant
cells, some of which are sensitive to PGE$_1$ but not to
RO20-1724, and vice versa. We have repeated the above
experiment using a clonal line (NBP$_2$). This clone is
relatively more sensitive to RO20-1724 than to PGE$_1$. In
order to suppress the tumorigenicity of differentiated
cells, we found it essential to treat the cells with both
PGE$_1$ and RO20-1724 for four days (Prasad, 1980a). More
recently, Anderson (personal communication) has observed
that the administration of PGE$_1$ (100 µg/mouse,
subcutaneous) and RO20-1724 (200 µg/mouse) in mice with
neuroblastoma caused objective regression of tumors. All
untreated mice with neuroblastoma died within 35 days;
however, all treated animals survived beyond 35 days.
Among survivors, 35% of the animals were free of tumor.
The transformation to ganglioneuroma was noted in treated
groups. This is a very exciting observation, because
this suggests that PGE$_1$ may act as an anticancer agent
in vivo by inhibiting the growth and by inducing

Table 5

Tumorigenicity of Mouse Neuroblastoma Cells
Treated with Prostaglandin (PG) E_1 and an
Inhibitor of Cyclic Nucleotide Phosphodiesterase

Treatment	No. of Animals	Incidence of Tumors (% of Total)
Control, untreated or treated with ethanol (1%)	30	100
PGE (10 μg/ml)	15	20
RO20-1724 (200 μg/ml)	15	50
PGE + RO20-1724	15	0

RO20-1724 = 4-(3-butoxy-4-methoxybenzyl)-2-imidazolidinone,
an inhibitor of cyclic nucleotide phosphodiesterase.
Uncloned neuroblastoma cells were treated with drugs for a
period of 4 days. These differentiated cells were injected
subcutaneously into male A/J mice, and the incidence of
tumors was determined. Data were taken from a previous
publication (Prasad, 1975).

differentiation, a phenomenon which is similar to that
observed *in vitro*.

MODULATION OF THE EFFECT OF PG BY VITAMIN E AND BUTYRIC ACID

It is becoming increasingly evident that vitamins,
especially vitamin A, vitamin C and vitamin E, not only by
themselves act as anticancer agents, but they can modify
the effect of pharmacological agents, including PG's, on
tumor cells in culture. Aquasol vitamin E (Prasad *et al.*,
1980) and butyric acid (Prasad, 1979) enhance the growth
inhibitory effect of PGE_1 on NB cells in a synergistic
fashion. These are preliminary observations and should be
further studied in order to optimize the anticancer
properties of PG's.

CONCLUSION AND COMMENTS

In vitro and some *in vivo* studies suggest that PG's

may act as anticancer agents by inducing growth inhibition and/or differentiation. These studies also suggest that only those tumor cells which have specific receptors for PGE_1 or PGA_2, and which would increase the intracellular level of cAMP after treatment of cells with PG's would respond to PG treatment. It should be kept in mind that the tumor cells may have PG-specific receptors, but these cells cannot raise the cAMP level after treatment with PG's because of a high cAMP phosphodiesterase activity. In such a situation, it would be necessary to combine PG with an inhibitor of cyclic nucleotide phosphodiesterase activity in order to produce an optimal antitumor activity. It is also possible that the extent of antitumor activity of PG's would depend upon the amount of the particular type of PG produced by tumor cells. Suppose a given type of tumor is producing an appreciable amount of the PGE series in the host, these prostaglandins may not be effective for that tumor, because cells may have developed resistance to the PGE series. However, in such conditions, the PGA series may be more effective than the PGE series in inhibiting the growth of tumors. Thus, the extent of the antitumor activity of PG's would depend upon several factors. Recent studies suggest that the PGE series may suppress the host's immune system and promote metastases in certain tumors (Goodwin *et al.*, 1980). It is not known whether the PGA series will inhibit the immune system and promote metastases. Further studies are needed to compare the effect of various types of PG's on tumor growth and differentiation, as well as on the host's immune system. Our *in vitro* studies show that the use of PG as an anticancer agent must be made on a biological rationale. At least we must know the following before selecting a particular type of prostaglandin for studying its anticancer property *in vivo*: (a) presence of receptors specific for a particular PG; (b) the PG must increase cellular cAMP; (c) type of PG produced by tumor; and (d) type of PG which does not interfere with the host's immune system.

Bottenstein JE, Sato GH (1979). Growth of rat neuroblastoma cell line in serum free supplemented medium. Proc Natl Acad Sci USA 76:514.

Burdman JA (1972). The relationship between DNA synthesis and the synthesis of nuclear proteins in rat brain during development. J Neurochem 19:1449.

Ehrlich YH, Brunngraber EG, Sinha PK, Prasad KN (1977).

Specific alterations in phosphorylation of cytosol proteins from differentiated neuroblastoma cells grown in culture. Nature 265:238.

Elgin SCR, Boyd JB, Hood LE, Wray, Wu FC (1973). A prologue to the study of the nonhistone chromosomal protein. Cold Spring Harbor Symposium. Quant Biol 38:821.

Gilman AG, Nirenberg MW (1971). Regulation of adenosine 3',5'-cyclic monophosphate metabolism in cultured neuroblastoma. Nature 234:356.

Goodwin JS, Husby G, Williams Jr RC (1980). Prostaglandin E and cancer growth. Cancer Immunol Immune Ther 8:3.

Gurley L, Walters R, Tobey R (1972). The metabolism of histone fractions. IV Synthesis of histones during the G_1-phase of the mammalian cell life cycle. Arch Biochem Biophys 148:633.

Gurley L, Walters R, Tobey R (1974). Cell cycle specific changes in histone phosphorylation associated with cell proliferation and chromosome condensation. J Cell Biol 60:356.

Hamprecht B, Jaffe BM, Philpott GW (1973). Prostaglandin production by neuroblastoma, glioma and fibroblast cell lines: Stimulation by N^6O^2-dibutyryl adenosine 3':5'-cyclic monophosphate. FEBS Letters 36:193.

Johnson GS, Pastan I (1971). Changes in growth and morphology of fibroblasts by prostaglandins. J. Natl Cancer Inst 47:1357.

Karmali RA (1980). Prostaglandins and cancer. Prostaglandins and Medicine 5:11.

Krause M, Inasi B (1974). Histones from exponential and stationary L-cells. Evidence for metabolic heterogeneity of histone fractions retained after isolation of nuclei. Arch Biochem Biophys 164:179.

Lazo JS, Prasad KN, Ruddon RW (1976). Synthesis and phosphorylation of chromatin associated proteins in cAMP-induced differentiated neuroblastoma cells in culture. Exp Cell Res 100:41.

Matsuzawa H, Nirenberg M (1975). Receptor-mediated shifts in cGMP and cAMP levels in neuroblastoma cells. Proc Natl Acad Sci USA 72:3472.

Naseem SM, Hollander VP (1973). Insulin reversal of growth inhibition of plasma cell tumor by prostaglandin or adenosine 3',5'-monophosphate. Cancer Res 33:2909.

Prasad KN (1972). Morphological differentiation induced by prostaglandins in mouse neuroblastoma cells in culture. Nature (New Biol) 236:49.

Prasad KN (1975). Differentiation of neuroblastoma cells in

culture. Biol Rev 50:129.

Prasad KN (1979). Effect of sodium butyrate in combination with x-irradiation, chemotherapeutic and cyclic AMP stimulating agents on neuroblastoma cells in culture. Experientia 35:906.

Prasad KN (1980a). Role of cyclic nucleotides in the expression of malignancy and differentiated functions in nerve cells. In Fox M (ed): "Advances in Medical Oncology Research and Education, Vol 4," New York: Academic Press, p 57.

Prasad KN (1980b). Control mechanisms of malignancy and differentiation in cultures of nerve cells. In Evans AE (ed): "Advances in Neuroblastoma Research," New York: Raven Press, p 135.

Prasad KN (1981). Expression of cyclic AMP-induced morphological differentiation in neuroblastoma cells. Presented at the International Meeting of Developmental Neurosciences, New York.

Prasad KN, Gilmer KN (1974). Demonstration of dopamine sensitive adenylate cyclase in malignant neuroblastoma cells and change in sensitivity of adenylate cyclase to catecholamines in differentiated cells. Proc Natl Acad Sci USA 71:2525.

Prasad KN, Kumar S (1973). Cyclic 3',5'-AMP phosphodiesterase activity during cyclic AMP-induced differentiation of neuroblastoma cells in culture. Proc Soc Exp Biol Med 142:406.

Prasad KN, Kumar S (1974). Cyclic AMP and the differentiation of neuroblastoma cells. In Clarkson B, Baserga R (eds): "Control of Proliferation in Animal Cells," Cold Spring Harbor: Cold Spring Harbor Laboratory, p 581.

Prasad KN, Sinha PK (1978). Regulation of differentiated functions and malignancy in neuroblastoma cells in culture. In Saunders GF (ed): "Cell Differentiation and Neoplasia," New York: Raven Press, p 111.

Prasad KN, Sinha PK, Sahu SK, Brown JL (1976). Binding of cyclic nucleotides with proteins in malignant and cyclic AMP-induced differentiated neuroblastoma cells in culture. Cancer Res 36:2290.

Prasad KN, Spuhler K, Arnold EB, Vernadakis A (1979). Modification of the response of mouse neuroblastoma cells in culture by serum type. In Vitro 15:807.

Prasad KN, Edwards-Prasad J, Ramanujam S, Sakamoto A (1980). Vitamin E increases the growth inhibitory and differentiating effects of tumor therapeutic agents on neuroblastoma and glioma cells in culture. Proc Soc Exp Biol Med 164:158.

Sahu SK, Prasad KN (1975). Effect of neurotransmitters and

prostaglandin E_1 on cyclic AMP levels in various clones
of neuroblastoma cells in culture. J Neurochem 24:1267.
Santoro MG, Philpott GW, Jaffe BM (1976). Inhibition of
tumor growth *in vivo* and *in vitro* by prostaglandin E.
Nature 263:777.
Santoro MG, Philpott GW, Jaffe BM (1977). Inhibition of
B-16 melanoma growth *in vivo* by a synthetic analog of
prostaglandin E_2. Cancer Res 37:3774.
Santoro MG, Benedetto A, Jaffe BM (1979). Prostaglandin A_1
induces differentiation in Friend erythroleukemia cells.
Prostaglandins 17:719.
Thomas DR, Philpott, Jaffe BM (1974). The relationship
between concentration of prostaglandin E and rates of
cell replication. Exp Cell Res 84:40.
Waymouth C (1977). Nutritional requirements of cells in
culture, with special reference to neural cells. In
Fedroff S, Hertz L (eds): "Cell, Tissue and Organ Culture
in Neurobiology," New York: Academic Press, p 631.
Yang T, Dale JB, Machanoff R (1976). Effects of prostaglandins E_1, E_2, and $F_{2\alpha}$ on the growth of leukemia cells
in culture. J Cell Science 20:199.

Prostaglandins and Cancer: First
International Conference, pages 453-464
© 1982 Alan R. Liss, Inc., 150 Fifth Avenue, New York, NY 10011

NORMAL AND METAPLASTIC SQUAMOUS
DIFFERENTIATION IN DIVERSE ORGANS IN VITRO

Sam Sorof, Frederick V. Schaefer
and R. Philip Custer
Institute for Cancer
Research, Fox Chase Cancer Center
Philadelphia, Pennsylvania 19111

Squamous (epidermoid) metaplasia is a common aberration of cellular development and differentiation in the
epithelia of many organs in animals and humans. The
epithelia normal to the site are replaced by cells that
resemble those of epidermis. The metaplastic cells
differentiate into flattened cells that may cornify into
keratin. The lesion often results in decreased normal
function. The metaplastic cells may regress, remain
benignly squamous, or they or related cells may progress
to epidermoid carcinoma (Anderson, Kissane 1977).

Squamous metaplasia has previously been brought
about in rodents by mechanical injury (McDowell et al.
1979), vitamin A deficiency (Wolbach, Howe 1925), chemical carcinogens (Bern, Levy 1952; Lasnitzski 1955, 1976;
Noyes 1975; Chopra, Wilkoff 1977; Müller-Salmin et al.
1979), and estrogen (Bern 1951, 1963). Retinoids can
prevent and reverse the metaplasia that arises from these
treatments (Lasnitzski 1955, 1976; Müller-Salmin et al.
1979). However, studies on these causal and preventive
factors do not provide a basis for understanding the
underlying physiological mechanism involved in the
induction of this common cellular aberration.

In search of the physiological mediators of this
lesion of abnormal development and differentiation, we
have found that the combination of dibutyryl cyclic AMP,
prostaglandins E_1, E_2 and B_1, and papaverine accelerates
normal epidermization in chick embryo skin, and also

induces metaplastic squamous cell development with keratin production in different organs.

The first system that we have studied is the mouse mammary gland (Schaefer et al. 1980). Fresh whole mammary glands of 3 to 4 weeks old BALB/c mice were cultured for 9 days in serum-free Waymouth MB 752/1 medium containing dibutyryl cyclic AMP at 10^{-4} M, papaverine at 10^{-6} M as a phosphodiesterase inhibitor, and insulin at 5 μg/ml. Under such conditions, 62% of the cultured mammary glands develop a few foci of epidermoid (squamous) metaplasia that occasionally differentiate to form keratin plaques (intensity grade ca. 1, on a scale of 1 to 4) (Table 1). However, when this medium is supplemented with a mixture of prostaglandins E_1, E_2 and B_1, each at 5 μg/ml, there is considerable enhancement of the ability of dibutyryl cyclic AMP to induce squamous metaplasia of the epithelium that lines both the mammary ducts and alveoli of the cultured mammary glands. Virtually all glands, i.e. 99%, then contain numerous foci of metaplasia with large keratin plaques (intensity grade 4). All three prostaglandins are necessary for maximal effect. Prostaglandins $F_{1\alpha}$ and $F_{2\alpha}$ are inactive, and dibutyryl cyclic GMP, 5'-adenylic acid, and sodium butyrate all fail to replace the dibutyryl cyclic AMP (Schaefer et al. 1980).

Figure 1 contains a histological section of mouse mammary gland cultured for 9 days in control medium lacking cyclic adenine nucleotide. Normal appearing ductules and lobuloalveoli are present. That appearance is in contrast to a section from glands cultured in medium containing dibutyryl cyclic AMP, papaverine, and PG E_1, E_2 and B_1, in addition to the insulin. Numerous areas of squamous metaplasia with central keratin plaques are evident. Mitotic figures are present in both the metaplastic and normal cells.

The continued presence of the inducers is necessary for the maintenance of the squamous metaplastic state. Their removal causes involution of the metaplastic cells (Figure 1d). Figure 2 diagrams a full cycle, consisting of abnormal mammary gland development evident as squamous metaplasia, aberrant differentiation marked by keratin production, and involution, i.e. regression.

Table 1. INDUCTION OF SQUAMOUS METAPLASIA IN CULTURED MAMMARY GLANDS

Supplements	No. of Glands	Squamous Metaplasia	
		Frequency %	Av. Stage ± S.E.M.
I+P+A+H	30	0	0
I	30	0	0
DbcAMP + pap + I	31	62	0.6 ± 0.1
DbcAMP + pap + I + PG E_1, E_2, B_1	114	99	4.0 ± 0
PG E_1, E_2, B_1 + I (control)	46	0	0

Whole mammary glands were incubated for 9 days in serum-free medium containing the listed supplements at the following concentrations: dibutyryl cyclic AMP (dbcAMP) at 10^{-4} M; papaverine (pap) at 10^{-6} M; prostaglandins (PG), insulin (I), prolactin (P), aldosterone (A), and hydrocortisone (H), each at 5 μg/ml.
Stages of metaplasia: Scale of 1 to 4.
Reprinted from Schaefer et al. 1980.

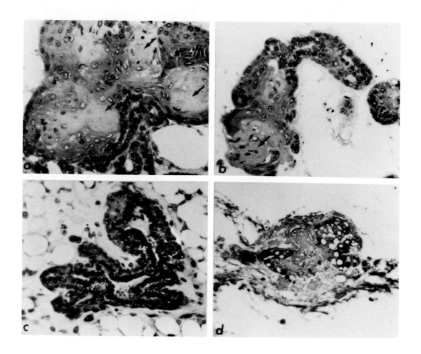

Figure 1. Microscopic details of squamous metaplastic and involuted mouse mammary glands. Arrows indicate parakeratotic and keratotic whorls surrounded by layers of differentiating squamous epithelium. (a) Section of gland that was incubated in metaplasia-inducing medium for 9 days. (b) Same preparation showing a distal ductule and alveolar buds with well developed keratinizing epidermoid metaplasia. (c) Section of a control gland that was incubated in the absence of dibutyryl cyclic AMP and papaverine in medium containing insulin and PG E_1, E_2 and B_1 for 9 days. (d) Section of a gland that was incubated in the metaplasia-inducing medium for 9 days, and then kept in medium supplemented only with

insulin for 15 days. The distal alveolar lobule that was partially metaplastic has involuted, leaving a residue of vacuolated secretory cells and a central plaque of keratin. All squamous cells have disappeared. (Reprinted from Schaefer et al. 1980).

ABNORMAL DEVELOPMENT AND DIFFERENTIATION

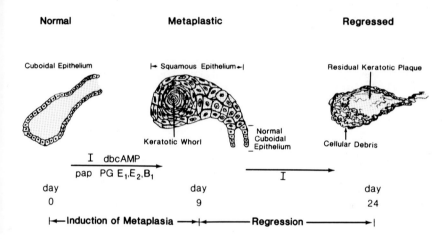

Figure 2. Abnormal development, differentiation and involution (regression) in mouse mammary glands in culture: induction of squamous metaplasia and keratin production by cyclic adenine nucleotide, prostaglandins and papaverine. (Reprinted from Schaefer et al. 1980).

The second organ system of study is the mouse prostate gland (Schaefer et al. in press). Fragments of mouse ventral prostate glands from 2 to 3 months old BALB/c mice can be cultured for a minimum of four weeks in CMRL-1066 medium supplemented with 5% horse serum.

Exposure of the prostate glands to the same combination of dibutyryl cyclic AMP at 10^{-4} M, papaverine, and PG E_1, E_2 and B_1 for 3 weeks induces extensive squamous metaplasia in the acinar epithelium (Figure 3). As with the mammary gland system, the components of the mixture act synergistically.

The addition of a ten-fold higher concentration of dibutyryl cyclic AMP, i.e. at 10^{-3} M, abrogates the requirement for the prostaglandins and papaverine in the induction of extensive squamous metaplasia in the cultured prostate glandular epithelium. At three weeks, there is near-maximal production of squamous metaplasia and keratin.

The production of the squamous metaplasia in the prostate glands specifically requires the cyclic adenine nucleotide. Sodium butyrate, dibutyryl cyclic GMP, and 5'-adenylic acid, all at the equivalent concentrations, do not replace the dibutyryl cyclic AMP.

The induction of squamous metaplasia in the cultured mouse prostate gland first becomes morphological evident as a hyperplasia of pre-existing epithelium, and then as focal proliferation of squamous cells within the annular structure that outlines the acini of the prostate gland. Keratin production in the cultured prostate gland is sparse.

Cyclic adenine nucleotide and specific prostaglandins thus synergistically bring about an extensive squamous metaplasia in mouse prostate gland in culture. This finding permits the possibility that these substances may be the physiological inducers of the analogous spontaneous lesion in prostate gland in animals and man.

The third system of study is human breast tissue (Schaefer FV, Custer RP, Sorof S, unpublished data). Fragments of human non-malignant breast biopsy tissue can be cultured for 11 days in serum-free Waymouth MB 752/1 medium under the same conditions as with the mouse mammary glands. The eight women donors studied to date were of ages ranging from 21 to 70 years.

Exposure of the human breast tissue to the same combination of dibutyryl cyclic AMP at 10^{-4} M,

ABNORMAL DEVELOPMENT AND DIFFERENTIATION
IN CULTURED MOUSE PROSTATE GLAND

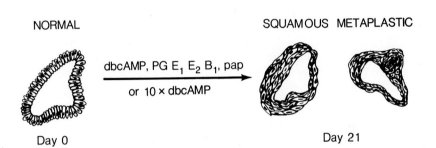

NORMAL   SQUAMOUS METAPLASTIC

dbcAMP, PG E_1 E_2 B_1, pap

or 10 × dbcAMP

Day 0   Day 21

Figure 3. Induction of squamous metaplasia in mouse prostate gland by cyclic adenine nucleotide, prostaglandins and papaverine in culture.

prostaglandins E_1, E_2 and B_1, and papaverine for 11 days induces a considerable amount of squamous metaplasia and a low level of keratin production. The use of dibutyryl cyclic AMP alone, without prostaglandins and papaverine, is under study. As with the mouse mammary and prostate glands, 5'-adenylic acid and dibutyryl cyclic GMP are unable to induce squamous metaplasia.

The fourth system of study is the skin of chick embryo (Schaefer et al. in press). The skin from the legs of the 13 day-old chick embryo can be cultured in BGJ_b medium containing 5% fetal bovine serum for at least 9 days. The cultured skin can develop and differentiate normally and fully in this unsupplemented control medium. At day 0, the skin is 6 to 7 cells thick, consisting of a one-cell layer of columnar basal cells, above which are 5 to 6 layers of polyhedral cells. At day 5, the control cultured skin is fully differentiated, with stratified cells that are overlaid by a condensed stratum corneum.

Five stages of skin development are discernible. The first four stages involve proliferation and development of the columnar basal cells to squamous cell morphology with early parakeratin production. The fifth stage involves the condensation of loose keratin to a cornified layer.

Exposure of the cultured skin to the same mixture of dibutyryl cyclic AMP at 10^{-4} M, prostaglandins E_1, E_2 and B_1, and papaverine significantly accelerates the rate of the first four stages of the normal development of the basal cells to squamous morphology, with production of parakeratin. At day 3, the development of the skin is accelerated by 1.5 days beyond that of the control cultures. The fifth stage of skin maturation, involving the condensation of the keratin, is unaffected.

The individual enhancing supplements act synergistically to accelerate the skin development. Dibutyryl cyclic AMP alone, or the mixture of only the three prostaglandins, or papaverine, or dibutyryl cyclic GMP, or the combination of dibutyryl cyclic GMP, papaverine and prostaglandins E_1, E_2 and B_1, is each weakly to moderately stimulatory over the normal activity of control skin. The maximum enhancement is achieved by the combination of dibutyryl cyclic AMP, papaverine and prostaglandins E_1, E_2 and B_1. Sodium butyrate, 5'-adenylic acid, and insulin produce insignificant effects.

We have also searched for agents that can prevent the squamous metaplasias. The production of metaplasia in the cultured mammary glands of mice is not prevented by the retinoid, retinylidene dimedone, up to 10^{-5} M concentration (Schaefer et al. 1980). However, the presence of the phorbol ester, phorbol-12,13-didecanoate, for the entire 9-day culture period totally prevents the induction of squamous metaplasia in the cultured mouse mammary glands. The inhibition is complete at 10^{-6} M phorbol ester (Table 2).

In contrast, the squamous metaplasia in cultured mouse prostate gland is prevented by the above cited retinoid (Schaefer FV, Custer RP, Sorof S, unpublished data). Retinoids have previously been found to prevent squamous metaplasia produced in rodent prostate glands by carcinogen, estrogen, or their combination (Lasnitzki

Table 2. PREVENTION OF SQUAMOUS METAPLASIA IN MOUSE MAMMARY GLANDS BY PHORBOL ESTER

Supplements	No. of Cultures	Stage of Metaplasia Av. $\pm$ S.E.M.
Insulin	30	0
DbcAMP, 10^{-4} M + pap + PG E_1, E_2, B_1 + insulin	26	3.7 ± 0.1
Same + phorbol didecanoate, 10^{-5} M	30	0.1 ± 0.1
Same + phorbol didecanoate, 10^{-6} M	28	0.3 ± 0.1
Same + phorbol didecanoate, 10^{-8} M	10	2.1 ± 0.3

Mouse mammary glands of BALB/c mice were cultured in serum-free Waymouth MB 752/1 medium for 9 days. Supplements: PG E_1, E_2, B_1 and insulin, each 5 µg/ml; papaverine (pap) 10^{-6} M.

Stages of metaplasia: Scale of 1 to 4.

1955, 1963, 1976; Müller-Salamin et al. 1979), and also
to prevent and even to reverse the metaplasia caused by
vitamin A deficiency and chemical carcinogens in other
organ systems (Wolbach, Howe 1925; Saffioti et al. 1967;
Grubbs et al. 1977; Tchao 1980). The mechanisms of these
actions by retinoid are unknown.

In addition, phorbol-12,13-didecanoate totally
prevents the squamous metaplasia induced in the cultured
mouse prostate glands (Schaefer FV, Custer RP, Sorof S,
unpublished data). The findings that retinoid and
phorbol ester can each prevent the onset of the metaplasia indicate that metaplastic squamous differentiation
can be blocked at at least two levels in its induction
process.

Cyclic adenine nucleotide appears to be the primary
mediator in the induction of the squamous metaplasias in
the cultured mammary and prostate glands, as well as in
the acceleration of normal development in cultured skin.
The cyclic adenine nucleotide, the specific prostaglandins, and papaverine are known to elevate the level
of intracellular cyclic AMP in other systems. Such
elevation in the cultured organs may result from three
synergistic actions: firstly by the entry of exogenous
dibutyryl cyclic AMP, secondly by the increased synthesis
of the cyclic nucleotide due to the stimulation of adenyl
cyclase by the prostaglandins, and thirdly by the inhibition by papaverine of the degradation of the nucleotide
by phosphodiesterase.

In summary, the findings in four organ culture
systems indicate that cyclic adenine nucleotide, in concert with the specific prostaglandins, may be general
physiological inducers of normal and metaplastic squamous
cell development in the epithelia of diverse organs.

These studies were supported in part by NIH grants
CA-30036, CA-21522, CA-05945, CA-06927, and RR-05539, and
appropriations from the Commonwealth of Pennsylvania.

Anderson WAD, Kissane JM (1977). Inflamation and healing.
    In "Pathology," Vol 1, 7th edn, St. Louis: Mosby, p 84.
Bern HA (1951). Estrogen and alkaline phosphatase activ-
    ity in the genital tract of the male mouse.
    Endocrinology 48:25.

Bern HA, Levy RS (1952). The effects of castration, estrogen administration, and methylcholanthrene carcinogenesis on phosphatase activities in the genital tract of male rats, guinea pigs, and rabbits. Am J Anat 90:131.

Bern HA (1963). Epithelial metaplasia in the prostate and other genital structures of male animals. In Vollmer EP, Kauffmann G (eds): "The Biology of Prostate and Related Tissues," National Cancer Institute Monograph 12, Washington, DC: US Gov, p 43.

Chopra DP, Wilkoff LJ (1977). Induction of hyperplasia and anaplasia by carcinogens in organ cultures of mouse prostate. In Vitro 13:260.

Grubbs CJ, Moon RC, Squire RA, Farrow GM, Stinson SF, Goodman DG, Brown CC, Sporn MB (1977). 13-cis-Retinoic acid: inhibition by bladder carcinogenesis induced in rats by N-butyl-N-(4-hydroxybutyl)nitrosamine. Science 198:743.

Lasnitzki I (1955). The influence of a hypervitaminosis on the effect of 20-methylcholanthrene on mouse prostate glands grown in vitro. Br J Cancer 9:434.

Lasnitzki I (1963). Growth pattern of the mouse prostate in organ culture and its response to sex hormones, vitamin A and 3-methylcholanthrene. In Vollmer EP, Kauffmann G (eds): "The Biology of the Prostate and Related Tissues," National Cancer Institute Monograph 12, Washington, DC: US Gov, p 381.

Lasnitzki I (1976). Reversal of methylcholanthrene-induced changes in mouse prostates in vitro by retinoic acid and its analogues. Br J Cancer 34:239.

McDowell EM, Beccì PJ, Schurch W, Trump BF (1979). Epidermoid metaplasia of hamster tracheal epithelium during regeneration following mechanical injury. J Natn Cancer Inst 62:995.

Müller-Salamin L, Matter A, Lasnitzki I (1979). Interaction of retinoic acid and 3-methylcholanthrene on the fine structure of mouse prostate epithelium in vitro. J Natn Cancer Inst 63:485.

Noyes WF (1975). Effect of 3-methylcholanthrene (NCS-21970) on human prostate in organ culture. Cancer Chemotherapy Reports 59:67.

Saffiotti U, Montesano R, Sellakumar AR, Borg SA (1967). Inhibition by vitamin A of the induction of tracheobronchial squamous metaplasia and squamous cell tumors. Cancer 20:357.

Schaefer FV, Custer RP, Sorof S (1980). Induction of abnormal development and differentiation in cultured mammary glands by cyclic adenine nucleotide and prostaglandins. Nature 286:807.

Schaefer FV, Custer RP, Sorof S Differentiation, in press.

Tchao R (1980). Keratinization and the effect of vitamin A in aggregates of a squamous carcinoma cell line NBT II. In Vitro 16:407.

Wolbach SB, Howe PR (1925). Tissue changes following deprivation of fat-soluble A vitamin. J Exp Med 42:753.

**Prostaglandins and Cancer: First
International Conference, pages 465–480
© 1982 Alan R. Liss, Inc., 150 Fifth Avenue, New York, NY 10011**

PROSTAGLANDINS INDUCE DIFFERENTIATION AND REDUCE THE
NEOPLASTIC POTENTIAL OF A RAT MAMMARY TUMOUR STEM CELL
LINE

P. S. Rudland
and
M. J. Warburton

Ludwig Institute for Cancer Research
(London Branch), Royal Marsden Hospital,
Sutton, Surrey, SM2 5PX, U.K.

INTRODUCTION

The mammary gland of mature rats consists of a
branching system of ducts which terminate in clusters of
alveoli that secrete lipid and milk-specific proteins,
notably caseins, during lactation. Three main types of
mammary epithelial cell are distinguishable; those lining
the alveoli, those lining the ducts and thirdly the myo-
epithelial cells which form a layer around both ducts and
alveoli (Kon & Cowie, 1961). These three cell types can
also be recognised in carcinogen-induced tumours (Young &
Hallowes, 1973). The development of the normal glandular
structures and the growth of the carcinogen-induced tumours
is controlled in part by the circulating levels of a series
of hormones, including prolactin, estrogens, glucocorticoids
and insulin (Lyons et al, 1958; Nandi, 1958; Huggins et al,
1959). We have isolated a clonal cuboidal epithelial cell
line, Rama 25, from a dimethylbenz(a)anthracene (DMBA)-
induced rat mammary adenocarcinoma (Bennett et al, 1978).
This cell line appears to be capable of differentiating into
either droplet and doming cultures (alveolar-like cells) or
into elongated (myoepithelial-like) cells (Rudland et al,
1979; Rudland et al., 1980a). The former process can be
accelerated by a combination of the agents which induce
differentiation in Friend erythroleukemic cells (Friend et al.,
1971; Reuben et al., 1976) including dimethyl sulphoxide
(DMSO) and the hormones prolactin, hydrocortisone and
insulin. Agents which accelerate the latter step are as
yet unknown. The original cell line Rama 25 readily forms

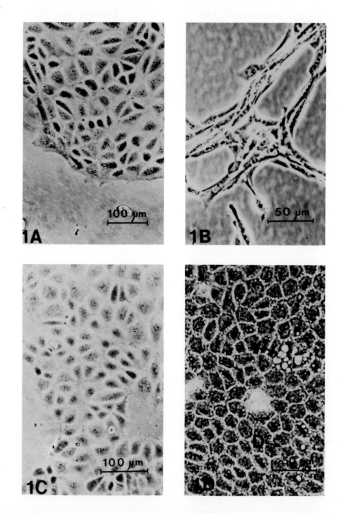

FIG. 1. <u>Morphology of Cells in Culture</u>. Living cells were
photographed with phase contrast optics. A. growing colony
of Rama 25 cuboidal cells. B. Criss-cross elongated cells
cloned from Rama 29, Rama 521. C. DMSO-resistant clone of
Rama 25, Rama 259. D. Confluent culture of Rama 25
treated for 2 days with DMSO and hormones showing droplet
cells (D) and vacuolated cells (V).

tumours in immunodeprived nude (nu-nu) mice whereas an
elongated myoepithelial-like cell line Rama 29 derived from
Rama 25 fails to form tumours under the same experimental

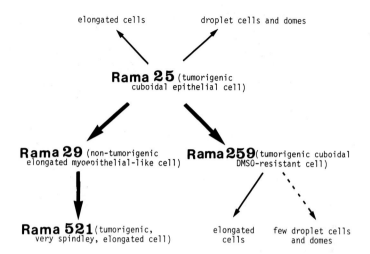

elongated cells   droplet cells and domes

Rama 25 (tumorigenic cuboidal epithelial cell)

Rama 29 (non-tumorigenic elongated myoepithelial-like cell)   **Rama 259** (tumorigenic cuboidal DMSO-resistant cell)

Rama 521 (tumorigenic, very spindley, elongated cell)   elongated cells   few droplet cells and domes

FIG. 2. Summary of the Isolation of Different Cell Lines and their Cellular Interconversions. Cell lines isolated from Rama 25 are shown by the thick arrows, the cellular interconversions of the individual cell lines are represented by the thin arrows. The hatched arrow indicates that although droplet cells and domes can be formed by Rama 259 cells this process is not accelerated with DMSO, unlike Rama 25.

conditions (Bennett et al., 1978; Rudland, et al., 1980b). Since the prostaglandins (PG's) can exert hormone-like actions (Pharriss et al., 1972; Lee, 1974) we have investigated the ability of the PG's to induce differentiation of our stem cell line to alveolar-like cells in culture and relate this to the concomitant change in its neoplastic potential when injected into nude mice.

ISOLATION OF TUMORIGENIC CELL VARIANTS FROM RAMA 25 AND RAMA 29

The original stem cell line from the DMBA-induced tumour, Rama 25 (Fig. la) yielded elongated (myoepithelial-like) cells at low frequency in culture (Bennett et al., 1978). Variant cells from one such elongated cell line, Rama 29, were isolated by repeatedly passaging Rama 29 at high densities and picking ring clones of the spindley, criss-cross cells which could be distinguished from the

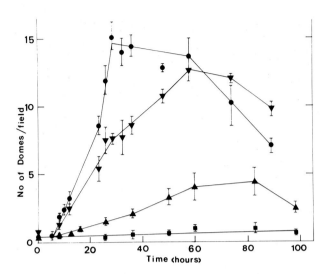

FIG. 3   Kinetics of "doming" after addition of PGE$_1$.   Rama 25 cultures were plated at 10^5 cells per 5 cms. petri dish and grown to confluency in Dulbecco's modified Eagles medium (DEM), 10% fetal calf serum (FCS), 50 ng/ml insulin (I), 50 ng/ml hydrocortisone (HC). The medium was changed on day 5 to Hams F12, 10% FCS, 50 ng/ml I, 50 ng/ml HC, 500 ng/ml prolactin (Pr) and an extra 4.2 mg/ml NaHCO$_3$. On day 7 the medium was removed and replaced with fresh Hams F12 containing HC, extra NaHCO$_3$, 500 ng/ml I, 5 μg/ml Pr, 2.7 ng/ml estradiol (E) and in addition 500 ng/ml (——), 200 ng/ml (——), 50 ng/ml (——) PGE$_1$. Fresh medium without PGE$_1$, but with hormones was also added (——). The number of "domes" per 14 mm^2 field was followed with time. Results are the average of 2 dishes +SEM, 4 microscopic fields were counted per culture dish.

closely aligned cells of the normal cultures. These variant cells were further cloned by picking single cells, and one such line was termed Rama 521 (Fig. 1b). Rama 25 cultures gave rise to variant cuboidal cells when the growth medium contained 1.8% DMSO. These variants were cloned by picking single cells, and one such cuboidal epithelial cell line was termed Rama 259 (Fig. 1c). Rama 259 cells would grow in medium without DMSO and not only formed elongated cells in sparse cultures but also formed droplet cells and domes in confluent cultures at a similar low rate to the parental

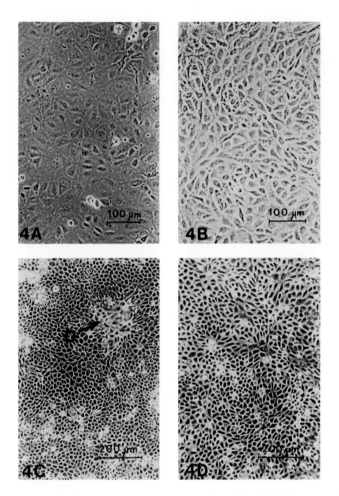

FIG. 4. Morphology of Cells treated with PGE_1. Living cells were photographed with phase contrast optics:A. Confluent culture of cuboidal Rama 25 cells treated with hormones but no PGE_1 for 2 days. B. Confluent culture of criss-cross, elongated Rama 521 cells treated with hormones and 0.5 μg/ml PGE_1 for 2 days. C. Confluent culture of Rama 25 cells treated for 2 days with hormones and PGE_1 showing droplet cells and a dome (D). D. Confluent culture of Rama 259 cells treated for 2 days with hormones and PGE_1.

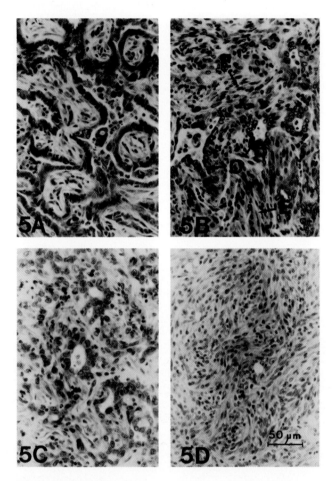

FIG.5. Histology of Tumours Formed in Nude Mice.
Haematoxylin and eosin stained histological sections from
tumours formed in 6 weeks in nude (nu-nu) mice are shown.
These tumours were caused by the injection of 2×10^6 cells
of confluent cultures of the following: A and B. Rama 25.
C. Rama 259. D. Rama 521. Most tumours from Rama 25 and
Rama 259 were of mixed cell types as in B comprising both
circular arrays of cuboidal cells (C) and elongated cells
(E).

cell line, Rama 25. However, 1.8% DMSO did not accelerate
the formation of droplet cells and domes in confluent
cultures as observed with confluent cultures of Rama 25

TABLE I. Effect of PG's and Serum on Rama 25 Cells

Additions	No 'domes' per field $\pm$SEM	Casein secreted (ng) $\pm$SEM	Labelled nuclei(%) $\pm$SEM
None	7+1	0.4 + 0.5	51+4
PGE_1	32+1	16.4 + 0.9	13+1
PGE_2	16+2	1.2 + 0.2	28+6
$PGF_{2\alpha}$	18+1	0.1 + 0.0	32+5
DMSO	34+1	23.2 + 0.1	14+5
PGE_1 -HC	17+2	0.0 + 0.4	-
PGE_1 - Pr	30+2	0.0 + 0.4	-
PGE_1 - E	31+1	0.0 + 0.4	-
PGE_1 - I	16+1	0.4 + 0.4	-
PGE_1 - HC-I-Pr	12+1	0.0 + 0.4	-
PGE_1 - S	16+1	0.4 + 0.6	-

Abbreviations: HC, hydrocortisone; Pr, prolactin;
E, estradiol, I, insulin; S, serum. Rama 25 cultures were
plated and grown initially as described in Fig. 3. However,
on day 4 the medium was changed to DEM, 10% FCS, 50 ng/ml I,
50 ng/ml HC, 500 ng/ml Pr, 2.7 ng/ml E and then on day 7
to Hams Fl2, 10% FCS, 50 ng/ml HC, 500 ng/ml I, 5 μg/ml
Pr, 2.7 ng/ml E, 4.2 mg/ml extra $NaHCO_3$. Finally on day 9
medium was again changed to that of day 7 omitting (-)
different agents and adding 500 ng/ml PGE_1, PGE_2, $PGF_{2\alpha}$
or 1.8% DMSO as indicated. The number of domes per $14mm^2$
field, the total immunoreactive casein (ng) in the medium
and the fraction (%) of cells in parallel cultures with
(^3H) thymidine radioactively labelled nuclei in 48 hours
were recorded. All results are the average of 2 dishes;
for 'doming' 4 fields per dish; for casein duplicate
samples per dish; and for (^3H) thymidine labelling 4 fields
per dish were recorded. Cellular protein content was approx.
constant at 0.5 mg in all cultures and thymidine labelling
was performed with 3 μCi/ml (^3H) thymidine at 1 μM.
(Rudland and Jimenez de Asua, 1979).

(Fig. 1d). Rama 521 and 259 cell lines formed tumours in
nu-nu mice at a high frequency, comparable to that observed
with the original parental line Rama 25. (Table 4). The
isolation and properties of the variant cell lines are
summarised diagramatically in Fig. 2.

TABLE 2. Effect of PGE$_1$ on Rama 25 cells in Serum-Free Medium

Additions		Time (hrs)		No domes/ field $\pm$SEM	Labelled nuclei (%) $\pm$SEM
None	⎫		⎧	0 $\pm$ 0	5 $\pm$ 1
PGE$_1$	⎬ 5	⎨	1 $\pm$ 0	5 $\pm$ 1
DMSO	⎭		⎩	0 $\pm$ 0	5 $\pm$ 1
None	⎫		⎧	1 $\pm$ 1	25 $\pm$ 2
PGE$_1$	⎬ 24	⎨	12 $\pm$ 2	18 $\pm$ 4
DMSO	⎭		⎩	14 $\pm$ 2	10 $\pm$ 3
None	⎫		⎧	1 $\pm$ 1	44 $\pm$ 2
PGE$_1$	⎬ 48	⎨	13 $\pm$ 2	16 $\pm$ 2
DMSO	⎭		⎩	17 $\pm$ 1	13 $\pm$ 2

Rama 25 cultures were grown as described in Table 1 except that on day 7 the cultures were washed twice with isotonic phosphate buffered saline (PBS) and then Hams F12 plus 4.2 mg/ml NaHCO$_3$ were added back. Finally on day 9 Hams F12 with extra NaHCO$_3$ and the hormones HC, I, Pr, E as before were added (None) together with either 500 ng/ml PGE$_1$ or 1.8% DMSO. The number of domes/14 mm^2 microscopic field and the fraction (%) of cells with (^{3}H) thymidine radioactively labelled nuclei were recorded after 5, 24 and 48 hours.

PG's ACCELERATE THE DIFFERENTIATION OF STEM CELLS IN CULTURE

The differentiation of confluent cultures of Rama 25 to alveolar-like cells can be followed by the appearance of two markers, the ability of the cultures to form hemispherical blisters or domes in the cell monolayer (McGrath, 1975) and the appearance of immunoreactive casein-like material in the tissue culture medium (Warburton et al., 1979). Domes may be produced as in the MDCK kidney epithelial cell line (Abaza et al., 1974) by increased activity of the Na$^+$/K$^+$ ATPase pumping water under and forcing up the cell monolayer by hydrostatic pressure (Rudland et al., 1980a). The material precipitated by the anti-casein serum has the same molecular weight as authentic β-casein (42,000), and a similar chromatographic 'fingerprint' of tryptic peptides (Warburton et al., in prep.). Treatment of Rama 25 with PGE$_1$ also resulted in increases in both rates of formation of domes and appearance of immunoreactive casein-like

TABLE 3. Effect of PG's on Variant Cell Lines

Cell Line	Additions	No domes/ Field+SEM	Casein secreted (ng) $\pm$ SEM	Labelled nuclei(%) $\pm$ SEM
Rama 259	None	0+0	0.0 $\pm$ 0.02	53+4
	PGE_1	0+0	0.0 $\pm$ 0.02	58+6
	$PGF_{2\alpha}$	0+0	0.0 $\pm$ 0.01	52+5
	DMSO	0+0	0.0 $\pm$ 0.01	44+5
Rama 521	None	0+0	0.0 $\pm$ 0.01	33+2
	PGE_1	0+0	0.0 $\pm$ 0.01	32+4
	$PGF_{2\alpha}$	0+0	0.0 $\pm$ 0.04	29+3
	DMSO	0+0	0.0 $\pm$ 0.01	20+1

Rama 259 and 521 cultures were seeded and grown exactly as
described in Table 1. On day 9 500 ng/ml PGE_1, PG $F_{2\alpha}$, or
1.8% DMSO were added to the F12 medium containing serum and
the hormones HC, I, Pr and E and after 48 hours the number
of domes/14 mm^2 field, the amount of casein secreted/dish
and the fraction of cells with (^3H) thymidine labelled
nuclei in parallel cultures were recorded exactly as
previously.

material. Increasing concentrations of PGE_1 (50-500 ng/ml)
in the presence of fresh 10% serum and the hormones, prolactin, hydrocortisone,estradiol, and insulin increased the
rate of formation of domes (Fig. 3). The kinetics of
producing   domes by PGE_1 showed two distinct phases.
Initially there was a lag phase of 6-8 hours, the duration
of which was independent of the concentration of PGE_1 added.
Thereafter there was an abrupt change to a new rate of
formation of domes, the new rate was dependent on the concentration of PGE_1 upto a maximum of 500 ng/ml (Fig. 3).
Above this concentration the rate was relatively independent
of the concentration of PGE_1 upto 5 μg/ml. At higher concentrations the rate of doming decreased with increasing
concentrations of PGE_1 (not shown). After about 2 days
exposure to the higher concentrations of PGE_1 (500 ng/ml
and above) the numbers of domes/field also started to
decline (Fig. 3).

The kinetics of the formation of domes with PGE_1 were
similar to those obtained previously with varying concentrations of DMSO, even to the duration of the 'lag' phase
(Rudland et al., 1980a). However, the maximum effect with

TABLE 4. Effect of PG's on Formation of Tumours in Nude Mice

Cell line injected	Treatment _in vitro_	Animals surviving	Tumour Incidence (%)
Rama 25	None	20	95%
	Hormones	20	80%
	PGE_1 + hormones	18	17%
	PGE_2 + hormones	19	42%
	$PGF_{2\alpha}$ + hormones	19	47%
	$DMSO$ + hormones	19	11%
Rama 259	None	20	90%
	PGE_1 + hormones	19	89%
Rama 521	None	19	84%
	PGE_1 + hormones	20	90%

All cultured cells were grown to confluency for 7 days as described in Table 1 except that 600 ml Falcon flasks were used to obtain the larger cultures. The medium was then changed to Hams F12, 10% FCS, 500 ng/ml I, 50 ng/ml HC, 4.2 mg/ml $NaHCO_3$ with no extra additions (none); 5 μg/ml Pr, 2.7 ng/ml E (hormones); and 0.5 μg/ml PG's or 1.8% DMSO as indicated. After 48 hours the medium was removed, the cell monolayer washed twice with PBS; incubated for 30 minutes at $37^{O}C$ with 0.5 mM EDTA in PBS and then removed by digestion with trypsin/EDTA solutions at $37^{O}C$ (Bennett et al., 1978). Cells were collected by centrifugation and inoculated at 2×10^6 in PBS through the skin into the right inguinal mammary gland of 4 to 8 week old female nu-nu mice (ICR, Fulham Road, London). Animals were killed after 6 weeks and tumours removed, sized, and fixed for histological examination.

the optimum concentration of DMSO (1.8%) was observed after 24 rather than 48 hours, and was roughly double (30 domes/field) than with the optimum concentration of PGE_1 (15 domes/field). However, altering the conditions of culture prior to adding PGE_1 or DMSO could alter the relative maximum effects on doming without altering the qualitative nature of the kinetic response. Thus if the cultures were maintained at confluency for a further 2 days with fresh serum and hormones before adding the inducers, then the basal and PGE_1 stimulated numbers of domes per microscopic field were both increased but those with DMSO remained unchanged. The effect with 500 ng/ml PGE_1 was then close to that observed with 1.8% DMSO after 48 hours (Table 1). PGE_2 and $PGF_{2\alpha}$ were both about half as effective as PGE_1 in stimulating doming

when added to either 7 day (not shown) or 9 day cultures
of Rama 25 (Table 1). Four hormones, prolactin, hydrocortisone, insulin, and estradiol, together with serum and
PGE_1 were required to yield maximum rates of formation of
domes and of production of immunoreactive casein (Table 1).
However the hormonal effects on the two parameters of
differentiation were different. Hydrocortisone and serum
were required for maximum production of domes, while all 4
hormones and serum were required for maximum production of
immunoreactive casein (Table 1). There was little effect
on doming when insulin was omitted for 24 hours (not shown)
but after 48 hours the numbers of domes/field were reduced
(Table 1). The fact that PGE_1 or DMSO and the hormones
could still stimulate the rate of formation of domes in the
absence of serum, albeit at about a 50% reduced rate, was
confirmed when they were added to confluent cultures of
Rama 25 which had previously been washed twice and incubated
with serum-free and hormone-free medium for 2 days (Table 2).
There was little production of casein under these conditions.
(not shown). The stimulatory effects of PGE_1 and $PGF_{2\alpha}$ on
the rate of production of both markers of differentiation,
was specific for the Rama 25 cell line, no increases were
observed in confluent cultures of Rama 29 (not shown) and
the variant cell lines, Rama 521 and Rama 259 (Table 3 and
Fig. 4).

PG's REDUCE DNA SYNTHETIC RATES ON DIFFERENTIATION OF STEM
CELLS

The addition of fresh medium, 10% fetal calf serum and
the hormones, prolactin, hydrocortisone, and insulin to confluent cultures of Rama 25 causes acceleration of the rate of
DNA synthesis. The rate remains constant for 6-8 hours and
reaches a maximum after 16 to 18 hours. (Rudland et al,
1980a). When PGE_1 was added with serum and hormones the
enhanced rate of cellular entry into S phase due to serum
and hormones alone was reduced after both 24 (not shown) and
48 hours (Table 1). The optimum concentration (0.5 μg/ml)
required to reduce the rate of cellular entry into S phase
was the same as that for promoting the increase in rate of
doming measured in parallel cultures   (not shown). This
reduction was about the same as that caused by 1.8% DMSO.
PGE_2 and $PGF_{2\alpha}$ at 0.5 μg/ml were about half as effective
as PGE_1, and this difference paralleled their relative
effects on inducing increased rates of doming. PGE_1 and DMSO
could also inhibit rates of cellular entry into S phase in

confluent cultures of Rama 25 previously maintained for two
days in serum and hormone-free medium. There was very little
effect for the first 5 hours but thereafter the rate was
greatly reduced (Table 2). PGE_1, $PGF_{2\alpha}$, and DMSO failed to
reduce the rates of cellular entry into S phase in the
variant cell lines Rama 259 and Rama 521. (Table 3).

PG's REDUCE THE INCIDENCE OF TUMOURS FORMED BY STEM CELLS
IN NUDE MICE

     Confluent cultures of Rama 25 were incubated with
fresh medium, prolactin, hydrocortisone, insulin, estradiol
and 500 ng/ml PGE_1 under the same conditions that produce
droplet and doming cultures and were then tested for neoplastic potential by inserting them into nude mice. The number
of tumours formed in six weeks was only 18% of those obtained
with cells incubated without PGE_1, and this reduction was
approximately the same as that with DMSO (Table 4). This
fractional decrease was maintained for animals kept upto
3 months, there was no indication that the incidence of
tumours increased with time beyond six weeks. PGE_2 and $PGF_{2\alpha}$
were only about 60% as effective as PGE_1 in reducing the
incidence of tumours at the same concentration. The optimum
concentration of PGE_1 for reducing the incidence of tumours
was 500 ng/ml, the same as that for inducing doming and
reducing DNA synthetic rates   (not shown). The effects of
PGE_1 and DMSO were not simply due to killing the confluent
cultures of Rama 25 cells since their effects could be
reversed. Thus the medium containing PGE_1 and DMSO was
removed, the cell monolayers were washed with fresh medium,
serum, and hormones and then incubated in this medium for
a further 2 days. When the resultant cells were injected
into nude mice 85% to 90% of the mice produced tumours in
6 weeks (not shown).

     The reduction in the incidence of tumours with PGE_1 was
specific for those cells in which PGE_1 stimulated both the
rate of alveolar-like cell production and in which it caused
a reduction in DNA synthetic rates. Thus Rama 259 and
Rama 521 when injected at the same dose as Rama 25 cells
formed tumours in nude mice just as readily as Rama 25 itself
(Table 4). PGE_1 at 500 ng/ml failed to reduce the incidence
of tumours caused by either variant cell line (Table 4).
The tumours formed from these three lines, however, differed
pathologically. Rama 25 and Rama 259 formed histologically
identical tumours which were predominantly composed of two
structures: circular rings of cells typical of adenocarcinoma

and spindle cell regions. Rama 521 formed tumours containing only spindle cells (Fig. 5) (Rudland et al., in prep.). The few tumours which arose from Rama 25 and those from Rama 259 and Rama 521 cultures which had all been treated with PGE_1 were identical to those tumours obtained with untreated cultures. Thus PGE_1 failed to cause either a major change in the histology of tumours induced by the PGE_1-unresponsive cell lines (Rama 259, Rama 521) or in the few tumours induced by the PGE_1-responsive cell line (Rama 25).

DISCUSSION

The mechanism of action of the PG's on Rama 25 stem cells is unclear. Two extremes may be considered; either the PG's behave rather non-specifically acting as lipophilic agents by dissolving to varying degrees in the plasma membrane (Clark & Ryan, 1980) or they act through specific receptors (Kuehl & Humes, 1972). Either mechanism then triggers changes in plasma membrane enzyme systems, ion fluxes, cyclic nucleotide concentrations etc. as reported for $PGF_{2\alpha}$ and PGE_1 on cultured 3T3 cells (Rudland & Jimenez de Asúa, 1979). The fact that diverse agents including DMSO, in addition to the PG's, accelerate the rate of differentiation of Rama 25 stem cells without affecting the rate of the DMSO-resistant stem cell line, Rama 259, may favour the non-specific mechanism. However, since the effects of the PG's can be achieved with near physiological concentrations (Lee, 1974; Samuelson, 1978), that in freshly confluent cultures DMSO and PGE_1 synergise together in promoting doming (unpublished results), and that another inducer, retinoic acid, also synergises with DMSO (Rudland et al, 1980a) suggests that the initial interaction of the PG's with the cells may be different from that of DMSO and more closely akin to that of the retinoids. Whatever the mechanism the "differentiation" of Rama 25 cells is reversible within a few days of the removal of the PG's from the culture medium. Thus the "differentiated" Rama 25 cells when injected into nude mice probably fail to establish themselves within this time period. If they survived for longer times then presumably they would revert to the original stem cells and produce tumours at the original frequency.

Previous reports have shown that PGA_1 can induce differentiation of cultured Friend erythroleukemic cells with a concomitant reduction in their rate of proliferation (Santoro et al., 1978). Moreover treatment of these cells

with 16, 16-dimethyl-PGE$_2$-methyl ester in vitro before
injecting them into DBA/2J mice increases the mice's median
survival time compared with mice injected with untreated cells.
(Santoro & Jaffe, 1979). We have now shown that PGE$_1$ and to
a lesser extent PGE$_2$ and PGF$_{2\alpha}$ can increase the rate at which
a rat mammary tumour stem cell line differentiates to alveolar-
like cells with a corresponding reduction in its DNA synthetic
rate and in its tumour-incidence in nude mice. However, the
PG's are not unique in being able to stimulate Friend and
mammary stem cells to differentiate since other agents
including DMSO behave similarly.Thus whether the PG's ever
perform this role in vivo is unclear. Nevertheless PG's are
produced by many diverse cells including those from murine
and human tumours (Sykes & Maddox, 1972; Williams et al., 1963;
Bhana et al., 1971) particularly of the breast (Tan et al., 197
Dowsett et al., 1976; Bennett et al., 1976) at concentrations
sufficient to elicit the changes reported in our rat mammary
system. Thus different PG's may influence the progression of
a tumour not only by increasing (Jimenez de Asua et al., 1975)
or decreasing (Otten et al., 1972) rates of cell replication
but also by promoting differentiation of the tumour stem cells
to new cell types with an altered neoplastic potential.

REFERENCES

Abaza NA, Leighton J, Shultz SG (1974). Effect of ouabain on
    the function and structure of a cell line (MDCK) derived
    from canine kidney. In Vitro 10:172.
Bennett A, Charlier EM, McDonald AM, Simpson JS, Stamford IF
    (1976). Bone destruction by breast tumours.
    Prostaglandins 11:460.
Bennett DC, Peachey L, Durbin H, Rudland PS (1978). A
    possible mammary stem cell line. Cell 15:283.
Bhana D, Hillier K, Karim SMM (1971). Vasoactive substances
    in Kaposi sarcoma. Cancer 27:233.
Clark GD, Ryan PJ (1980). Tranquillizers can block mito-
    genesis in 3T3 cells and induce differentiation in
    Friend cells. Nature 287:160.
Dowsett M, Easty GC, Powles TJ, Easty DM, Neville AM (1976).
    Human breast tumour-induced oestolysis and prostaglandins.
    Prostaglandins 11:447.
Friend C, Scher W, Holland JG, Sato T (1971). Hemoglobin
    synthesis in murine virus-induced leukemic cells in
    vitro: stimulation of erythroid differentiation by
    dimethyl sulphoxide. Proc. Natl. Acad. Sci. USA 63:378.

Huggins C, Briziarelli G, Sutton H (1959). Rapid induction
    of mammary carcinoma in the rat and the influence of
    hormones on the tumours. J. Expt. Med. 109:25.
Jimenez de Asua L, Clingan D, Rudland PS (1975). Initiation
    of cell proliferation in cultured mouse fibroblasts by
    prostaglandin $F_{2\alpha}$. Proc. Natl. Acad. Sci. USA 72:2724.
Kon SK, Cowie AT (1961). "Milk: the Mammary Gland and its
    Secretion. I". New York: Academic Press p.3.
Kuehl FA, Humes JL (1972). Direct evidence for a prosta-
    glandin receptor and its applications to prostaglandin
    measurements. Proc. Natl. Acad. Sci. 69:480.
Lee JB (1974). Prostaglandins and the Renal Antihypertensive
    and Natriuretic Endocrine Function. Recent Prog. Horm.
    Res. 30:481.
Lyons RW, Li CH, Johnson RE (1958). The hormonal control of
    mammary growth and lactation and the growth of tumours.
    Recent Prog. Horm. Res. 14:219.
McGrath CM (1975). Cell organisation and responsiveness to
    hormones in vitro: genesis of domes in mammary cell
    cultures. Amer. Zool. 15:231.
Nandi SJ (1958). Endocrine control of mammary gland
    development and function in the C3H/He Crgl mouse.
    J. Natl. Cancer Inst. 21:1039.
Otten J, Johnson GS, Pastan I (1972). Regulation of cell
    growth by cyclic adenosine 3', 5' - monophosphate.
    J. Biol. Chem. 247:7082.
Pharriss BB, Tillson SA, Erickson RR (1972). Prostaglandins
    and Luteal Function. Recent Prog. Horm. Res. 28:51.
Reuben RC, Wife RL, Breslow R, Rifkind RA, Marks PA (1976).
    A new group of potent inducers of differentiation in
    murine erythroleukemic cells. Proc. Natl. Acad. Sci.
    USA 73:862.
Rudland PS, Bennett DC, Warburton MJ (1979). Hormonal control
    of growth and differentiation of cultured rat mammary
    gland epithelial cells. Cold. Spr. Hb. Conferences on
    Cell Proliferation 6:677.
Rudland PS, Jimenez de Asua L (1979). Action of growth
    factors in the cell cycle. Biochim. Biophys. Acta 560:91.
Rudland PS, Bennett DC, Ritter MA, Newman RA, Warburton MJ
    (1980a). Differentiation of a rat mammary stem cell line
    in culture. In Jimenez de Asua L et al (eds) "Control
    Mechanisms in Animal Cells". New York: Raven Press p.341.
Rudland PS, Ormerod EJ, and Paterson F (1980b). Stem cells
    in rat mammary development and cancer: a review.
    J. Royal Soc. Med. 73:437.
Samuelsson B (1978). Prostaglandins and Thromboxanes. Recent
    Prog. Horm. Res. 34:239.

Santoro MG, Benedetto A, Jaffe BM (1978). Prostaglandin A$_1$ induces differentiation in Friend erythroleukemic cells. Prostaglandins 17:719.
Santoro MG, Jaffe BM (1979). Inhibition of Friend erythro-leukemia-cell tumours in vivo by a synthetic analogue of prostaglandin E$_2$. Brit. J. Cancer 39:408.
Sykes JAC, Maddox IS (1972). Prostaglandin production by experimental tumours and effects of anti-inflammatory compounds. Nature New Biol. 237:59.
Tan WC, Privett OS, Goldyne ME (1974). Studies of prosta-glandins in rat mammary tumours induced by 7,12-dimethyl-benz(a)anthracene. Cancer Res. 34:3229.
Warburton M, Head L, Rudland PS (1979). Induction of casein synthesis in a rat mammary tumour epithelial cell line by dimethyl sulphoxide. Biochem. Soc. Trans. 7:115.
Williams ED, Karim SMM, Sandler M (1968). Prostaglandin secretion by medullary carcinoma of the thyroid. A possible cause of the associated diarrhoea. Lancet i:22.
Young S, Hallowes RC (1973). "Pathology of Tumours in Laboratory Animals I - Tumours of the rat". Lyon: IARC p. 31.

ACKNOWLEDGEMENTS

We thank Anna Bruton, Sharon Heath, Karin Dawson for expert technical assistance, Geoffrey Webby, Linda Lovell for animal care, and Dr. J. Pike, UpJohn Company for gifts of the PG's used.

Prostaglandins and Cancer: First
International Conference, pages 481–485
© 1982 Alan R. Liss, Inc., 150 Fifth Avenue, New York, NY 10011

EVIDENCE FOR INVOLVEMENT OF THE LIPOXYGENASE PATHWAY IN
CSF-INDUCED HUMAN AND MURINE MYELOID COLONY FORMATION

Alan M. Miller, Vincent A. Ziboh[1] & Adel A. Yunis

Departments of Medicine, Oncology and Dermatology, University
of Miami School of Medicine, and the Howard Hughes Medical
Institute, P.O. Box 016960 (R-38), Miami, FL 33101

[1] Currently University of California at Davis

INTRODUCTION

Continuous presence of a glycoprotein termed colony stimulating factor (CSF) is
necessary for the *in vitro* clonal growth of the committed granulocyte-macrophage
progenitor cell (CFU-C) (Metcalf, 1970). Various small molecules, including prostaglandins, have been shown to either augment or inhibit CSF-induced colony formation
(Kurland & Moore, 1977, Kurland et al 1978, Miller et al 1978).

Recently, we have reported that CSF can stimulate the release of ^{14}C-arachidonic
acid from membrane phospholipids of rat bone marrow cells. Subsequently, products of
both cyclooxygenase and lipoxygenase metabolism are generated (Ziboh et al 1981).
Hydroxy-eicosatetraenoic acids (HETEs) have been reported to exert a variety of
effects on differentiated functions of mature granulocytes (Goetzel et al 1980,
Klickstein et al 1980, Lewis et al 1980).

In the present studies we have examined the role of the lipooxygenase pathway of
arachidonic acid in the stimulation of granulopoiesis.

METHODS

3-amino-1 [m-(trifluoromethyl)-phenyl] 2-pyrazoline (BW755C) and indomethacin
were gifts from Dr. Shen of Merck, Sharp and Dohme, Rahway, New Jersey. Nordi-
hydroguariretic acid (NDGA) was a gift from Dr. James Hamilton, Hoffman La Roche,
Nutley, New Jersey. Calcium Inophore (23187) was purcharsed from Calbiochem, San
Diego, California. 5,8,11,13-eicosatetraenoic acid (15-HETE) was a gift from Dr. Robert
Bryant of George Washington University, Washington, D.C. All the compounds with the
exception of the calcium ionophore were added in ethanol at a concentration of 0.1% of
the incubation medium. Ethanol at this concentration had no effects on the growth of

the colonies or on the incubating cells. Calcium ionophore was dissolved in dimethylsulf-oxide (DMSO) and used in the incubation medium at a concentration of 0.1%. DMSO alone at this concentration had no effect.

Preparation of Human Bone Marrow Cells

Marrow was obtained by needle aspiration from the posterior iliac crest of normal donors (informed consent was obtained according to the principles of the Declaration of Helsinki). Approximately 10 ml of marrow was collected from each of two sites and mixed with phenol-free heparin (10 U/ml). The marrow was diluted 1:1 with physiological saline, gently layered on top of a Hypaque-Ficoll solution with a specific gravity of 1.078 (LSM, Bionetics), and centrifuged at 400 X G for 40 min. The light density inter-face cells were collected and washed twice in media.

Mouse CFU-C Assay

C57Bl/6J mice (6—8 wk, male) were obtained from Jackson Laboratories (Bar Harbor, Maine). Murine bone marrow myeloid colony formation was assayed according to the method of Bradley and Metcalf (1966) as previously described (Ratzan et al 1974). Enzyme inhibitors, lipoxygenase extracts and colony stimulating factor were added directly to plates prior to plating. The source of colony stimulating factor used was mouse lung conditioned media, prepared as described (Ratzan et al 1974). Plates were incubated for six days and colonies of 50 or more cells were counted.

Human CFU-C Assay

The method used to culture human marrow was similar to that used in mouse with the following modifications. 1 X 10^5 Hypaque-Ficoll interface cells, were plated with human lung conditioned media as a source of CSF (Miller et al 1978a). Plates were incubated for seven days and colonies of 30 or more cells counted.

Generation of Lipoxygenase Products

Peritoneal neutrophils (>80%) were collected from rats according to the method of Gemsa et al (1973). Rat neutrophil lipoxygenase products were generated as described by Walker and Dawson (1979).

RESULTS

Effects of Lipoxygenase and Cyclooxygenase Inhibitors

Mouse bone marrow cells were incubated with CSF and various inhibitors of lipoxy-genase and cyclooxygenase. As can be seen in Figure 1, inhibitors of both enzymes, NDGA and BW755C (Walker 1980, Higgs et al 1979) inhibited colony formation in a dose dependent manner with near total inhibition at 10 μg/ml. Indomethacin which selectively inhibits cyclooxygenase at low concentrations (Higgs et al 1979) causes relatively little inhibition. In a single experiment 5,8,11,13-eicosatetraenoic acid (15-HETE) which selectively inhibits lipoxygenase (Vanderhock et al 1980) was more inhibitory than either NDGA or BW755C. In preliminary experiments, the effects of crude neutrophil lipoxygenase products partially reversed NDGA inhibition, (data not shown).

NDGA at 5 μg/ml inhibited both granulocyte and macrophage colonies equally.

Human bone marrow colony growth appears to be even more sensitive than mouse marrow to inhibition by NDGA and BW755C with 100% and 70% inhibition respectively by 5 μg/ml of those compounds (Figure 2). As with mouse marrow, little inhibition was seen with indomethacin (<10%).

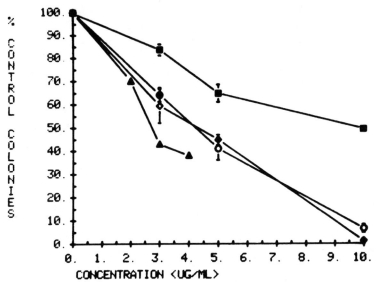

Figure 1. Effect of cycloxygenase and lipoxygenase inhibitors on murine bone marrow formation. Results are the sum of 11 (NDGA), 5 (BW755C and indomethacin) and 1 (15-HETE) individual experiment(s) with duplicate or triplicate plates in each experiment and are expressed as percentage of control plates which averaged 130.1 ± 5.8 colonies/ 100,000 cells. All plates contained .05 ml mouse lung conditioned media. —o— NDGA, — — BW755C, —△— 15-HETE, —□—indomethacin.

DISCUSSION

Data in these studies suggest that CSF stimulation may involve the generation of products of the lipoxygenation of arachidonic acid. NDGA and BW755C compounds reported to inhibit both the lipoxygenase and cylcooxygenase pathways (Walker 1980, Higgs et al 1979) and 15-HETE, a selective inhibitor of mammalian lipoxygenase (Vanderhock et al 1980) inhibited CSF induced colony formation in mouse and human marrow. Inhibition of cyclooxygenase activity in this and previous studies did not prevent colony formation to an appreciable extent (Kurland et al 1978).

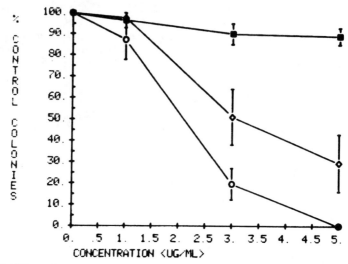

Figure 2. Effect of cycloxygenase and lipoxygenase inhibitors on day seven human bone marrow colony formation. Results are the sum of three individual experiments with triplicate plates in each experiment and are expressed as percentage of control ± standard error of the mean. Control plates averaged 48.8 ± 7.0 colonies/100,000 light density (<1.078 s.g.) cells. All plates contained .01 ml human lung conditioned media. —o— NDGA, — — BW755, —□—indomethacin.

Addition of small amounts of lipoxygenase products partially reversed the reduction in colonies caused by NDGA. Goetzl and co-workers similarly have demonstrated that NDGA inhibition of granulocyte random migration and chemotaxis could be completely reversed by addition of small quantities of the lipoxygenase product 5-HETE (Goetzl et al 1980, Klickstein et al 1980).

The products of lipoxygenation of arachidonic acid, the monohydroxyeicosatetraenoic acids (HETEs) and the leukotrienes have been shown to have a variety of activities on the differentiated cells of the myeloid series (Goetzl et al 1980, Klickstein et al 1982, Lewis et al 1980). The activities on mature granulocytes include their recruitment and expression of enzymatic activity. It would therefore appear to be biologically economical for similar compounds to exert activities to replace and provide additional cells.

Prostaglandins, products of cyclooxygenase metabolism of arachidonic acid, appear to be involved in myeloid colony formation, primarily as modulators (Kurland and Moore 1977, Kurland et al 1978, Miller et al 1978). Lipoxygenase products appear to have a more central role in the production of granulocytes and macrophages from their committed precursors. Further investigation of these molecules in normal and disordered hemato-poiesis is currently underway.

ACKNOWLEDGMENTS

We would like to thank Ms. L. Planas, Mr. J. Jimenez and Mrs. L. Lo for their expert help in these experiments.

This study was supported in part by USPHS grants GM28892, CAl4395 and AM26207.

REFERENCES

Bradley, T.R. and Metcalf, D., 1966: The Growth of Mouse Marrow Cells *In Vitro. Aust. J. Exp. Biol. Md. Sci.* 55:287–299.

Gemsa, D., Woo, C.H., Fudenberg, H.H. and Schmid, R.,1973: Erythrocyte Catabolism by Macrophages *In Vitro*: The Effect of Hydrocortisone on Erythrophagocytosis and on the Induction of Heme Oxygenase. *J. Clin. Invest.* 52:812–822.

Goetzl, E.J., Brash, A.R., Tauber, A.I., Oates, J.A. and Hubbard, W.C., 1980: Modulation of Human Neutrophil Function by Monohydroxy-Eicosatetraenoic Acids. *Immunol.* 39:491–501.

Higgs, G.A., Flower, R.J. and Vane, J.R., 1979: A New Approach to Anti-Inflammatory Drugs. *Biochem. Pharm.* 28:1959–1961.

Klickstein, L.B., Shapleigh, C. and Goetzl, E.J., 1980: Lipoxygenation of Arachidonic Acid as a Source of Polymorphonuclear Leukocyte Chemotactic Factor in Synovial Fluid and Tissue in Rheumatic Arthritis and Spondyloarthritis. *J. Clin. Invest.* 66: 1166–1170.

Kurland, J. and Moore, M.A.S., 1977: Modulation of Hemopoiesis by Prostaglandins. *Exp. Hemat.* 5:357–373.

Kurland, J., Bockman, R.S., Broxmeyer, H.E. and Moore, M.A.S.,1978: Limitation of Excessive Myelopoiesis by the Intrinsic Modulation of Macrophage-Derived Prostaglandin E. *Science* 199:552–555.

Lewis, R.A., Austen, K.F., Drazen, J.M., Clark, D.A., Marfat, A. and Corey, E.J., 1980: Slow Reacting Substances of Anaphylaxis: Identification of Leukotrienes C-1 and D from Human and Rat Sources. *Proc. Natl. Acad. Sci.* 77:3710–3714.

Metcalf, D., 1970: Studies on Colony Formation *In Vitro* by Mouse Bone Marrow Cells. II. Action of Colony Stimulating Factor. *J. Cell Physiol.* 76:89–99.

Miller, A.M., Russell, T.R., Gross, M.A. and Yunis, A.A., 1978: Modulation of Granulopoiesis: Opposing Roles of Prostaglandins F and E. *J. Lab. Clin. Med.* 92:983–990.

Miller, A.M., Gross, M.A. and Yunis, A.A., 1978a: Heterogeneity of Human Colony-Forming Cells (CFU-C): Difference in Size, Rate of Colony Formation, and Responsiveness to Colony Stimulating Factor. *J. Lab. Clin. Med.* 92:3844.

Ratzan, R.J., Moore, M.A.S. and Yunis, A.A., 1974: Effect of Chloramphenicol and Thiamphenicol on the *In Vitro* Colony Forming Cell. *Blood* 43:363–369.

Vanderhock, J.Y., Bryant, R.W. and Bailey, J.M., 1980: 15-Hydroxy-5,8,11-13-Eicosatetraenoic Acid: A Potent and Selective Inhibitor of Platelet Lipoxygenase. *J. Biol. Chem.* 255:5996–5998.

Walker, J.R. and Dawson, W., 1979: Inhibition of Rabbit PMN Lipoxygenase Activity by Benoxaprofen. *J. Pharm. Pharmacol.* 31:778–780.

Walker, J.R., 1980: Interrelationship of SRS-A Production and Arachidonic Acid Metabolism in Human Lung Tissue. In Advances in Prostaglandin and Thromboxane Research, Vol. 6, B. Samuelsson, P. Ramwell and R. Paoletti, eds.

Ziboh, V., Miller, A.M., Wu, M.-C and Yunis, A.A., 1981: Colony Stimulating Factor (CSF)-Induced Release of Archidonic Acid in Myeloid Cells. *Clin. Res.* 29:354A Abs.

**Prostaglandins and Cancer: First
International Conference, pages 487–491**
© **1982 Alan R. Liss, Inc., 150 Fifth Avenue, New York, NY 10011**

RELATIONSHIP OF DIFFERENTIATION AND PROSTAGLANDIN PRODUCTION
IN HUMAN PROMYELOCYTIC LEUKEMIA

David T. Dudley, Ann Louise Olson and
C. Patrick Burns
Department of Medicine, University of Iowa
College of Medicine
Iowa City, Iowa   52242

INTRODUCTION

The human promyelocytic leukemia cell line, HL-60, was
established by Collins and co-workers from the blood of a
patient with acute promyelocytic leukemia (1977). This cell
line grows continuously in suspension culture and undergoes
myeloid differentiation in response to a wide variety of
compounds. Since leukemia is thought to originate from a
defect in the process of differentiation, the HL-60 affords
a useful model to study various aspects of the leukemic
process. We have studied the effect of differentiation on
prostaglandin production by this cell line. Furthermore,
we have compared two differentiation inducing compounds,
DMSO and retinoic acid, in respect to morphologic and biochemical indicators of differentiation and prostaglandin
production.

METHODS

HL-60 cells were maintained in suspension culture in
RPMI-1640 media supplemented with gentamicin (40 µg/ml) and
10% fetal bovine serum. To induce differentiation, cells
were seeded at 1 x 10^5/ml in media containing either 1.3%
DMSO or 10^{-6}M retinoic acid (all trans, Sigma Chemical Co.,
St. Louis, MO). To determine superoxide anion (O_2^-) production, an assay was employed which measured the amount of
cytochrome c reduced in response to 12-0-tetradecanoylphor-
bol-13-acetate (TPA) (Mendelsohn et al., 1980). Superoxide
dismutase (Sigma) was used in control samples so that the

reported values reflect reduction due to O_2^-. Prostaglandin production was determined by incubating 2 x 10^7 cells at 37° for 1 hr in the presence of $[1-{}^{14}C]$arachidonic acid (1.5 μM, 3.7 x 10^5 cpm, New England Nuclear). Control cells were preincubated with 2 mM acetylsalicylic acid to irreversibly inhibit cyclooxygenase activity. After the incubations, cells were centrifuged and the oxygenated arachidonic acid products were extracted from the supernatant with ethyl acetate. The extract was dried and chromatographed on silica gel G thin layer chromatography plates using ethyl acetate/2,2,4-trimethylpentane/acetic acid/water (11:5:2:10, v/v). Bands corresponding to authentic standards (Sigma) were removed and counted for radioactivity in a liquid scintillation counter.

RESULTS AND DISCUSSION

As seen in Figure 1, both DMSO and retinoic acid produced a time dependent increase in the proportion of morphologically differentiated HL-60 cells. Furthermore, both concentrations of retinoic acid resulted in about 25% more differentiation by day 6 as compared to DMSO. This is

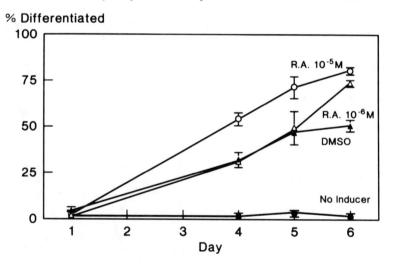

Fig. 1. Differentiation induced in HL-60 as measured by differential counts of Wright-stained Cytospin preparations. RA - retinoic acid.

similar to reports of Breitman, et al., (1980). Concentrations of 10^{-6}M retinoic acid were chosen for further studies since growth rate was depressed and viability was lower in cells treated with 10^{-5}M (data not shown).

A convenient measure of the respiratory burst of granulocytes is the amount of superoxide anion produced upon exposure to TPA (Newburger, et al., 1980). We employed this assay to compare HL-60 cells treated with either retinoic acid or DMSO in their ability to produce O_2^-. O_2^- production by the untreated HL-60 was 3.6 nmol/hr/10^6 cells. DMSO treated cells had a 5-fold greater production of O_2^- at day 6 (17.9 nmol/hr/10^6 cells) than untreated cells. However, retinoic acid treated cells produced almost twice as much O_2^- at day 6 as the DMSO treated cells (32.3 nmol/hr/10^6 cells).

Prostaglandin production results are detailed in Figure 2. Untreated HL-60 cells had less than 200 cpm appearing in the prostanoid bands. This corresponds to less than 0.05% conversion of the added substrate to any prostaglandin. Cells treated with DMSO also produced only a minimal amount of prostaglandin. The heaviest labeled band was PGE_2 which contained 3620 $\pm$ 295 cpm. However, these counts amount only to about 1% conversion of the arachidonic acid to PGE_2. Less than 200 cpm appeared in the TXB_2 band. This is in contrast to Bonser, et al. who found TXB_2 to be the main prostanoid produced by HL-60 cells treated with DMSO (1981). The greatest prostaglandin production was by cells treated with retinoic acid. As with DMSO treated cells, the main product was PGE_2. With retinoic acid treated cells, however, the PGE_2 produced (30,750 $\pm$ 2580 cpm) amounted to an 8.3% conversion of the added label. This is an 8-fold increase over DMSO treated cells, and a 175-fold increase over untreated cells.

These results indicate that prostaglandin production in the HL-60 cell is dependent upon maturity. We can offer several possible explanations for this observation. Prostaglandins may be required for the specialized function of the terminally differentiated myeloid cell, but not for its promyelocyte precursor. Alternately, the leukemic phenotype of the undifferentiated promyelocyte may be characterized by a loss of the capacity for prostaglandin biosynthesis. Such a metabolic defect may be corrected as the leukemic block in differentiation is overcome by retinoic acid.

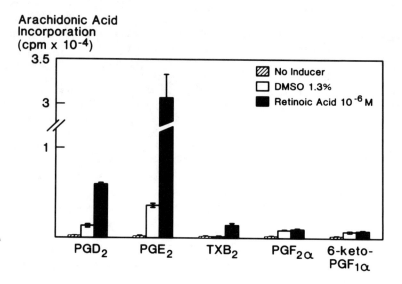

Fig. 2. Prostaglandin production from [1-^{14}C]arachidonic
acid by HL-60 and effect of differentiation inducers at day
6. Values shown are per 2 x 10^7 cells.

Retinoic acid appears to be a more effective inducer of
myeloid differentiation in this cell line as compared to
DMSO. The greater production of PGE2 after retinoic acid may
be due simply to quantitatively more effective differentiation. However, the degree of differentiation induced by
retinoic acid resulted in only a 2-fold greater generation
of O$_2^-$ and a 1.5-fold higher proportion of morphologically
mature cells. Since these measures of differentiation are
much less than the 8.5-fold greater production of prostaglandin, there may be qualitative differences in the manner
that retinoic acid affects the cell. Furthermore, these
data suggest that there is not necessarily close coupling of
metabolic and morphologic events during differentiation.

ACKNOWLEDGMENTS

This investigation was supported by Grant CA 17283
awarded by the National Cancer Institute, Department of

Health and Human Services. C. Patrick Burns is recipient of
a USPHS Research Career Development Award CA 00324. HL-60
was a gift from Dr. Robert Gallagher.

REFERENCES

Bonser RW, Siegel MI, McConnell RT, Cuatrecasas P (1981).
    The appearance of phospholipase and cyclo-oxygenase ac-
    tivities in the human promyelocytic leukemia cell line
    HL60 during dimethyl sulfoxide-induced differentiation.
    Biochem Biophys Res Commun 98:614-620.
Breitman TR, Selonick SE, Collins SJ (1980). Induction of
    differentiation of the human promyelocytic leukemia cell
    line (HL-60) by retinoic acid. Proc Natl Acad Sci USA
    77:2936-2940.
Collins SJ, Gallo RC, Gallagher RE (1977). Continuous
    growth and differentiation of human myeloid leukaemic
    cells in suspension culture. Nature 270:347-349.
Mendelsohn N, Gilbert HS, Christman JK, Acs G (1980). Ef-
    fect of maturation on the response of human promyelocytic
    leukemia cells (HL-60) to the tumor promoter 12-0-tetra-
    decanoylphorbol-13-acetate. Can Res 40:1469-1474.
Newburger PE, Chovaniec ME, Cohen HJ (1980). Activity and
    activation of the granulocyte superoxide-generating sys-
    tem. Blood 55:85-92.

**Prostaglandins and Cancer: First
International Conference, pages 493–497
© 1982 Alan R. Liss, Inc., 150 Fifth Avenue, New York, NY 10011**

INDUCTION OF GLUCAGON RECEPTORS AND RESPONSIVENESS IN TRANS-
FORMED KIDNEY CELLS BY PROSTAGLANDINS

Michael C. Lin, Sue-May Wang & Suzanne K. Beckner

National Institutes of Health
Bethesda, Maryland 20205

The appearance of differentiated characteristics during
cellular development is a highly regulated event. Sensitivity
of tissues toward hormones, particularly peptide hormones, is
one function closely associated with a more differentiated
state. Our aim is to identify factors in the cellular environment which govern the development of hormone responsiveness
by examining the hormone-sensitive adenylate cyclase system
during differentiation. We have found that in a dog kidney
cell line (MDCK cells), glucagon receptors and responsiveness
are selectively abolished by viral transformation and can be
restored by differentiation inducers and prostaglandins.

Materials and Methods

Cell culture – MDCK cells (Madin-Darby canine kidney) were
maintained as a monolayer culture in Dulbecco's modified
Eagle medium (DMEM) containing 5% heat-inactivated fetal
bovine serum and antibiotics. A cloned line of MDCK (T) cells
transformed by Harvey murine sarcoma virus was also grown
under the same culture conditions. This transformed line has
been characterized and shown to produce a specific viral
protein (Shih et al., 1979). For some experiments, transformed cells were also maintained in a chemically-defined
medium containing insulin, transferrin, hydrocortisone, tri-
iodothyronine, selenium dioxide, prostaglandin E_1 (PGE_1) and
HEPES buffer, pH 7.4, as reported for the parental MDCK line
(Taub et al, 1979).

Assay for cyclic AMP-mediated hormone sensitivity – Hormone
responsiveness was measured as described in Table I. Stimu-

lation time was kept to 3 min to allow linear production of intracellular cyclic AMP without its leakage into the medium. All hormone concentrations were saturating.

Assay for glucagon receptors - The receptor concentration was estimated by binding of (^{125}I)-glucagon (supplied by Meloy Lab, specific activity was about 4×10^5 cpm/pmol) (Lin et al., 1976). Monolayer cultures were incubated with 1 nM (^{125}I)-glucagon (in the absence or presence of 2 μM unlabeled glucagon for the estimation of non-specific binding) in DMEM containing 20 mM HEPES buffer, pH 7.4, 0.5% bovine serum albumin (BSA) and 1 mM bacitracin for 15 min at 37°. After washing, the radioactivity bound was determined.

Determination of prostaglandin production in MDCK cells - Various aspects of prostaglandin production were measured as indicated in Table 2. Concentrations of PGE_2 and $F_{2\alpha}$ were quantitated by radioimmunoassay (Sigma). Approximately 90% of ^{14}C-arachidonic acid taken up by both cell types was incorporated into cellular phospholipids. The release of arachidonic acid and PGE_2 from cells was maximal at 8 and 3 hr, respectively.

Results and Discussion

Loss of glucagon receptors and responsiveness upon viral transformation - The adenylate cyclase of the parental MDCK line is responsive to glucagon, vasopressin, β-adrenergic agonists and PGE_1 (Rindler et al., 1979). Following transformation with Harvey murine sarcoma virus, a clone of MDCK cells selectively lost glucagon sensitivity, while maintaining responsiveness to other hormones (Table I). This loss of glu-

Table 1. Hormone responsiveness of different types of MDCK cells.

Hormone[a]	Type of MDCK cells			
	Parental	T	T+Butyrate[b]	T+PGE$_1$[b]
Glucagon	+++	–	++	++
Vasopressin	+++	+	++	++
Isoproterenol	++++	+++	+++	+++
PGE$_1$	++++	++++	+++	+++

a. Monolayer cultures were incubated at 25° for 30 min in DMEM containing 20 mM HEPES, 20 μM Ro20-1724 (a phosphodiesterase inhibitor); hormone (glucagon 2 µM, vasopressin 1 µM, isoproterenol 1 µM or PGE_1 1 µM) was then added. The reaction was terminated by removal of the medium and cyclic AMP extracted with boiling water (Lin 1980). Cyclic AMP was measured by a radioimmunoassay (NEN).

b. Transformed MDCK cells were cultured in the absence or presence of butyrate (3 mM) for 3 days or PGE_1 (0.1 µM) for 6 days before assaying for hormone sensitivity.

cagon sensitivity was paralleled by a loss of glucagon receptors, measured both in intact cells as well as isolated plasma membranes (data not shown). Glucagon receptors and responsiveness could be restored to transformed MDCK cells by sodium butyrate (a differentiation inducer) (Leder & Leder, 1975; Lin et al., 1979). This induction was completely blocked by tunicamycin (a glycosylation inhibitor) or cycloheximide (an inhibitor of protein synthesis) and partially blocked by α-amanitin (an inhibitor of RNA polymerase). These findings suggest that transformation leads to a selective loss of glucagon receptors, but has no effect on other components of the adenylate cyclase system, and that the restoration of glucagon sensitivity by sodium butyrate involves de novo synthesis of glucagon receptors.

Induction of glucagon response by PGE_1 - When adopting a chemically-defined medium for the growth of the transformed line, we discovered that glucagon sensitivity developed after several days of culture. The omission of PGE_1 from the defined medium essentially abolished the appearance of glucagon sensitivity suggesting that PGE_1 is also capable of inducing glucagon responsiveness. The mechanism of glucagon receptor induction by such diverse agents as butyrate and PGE_1 is currently under investigation. Whether these agents share a common pathway is unknown.

Loss of prostaglandin production in transformed MDCK cells - It is well known that MDCK cells produce prostaglandins. The fact that exogenously added PGE_1 induced glucagon sensitivity in transformed cells prompted an examination of prostaglandin production in these cell lines. We found that production of PGE_2 and $F_{2\alpha}$ were reduced by more than 90% in transformed cells as compared to the normal line (Table II). The inability of the transformed line to produce prostaglandins does not seem to be due to any defect in the uptake of arachidonic acid, since the incorporation of ^{14}C-arachidonic acid into cellular

phospholipid was unchanged in transformed cells. When the
release of ^{14}C-arachidonic acid from cells was followed as
a measure of phospholipase activity, we found that the ability of transformed cells to release this precursor for pros-
tanglandins was reduced by 85% as compared to that of normal

Table 2. Production of prostaglandins in MDCK cells.

| | Type of MDCK cells | |
	Parental	Transformed
Phospholipase activity:[a] (% release of total radio- activity incorporated)	28	4.2
PGE$_2$ synthetase activity:[b] (pmol/mg protein/min)	59	18
PGE$_2$ secretion:[c] (pmol/10^6 cells/3 hr)	83	1

a. MDCK cells were prelabeled for 16 hr with ^{14}C-arachi-
    donic acid. The release of radioactivity in DMEM con-
    taining essential fatty acid-free BSA was followed for
    8 hr as an indirect measurement of phospholipase activity.
b. The formation of PGE$_2$ from arachidonic acid as substrate
    was measured in an 8000 xg pellet from MDCK cells.
c. Intact cells were incubated in DMEM containing essential
    fatty acid-free BSA for 3 hr and the amount of PGE$_2$ in
    the media quantitated.

cells. Furthermore, when prostanglandin synthetase activity was measured in broken cell preparations, the ability of
the transformed line to utilize arachidonic acid for PGE$_2$
synthesis was also decreased by 70%. MDCK cells transformed
by Harvey murine sarcoma virus are known to produce a specific
viral protein carrying phosphorylating activity (Shih et al.,
1980). Whether any of these defects is a direct consequence
of viral protein production remains to be elucidated.

It is tempting to speculate that the decreased prostaglandin production in transformed cells might be responsible
for the loss of glucagon receptors upon transformation.
Whether these effects are directly mediated by PGE$_2$, PGF$_{2\alpha}$,
their metabolites or some unknown intermediates awaits further studies. Our preliminary results indicate that cellular
conditions favoring prostaglandin production facilitate the
appearance of glucagon sensitivity. These observations are

consistent with the role of prostaglandins as local development hormones essential for the evolution of glucagon receptors
and responsiveness in these kidney cells.

Leder A, Leder P (1975). Butyric acid, a potent inducer of
erythroid differentiation in cultured erythroleukemic cells.
Cell 5:319.

Lin MC, Nicosia S, Rodbell M (1976). Effects of iodination
of tyrosyl residues on the binding and action of glucagon
at its receptor. Biochemistry 15:4537.

Lin MC, Lin C-S, Whitlock JP (1979). Reduction of GTP activation of adenylate cyclase system by its coupling to hormone receptor. J. Biol. Chem. 254:4684.

Lin MC (1980). Long term maintenance of hormone responsiveness
in primary hepatocyte culture. Ann. N.Y. Acad. Sci. 349:
383.

Rindler MJ, Chuman LM, Shaffer L, Saier MH (1979). Retention
of differentiated properties in an established dog kidney
epithelial cell line (MDCK). J. Cell Biol. 81:635.

Shih TY, Weeks MD, Young HA, Scolnick EM (1979). Identification of a sarcoma virus-coded phosphoprotein in nonproducer
cells transformed by Kirsten or Harvey murine sarcoma virus.
Virology 96:64.

Shih TY, Papageorge AG, Stokes PE, Weeks MO, Scolnick EM
(1980). Guanine nucleotide-binding and autophosphorylating
activities associated with the p21^{src} protein of Harvey
murine sarcoma virus. Nature 287:686.

Taub M, Chuman L, Saier MH, Sato G (1979) Growth of Madin-
Darby canine kidney epithelial cell line in hormone-supplemented, serum-free medium. Proc. Natl. Acad. Sci. USA 76:
3338.

PROSTAGLANDINS, BONE METASTASES, AND HYPERCALCEMIA

Prostaglandins and Cancer: First International Conference, pages 501–511
© 1982 Alan R. Liss, Inc., 150 Fifth Avenue, New York, NY 10011

INVOLVEMENT OF PROSTAGLANDIN SYNTHESIS IN MECHANISMS OF
MALIGNANT HYPERCALCEMIA

Gregory R. Mundy, M.D.

University of Texas Health Science Center
7703 Floyd Curl Drive
San Antonio, TX 78284

Increased bone resorption and hypercalcemia are common
concomitants of malignant disease. The cellular and molecular mechanisms responsible for causing the increase in bone
resorption which is the primary cause of hypercalcemia in
patients with malignancy are still not clear. Interest has
been shown in the prostaglandins as potential mediators of
hypercalcemia of malignancy since they were first shown to
stimulate bone resorption by Klein and Raisz over 10 years
ago (Klein and Raisz, 1970). Since that time, there have
been a plethora of studies in both animal models and in
patients with hypercalcemia which have attempted to define
their role. Unfortunately it is still not clear just what
role prostaglandins play in the pathogenesis of hypercalcemia. In this review I will attempt to cover (outline) the
studies relevant to the role of prostaglandins in the hypercalcemia of malignancy.

EFFECTS OF PRODUCTS OF ARACHIDONIC ACID METABOLISM ON BONE
RESORPTION.

The initial study which showed that prostaglandins
could stimulate bone resorption in vitro was performed by
Klein and Raisz (1970). Since that time a series of prostaglandin metabolites have been shown to affect bone metabolism. Prostaglandins of the E series are the most potent
bone resorbing metabolites although other prostaglandins,
including $PGF2_\alpha$ and PGA_2 are also bone resorbing factors
(Dietrich and Raisz, 1975). More recently Tashjian et al.
(1977) and Raisz et al. (1977) have shown that other

arachidonic acid metabolites including prostaglandin endoperoxides, prostacyclin and prostaglandin E metabolites are
also stimulators of bone resorption (Raisz et al., 1977;
Tashjian et al., 1977; Martin and Partridge, 1980). The
effect of prostaglandins on bone cell cultures has also been
examined (Atkins and Martin, 1977a; Crawford et al., 1978;
Yu et al., 1976; Rao et al., 1977). The prostaglandins
activate adenylate cyclase which in turn causes an increase
in bone cell cyclic AMP content, but the prostaglandin
receptor seems to be separate from the parathyroid hormone
receptor. Thus it is clear that prostaglandins have effects
on bone cell metabolism to stimulate bone resorption.
Studies of the effects of prostaglandins on bone formation
in organ culture systems suggest that they inhibit collage-
nase-digestible protein synthesis (Raisz and Kooemans-
Beynen, 1974a). The effects of prostaglandin-E_2 on osteoclast ultrastructure have been studied in organ cultures of
bone by Holtrop et al. (1978). Prostaglandin E_2, like PTH,
causes an increase in the area of ruffled borders and clear
zones of osteoclasts associated with the resorption of the
bones.

POTENTIAL MECHANISMS OF THE INCREASED BONE RESORPTION AND
HYPERCALCEMIA IN MALIGNANCY.

There is clearly no single unifying mechanism for the
hypercalcemia which occurs in either patients or animals
with malignant disease. For purposes of simplicity we pre-
fer to divide the patients with the hypercalcemia of malignancy into three clinical categories - those patients with
solid tumors without bone metastases, those patients with
solid tumors with bone metastases and those patients with
myeloma and other hematologic disorders. It appears likely
that the pathogenetic mechanism for bone resorption is
different in each of these categories. It is also possible
that even within these individual categories that different
mediators are responsible for causing hypercalcemia.

Solid Tumors Without Bone Metastases.

This group has been called the humoral hypercalcemia of
malignancy (Martin and Atkins, 1979; Stewart et al., 1980)
and is presumably due to the production of a humoral circulating stimulator of bone resorption by the tumor cells.

The factor which is responsible for causing increased bone resorption is unknown but the prostaglandins have been suggested as candidates since the demonstration that prostaglandins of the E series were responsible in several animal models (Tashjian et al., 1972; Voelkel et al., 1975; Galasko and Bennett, 1976). Patients (Stewart et al., 1980; Rude et al., 1981) and animals (Saxe et al., 1981; Sica et al., 1981; Schmidt-Gayk et al., 1979) with this syndrome have other characteristic abnormalities. They have decreased circulating immunoreactive parathyroid hormone concentrations, increased nephrogenous cyclic AMP (in some studies, although not in others), and increased renal phosphate clearance. It is likely that some of these patients have increased urinary excretion of prostaglandins and metabolites of prostaglandins of the E series and this has led to the suggestion by Seyberth et al. (1975; 1976) that prostaglandins are responsible for the hypercalcemia. Seyberth's patients responded to indomethacin or aspirin, drugs which inhibit prostaglandin synthesis. However, in one of the animal models of this syndrome, indomethacin had no effect on the serum calcium but reduced the urinary prostaglandin metabolite excretion markedly (Seyberth et al., 1980). The patients of Seyberth et al. (1975; 1976) with the humoral hypercalcemia of malignancy did not have increased nephrogenous cyclic AMP generation, unlike those of Stewart et al. (1980) and Rude et al. (1981). It is not clear whether the prostaglandins which appear in the urine in patients with this syndrome are responsible for the hypercalcemia or whether they are "innocent bystanders." It is possible in some cases that they are not responsible for the hypercalcemia because indomethacin is not usually effective in the treatment of patients with hypercalcemia. Nevertheless it is also possible that indomethacin is not getting to the bone sites where osteoclasts are being stimulated to cause increased bone resorption and hypercalcemia. In one patient studied by Seyberth et al. (1976), hypercalcemia was not relieved by indomethacin but was later relieved by aspirin.

An argument against prostaglandins being responsible for this type of hypercalcemia is that there is no currently identified circulating product of arachidonic acid metabolism which is a potent bone resorber. Prostaglandins of the E series do not circulate in appreciable amounts. The most stable circulating metabolite of PGE is 13,14-dihydro, 15-keto prostaglandin E, which is a weak bone resorbing factor (Raisz et al., 1977; Tashjian et al., 1977). A more potent

bone resorbing factor is 13,14-dihydro PGE2, but it is not
known if this compound circulates in patients or animals
with tumors. It is also possible that other circulating
factors or mediators cause bone resorption by generating
prostaglandin synthesis locally in bone. Raisz et al.
(1974b) showed that prostaglandin synthesis could be generated in bone by complement-sufficient serum. Later Tashjian
et al. (1978) showed that phorbol esters and epidermal
growth factor (1979) could stimulate prostaglandin synthesis
in bone cultures, although this latter finding could not be
confirmed by Raisz et al. (1980). Bockman (1981) has
suggested that lymphokine-mediated bone resorption is dependent on prostaglandin synthesis in bone, but others have not
been able to demonstrate this (Raisz et al., 1975; Yoneda
and Mundy, 1979a,b; Josse et al., 1981). Recently, Minkin
et al. (personal communication) have found that tumor extracts may generate prostaglandin synthesis by bone cultures.

Solid Tumors With Metastases.

     The majority of patients with the hypercalcemia of malig-
nancy have solid tumors which have metastasized to bone
(Myers, 1960). This is most frequently seen with breast
cancer and lung cancer. In this situation the mechanism of
bone destruction may be very complex and involve complicated
cell-cell interactions between tumor cells, monocytes,
lymphocytes and osteoclasts. Monocytes and lymphocytes
frequently accumulate in metastatic tumor deposits and could
stimulate osteoclastic bone resorption by releasing cytokines or lymphokines and in particular the lymphokine osteoclast activating factor (Mundy et al., 1974a,b). Both
prostaglandins and osteoclast activating factor could in
turn lead to osteoclast activation and bone resorption.
Tumor cells also could cause bone resorption by direct
release of local mediators of bone resorption such as prostaglandins. We have found that some tumor cells in culture
will release prostaglandins when they are exposed to
estrogens (Eilon and Mundy, 1980). A number of workers have
co-cultured fresh slices or cores of tumor cells with bones
and found that bone resorption is stimulated and this effect
is inhibited by indomethacin (Powles et al., 1973, 1976;
Bennett et al., 1977; Atkins et al., 1977b). These results
are difficult to interpret however since fresh human tumors
in liquid culture contain a large number of dying cells
which release prostaglandins agonally (Hong et al., 1976).

In addition these plugs of tumor contain other cells such as monocytes and fibroblasts and it is not clear which cells are releasing the prostaglandins. Studies in patients with these disorders in which indomethacin or aspirin have been used have not been effective in either decreasing bone metastases or relieving the hypercalcemia (Coombes et al., 1976) although in an animal model in which tumor cells were injected directly into the aorta, bone resorption was inhibited by prostaglandin synthesis inhibitors (Powles et al., 1973). Recently we have used fresh human tumor cells cultured in semi-solid agar in which the fibroblasts are removed. There are considerable amounts of prostaglandins in these cultures and we are in the process of separating the tumor cells from the monocytes to determine which cells are responsible for producing the prostaglandins.

Myeloma and Other Hematologic Malignancies.

Bone destruction is almost invariable in patients with myeloma and is frequently associated with hypercalcemia. The cellular mechanism of bone resorption in myeloma is osteoclastic (Mundy et al., 1974b; Meunier et al., 1977) and appears to be due to the production of a lymphokine by the myeloma cells which we have called osteoclast activating factor (Mundy et al., 1974a,b; Mundy and Raisz, 1977). Osteoclast activating factor is also produced by normal activated lymphocytes (Horton et al., 1972; Yoneda and Mundy, 1979a,b). We have studied the role of prostaglandins in the production of osteoclast activating factor and found that it is dependent on prostaglandin synthesis. The activated lymphocyte is the cell source of origin of osteoclast activating factor (Yoneda and Mundy, 1979a,b). However the lymphocyte will not produce osteoclast activating factor unless it is cultured in the presence of monocytes which are synthesizing prostaglandins. When lymphocytes and monocytes are cultured with inhibitors of prostaglandin synthesis such as indomethacin, then OAF production is reduced. OAF production can be restored by the addition of exogenous prostaglandins to the lymphocyte cultures. OAF production is also restored by the addition of monocytes, monocyte-conditioned medium and agents which increase lymphocyte cyclic AMP content such as dibutyryl cyclic AMP, isobutyl methyl zanthine and isoproterenol (Yoneda and Mundy, 1981). Recently Josse et al. (1981) have shown that cultured myeloma cells also depend on prostaglandin synthesis

for the production of osteoclast activating factor. When
fresh human myeloma cells were cultured in the presence of
indomethacin, no OAF production was produced. Bockman has
found similar results with a factor produced by cultured
lymphoma cells (Bockman, 1981). Although it appears that
prostaglandin synthesis is necessary for OAF production in
vitro, drugs which inhibit prostaglandin synthesis such as
indomethacin have no effect on hypercalcemia in patients
with myeloma. Possible reasons for the failure of prostaglandin synthesis inhibitors to decrease bone resorption in
myeloma are that the drugs do not reach the site of OAF production in the marrow by myeloma cells, or that the myeloma
cell, unlike the normal activated lymphocyte, does not require prostaglandins for its production. OAF is a local
mediator of bone resorption (Mundy et al., 1974b).

EFFECTS OF INHIBITORS OF PROSTAGLANDIN SYNTHESIS ON HYPER-
CALCEMIA.

Inhibitors of prostaglandin synthesis such as indomethacin have been tried enthusiastically in patients with
hypercalcemia since the early reports of ten years ago that
they were effective in several animal models of hypercalcemia and that they were also effective in several patients
with hypercalcemia (Brereton et al., 1974; Robertson et al.,
1974; Ito et al., 1975). In general, however, they have
been very disappointing. Although they may be effective at
relieving bone pain in patients with osteolytic bone destruction (Brodie, 1974), they are usually ineffective in lowering
the serum calcium. This has been demonstrated by a number
of workers including Coombes et al. (1976) and Tashjian
(1975). In our experience, indomethacin is effective in
less than 20% of all patients with the hypercalcemia of
malignancy.

SUMMARY

The role of prostaglandins in the hypercalcemia of
malignancy is still unclear. There is very good evidence in
some animal models that they are responsible, but these
tumors are associated with very large bulk and they may not
be relevant to the human situation. The evidence supporting
their role in human hypercalcemia of malignancy is much less
satisfactory. It is particularly difficult to determine

their importance because there are probably multiple mechanisms responsible for the human hypercalcemia of malignancy.
In some situations prostaglandins may be primarily responsible, in some situations they may be partly responsible or
work as co-factors with other mediators of bone resorption,
and in some situations they may be secreted in large amounts
but be innocent bystanders and not primarily responsible for
the hypercalcemia. Continued research using techniques of
cell and organ culture combined with in vivo studies in
animal models and clinical observations in patients with
hypercalcemia and increased bone resorption will be necessary
to clarify their role. It is clear at the present time that
the currently available prostaglandin synthesis inhibitors
such as indomethacin are not warranted as routine first-line
agents in the treatment of hypercalcemia.

REFERENCES

Atkins D, Ibbotson KJ, Hillier K, Hunt NH, Hammonds JC,
    Martin TJ (1977). Secretion of prostaglandins as bone
    resorbing agents by renal corticocarcinoma in culture. Br
    J Cancer 36:601.
Atkins D, Martin TJ (1977). Effects of some prostaglandins,
    their metabolites, and analogues on cyclic AMP production.
    Prostaglandin 13:861.
Bennett A, Charlier EM, McDonald AM, Simpson JS, Stamford IF,
    Zebro T (1977). Prostaglandins and breast cancer. Lancet
    2:624.
Bockman R (1981)."Proceedings of the Third Annual Meeting of
    the American Society for Bone and Mineral Research."
    Calcif Tiss Intern (in press).
Brereton HD, Halushka PV, Alexander RW, Mason DM, Keiser HO,
    DeVita VT Jr. (1974). Indomethacin - responsive hyper-
    calcemia in a patient with renal-cell adenocarcinoma. N
    Engl J Med 291:83.
Brodie (1974). Indomethacin and bone pain. Lancet 1:1160.
Coombes RC, Neville AM, Bondy PK (1976). Failure of
    indomethacin to reduce hydroxyproline excretion or hyper-
    calcemia in patients with breast cancer. Prostaglandins
    12:1027.
Crawford A, Atkins D, Martin TJ (1978). Rat osteogenic
    sarcoma cells: Comparison of the effects of prostaglandins
    E1, E2, I2 (prostacyclin), 6Keto, F-1-alpha and thromboxane
    B2 on cyclic AMP production and adenylate cyclase activity.
    Biochem Biophys Res Comm 82:1195.

Dietrich JW, Raisz LG (1975). Prostaglandin and calcium in bone metabolism. Clin Ortho Rel Res 111:228.

Dietrich JW, Goodson JM, Raisz LG (1975). Stimulation of bone resorption by various prostaglandins in organ culture. Prostaglandins 10:231.

Eilon G, Mundy GR (1980). Production of bone resorbing activity by human breast cancer cells. Proc Am Soc Bone Min Res 24A.

Galasko CSB, Bennett A (1976). Relationship of bone destruction in skeletal metastases to osteoclast activation and prostaglandins. Nature 263:508.

Heersche JNM, Jez DH, Aubin J, Sodek J (1981). Regulation of hormone responsiveness of bone in vitro by corticosteroids, PTH, PGE2 and calcitonin. In Cohn DV, Talmage RV, Matthews JL (eds): "Hormonal Control of Calcium Metabolism," Amsterdam, Excerpta Medica, p 157.

Holtrop ME, King GJ, Raisz LG (1978). Factors influencing osteoclast activity as measured by ultrastructural morphometry. In Copp DH, Talmage AR (eds): "Endocrinology of Calcium Metabolism," Amsterdam, Excerpta Medica, p 91.

Hong SL, Polsky-Cynkin R, Levine L (1976). Stimulation of prostaglandin biosynthesis by vasoactive substances in methylcholanthrene-transformed mouse BALB/3T3. J Biol Chem 251:776.

Horton JE, Raisz LG, Simmons HA, Oppenheim JJ, Mergenhagen SE (1972). Bone resorbing activity in supernatant fluid from cultured human peripheral blood leukocytes. Science 177:793.

Ito H, Sanada T, Katayama T, Shimaryaki J (1975). Indomethacin responsive hypercalcemia. N Engl J Med 293:558.

Josse RG, Murray TM, Mundy GR, Jez D, Heersche JNM (1981). Observations on the mechanism of bone resorption induced by multiple myeloma marrow culture fluids and partially purified osteoclast activating factor. J Clin Invest 67: 1472.

Klein DC, Raisz LG (1970). Prostaglandins: stimulation of bone resorption in tissue culture. Endocrinology 86:1436.

Martin TJ, Atkins D (1979). Biochemical regulators of bone resorption and their significance in cancer. Essays Med Biochem 4:49.

Martin TJ, Partridge NC (1980). Prostaglandins, cancer and bone: Pharmacological considerations. Metab Bon Dis Rel Res 2:167.

Meunier P, Edouard C, Bressot C, Bernard J, Valat JN (1977). Retentissement sur le tissu osseux de la proliferation plasmocytaire myelomateuse: Bonnees histomorphometriques.

Lyon Medical 237:187.
Minkin C, Fredericks RS, Pokress S, Rude K, Sharp E, Tong M, Singer FR. Personal Communication.
Mundy GR, Luben RA, Raisz LG, Oppenheim JJ, Buell DR (1974a). Bone-resorbing activity in supernatants from lymphoid cell lines. N Engl J Med 290:867.
Mundy GR, Raisz LG, Cooper RA, Schechter GP, Salmon SE (1974b). Evidence for the secretion of an osteoclast stimulating factor in myeloma. N Engl J Med 291:1041.
Mundy GR, Raisz LG (1977). Big and little forms of osteoclast activating factor. J Clin Invest 60:122.
Myers WPL (1960). Hypercalcemia in neoplastic disease. Arch Surg 80:308.
Powles TJ, Clark SA, Easty DM, Easty GC, Neville AM (1973). The inhibition by aspirin and indomethacin of osteolytic tumor deposits and hypercalcemia in rats with Walker tumour, and its possible application to human breast cancer. Br J Cancer 28:316.
Powles TJ, Dowsett M, Easty DM, Easty GC, Neville AM (1976). Breast cancer osteolysis, bone metastases and anti-osteolytic affect of aspirin. Lancet I:608.
Raisz LG, Kooenans-Beynen AR (1974). Inhibition of bone collagen synthesis by prostaglandin E2 in organ culture. Prostaglandins 10:377.
Raisz LG, Luben RA, Mundy GR, Dietrich JW, Horton JE, Trummel CL (1975). Effects of osteoclast activating factor from human leukocytes on bone metabolism. J Clin Invest 56:408.
Raisz LG, Dietrich JW, Simmons HA, Seyberth HW, Hubbard WN, Oates JA (1977). Effects of prostaglandin endoperoxides and metabolites and bone resorption in vitro. Nature 267:532.
Raisz LG, Sandberg AL, Goodson GM, Simmons HA, Mergenhagen SE (1974). Complement-dependent stimulation of prostaglandin synthesis in bone resorption. Science 185:789.
Raisz LG, Simmons HA, Sandberg AL, Canalis E (1980). Direct stimulation of bone resorption by epidermal growth factor. Endocrinology 107:270.
Rao LG, NG, Brunette DM, Heersche JNM (1977). Parathyroid hormone and prostaglandin E1 - response in a selected population of bone cells after repeated sub-culture and storage at -80°C. Endocrinology 100:1233.
Robertson RP, Baylink DJ, Marini JJ, Adkinson HW (1975). Elevated prostaglandins and suppressed parathyroid hormone associated with hypercalcemia and renal cell carcinoma. J Clin Endocrinol Metab 41:164.

Rude RK, Sharp CF Jr, Fredericks RS, Oldham SB, Elbaum N,
Link J, Irwin L, Singer FR (1981). Urinary and the nephro-
genous adenosine 3', 5'-monophosphate in the hypercalcemia
of malignancy. J Clin Endocrinol Metab 52:765.
Saxe A, Brennan M, Deftos L, Spiegel (1981). Humoral hyper-
calcemia caused by a rat leydig cell tumor is associated
with increased urine cyclic AMP and suppressed PTH. In
"Proceedings of the Third Annual Scientific Meeting of the
American Society for Bone and Mineral Research," p 39A.
Schmidt-Gayk H, Lohrke H, Fischkal A, Goerttler K, Hofmann
F (1979). Urinary cyclic AMP and bone histology in Walker
carcinosarcoma: evidence of parathyroid hormone-like
activity. Eur J Canc 15:1211.
Seybeth HW, Segre GV, Morgan JL, Sweetman BJ, Potts Jr JT,
Oates JA (1975). Prostaglandins as mediators of hyper-
calcemia associated with certain types of cancer. N Engl
J Med 293:1278.
Seyberth HW, Segre GV, Hamet P, Sweetman BJ, Potts Jr JT,
Oates JA (1976). Characterization of the group of patients
with the hypercalcemia of cancer who respond to treatment
with prostaglandin synthesis inhibitors. Trans Assoc Am
Physicians 89:92.
Seyberth HW, Bonsch G, Muller H, Minne HW, Erlenmaier T,
Strein K, Imbeck H, Nrongovius R (1980). Prostaglandin-E
production and hypercalcemia in rats bearing the Walker
carcinosarcoma. Brit J Canc 42:455.
Sica D, Martodam R, Aronow J, Mundy G (1981). The relationship between hypercalcemia and urinary cyclic AMP in the
humoral hypercalcemia of malignancy. In "Proceedings of
the Third Annual Scientific Meeting of the American
Society for Bone and Mineral Research," p 30A.
Stewart AF, Horst R, Deftos LJ, Cadman EC, Lang R, Broadus
AE (1980). Biochemical evaluation of patients with cancer
associated with hypercalcemia: Evidence for humoral and
non-humoral groups. N Engl J Med 303:1377.
Tashjian AJ Jr (1975). Prostaglandins, hypercalcemia and
cancer. N Engl J Med 293:1317.
Tashjian AH Jr, Tice JE, Sides SA (1977). Biological
activities of prostaglandin analogues and metabolites on
bone in organ culture. Nature 266:645.
Tashjian AH Jr, Levine L (1979). Epidermal growth factor
stimulates prostaglandin production and bone resorption in
cultured mouse calvaria. Biochem Biophys Res Comm 85:966.
Tashjian AH Jr (1978). Prostaglandins as local mediators of
bone resorption. In Horton JVE, Tarpley TM, Davis WF (eds):
"Mechanisms of Localized Bone Loss - A Special Supplement

to Calcified Tissue Abstracts," Washington: Information Retrieval, Inc., p 173.

Tashjian AH Jr, Voelkel EF, Levine L, Goldhaber P (1972). Evidence that the bone resorption-stimulating factor produced by mouse fibrosarcoma cells is prostaglandin E2: A new model for the hypercalcemia of cancer. J Exp Med 136: 1329.

Tashjian AH Jr, Tice JE, Sides K (1977). Biological activities of prostaglandin analogues and metabolites on bone in organ culture. Nature 266:645.

Voelkel EF, Tashjian AH Jr, Franklin R, Wasserman E, Levine L (1975). Hypercalcemia and tumor-prostaglandins: The VX2 carcinoma model in the rabbit. Metabolism 24:973.

Yoneda T, Mundy GR (1979a). Prostaglandins are necessary for osteoclast activating factor (OAF) production by activated peripheral blood leukocytes. J Exp Med 149:279.

Yoneda T, Mundy GR (1979b). Monocytes regulate osteoclast activating factor production by releasing prostaglandins. J Exp Med 150:338.

Yoneda T, Mundy GR (1981). Release of the lymphokine osteoclast activating factor requires cyclic AMP accumulation. Calcif Tiss Int (in press).

Yu JH, Wells H, Ryan WJ, et al. (1976). Effects of prostaglandins and other drugs on the cyclic AMP content of cultured bone cells. Prostaglandins 12:501.

**Prostaglandins and Cancer: First
International Conference, pages 513–523
© 1982 Alan R. Liss, Inc., 150 Fifth Avenue, New York, NY 10011**

PROSTAGLANDINS, TUMOR CELLS AND BONE METABOLISM

Armen H. Tashjian, Jr., Edward F. Voelkel and
Lawrence Levine

Laboratory of Toxicology, Harvard School of
Public Health and Department of Pharmacology,
Harvard Medical School, Boston, MA 02115; and
Department of Biochemistry, Brandeis University,
Waltham, MA 02254

INTRODUCTION

The purpose of this report is to summarize some of our
studies on the interrelationships between prostaglandins,
tumor cells and bone metabolism. Altered bone remodeling
and hypercalcemia often occur in patients with cancer. The
pathophysiology is complex but usually appears to result
either from deposits of metastatic tumor in bone or from
humoral factors produced by tumor cells and secreted into
the systemic circulation where they are then transported to
the skeleton. The postulated mediators of altered bone
remodeling produced by tumor cells either locally in bone or
at distant sites include parathyroid hormone, vitamin D or
its metabolites, osteoclast activating factor, a variety of
proteolytic enzymes including collagenase, metabolites of
arachidonic acid, and several growth factors. This list is
undoubtedly incomplete, and by no means have all the factors
listed been proven to play a role in human disease. In this
discussion we plan to focus on arachidonic acid metabolites
and growth factors as mediators of altered bone metabolism
that occurs in association with cancer. We shall present
two different but interrelated mechanistic pathways. The
first involves the production of prostaglandin E_2 (PGE_2)
by tumor cells; the second involves the actions of peptide
growth factors on bone cells which result in the local
production of PGE_2.

MODEL SYSTEMS

Production of PGE$_2$ by Tumor Cells

The evidence that tumors can produce and secrete
excessive quantities of PGE$_2$, which then act on the skeleton to induce a generalized abnormality of mineral metabolism and hypercalcemia, is derived from studies in two animal models. It has been established that PGE$_2$ is the most
potent tested metabolite of arachidonic acid as a direct-
acting bone resorption-stimulating agent (Klein and Raisz,
1970; Tashjian et al., 1972; Tashjian et al., 1977a; Raisz
et al., 1977). The animal and cell culture model systems
which we have studied are the HSDM$_1$ murine fibrosarcoma
and the rabbit VX$_2$ carcinoma. In brief, the findings are
as follows: 1. Both tumors induce a hypercalcemic syndrome
in the host (Tashjian et al., 1972; Voelkel et al., 1975).
Accompanying or preceding the hypercalcemia there is a small
increase in the concentration of PGE$_2$ in plasma and a much
larger (up to 50 times the normal value) increase in the
concentration of the PGE$_2$ metabolite 13,14-dihydro-15-
keto-PGE$_2$ (Tashjian et al., 1972; Voelkel et al., 1975;
Tashjian et al., 1977b, 1977c; Alam et al., 1980). There
are no statistically significant increases in the plasma
levels of 6-keto-PGF$_{1\alpha}$, TXB$_2$, 13,14-dihydro-PGE$_2$ or
15-keto-PGE$_2$ (Alam et al., 1980). 2. The tumor tissue
contains ether-extractable bone resorption-stimulating activity (assayed on mouse calvaria in organ culture) which is
completely accounted for by the PGE$_2$ content of the extracts (Tashjian et al., 1972; Voelkel et al., 1975).
3. Clonal strains of HSDM$_1$ and VX$_2$ cells in culture produce and secrete into medium bone resorption-stimulating
activity and PGE$_2$. The synthesis of both the biological
activity and PGE$_2$ is inhibited in parallel by indomethacin, hydrocortisone and 5,8,11,14-eicosatetraynoic acid
(Tashjian et al., 1972; Tashjian et al., 1974; Tashjian et
al., 1975; Voelkel et al., 1975). 4. In animals, treatment
with indomethacin or hydrocortisone can prevent or reverse
the hypercalcemia and reduce the concentrations of 13,14-
dihydro-15-keto-PGE$_2$ in plasma (Tashjian et al., 1973;
Voelkel et al., 1975). 5. The venous drainage of the tumor
contains high concentrations of PGE$_2$ (Voelkel et al.,
1975). 6. Histopathologic and morphometric analyses of the
skeletons of normal and tumor-bearing rabbits demonstrate
two distinctive abnormalities: a diffuse decrease in bone
formation, and a generalized increase in bone resorption and

numbers of osteoclasts (Hough et al., 1977; Wolfe et al., 1978). It should be emphasized that no skeletal metastases were found as evidence of direct invasion of bone by tumor cells. The bone pathology was at sites distant (vertebral bodies and iliac crest) from tumor implantation (distal hind leg). These findings have led us to propose that these two animal tumors synthesize and secrete large amounts of PGE$_2$, which although short-lived in plasma, accumulates in sufficient quantity and for a sufficient period of time to stimulate bone cells to resorb skeletal mineral and release it in excessive quantities into extracellular fluid and plasma thus producing the hypercalcemic syndrome.

Because the VX$_2$ and HSDM$_1$ tumor cells can metabolize arachidonic acid to products other than PGE$_2$ and because these tumor cell products can be metabolized further in other tissues, it is important to consider potential medi-ators other than PGE$_2$. We have approached this problem in two ways. First, we have examined the bone resorption-stimulating activity of a variety of arachidonate metabo-lites or analogs including endoperoxide analogs, TXB$_2$, PGI$_2$, 6-keto-PGF$_{1\alpha}$, 10,10-difluoro-dehydro-PGI$_2$, 13,14-dihydro-15-keto-PGE$_2$, 15-keto-PGE$_2$ and 13,14-dihydro-PGE$_2$ (Tashjian et al., 1977a; and unpublished data). None of these appears to have sufficient intrinsic bone resorption-stimulating activity to account for the bio-logical response observed in vivo. Preliminary results with 5-, 8+9-, 11-, 12-, and 15-HETEs also suggest that these products are not likely to be mediators of the hypercalcemic syndrome. Secondly, we have measured the concentrations of several metabolites in the plasma of control and tumor-bearing rabbits using high performance liquid chromatography and radioimmunoassay (Alam et al., 1980). Only 13,14-dihydro-15-keto-PGE$_2$ and 13,14-dihydro-15-keto-PGF$_{2\alpha}$ were elevated in tumor-bearing animals; the concentrations of 6-keto-PGF$_{1\alpha}$, TXB$_2$, 13,14-dihydro-PGE$_2$ and 15-keto-PGE$_2$ were normal. These results offer no support for the possibility that arachidonate metabolites other than PGE$_2$ are the mediators of altered bone remodeling in these animal models.

Further confirmation of our hypothesis that PGE$_2$ is a mediator was obtained from immunoprecipitation experiments. We have incubated PGE$_2$, crude extracts of tumor tissue, and conditioned medium from tumor cells with normal rabbit serum or rabbit anti-PGE$_2$ and then precipitated the gamma

globulins by incubation with goat anti-rabbit IgG. The
supernatant solutions were then assayed in vitro for bone
resorption-stimulating activity. The results in Fig. 1
(left panel) show that about 80% of the [^{3}H]PGE$_2$ tracer
was precipitated by anti-PGE$_2$ by the procedure used.

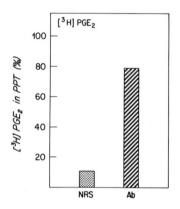 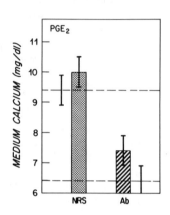

Fig. 1. Immunoprecipitation of [^{3}H]PGE$_2$ and the bone
resorption-stimulating activity of PGE$_2$ by incubation with
anti-PGE$_2$. A mixture of [^{3}H]PGE$_2$ tracer (15,000 cpm)
and PGE$_2$ (60 ng) were incubated with 60 μl of rabbit anti-
PGE$_2$ (Ab) or 60 μl of normal rabbit serum (NRS) for 1 hour
at 37°C and then for 1 hour at 4°C. Thereafter, 1.2 ml of
goat anti-rabbit IgG was added and the mixtures incubated
overnight at 4°C. After centrifugation for 45 minutes at 4°
C, the supernatant solutions and precipitates were separated
for measurements of radioactivity and bone resorption-stimulating activity. Left panel. Radioactivity in the supernatant solutions and precipitates was determined by liquid
scintillation counting. The bars give the percentages of
total radioactivity in the precipitates obtained with normal
rabbit serum (NRS) and anti-PGE$_2$ (Ab). Right panel. The
supernatant solutions were assayed for bone resorption-
stimulating activity using neonatal mouse calvaria at a dose
equivalent to 5 ng PGE$_2$/ml bone culture medium. The lower
horizontal dashed line gives the medium calcium of control
bones. The upper dashed horizontal line gives the medium
calcium of bones incubated with 5 ng/ml PGE$_2$ standard.
The bars give the mean values for solutions of PGE$_2$ incubated with NRS or anti-PGE$_2$. The brackets give the SE of
groups of 5 bones. The residual biological activity in the
antiserum-treated sample was not significantly different
from control (p > 0.05).

This value varied from 65 to 85% in 5 separate experiments.
The right panel shows that coprecipitation by anti-PGE$_2$,
but not by normal rabbit serum, markedly reduced the bone
resorption-stimulating activity of authentic PGE$_2$. The
results in Fig. 2 show the bone resorption-stimulating
activities in crude extracts of HSDM$_1$, and VX$_2$ tumors

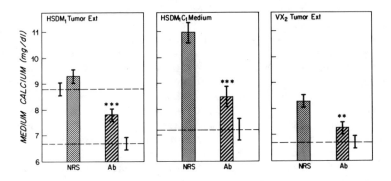

Fig. 2. Effect of immunoprecipitation with anti-PGE$_2$ on
the bone resorption-stimulating activity in extracts of
HSDM$_1$ and VX$_2$ tumors and conditioned medium from
HSDM$_1$C$_1$ cells in culture. Tumor tissue was homogenized
with Gey's balanced salt solution (5 ml/g) for 1 minute in a
Waring blender. The homogenate was centrifuged at 10,000 x
g for 30 minutes at 4°C, and the crude supernatant solution
used for these experiments. The dose equivalents used in
the bone culture assay were 20 μl/ml and 2.5 μl/ml culture
medium for the VX$_2$ and HSDM$_1$ tumor extracts, respectively. Conditioned medium from HSDM$_1$C$_1$ cells in culture
(about 500 μg cell protein, 3 ml medium, 5 days) was assayed
at a dose equivalent of 20 μl/ml bone culture medium. The
dashed horizontal lines between 6.5 and 7.5 mg/dl give the
medium calcium values for control bones; the upper dashed
horizontal line (left panel only) gives the medium calcium
value of unincubated HSDM$_1$ tumor extract. Unincubated
controls were not used for the HSDM$_1$C$_1$ medium and VX$_2$
tumor extract experiments. The bars give the mean values,
and the brackets give the SE for 4 or 5 bones per group.
The statistical significance of the difference between NRS
and Ab is given by the stars (*** = p < 0.001 and ** = p <
0.01).

and in conditioned medium from $HSDM_1C_1$ cells in culture were, in each case, markedly reduced by incubation with anti-PGE_2 but not with normal rabbit serum. Preliminary results using anti-$PGF_{2\alpha}$ and anti-5,6-dihydro-PGI_2 as control antisera showed no removal of the biological activity.

From the various lines of evidence cited above we have proposed that PGE_2 is the mediator of altered bone remodeling produced by the $HSDM_1$ and VX_2 tumors. However, we acknowledge several sorts of findings that are not entirely consistent with this hypothesis. First, it has been difficult to reproduce a hypercalcemic syndrome in vivo by administration of exogenous PGE_2 in all animal models studied (Beliel et al., 1973; Robertson and Baylink, 1977; Santoro et al., 1977; Vanderwiel and Talmage, 1979). Nevertheless, we have shown that the constant intravenous infusion of PGE_2, but not $PGF_{2\alpha}$, in intact, conscious, unanesthetized rats elevates the plasma calcium concentration (Franklin and Tashjian, 1975). It is clear that these important experiments need to be extended to the mouse and rabbit using infusion methods and timing which mimic as closely as possible the effects of implanted tumor and which maintain plasma levels of PGE_2 and its metabolites comparable to those in tumor-bearing animals. Secondly, Hubbard et al. (1980a) have reported that implantation of the VX_2 tumor intraperitoneally did not cause hypercalcemia despite high levels of 13,14-dihydro-15-keto-PGE_2 in plasma. We believe this result is likely to be due to single pass metabolism of tumor-derived PGE_2 by the liver; alternatively, the mediator of hypercalcemia might be an unidentified polyenoic acid metabolite other than PGE_2. Thirdly, Hubbard and his colleagues (1980b) have shown in vitro that VX_2 tumor tissue converts 3-8% of arachidonic acid to 11-HETE and 15-HETE and converts linoleic acid to a mixture of 9- and 13-hydroxy octadecanoic acids. The bone resorption-stimulating activity of the monohydroxy C-18 fatty acids have not been reported.

Peptide Growth Factor and Bone Metabolism

We should now like to consider a different hypothesis for the mechanism by which certain tumors may affect bone cell metabolism. This hypothesis also involves arachidonic acid metabolites, but in this case, not the production and secretion of metabolites of arachidonate by the tumor, but rather the enhanced production of such metabolites locally in bone leading to increased bone resorption.

Using high performance liquid chromatography to separate and radioimmunoassay to quantitate, we have shown that mouse bone in organ culture produces the following metabolites of arachidonic acid: cyclooxygenase products including PGE_2, $PGF_{2\alpha}$, PGI_2, and TXA_2; metabolites or stable derivatives including 13,14-dihydro-15-keto-PGE_2, 13,14-dihydro-15-keto-$PGF_{2\alpha}$, 6-keto-$PGF_{1\alpha}$, 6,15-diketo-$PGF_{1\alpha}$ and TXB_2 (Voelkel et al., 1980). Similar results have been reported by Raisz et al. (1979) using rat bone. Of particular interest are the findings that arachidonic acid metabolism in bone is enhanced markedly by certain polypeptide growth factors at concentrations at which they are found in human plasma or serum. Furthermore, this local production of arachidonic acid metabolites leads to enhanced bone resorption.

The two factors we have studied extensively are epidermal growth factor (Carpenter and Cohen, 1979) and platelet-derived growth factor (Ross and Vogel, 1978; Scher et al., 1979). The actions of epidermal growth factor (EGF) on bone are as follows: 1. EGF stimulates bone resorption and the ED_{50} is 0.4 ng/ml (7×10^{-11} M). 2. EGF stimulates the production of PGE_2 by bone (Tashjian and Levine, 1978). 3. The EGF-induced increases in bone resorption and PGE_2 production are inhibited in parallel by indomethacin and hydrocortisone. 4. The actions of EGF on bone are mediated via a single class of high affinity ($K_d = 2 \times 10^{-9}$ M), saturable receptors (Shupnik et al., 1980; Shupnik and Tashjian, 1981). Although EGF down-modulates its own receptor number on bone cells, EGF binding in bone differs from that in several other systems in that a prolonged plateau phase (lasting 6-8 hours) of maximal binding is observed in calvaria and bone cells, while maximal binding begins to decrease after 1-2 hours in most other systems (Carpenter and Cohen, 1979).

Platelet-derived growth factor (PDGF) also stimulates the production of PGE_2 by bone cells and bone resorption in mouse calvaria with an ED_{50} of 10 ng/ml (Hohmann et al., 1981). Like the actions of EGF, the effects of PDGF on PGE_2 production and bone resorption are inhibited in parallel by indomethacin. However, unlike EGF, a brief exposure (5-15 minutes) to PDGF can trigger a prolonged resorptive response in bone. PDGF increases cyclic AMP production by bone, and this effect of PDGF is completely blocked by indomethacin, while the action of exogenous PGE_2 on the production of cyclic AMP is not blocked by indomethacin. The effect of a low concentration of PDGF (1 ng/ml), which does not stimulate bone resorption alone, is potentiated by the phosphodiesterase inhibitor isobutyl-methylxanthine (Hohmann et al., 1981 and unpublished data).

These findings taken together demonstrate the following: 1. bone cells can metabolize arachidonic acid to PGE_2; 2. the locally produced PGE_2 can stimulate bone resorption; and 3. production of PGE_2 by bone cells is enhanced by EGF and PDGF. These data suggest, therefore, a possible new mechanism by which tumors may alter bone metabolism. Namely, the production by the tumor either locally in bone or systemically at sites distant from bone, of EGF, PDGF or analogous factors which alter bone remodeling by stimulating the metabolism of arachidonic acid in bone cells.

SUMMARY

We have emphasized results from our own laboratories from studies in model systems in animals or in vitro. These data give clues regarding the diversity of mechanisms by which tumors alter bone metabolism. On the other hand, much new information needs to be learned about hypercalcemic syndromes associated with human cancer for the available clinical data indicate that the most important mediators in man have probably not yet been discovered. That discovery will be an important milestone in endocrinology and oncology.

ACKNOWLEDGMENTS

Much of the original research which is summarized in this report was supported by research grants from the USPHS (AM 10206, AM 11011 and CA 17309). L.L. is an American Cancer Society Research Professor of Biochemistry (Award PRP-21).

REFERENCES

Alam I, Voelkel EF, Tashjian AH Jr, Levine L (1980).
Analysis by high performance liquid chromatography of
cyclooxygenase products of arachidonic acid metabolism in
plasma of rabbits bearing the VX_2 carcinoma.
Prostaglandins and Med 4:227.
Beliel OM, Singer FR, Coburn JW (1973). Prostaglandins:
effect on plasma calcium concentration. Prostaglandins
3:237.
Carpenter G, Cohen S (1979). Epidermal growth factor. Ann
Rev Biochem 48:193.
Franklin RB, Tashjian AH Jr (1975). Intravenous infusion
of prostaglandin E_2 raises plasma calcium concentra-
tion in the rat. Endocrinology 97:240.
Hohmann E, Levine L, Antoniades HN, Tashjian AH Jr (1981).
Platelet-derived growth factor stimulates bone resorp-
tion via a prostaglandin-mediated mechanism. Prog 63rd
Ann Meeting of The Endocrine Society, p 237, Abstract no.
619.
Hough A Jr, Seyberth H, Oates J, Hartmann W (1977).
Changes in bone and bone marrow of rabbits bearing the
VX_2 carcinoma. Am J Pathol 87:537.
Hubbard WC, Hough AJ, Johnson RM, Oates JA (1980a). The
site of VX_2 tumor transplantation affects the development of hypercalcemia in rabbits. Prostaglandins 19:881.
Hubbard WC, Hough AJ, Brash AR, Watson JT, Oates JA
(1980b). Metabolism of linoleic and arachidonic acid in
VX_2 carcinoma tissue: identification of monohydroxy
octadecadienoic acids and monohydroxy eicosatetraenoic
acids. Prostaglandins 20:431.
Klein DC, Raisz LG (1970). Prostaglandins: stimulation of
bone resorption in tissue culture. Endocrinology 86:1436.
Raisz LG, Dietrich JW, Simmons HA, Seyberth HW, Hubbard W,
Oates JA (1977). Effects of prostaglandin endoperoxides
and metabolites on bone resorption in vitro. Nature
267:532.
Raisz LG, Vanderhoek JY, Simmons HA, Kream BE, Nicolaou KC
(1979). Prostaglandin synthesis by fetal rat bone in
vitro: evidence for a role of prostacyclin.
Prostaglandins 17:905.
Robertson RP, Baylink DJ (1977). Hypercalcemia induced by
prostaglandin E_2 in thyroparathyroidectomized, but not
intact rats. Prostaglandins 13:1141.
Ross R, Vogel A (1978). The platelet-derived growth
factor. Cell 14:203.

Santoro MG, Jaffe BM, Simmons J (1977). Bone resorption in vitro and in vivo in PGE-treated mice. Proc Soc Exp Biol Med 156:373.

Scher CD, Shepard RC, Antoniades HN, Stiles CD (1979). Platelet-derived growth factor and the regulation of the mammalian fibroblast cell cycle. Biochim Biophys Acta 560:217.

Shupnik MA, Ip NY-Y, Tashjian AH Jr (1980). Characterization and regulation of receptors for epidermal growth factor in mouse calvaria. Endocrinology 107:1738.

Shupnik MA, Tashjian AH Jr (1981). Functional receptors for epidermal growth factor on human osteosarcoma cells. J Cell Physiol, in press.

Tashjian AH Jr, Voelkel EF, Levine L, Goldhaber P (1972). Evidence that the bone resorption-stimulating factor produced by mouse fibrosarcoma cells is PGE_2: a new model for the hypercalcemia of cancer. J Exp Med 136:1329.

Tashjian AH Jr, Voelkel EF, Goldhaber P, Levine L (1973). Successful treatment of hypercalcemia by indomethacin in mice bearing a prostaglandin-producing fibrosarcoma. Prostaglandins 3:515.

Tashjian AH Jr, Voelkel EF, Goldhaber P, Levine L (1974). Prostaglandins, calcium metabolism and cancer. Federation Proc 33:81.

Tashjian AH Jr, Voelkel EF, McDonough J, Levine L (1975). Hydrocortisone inhibits prostaglandin production by mouse fibrosarcoma cells. Nature 258:739.

Tashjian AH Jr, Tice JE, Sides S (1977a). Biological activities of prostaglandin analogs and metabolites on bone in organ culture. Nature 266:645.

Tashjian AH Jr, Voelkel EF, Levine L (1977b). Effects of hydrocortisone on the hypercalcemia and plasma levels of 13,14-dihydro-15-keto-prostaglandin E_2 in mice bearing the $HSDM_1$ fibrosarcoma. Biochem Biophys Res Commun 74:199.

Tashjian AH Jr, Voelkel EF, Levine L (1977c). Plasma concentrations of 13,14-dihydro-15-keto-prostaglandin E_2 in rabbits bearing the VX_2 carcinoma: effects of hydrocortisone and indomethacin. Prostaglandins 14:309.

Tashjian AH Jr, Levine L (1978). Epidermal growth factor stimulates prostaglandin production and bone resorption in cultured mouse calvaria. Biochem Biophys Res Commun 85:966.

Vanderwiel CJ, Talmage RV (1979). Comparison of the effects of prostaglandin E_2 and parathyroid hormone on plasma calcium concentration and osteoclast function. Endocrinology 105:588.

Voelkel EF, Tashjian AH Jr, Franklin R, Wasserman E, Levine L (1975). Hypercalcemia and tumor prostaglandins: the VX_2 carcinoma model in the rabbit. Metabolism 24:973.

Voelkel EF, Tashjian AH Jr, Levine L (1980). Cyclooxygenase products of arachidonic acid metabolism by mouse bone in organ culture. Biochim Biophys Acta 620:418.

WolfeHJ, Bitman WR, Voelkel EF, Griffiths HJ, Tashjian AH Jr (1978). Systemic effects of the VX_2 carcinoma on the osseous skeleton: a quantitative study of trabecular bone. Lab Invest 38:208.

**Prostaglandins and Cancer: First
International Conference, pages 525-540**
© **1982 Alan R. Liss, Inc., 150 Fifth Avenue, New York, NY 10011**

PROSTAGLANDINS AND CELLULAR BONE RESORPTION

T.J. Martin and N.C. Partridge

University of Melbourne, Department of Medicine,

Repatriation General Hospital, Victoria, Australia

The demonstration by Klein and Raisz (1970) that
prostaglandins were able to resorb bone directly *in vitro*
followed the observation (Chase and Aurbach, 1969) that
prostaglandins, like parathyroid hormone, stimulated
adenylate cyclase activity in bone cell membranes. The
direct resorbing action of prostaglandins has been amply
confirmed in several laboratories, and the prostaglandins
are thought to have important effects on bone in normal and
in disease states.

There are many similarities between the actions of
prostaglandins and parathyroid hormone upon bone. They
each increase adenylate cyclase activity in bone cell
membranes and increase cyclic AMP production in osteoblasts
(Partridge et al, 1981 a & b; Atkins et al, 1977; Rao et
al, 1977; Heersche and Ng, 1978), and with each of these
agents there is an increase in the activity and numbers of
osteoclasts (Schelling et al, 1980). The fact that they
each stimulated cyclic AMP formation in bone, together with
the known resorptive effect of dibutyryl cyclic AMP (Klein
and Raisz, 1971) pointed to a role of cyclic AMP in
mediating the actions of parathyroid hormone and prostaglandins on bone resorption. The significance of cyclic
AMP generation in bone is controversial (Peck, 1979).
Calcitonin, which acts by inhibiting osteoclastic bone
resorption, increases cyclic AMP formation in osteoclast-
rich populations of mouse bone cells (Luben et al, 1976),
and wherever specific calcitonin receptors have been found
in tumor cells they are associated with a calcitonin
responsive adenylate cyclase (Marx et al, 1974; Hunt et al

1977; Findlay et al, 1980), suggesting that calcitonin action is mediated via cyclic AMP. In bone the paradox may be explained by the fact that the bone resorbing hormones, prostaglandin E_2 (PGE_2) and parathyroid hormone, exert their cyclic AMP effects on one population (the osteoblasts), and calcitonin on another (the osteoclasts).

The major difference between parathyroid hormone and PGE_2 in their actions upon bone is that parathyroid hormone is clearly capable of elevating the serum calcium when administered to animals whereas data with PGE_2 is conflicting. Prostaglandins are metabolized in the tissues which produce them and in virtually all organs, but particularly the lungs and the liver. This breakdown into inactive metabolites occurs rapidly, and an intravenously administered dose of a prostaglandin is cleared almost completely by one circulation through the pulmonary vascular bed (Ferreira and Vane, 1967; McGiff et al, 1969; Piper et al, 1970). This probably explains the considerable difficulty which has been experienced in raising blood calcium in experimental animals by infusing PGE_2 (Robinson and Parsons, 1974; Franklin and Tashjian, 1975). These observations are relevant to any consideration of a role for prostaglandins as circulating agents acting upon bone. In general it seems more likely that they are important as local mediators.

CELLULAR ASPECTS OF BONE RESORPTION

Resorption of bone mineral and matrix results from a complex series of interactions between the cells of bone, influenced by the resorbing hormones. The major cells are:
(i) the osteoblast, traditionally thought to be dedicated to the laying down of the organic matrix and possibly to its subsequent mineralization,
(ii) the osteocyte, which is effectively an osteoblast trapped within the bone matrix, occupying spaces known as lacunae, and
(iii) the osteoclast, whose function is to resorb bone. The osteoclast is believed to be derived from blood forming cells, probably of the monocyte-macrophage series (Teitelbaum and Kahn, 1980) and in its activated and recognizable form is a large multinucleate cell with a characteristic "ruffled border", which consists of a series of fine cyto-

plasmic projections fanning out from the cell to end on the
bone surface.   In addition to its role as an osteoclast
precursor, the monocyte may itself resorb bone, and may
exert a "helper" function in modulating osteoclastic
resorption (Teitelbaum and Kahn, 1980).   A further link
between monocytes and resorption control mechanisms is
provided by the observation of Yoneda and Mundy (1979) that
monocyte production of prostaglandins is necessary to allow
transformed lymphocytes to produce the bone resorbing
lymphokine, osteoclast activating factor.

Although the bone resorbing hormones, including parathyroid hormone and the prostaglandins, are known to increase
the numbers and activity of osteoclasts following treatment
of bone *in vitro*, there is no evidence that these hormones
act directly upon the osteoclast itself.   As yet no suitable
preparations of isolated osteoclasts have been developed
which would allow any attempt to demonstrate this.   On the
other hand there is very convincing evidence that these
hormones act upon the osteoblast, and this will be reviewed
below.

BONE RESORPTION PRODUCED BY ARACHIDONIC ACID METABOLITES

Of the metabolites of arachidonic acid studied so far,
it is clear that PGE_2 is the most potent in stimulating bone
resorption (Raisz et al, 1979;   Tashjian et al, 1977b;
Greaves et al, 1980;   Table 1), whether the effects are
studied in cultured fetal rat long bones or in mouse calvaria.

There are several important features to note from these
studies of relative bone resorbing potencies of prostaglandins.
First, oxidation of the 15-hydroxyl group leads to virtually
complete loss of bone resorbing activity, an observation all
the more significant because of the predominance of 15-keto
metabolites as major circulating forms of biologically active
prostaglandins.   Thus 13,14-dihydro, 15-keto PGE_2 is a
relatively ineffective bone resorber, but is the major
circulating metabolite of PGE_2, a fact which must be borne
in mind in assessing the importance of <u>circulating</u> PGE_2 as a
bone resorbing substance.   On the other hand the 13,14-
dihydro metabolites of PGE and PGF are relatively potent, but
it is uncertain whether these substances are generated *in
vivo*.   It is possible to demonstrate formation of 13,14-
dihydro PGE_2 from 13,14-dihydro, 15-keto PGE_2 precursor

perfused through liver (Hamberg and Samuelsson, 1971) but there is no evidence yet that it circulates. Finally the two endoperoxide analogues (U44069 and U46619), which probably function effectively as agents which mimic the action of thromboxane A_2, are relatively ineffective as bone resorbing agents.

TABLE 1. Comparison of the effects of various prostanoids on bone resorption in organ culture or on cyclic AMP accumulation in bone tumor cells.

	Bone Resorption	Cyclic AMP
PGE_2	100	100
PGE_1	50	80
PGI_2		10
$PGF_{2\alpha}$	10	10
13,14-dihydro PGE_2	10-20	50
13,14-dihydro PGE_1	10-20	
13,14-dihydro $PGF_{2\alpha}$		0
6-keto $PGF_{1\alpha}$	5*	10
15-keto PGE_2	1-2*	1-2*
13,14-dihydro, 15-keto PGE_2	1-2*	1-2*
13,14-dihydro, 15-keto $PGF_{2\alpha}$		0
U44069 (endoperoxide analogue)	5*	1-2*
U46619 (endoperoxide analogue)	5*	1-2*
PGA_2	5*	
TxB_2	0	1-2*
PGB_2	0	
PGD_2	0	

PGE_2 = 100 arbitrary units

* non-parallel and partial responses.

Data from Greaves et al (1980) and Martin and Partridge, (1980).

The difficulty with these bone culture systems which

required 48 to 72 hour incubation periods is that they are
not suitable for estimating the activity of labile compounds.
For that reason thromboxane A_2 itself has not been tested,
and indeed the experimental data obtained with 13,14-dihydro,
15-keto PGE_2 must be viewed with the reservation that this
substance is chemically very unstable (Granstrom et al,
1980). However the equivalent metabolite of $PGF_{2\alpha}$ is much
less unstable, and oxidation of the 15-hydroxyl group of
that substance is also associated with marked loss of bone
resorbing activity. The very important labile prostanoid,
prostacyclin (PGI_2) has been shown by Raisz et al (1979) to
be produced by fetal rat long bones in culture and also to
stimulate resorption by those bones when synthetic prostacyclin was added at repeated intervals over a 24 hour
period. The nature of that experiment was such that it
was not possible to ascribe an accurate potency to prostacyclin, but it seems likely that it is less effective in
stimulating resorption than PGE_2. To the present time
there is no information relating to the effects of any
lipoxygenase products of arachidonic acid metabolism upon
bone resorption. This will be important to resolve
particularly if the major function of arachidonic acid
metabolites in bone is as locally active agents.

Indeed the lability of prostaglandins in the
circulation together with the fact that they are known to
be local mediators of physiological and pathological
effects in many tissues makes it likely that they are more
important in this regard in bone than they are as
circulating factors acting generally upon the skeleton to
promote resorption. The only good evidence for an
important role of circulating prostaglandins as mediators
of resorption effects on the whole skeleton comes from the
work of Tashjian and his colleagues, who have found that in
two animal models of malignant hypercalcemia, the $HSDM_1$
fibrosarcoma in the mouse (Tashjian et al, 1972) and the
VX_2 carcinoma in the rabbit (Voelkel et al, 1975) a
circulating prostaglandin is the major factor in mediating
the excessive bone resorption. A difficulty with this is
that very little PGE_2 circulates but there are large amounts
of 13,14-dihydro, 15-keto PGE_2 (Tashjian et al, 1977 a & b;
Seyberth et al, 1977), a relatively ineffective bone resorber. Furthermore the VX_2 carcinoma causes hypercalcemia
when transplanted subcutaneously, but not intraperitoneally
(Hubbard et al, 1980a), despite the fact that the PGE_2
metabolite levels are the same in the two situations. This

raises the possibility that some other arachidonic acid
metabolite may be responsible.   It might be relevant that
Hubbard et al (1980b) have discovered that lipoxygenation
of linoleic acid in VX_2 carcinoma homogenates provides
constant yields of a monohydroxy acid, which should be
investigated as a possible resorbing agent.

A number of agents have been shown to stimulate
resorption by a mechanism requiring the synthesis within
bone of prostaglandins.   Mergenhagen et al (1969) and
Hausmann et al (1972) demonstrated that complement could
resorb bone *in vitro*, and Raisz et al (1974) showed that
complement sufficient serum stimulated resorption and
prostaglandin production in fetal rat bone in culture.
Antibodies reacting with certain cell surface antigens and
able to activate complement (Sandberg et al, 1977) also
stimulate resorption, and experiments in the cat have shown
that immune complexes stimulate resorption by a prostaglandin dependent mechanism (Torbinejad et al, 1979).   Both
melittin, a peptide constituent of bee venom, and tumor
promoting phorbol diesters appear to resorb bone by a
prostaglandin mediated mechanism (Tashjian et al, 1978).
Epidermal growth factor (EGF) has been shown to have a
similar action in experiments with mouse calvaria (Tashjian
and Levine, 1978), but Raisz et al (1980) in demonstrating
a bone resorbing effect of EGF in fetal rat long bones found
that this effect did not require the synthesis of prostaglandins.   This discrepency is not yet resolved.   In
considering the involvement of prostaglandins in the pathogenesis of hypercalcemia in cancer it is possible that
humoral factors or immune processes resulting from certain
human cancers could stimulate bone resorption by mechanisms
requiring the synthesis within bone of prostaglandins
(Martin and Partridge, 1980).   Evidence consistent with
such a possibility is provided by the work of Minkin et al
(in press), who showed that extracts of hypercalcemic
cancers promoted bone resorption *in vitro* and that this
required intra-osseous synthesis of prostaglandins.

It may be that other agents also act upon bone by
mechanisms requiring the metabolism of arachidonic acid.
The application of more specific inhibitors of metabolic
pathways and of newer methods of analysis of these
metabolites will be helpful in this area.   Many experiments
in the past have relied upon the use of inhibitors of cyclo-
oxygenase, and this may explain some of the conflicting

results.   Thus for example Powles et al (1973) found that
aspirin inhibited resorption stimulated by parathyroid
hormone or PGE$_1$, an observation not substantiated by others.
Similarly the demonstration that prostaglandins mediate the
effect of collagenase on bone resorption (Dowsett et al,
1976) will require testing by more direct experiments.

PROSTAGLANDIN EFFECTS ON BONE CELLS

     While we and others were studying the effect of the
various prostaglandins, metabolites and analogues upon bone
resorption *in vitro* we were also investigating the regulation of cyclic nucleotide metabolism in a transplantable
osteogenic sarcoma in the rat which we showed to be a tumor
of cells which were of the osteoblast phenotype (Martin et
al, 1976;   Ingleton et al, 1977;   Martin et al, 1979).   In
this work we noted that the relative potencies of the
prostaglandins in stimulating either adenylate cyclase
activity in membrane preparations of the tumor or cyclic
AMP accumulation in isolated cells in experiments requiring
very short incubation periods closely parallelled their
relative potencies as stimulators of bone resorption (Atkins
and Martin, 1977;   Table 1).   This was despite the fact
that we were dealing with cells which were of the osteoblast
phenotype, and yet bone resorption effects are thought to
be due to the actions of resorbing hormones upon osteoclasts.
This led us to suspect that the osteoblast might be the
primary target of the bone resorbing hormones, and that the
osteoblasts might direct the resorbing activity of the
osteoclast.   On this basis we proposed (Crawford et al,
1978) that prostacyclin might be a bone resorbing factor,
but probably less potent than PGE$_2$, a prediction substantiated by Raisz et al, 1979.   Indeed in our subsequent work
with cell cultures established from the osteogenic sarcoma
and with clonal lines derived from it, enriched in the
osteoblast phenotype, and also in studies of osteoblast-
rich normal rat bone cells in culture (Partridge et al,
1981 a & b) we obtained further evidence that the relative
efficacies of prostanoids, their metabolites and analogues
upon cyclic AMP formation in osteoblasts resembled their
potencies as stimulators of resorption.   Moreover the
osteoblast-like cells, whether of benign or malignant type,
contained receptors or responses for the other bone
resorbing hormones, parathyroid hormone, 1,25(OH)$_2$- vitamin
D and epidermal growth factor (Partridge et al, 1980;   Ng

et al, in press).   There is not yet any evidence that any
of the bone resorbing hormones are capable of acting
<u>directly</u> upon the osteoclast.   Thus whether or not osteo-
clasts contain receptors for these hormones, the osteoblasts
clearly do, and the suggestion that osteoblasts mediate the
actions of resorbing hormones is a testable hypothesis
which fits with known facts about the cellular regulation of
bone resorption (Rodan and Martin, 1981;   Martin and
Partridge, 1981).

The cellular actions of PGE_2 upon the osteoblast
resemble those of parathyroid hormone.   Both PGE_2 and prostacyclin stimulate adenylate cyclase activity in osteoblasts,
with PGE_2 being more potent (Fig. 1) and each of these hormones rapidly activates cyclic AMP-dependent protein kinase.

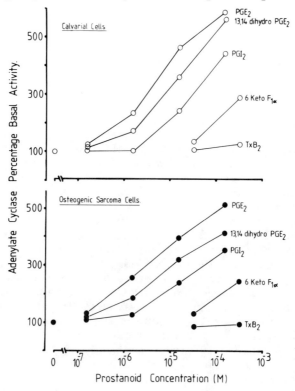

Figure 1.   Adenylate cyclase response to prostanoids in
bone cell and osteogenic sarcoma cell homogenates.
Reproduced with permission of the editors from Partridge
et al (1981a).

As with parathyroid hormone, the activation of protein kinase by prostaglandin requires only a small percentage of the generated cyclic AMP for its effect, the remainder being "spare" (Fig. 2).

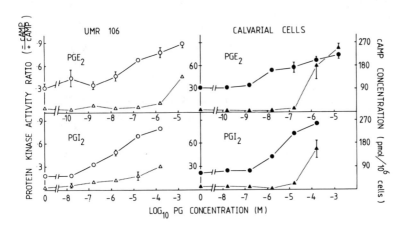

Figure 2.   Effect of increasing concentrations of PGE_2 and PGI_2 on cyclic AMP-dependent protein kinase activation and cyclic AMP concentrations in cloned osteoblast-like osteogenic sarcoma cells (UMR 106) and osteoblast-rich normal rat calvarial cells.   Cell samples were removed 1 min after addition of hormones for preparation of extracts for enzyme and cyclic AMP assay.   O, ●, protein kinase activity; Δ, ▲, cyclic AMP concentrations.

The nature of subsequent events in prostaglandin action upon osteoblasts is quite unknown, just as it is for parathyroid hormone.   The fact that PGE_2 is more effective than prostacyclin in stimulating cyclic AMP formation in osteoblasts suggests that the osteoblast does respond specifically to PGE_2 rather than to prostacyclin.   If it contained a genuine prostacyclin receptor, such as exists in e.g. the platelet, then it might be expected that the responsiveness to prostacyclin would be greater than that to PGE_2.   The fact that there is any response at all to prostacyclin may simply be due to a PGE_2-like agonist activity in that molecule.

ARACHIDONIC ACID METABOLISM IN BONE

The cyclooxygenase products of arachidonic acid
metabolism have been characterised in the clonal malignant
osteoblasts and in osteoblast-rich normal rat bone cells in
culture (Nolan et al, in press) and prostacyclin has been
shown to be the major product as measured by its stable
breakdown product 6-keto-PGF$_{1\alpha}$, with lesser amounts of PGE$_2$,
still less PGF$_{2\alpha}$ and no detectable thromboxane (Table 2).

TABLE 2. Cyclooxygenase products of arachidonic acid
metabolism in osteoblast-like cells.

Cells	Prostanoid Production (ng per 10^6 cells in 4h)			
	6-keto PGF$_{1\alpha}$	PGE$_2$	PGF$_{2\alpha}$	TxB$_2$
UMR 104	1.68	0.56	0.41	<0.05
UMR 105	0.95	1.39	0.68	<0.05
UMR 106	1.56	0.78	0.76	<0.05
UMR 108	2.11	0.63	0.11	<0.05
Osteoblast-rich calvarial cells	29.5	4.9	0.34	<0.05

Data from Nolan et al (in press).

In organ culture of resorbing mouse bone Voelkel et al
(1980) also found that prostacyclin was the major cyclo-
oxygenase product, but that most of the 6-keto PGF$_{1\alpha}$ was
metabolised further to 6,15-diketo PGF$_{1\alpha}$ at the end of 48
hour culture periods.   They also demonstrated PGE$_2$
production and significant amounts of thromboxane B$_2$.

The fact that the osteoblasts produce these metabolites
of arachidonic acid suggests that they are available either
for action upon other cells in bone or to act back on the
osteoblasts themselves (see Fig. 3), analogous with the
production by endothelial cells of prostacyclin which then
acts on the same cell (Hopkins and Gorman, 1981).   However
as discussed above, the nature of the response in osteoblasts indicates that this cell may not be specifically
responsive to prostacyclin.   The latter may have a separate
action in bone, perhaps upon vascular tissue as part of a
function in regulating bone blood flow, leaving PGE$_2$ to play

a part in the control of bone resorption.   Finally, it is possible that PGE_2 produced by the osteoblast exerts its local function in bone by acting directly upon the osteoclast.   We think that this is unlikely, but are unable to exclude the possibility with available methods.

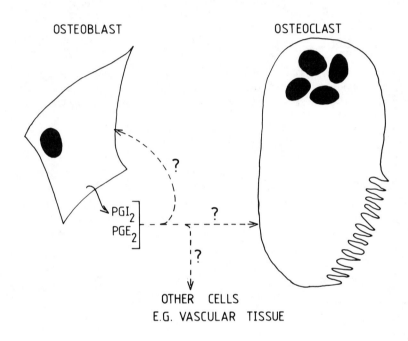

Figure 3.   Possible actions of prostaglandins produced by osteoblasts.

CONCLUSION

Thus metabolites of arachidonic acid are produced locally in bone, and they also act upon bone to cause it to resorb.   It seems likely that they are more important as local products than as humoral factors, and it is possible that arachidonic acid metabolites may have a part to play in normal bone remodelling.   Until now no information has been available on the lipoxygenase products of arachidonic acid metabolism, and it would be wise to consider this pathway in future studies of arachidonic acid and bone resorption, either because lipoxygenase products might influence formation of cyclooxygenase products or because they might influence resorption themselves. Certainly much direct and indirect evidence points to the likelihood of an important role for arachidonic acid metabolites in bone resorption in physiological and pathological states.

ACKNOWLEDGEMENTS

Work from the authors' laboratory was supported by grants from the Anti Cancer Council of Victoria and the Australian Government Department of Veterans' Affairs.

REFERENCES

Atkins D, Hunt NH, Ingleton PM, Martin TJ (1977). Rat osteogenic sarcoma cells. Isolation and effects of hormones on the production of cyclic AMP and cyclic GMP. Endocrinology 101:555.

Atkins D, Martin TJ (1977). Rat osteogenic sarcoma cells: effects of some prostaglandins, their metabolites and analogues on cyclic AMP production. Prostaglandins 13: 861.

Chase LR, Aurbach GD (1970). The effect of parathyroid hormone on the concentration of adenosine 3',5'-monophosphate in skeletal tissue, in $vitro$. J Biol Chem 245:1520

Crawford A, Atkins D, Martin TJ (1978). Rat osteogenic sarcoma cells: comparison of the effects of prostaglandin E_1, E_2, I_2 (prostacyclin), 6-keto $F_{1\alpha}$ and thromboxane B_2 on cyclic AMP production and adenylate cyclase activity. Biochem Biophys Res Commun 82:1195.

Dowsett M, Eastman AR, Easty DM, Easty GC, Powles TJ, Neville AM (1976). Prostaglandin mediation of collagenase-induced bone resorption. Nature 63:72.

Ferreira SH, Vane JR (1967). Prostaglandins, their disappearance from and release into the circulation. Nature 216:868.

Findlay DM, Michelangeli VP, Eisman JA, Frampton RJ, Moseley JM, MacIntyre I, Whitehead R, Martin TJ (1980). Calcitonin and 1,25-dihydroxyvitamin D_3 receptors in human breast cancer cell lines. Cancer Res 40:4764.

Franklin RB, Tashjian AH Jr (1975). Intravenous infusion of prostaglandin E_2 raises plasma calcium concentration in the rat. Endocrinology 97:240.

Granstrom E, Hamberg M, Hansson G, Kindahl H (1980).
Chemical instability of 15-keto-13,14-dihydro PGE_2: the
reason for low assay reliability. Prostaglandins 19:933.

Greaves M, Ibbotson KJ, Atkins D, Martin TJ (1980).
Prostaglandins as mediators of bone resorption in renal
and breast tumors. Clin Sci 58:210.

Hamberg M, Samuelsson B (1971). Metabolism of prostaglandin E_2 in guinea pig liver. J Biol Chem 246:1073

Hausmann E, Weinfeld E, Miller WA (1972). Effects of
lipopolysaccharides on bone resorption in tissue culture.
Calc Tiss Res 9:272.

Heersche JNM, Ng B (1978). Hormone specific suppression of
cyclic AMP responses in bone *in vitro*. In Copp DH,
Talmage RV (eds): "The Endocrinology of Calcium
Metabolism", Exc Med Int Congr Ser, p 270.

Hopkins NK, Gorman RR (1981). Regulation of endothelial
cell cyclic nucleotide metabolism by prostacyclin. J
Clin Invest 67:540.

Hubbard WC, Hough A, Johnson RM, Oates JA (1980a). The
site of VX_2 tumor transplantation affects the development
of hypercalcemia in rabbits. Prostaglandins 19:881.

Hubbard WC, Hough AJ Jr, Brash AR, Watson JT, Oates JA
(1980b). Metabolism of linoleic and arachidonic acids
in VX_2 carcinoma tissue: identification of monohydroxy
octadecadienoic acids and monohydroxy eicosatetraenoic
acids. Prostaglandins 20:431.

Hunt NH, Ellison M, Underwood JCE, Martin TJ (1977).
Calcitonin-responsive adenylate cyclase in a calcitonin-
producing human cancer cell line. Brit J Cancer 35:777.

Ingleton PM, Underwood JCE, Hunt NH, Atkins D, Giles B,
Coulton LA, Martin TJ (1977). Radiation induced
osteogenic sarcoma in the rat as a model of hormone-
responsive differentiated cancer. Lab Animal Sci 27:748.

Klein DC, Raisz LG (1970). Prostaglandins: stimulation
of bone resorption in tissue culture. Endocrinology 85:
657.

Klein DC, Raisz LG (1971). Role of adenosine-3'5'-mono-
phosphate in the hormonal regulation of bone resorption:
studies with cultured fetal bone. Endocrinology 89:818.

Luben RA, Wong GL, Cohn DV (1976). Biochemical
characterization with parathormone and calcitonin of
isolated bone cells; provisional identification of
osteoclasts and osteoblasts. Endocrinology 99:526.

McGiff JC, Terrange NA, Strand JC, Lee JB, Lonigro AJ, Ng
KK (1969). Selective passage of prostaglandins across
the lung. Nature 223:742.

Martin TJ, Ingleton PM, Underwood JCE, Michelangeli VP, Hunt NH, Melick RA (1976). Parathyroid hormone-responsive adenylate cyclase in induced transplantable osteogenic rat sarcoma. Nature 260:436.

Martin TJ, Ingleton PM, Coulton LA, Melick RA (1979). Metabolic properties of hormonally responsive osteogenic sarcoma cells. Clin Orthop Rel Res 140:247.

Martin TJ, Partridge NC (1980). Prostaglandins, cancer and bone: pharmacological considerations. Metab Bone Dis Rel Res 2:167.

Martin TJ, Partridge NC (1981). Initial events in the activation of bone cells by parathyroid hormone, prostaglandins and calcitonin. In Cohn DV, Talmage RV, Matthews JL (eds): "Hormonal Control of Calcium Metabolism", Int Congr Ser No. 511, Amsterdam, Oxford, Princeton, p 147.

Marx SJ, Aurbach GD, Gavin JR, Buell DW (1974). Calcitonin receptors on cultured human lymphocytes. J Biol Chem 249:6812.

Mergenhagen SE, Syderman R, Gewurz H, Shin HS (1969). Significance of complement to the mechanism of action of endotoxin. Current Topics in Microbiol Immunol 50:37.

Minkin C, Fredericks RS, Pokress S, Rude RK, Sharp CF Jr, Tong M, Singer FR (in press). Bone resorption and hypercalcemia of malignancy: stimulation of bone resorption *in vitro* by tumor extracts is inhibited by prostaglandin synthesis inhibitors. J Clin Endocrinol Metab.

Ng KW, Partridge NC, Niall M, Martin TJ. Epidermal growth factor receptors in clonal lines of a rat osteogenic sarcoma and in osteoblast-rich rat bone cells. (submitted for publication).

Nolan RD, Partridge NC, Godfrey HM, Martin TJ. Cyclo-oxygenase products of arachidonic acid metabolism in rat osteoblasts (submitted for publication).

Partridge NC, Frampton RJ, Eisman JA, Michelangeli VP, Elms E, Bradley TR, Martin TJ (1980). Receptors for $1,25(OH)_2$ - vitamin D_3 in cloned osteoblast-like rat osteogenic sarcoma cells. FEBS Lett 115:139.

Partridge NC, Alcorn D, Michelangeli VP, Kemp BE, Ryan GB, Martin TJ (1981a). Functional properties of hormonally responsive cultured normal and malignant rat osteoblastic cells. Endocrinology 108:213.

Partridge NC, Kemp BE, Veroni MC, Martin TJ (1981b). Activation of adenosine 3'5'-monophosphate-dependent protein kinase in normal and malignant bone cells by parathyroid hormone, prostaglandin E$_2$ and prostacyclin. Endocrinology 108:220.

Peck WA (1979). Cyclic AMP as a second messenger in the skeletal actions of parathyroid hormone: a decade-old hypothesis. Calc Tiss Int 29:1.

Piper PJ, Vane JR, Wyllie JH (1970). Inactivation of prostaglandins by the lung. Nature 225:600.

Powles TJ, Clark SA, Easty DM, Easty GC, Neville AM (1973). The inhibition by aspirin and indomethacin of osteolytic tumor deposits and hypercalcemia in rats with Walker tumor and its possible application to human breast cancer. Brit J Cancer 28:316.

Rao LG, Ng B, Brunette DM, Heersche JNM (1977). Parathyroid hormone- and prostaglandin E$_1$- response in a selected population of bone cells after repeated subculture and storage at -80°C. Endocrinology 100:1233.

Raisz LG, Sandberg AL, Goodson JM, Simmons HA, Mergenhagen SE (1974). Complement-dependent stimulation of prostaglandin synthesis and bone resorption. Science 185:789.

Raisz LG, Dietrich JW, Simmons JA, Seyberth HW, Hubbard E, Oates JA (1977). Effects of prostaglandin endoperoxides and metabolites on bone resorption *in vitro*. Nature 267:532.

Raisz LG, Vanderhoek JY, Simmons HA, Kream BE, Nicolau KC (1979). Prostaglandin synthesis by fetal rat bone *in vitro*: evidence for a role of prostacyclin. Prostaglandins 17:905.

Raisz, LG, Simmons HA, Sandberg AL, Canalis E (1980). Direct stimulation of bone resorption by epidermal growth factor. Endocrinology 107:270.

Robinson CJ, Parsons JA (1974). Lack of hypercalcaemia on infusing prostaglandin E$_2$ to rats argues against its suggested role in the "non-parathyroid hypercalcaemic tumour" syndrome. J. Endocrinology 64:14.

Rodan GA, Martin TJ (1981). Hormonal control of bone resorption - a hypothesis. Calc Tiss Int (in press).

Sandberg AL, Raisz LG, Goodson JM, Simmons HA, Mergenhagen SE (1977). Initiation of bone resorption by the classical and alternative complement pathways and its mediation by prostaglandins. J. Immunol 119:1378.

Schelling SH, Wolfe HJ, Tashjian AH Jr (1980). Role of the osteoclast in prostaglandin E$_2$-stimulated bone resorption. A correlative morphometric and biochemical analysis. Lab Invest 42:290.

Seyberth HW, Hubbard WC, Oelz O, Sweetman BJ, Watson JT, Oates JA (1977). Prostaglandin-mediated hypercalcemia in

the VX_2 carcinoma-bearing rabbit.   Prostaglandins 14:319.
Tashjian AH Jr, Voelkel EF, Levine L, Goldhaber P (1972).
Evidence that the bone resorption-stimulation factor
produced by mouse fibrosarcoma cells is prostaglandin E_2:
a new model for the hypercalcemia of cancer.   J Exp Med
136:1329.
Tashjian AH Jr, Voelkel EF, Levine L (1977a).   Plasma
concentrations of 13,14-dihydro-15-keto-prostaglandin E_2
in rabbits bearing the VX_2 carcinoma.   Effects of
hydrocortisone and indomethacin.   Prostaglandins 14:309.
Tashjian AH Jr, Tice JE, Sides R (1977b).   Biological
activities of prostaglandin analogues and metabolites on
bone in organ culture.   Nature 266:645.
Tashjian AH Jr, Levine L (1978).   Epidermal growth factor
stimulates prostaglandin production and bone resorption
in cultured mouse calvaria.   Biochem Biophys Res Commun
85:966.
Tashjian AH Jr, Ivey JL, Delclos B, Levine L (1978).
Stimulation of prostaglandin production in bone by phorbol
diesters and melittin.   Prostaglandins 16:221.
Teitelbaum SL, Kahn AJ (1980).   Mononuclear phagocytes,
osteoclasts and bone resorption.   Min Elec Metab 3:2.
Torbinejad M, Clagett J, Engel D (1979).   A cat model for
the evaluation of mechanisms of bone resorption;
induction of bone loss by stimulated immune complexes and
inhibition by indomethacin.   Cal Tiss Int 29:207.
Voelkel EF, Tashjian AH Jr, Franklin R, Wasserman E,
Levine L (1975).   Hypercalcemia and tumor-prostaglandins:
the VX_2 carcinoma model in the rabbit.   Metabolism 24:973.
Voelkel EF, Tashjian AH Jr, Levine L (1980).   Cyclo-
oxygenase products of arachidonic acid metabolism by
mouse bone in organ culture.   Biochim Biophys Acta 620:418.
Yoneda T, Mundy GR (1979).   Monocytes regulate osteoclast
activating factor production by releasing prostaglandins.
J Exp Med 150:338.

**Prostaglandins and Cancer: First
International Conference, pages 541-553**
© 1982 Alan R. Liss, Inc., 150 Fifth Avenue, New York, NY 10011

MECHANISMS FOR DEVELOPMENT OF BONE METASTASES AND EFFECTS OF
ANTI-INFLAMMATORY DRUGS.

T.J. Powles, J. Muindi, R.C. Coombes

Medical Breast Unit, Division of Medicine,
Royal Marsden Hospital,
Sutton, Surrey SM2 5PX, U.K.

The basic structure of bone consists of complexed
calcium phosphate crystals dispersed throughout an organic
collagen matrix. Osteolysis, an essential part of the
process of bone turnover, involves breakdown of both the
organic and mineral components by bone cells.

For example, parathyroid hormone (PTH) will cause
osteolysis by stimulating release of osteolytic lysosomal
enzymes and organic acids from osteocytes, followed by
recruitment of macrophage-like osteoclasts, which also
release osteolytic enzymes and acid, and can phagocytose
small pieces of bone to complete the solubilisation process
(Vaes, 1969).

Involvement of cyclic nucleotide metabolism in
mechanisms of osteolysis is supported by the observation
that PTH will stimulate adenyl cyclase and accumulation of
cAMP in bone (Chase et al, 1970) and exposure of bone
in vitro to low concentrations of the dibutyral derivative
of cAMP will cause osteolysis (Raisz and Klein, 1969).
Similarly, PGE will stimulate adenyl cyclase in bone
(Chase and Aurbach, 1970) and cause in vitro osteolysis
(Klein and Raisz, 1970) as will other PG's (Dowsett et al,
1976; Bennett et al, 1980).

The possibility that PG's may be involved in mechanisms
of osteolysis is suggested by the observed synthesis of PG's
by bone when stimulated by osteolytic agents such as
collagenase or complement (Raisz et al, 1974; Dowsett et al
1976). Aspirin will inhibit, in part, osteolysis stimulated

by collagenase (Powles et al, 1975) and PTH (Powles et al, 1973), although indomethacin seems unable to affect PTH stimulated osteolysis (Goldhaber and Rabadjijih, 1974).

The ability of bone metastases to develop in hard cortical bone depends, at least in part, on the ability of the tumour cells to release osteolytic substances and cause local destruction of bone (Powles et al, 1973) associated with pain, hypercalcaemia and hydroxyprolinuria (Powles, T.J., 1977). P.G. synthesis and release by tumour cells, which is generally more than for normal tissues (Sykes and Maddox, 1972; Levine et al, 1972; Thomas et al, 1974) may be involved in mechanisms for local osteolysis by developing bone metastases and some breast cancers particularly those from patients with bone metastases, can synthesize materials with PG-like biological activity in vitro (Bennett et al, 1975). Furthermore, it has been shown that 60% of human breast cancers can cause lysis of bone in organ culture (Powles, Dowsett, Easty et al, 1976) a property which is related to the ability of the tumours to release PG's and other non-dialisable osteolytic agents (Dowsett, Easty Powles et al, 1976).

In vitro PG synthesis and osteolysis by these tumours can be inhibited, in part, by drugs like aspirin and indomethacin as can in vitro osteolysis caused by the Walker rat tumour (Powles, Clark, Easty et al, 1973; Dowsett, Easty, Powles et al, 1976). Development of osteolytic bone metastases and hypercalcaemia caused by this tumour can be prevented by administration of aspirin, indomethacin or benorylate to the rats. Similarly, development of the osteolytic VX2 tumour in the rabbit femur can be inhibited by indomethacin provided it is given during the early phase of osteoclastic bone resorption stimulated by the tumour cells. Administration of the drug in the later non-osteoclastic phase fails to prevent further development. Mechanisms other than PG synthesis may be involved, because dosage of drug sufficient to inhibit the excessive PG production by the tumour in the early osteoclastic phase, is not sufficient to inhibit tumour development in bone which requires approximately twice this dose (Galasko and Bennett, 1976 Galasko, 1976).

To determine whether aspirin-like drugs could influence development of bone metastases we have given benorylate to patients with primary bad risk breast cancer. To examine the effect of anti-inflammatory drugs on osteolysis, we have given aspirin, indomethacin, flurbiprofen or benoxaprofen to patients with osteolytic bone metastases. To test whether anti-inflammatory drugs will influence the therapeutic effects of chemotherapy on bone metastases, we have given flurbiprofen to patients receiving this type of treatment.

PATIENTS AND METHODS

1. Primary breast cancer/benorylate trial

From January 1975 - August 1977, 160 patients with primary breast cancer who had an increased risk of relapse after mastectomy, either because of local lymph node metastases or anaplastic primary tumours were entered into the trial. They were stratified according to prognostic criteria and then randomised to receive either benorylate (Benoral, Winthrop) 4 gms (10 mls) twice per day, or placebo, for 18 months. All patients were clinically staged at the time of primary treatment and subsequently every six months, and were clinically reviewed at two month intervals between staging. None have been lost to follow up and all relevant data has been continually updated and stored on the PDP 11 computer data storage system at the Royal Marsden Hospital.

Early follow up results for this trial have previously been reported (Powles, Dady, Williams et al, 1980) and this paper will report the results of recent analysis (14/8/81).

2. Osteolytic bone metastases/anti-inflammatory studies

Twenty six patients with histologically confirmed breast cancer and radiological evidence of osteolytic bone metastases were studied for periods ranging from 5-51 days. Eight patients received soluble aspirin 2700 mg/day and indomethacin 75 mg/day, two received indomethacin 300mg per day, nine received flurbiprofen 300 mg/day and seven received benoxaprofen 300 mg/day.

Serum calcium and urinary hydroxyproline excretion (estimated as hydroxyproline, creatinine ratio) were estimated before and at weekly intervals during the studies. Pain and analgesic requirements were assessed weekly by an independent observer. All patients had previously received endocrine or chemotherapy but not for at least four weeks before these studies commenced. Paracetamol or opiates were used for pain control, and these analgesic requirements were taken into consideration for assessment of pain relief by the agents under study.

3. Chemotherapy/flurbiprofen trial

All patients with assessable metastases or locally advanced breast cancer with a life expectancy greater than 3 months and who have not previously received chemotherapy were considered eligible for this trial. Patients were treated with adriamycin 40mg/M^2 and vindesine 3 mg/M^2 or vincristine 1.4mg/M^2 on days 1 and 8 of a 28 day cycle. They also received either flurbiprofen 100mg t.d.s. or placebo for at least two weeks of each cycle. Between 1/4/79 and 1/4/81, 101 patients were randomised, 96 of whom are assessable for toxicity and 83 for response (according to UICC criteria).

The preliminary results of this trial will be presented in this paper, although more patients with a longer follow up time are necessary for proper assessment of effect.

RESULTS

1. Primary breast cancer/Benorylate trial

We have previously reported the early follow up data of this trial which showed that benorylate had no effect on the rate of development of bone metastases after primary treatment of 'poor-risk' breast cancer, even though the benorylate patients had sufficient medication to reduce plasma thromboxane B$_2$ to very low levels (Powles, Dady, Williams et al, 1980).

These results have been confirmed in this later analysis. The rate of development of bone metastases, any metastases and overall survival is the same for the patients who received benorylate or placebo (Figures 1, 2 and 3).

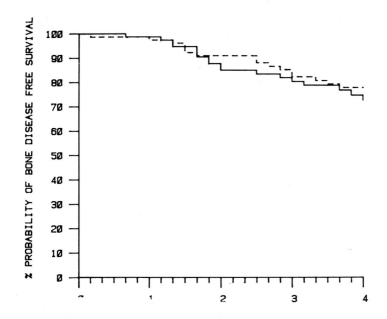

<u>Figure 1.</u> Probability of developing bone metastases after
primary treatment of breast cancer for 160 patients
who received benorylate 4 gms per day (——) or
placebo (---).

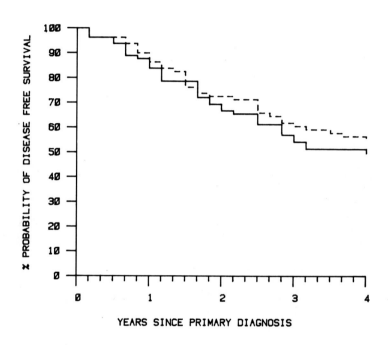

Figure 2. Probability of developing any metastases after primary treatment of breast cancer for 160 patients who received benorylate 4 gms per day (———) or placebo (———).

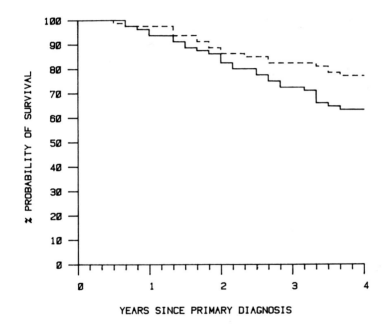

<u>Figure 3.</u> Probability of survival after primary treatment
of breast cancer for 160 patients who received
benorylate 4 gms per day (——) or placebo (---).

2. Osteolytic bone metastases/anti-inflammatory studies

The results are summarised in Table 1. Although aspirin/indomethacin, flurbiprofen and benoxaprofen relieved bone pain in some patients, they generally were unable to influence osteolysis. Serum calcium was significantly but not markedly reduced in two patients who had flurbiprofen and one who had benoxaprofen. Growth of soft tissue metastases remained clinically unaffected by these agents.

TABLE 1. The effects of administration of anti-inflammatory agents to patients with osteolytic bone metastases.

	Indomethacin 75 - 300 mg (2) $^+/_-$ Aspirin 2700 mg/day (8)	Flurbiprofen 300 mg/day	Benoxaprofen 300 mg/day
No.of patients	10	9	7
No. with hypercalcaemia	4	4	2
Duration of treatment	5 - 8	21 - 28	8 - 51
Reduction in bone pain	2/10	2/9	2/7
Reduction in serum calcium	0/4	2/4	1/2
Reduction in OHP	0/10	2/8	0/5
Radiological sclerosis	0/10	0/7	0/7

3. Chemotherapy/Flurbiprofen Trial

Early follow up data indicates that flurbiprofen failed to influence the response rate of bone or other metastases to chemotherapy (Table 2). The median survival of patients who received flurbiprofen with chemotherapy (10.2 months) was the same as for those patients who had placebo with chemotherapy (10.6 months) (p = 0.76). Although generally toxicity for the two groups of patients was similar leucopenia and peripheral neuropathy occurred less frequently in the flurbiprofen group (Table 3) even though dosage of chemotherapy for these two groups was the same. (Table 4).

TABLE 2 Response of metastatic breast cancer to Vinca/ adriamycin chemotherapy with flurbiprofen (VAF) or Placebo (VAP)

		Objective response	Stabilisation	Progressive Disease
All sites	VAF (43)	23	8	12
	VAP (40)	24	5	11
Bone	VAF (9)	3	4	2
	VAP (11)	1	4	6

TABLE 3. Toxicity of Vinca/adriamycin chemotherapy with flurbiprofen (VAF) or placebo (VAP)

	VAP (45)	VAF (51)
Leucopenia 3,000	29 (64%)	21 (41%)
Thrombocytopenia 100,000	5 (11%)	4 (7%)
Nausea/Vomiting	28 (62%)	22 (40%)
Peripheral neuropathy	28 (62%)	21 (41%)

TABLE 4. Dosage of adriamycin used in Vinca/adriamycin combination with flurbiprofen (VAF) or placebo (VAP)

	VAF	VAP
No. of patients	51	45
(1) ADRIAMYCIN		
Total dose/patient	438	415
Dose/injection	48.3	47.1
Total dose/patient (1st 2 courses)	170	189
(2) VINCRISTINE		
Total dose/patient (1st 2 courses)	5.8	6.1
(3) VINDESINE		
Total dose/patient (1st 2 courses)	15.16	17.35

DISCUSSION

Although experimental data indicates that anti-inflammatory drugs will inhibit tumour osteolysis, we have failed to show similar effects in patients with cancer. Benorylate given for 18 months to patients with primary breast cancer failed to influence subsequent development of bone metastases. It is possible that this medication although sufficient to reduce plasma TxB_2 levels was insufficient to inhibit local tumour P.G. synthesis. Alternatively, as indicated in the Vx2 tumour experiments of Galasko, higher dosages than are necessary to inhibit PG synthesis are required to prevent development of osteolytic bone deposits (Galasko, Rawlins and Bennett, 1979). Alternatively, the different rates of growth and development of experimental osteolytic tumour deposits transplanted directly into bone may bear little resemblance to development of bone metastases in patients with cancer and therefore successful therapy in animals may be inappropriate for man.

In patients with established bone metastases, the failure to influence osteolysis with anti-inflammatory drugs may relate to the extent of disease. It has been shown with the VX2 tumour that although anti-inflammatory drugs will inhibit the early development of osteolysis, the later more extensive non-osteoclastic phase is unaffected by these agents (Galasko and Bennett, 1976). Similarly, administration of flurbiprofen with chemotherapy failed to improve the response of bone or other metastases or improve survival. However, the number of patients with bone metastases is small at present and further follow up of more patients is required.

In conclusion, it is disappointing that we have failed to confirm in patients with cancer, the experimental findings that anti-inflammatory drugs will inhibit development of bone metastases. Whether higher doses, or combinations with other anti-osteolytic agents such as mithramycin, diphosphonates or calcitonin will have significant anti-osteolytic effects on established bone metastases remains to be seen.

REFERENCES

Bennett A, Edwards D, Ali N, Auger D, Harris M (1980)
Advances in Prostaglandin and Thromboxane Research 6, 547.

Bennett A, McDonald AM and Simpson JS (1975)
Lancet 1, 1218.

Chase LR, and Aurbach GD (1970)
J. Biol. Chem. 245, 1520.

Dowsett M, Easty GC, Powles TJ, Easty D and Neville AM (1976)
Prostaglandins 11, 447.

Dowsett M, Eastman AR, Easty DM, Easty GC, Powles TJ (1976)
Nature 263, 72.

Galasko CSB (1976)
Nature 263, 507

Galasko, CSB and Bennett A (1976)
Nature 263, 508

Galasko, CSB, Rawlins R, and Bennett A (1979)
Br. J. Cancer 40, 360.

Galasko CSB (1981)
Clin.Orth. Related Res. 155, 269.

Galasko CSB, Rawlins R and Bennett A (1979)
Br. J. Cancer 40, 360.

Galasko CSB (1981)
Clin Orth. Related Res. 155, 269.

Goldhaber P and Rabadjijeg L (1974)
J. Dent Res. 53, 139

Klein DG and Raisz LG (1970)
Endocrinology 86, 1436.

Powles TJ (1975)
Ph.D. Thesis, University of London.

Powles TJ, Easty GC. Easty GC, Bondy PK and Neville AM (1973)
Nature 245, 83.

Powles, TJ Clark SA, Easty DM, Easty GC, and Neville AM (1973)
B.J. Cancer 28, 316.

Powles TJ (1977)
In Secondary Spread in Breast Cancer. Ed. BA Stoll,
Pub. Heinemann pp 81-93.

Powles TJ, Dowsett M, Easty GC, Easty DM and Neville AM (1976)
Lancet 1, 508.

Powles TJ, Dady PJ, Williams J, Easty GC, Coombes RC (1980)
Adv. in Prostaglandin and Thromboxane Res.

Raisz LG and Klein DG (1969)
Fed. Proc. 28, 320.

Raisz LG (1974)
Science 185, 789.

Sykes JAC and Maddox IS (1972)
Nature N.B. 237, 59.

Thomas DR, Philpott GW, Jaffe BM (1974)
Expl. Cell Res. 84, 40.

Vaes G (1969).
In Lysosomes in Biology and Pathology Vol 1, p 217,
North Holland, Amsterdam.

ACKNOWLEDGEMENTS

We thank the Boots Company for their help with the
flurbiprofen studies, Eli Lilly for their help with the
Benoxaprofen study, Sterling Winthrop for their help with
the benorylate study and Dr. J. Milan for computer and
statistical services at the Royal Marsden Hospital/Institute
of Cancer Research.

Prostaglandins and Cancer: First
International Conference, pages 555-559
© 1982 Alan R. Liss, Inc., 150 Fifth Avenue, New York, NY 10011

LYMPHOKINE MEDIATED BONE RESORPTION REQUIRES PROSTAGLANDIN
SYNTHESIS

R.S. Bockman

Memorial Sloan-Kettering Cancer Center

]275 York Avenue, New York, New York, 10021

Localized bone loss can be associated with certain
inflammatory, hypermetabolic and neoplastic diseases. The
pathogenesis of osteolytic lesions in most of the latter
conditions has not been elucidated. Recent studies have
identified immune cell derived factors as possible mediators
of bone resorption in such diverse pathological conditions
as osteomyelitis (Corbett et al., 1979), gingivitis (Goldhaber, 1971; Goodson et al., 1974), multiple myeloma and
certain lymphomas (Mundy et al., 1974a, 1974b). Lymphocytes
from normal individuals have been shown to release factor(s)
with osteolytic activity (Horton et al., 1972). One lymphokine, osteoclast activating factor (OAF), a product of T or
B lymphocytes, has in part been chemically characterized
(Horton et al., 1974; Chen et al., 1976; Luben et al., 1974;
Mundy et al., 1977). Bioassays have not been able to distinguish osteoclast-mediated bone resorption initiated by
parathyroid hormone (PTH) from that caused by OAF. Both
agents cause the release of calcium from bone with similar
dose dependency curves (Bockman & Myers, 1977), both cause
osteoclast activation as measured by increased cell number
and size (Holtrop & Raisz, 1979), and both agents activate
adenylate cyclase in bone cells (Aurbach & Chase, 1970;
Luben et al., 1979). We therefore decided to look more
closely at the sequence of biochemical events which occurs
during lymphokine-mediated bone resorption. In particular,
we examined endogenous bone synthesis and release of prostaglandins following exposure to a lymphokine preparation
prepared from lymphocyte conditioned media of normal subjects
in the presence of phytohemagglutinin or media conditioned
by malignant B cells derived from a patient with a non-Hodgkin

lymphoma. This latter patient had accelerated bone loss
manifested by progressive osteoporosis and hypercalciuria.

Lymphokine preparations prepared from normal lymphocytes as well as the malignant lymphocytes caused the prompt
release of tritiated PGE_2 from fetal rat bones that had been
prelabelled with tritiated arachidonic acid. By 2-D thin
layer chromatography, PGE_2 was clearly the major product of
bone cyclooxygenase. A dose dependent increase in PGE_2
release was seen when increasing amounts of lymphokine were
added to bone cultures, table 1.

Table 1

Bone release of Prostaglandin E [1]

	Amount[2]	ngPGE released/bone[3]	P[4]
Lymphocyte conditioned media			
—	0.1ml	2.8 ± 0.2	0.001
—	0.2ml	3.6 ± 0.8	0.001
—	0.3ml	4.8 ± 0.6	0.001
—	0.4ml	12.6 ± 1.2	0.001
Parathyroid hormone			
—	0.01uM	0.9 ± 0.1	NS
—	1.0uM	1.3 ± 0.2	NS
—	10.0uM	1.3 ± 0.2	NS
Control	0	0.9 ± 0.1	—

1) Prostaglandin E release from individual fetal rat bones measured by radioimmunoassay.

2) Amount of test substance added (conditioned media from 5 million cells/ml or final molar concentration of PTH).

3) Mean ± SEM, n=4. For the control bones, n=16.

4) Significance of the difference compared to controls determined by the two tailed t-test.

No increase in bone PGE synthesis was noted when increasing concentrations of parathyroid hormone (0.1 to 10 μM) were tested. Both lymphokine and PTH were found to cause similar dose dependent curves of calcium release when bones that had been labelled with ^{45}Ca in utero were examined. The release of ^{45}Ca from the explanted bones in response to lymphokine occurred after the burst release of PGE_2. Inhibitors of cyclooxygenase abrogated lymphokine mediated ^{45}Ca release, table 2. by control bones.

Table 2		
Inhibition of lymphokine induced bone resorption [1]		
Concentration(μM)[2]	ngPGE release/bone	E/C [3]
0	22.6 + 4.3	1.38 + .11
0.1	21.6 + 8.8	1.44 + 0.07
1.0	1.86 + 0.45	0.91 + 0.07
10.0	0.67 + .09	0.89 + 0.08

1) 0.3ml of lymphocyte conditioned media was added to all test bone cultures and PGE levels measured by radioimmunoassay. PGE release by control bones that had not received lymphocyte conditioned media was 3.2 + 0.7 ngPGE/bone. Each data point represents the mean + SEM, n=4.

2) Concentration of the cyclooxygenase inhibitor flurbiprofen in bone culture.

3) E/C = cpm of ^{45}Ca released from test bones/cpm of ^{45}Ca released by control bones.

These same inhibitors had no effect on PTH induced bone ^{45}Ca release. These data suggest that PTH and lymphokine induced bone resorption follow distinct biochemical pathways; lymphokine mediated bone resorption appears to require endogenous bone PGE synthesis while PTH induced resorption does not. The bone resorbing activity that was derived from the malignant cells of the patient with non Hodgkin's lymphoma had many physical properties in common with that of OAF; in addition, the activity induced bone PGE synthesis. Bone resorption induced by this agent could be blocked by inhibitors of PG synthesis.

Others have shown that the secretion of OAF requires endogenous synthesis of PGE (Yoneda & Mundy, 1979). Our data would suggest that bone responds to lymphokine administration by synthesizing PGE. Such a response may represent an example of positive feedback that amplifies lymphokine release. Endogenous bone PGE production may also serve to initiate the sequence of biochemical events, e.g. the release of enzymes necessary for osteolysis.

References

Aurbach, G.D. and L.R. Chase. 1970. Cyclic 3'5' Adenylic Acid in bone and the mechanism of action of parathyroid hormone. Fed. Proc. 29 :1179-1182.

Bockman, R.S. and W.P.L. Myers. 1977. Osteotropism of human breast cancer.
In Cancer Invasion and Metastasis: Biologic Mechanisms and Therapy. S.B. Day et al., editors. Raven Press, New York, 431.

Corbett, M., S. Dekel, B. Puddle, R.A. Dickson and M.J.O. Francis. 1979. The production of prostaglandins in response to experimentally induced osteomyelitis in rabbits. Prostaglandins and Medicine. 2 :403.

Goldhaber, P. 1971. Tissue culture studies of bone as a model system for periodontal research. J. Dent. Res. 50 :278.

Goodson, J.M., F.E. Dewhirst and A. Brunetti. 1974. Prostaglandin E_2 levels in human periodontal disease. Prostaglandins. 6 :81-85.

Horton, J.E., L.G. Raisz, H.A. Simmons, J.J. Oppenheim and D.N. Buell. S.E. Mergenhagen. 1972. Bone resorbing activity in supernatant fluid from cultured human peripheral blood leukocytes. Science. 177 :793-795.

Luben, R.A., M.C-Y. Chen, D.M. Rosen and M.A. Mohler. 1979. Effects of osteoclast activating factor from human lymphocytes on cyclic AMP concentrations in isolated mouse bone and bone cells. Calcif. Tis. Int. 28 :23-32.

Mundy, G.R., L.G. Raisz, R.A. Cooper, G.P. Schecter and S.E. Salmon. 1974. Evidence for the secretion of an osteoclast stimulating factor in myeloma. N. Engl. J. Med. 291 :1041-1046.

Mundy, G.R., R.A. Luben, L.G. Raisz, J.J. Oppenheim and D.N. Buell. 1974. Bone resorbing activity in supernatants from lymphoid cell lines. N. Engl. J. Med. 290 :867-871.

Yoneda, T. and G.R. Mundy. 1979. Monocytes regulate osteoclast-activating factor by releasing prostaglandins. J. Exp. Med. 150 :338-350.

Acknowledgments:

This work was supported in part by grants CA 23500 from the National Institutes of Health and a Thomas Nichol, Jr. Memorial Grant for Cancer Research from the American Cancer Society.

**Prostaglandins and Cancer: First
International Conference, pages 561–565**
© **1982 Alan R. Liss, Inc., 150 Fifth Avenue, New York, NY 10011**

MORPHOLOGICAL PATTERNS OF BONE DESTRUCTION BY INFILTRATING
TUMOURS

R.L. Carter

Haddow Laboratories, Royal Marsden Hospital, Sutton, Surrey,
United Kingdom.

There is some evidence from clinical material that bone invasion by metastatic
tumour is a biphasic process, partly mediated by osteoclasts. The original studies[1,2] were
based on vertebrae from a series of autopsies performed on patients with various disseminated malignancies. Morphological evidence of a two-stage process of bone destruction is not readily confirmed in the usual range of tumour material submitted to the
surgical pathologist, and the histological patterns of bone destruction in cancer patients
is not well documented. Studies of *direct* bone invasion by squamous carcinomas of the
head and neck have, however, provided a useful model for examining both the patterns
and mechanisms[3–7] of bone destruction in man.

MATERIALS AND METHODS

22 tumours invading local bone were studied in detail from a series of 200 consecutive
major surgical resections. The tissues were decalcified in 10% formic acid and then
processed, cut and stained by standard procedures.

RESULTS

The sites of the primary tumours, the numbers invading bone and the bones involved
are shown in Table 1.

SITES OF PRIMARY TUMOUR	NOS.	BONES INVOLVED
Buccal cavity	14	Mandible, Maxilla
Paranasal sinuses	6	Maxilla, Nasal, Zygoma
nasal cavity		Frontal, Ethmoids
Miscellaneous		
External auditory meatus	1	Temporal, Zygoma
Lacrimal sac	1	Lacrimal, Nasal, Ethmoids

The main route of access is by direct spread from the adjacent primary lesion or from a contiguous nodal mass. Infiltration of perineural spaces is an important mode of indirect spread at some sites. In all instances the pattern of spread into the bone is *OUTWARDS →INWARDS* — the reverse of true metastatic bone disease.

The invasive process is conveniently considered in three stages (Figs. 1 to 3).

Breaching of Periosteum.

The normally smooth bone-soft tissue interface is variably distorted by local inflammation, fibrosis, and subperiosteal new bone formation. Tumour cells spreading onto these roughened regions gain access to the outermost cortical layer, often following the course of small blood vessels.

Stimulation of Osteoclasts.

Local osteoclastic activation is seen as soon as tumour cells are lodged in the bone cortex, and this reaction increases progressively in the deeper parts of the cortex and (particularly) around bone trabeculae. Large numbers of osteoclasts erode bone *in front of* the advancing tumour, a spatial relationship which is consistently maintained. There is a parallel, smaller increase in osteoblasts with some laying down of osteoid and new bone; this response is most marked in association with slowly invading tumours.

Destruction by Tumour Cells Alone.

Osteoclasts eventually disappear and tumour cells are now seen in direct contact with eroding bone substance.

The three stages described here form a continuous process and they may co-exist in different parts of the same involved bone. An identical sequence of events occurs when squamous carcinomas invade the foci of *metaplastic* bone which regularly develop in the larynx — a feature observed in 32 out of the first 60 consecutive laryngectomies in the present series.

DISCUSSION

These results show that osteoclasts are a prominent feature in bone invaded by squamous carcinomas of the head and neck. There is no evidence that the morphological findings are modified by previous radiotherapy or chemotherapy as appearances were similar in patients treated by surgery alone. Local infection at the time of operation cannot be implicated as no pathogenic micro-organisms were grown from swabs taken routinely from all the freshly excised tumours.

The consistency of the morphological changes described here can be adequately explained. Invasion of bones such as the mandible and maxilla can usually be detected at a relatively early stage, and the pathologist often has the opportunity to examine relatively early lesions, completely excised, in which osteoclasts are still a major feature. By contrast, distant skeletal deposits will often have been present for indeterminate

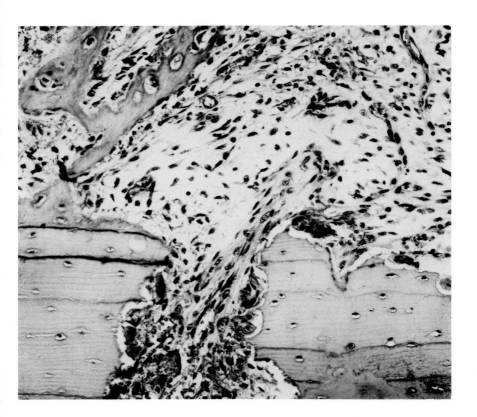

Fig. 1. Bone-soft tissue interface. The bone surface is irregular and the soft tissues are inflamed and fibrotic. Squamous carcinoma cells are infiltrating through a deficiency in the bone surface: the edges are scalloped and lined by multinucleate osteoclasts. H&E X240.

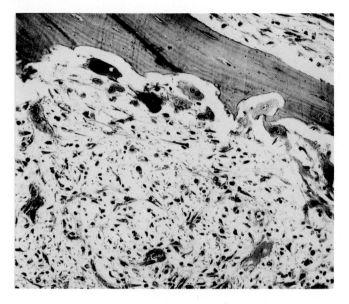

Fig. 2. A line of multinucleated osteoclasts is eroding bone in front of the irregular advancing edge of a squamous carcinoma. H&E ×300.

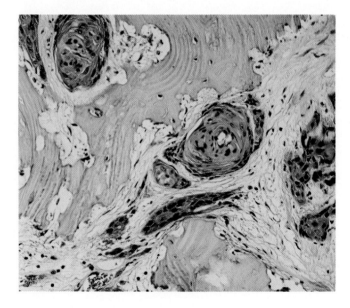

Fig. 3. Bone trabeculae invaded by squamous carcinoma. Note that osteoclasts are no longer present. H&E ×240.

periods of time and are likely to be sampled only by one small biopsy to confirm the diagnosis.

The importance of the time-factor in the sequential changes associated with bone destruction is borne out when the previous literature is assessed. Earlier clinical studies, usually based on autopsy material, regarded the osteoclast as an incrustant feature playing little or no part in bone resorption[8,9]. Contemporary experimental investigations, in which tumour fragments were implanted directly into marrow spaces, came to similar conclusions[10]. Only when these experiments were repeated and the early stages (during the first 2 weeks) were examined, was it apparent that a phase of osteoclastic resorption was a regular initial feature of tumour-associated bone destruction[11,12].

REFERENCES

1. Galasko, G.S.B. 1976. Mechanisms of bone destruction in the development of skeletal metastases. *Nature* 263, 507–508.
2. Galasko, C.S.B. 1975. The pathological basis for skeletal scintigraphy. *Journal of Bone and Joint Surgery* 57B, 353–359.
3. Carter, R.L., Tanner, N.S.B., Clifford, P., Shaw, H.J. 1980. Direct bone invasion by squamous carcinomas of the head and neck: a clinopathological study. *Clinical Otolaryngology* 5, 107–116.
4. Carter, R.L., Tanner, N.S.B. 1979. Local invasion by laryngeal carcinoma – the importance of focal (metaplastic) ossification within laryngeal cartilage. *Clinical Otolaryngology* 4, 283–290.
5. Carter, R.L., Pittam, M.R. 1980. Squamous carcinomas of the head and neck: some patterns of spread. *Journal of the Royal Society of Medicine* 73, 420–427.
6. Bennett, A., Carter, R.L., Stamford, I.F., Tanner, N.S.B. 1980. Prostaglandin-like material extracted from squamous carcinomas of the head and neck. *British Journal of Cancer* 41, 204–208.
7. Tsao, S-W., Burman, J.F., Easty, D.M., Easty, G.C., Carter, R.L. 1980. Some mechanisms of local bone destruction by squamous carcinomas of the head and neck. *British Journal of Cancer* 43, 392–401.
8. Milch, R.A., Changus, G.W. 1956. Response of bone to tumour invasion. *Cancer* 9, 340–351.
9. Jaffe, H.L. 1958. Tumors and tumorous conditions of the bones and joints. C.V. Mosby, Philadelphia.
10. Shivas, A.A., Black, J.W., Finlayson, N.D. 1963. The growth of Brown-Pearce carcinoma in the medullary cavity of the rabbit femur. *British Journal of Cancer* 17, 711–714.
11. Hulth, A., Olerud, S. 1965. The reaction of bone to experimental cancer. *Acta Orthopaedica Scandinavica* 36, 230–240.
12. Faccini, J.M. 1974. The mode of growth of experimental metastases in rabbit femora. *Virchow's Archives (A). Pathological anatomy and histology* 364, 249–263.

**Prostaglandins and Cancer: First
International Conference, pages 567–572**
© **1982 Alan R. Liss, Inc., 150 Fifth Avenue, New York, NY 10011**

IN VITRO PROSTAGLANDIN PRODUCTION BY METASTATIC BREAST
CANCER

G.N. Hortobagyi, P. Schultz, R. Cailleau,
N. Samaan, and G. Blumenschein

The University of Texas System Cancer Center
M.D. Anderson Hospital and Tumor Institute
Houston, Texas   77030

INTRODUCTION

More than 70% of patients presenting with stage IV
breast cancer exhibit osseous metastasis. This incidence
may be even higher in autopsy series. Prostaglandins (PG),
especially the E_2 subgroup, have been implicated in the
osteolytic process by in vitro experiments with a variety
of tumors and especially with breast cancer (1,2). PG-
mediated immunosuppression also has been described (3), and
it is of interest since immunosuppression is directly related to the extent of metastatic disease and inversely
correlated with response to therapy and length of survival
(4). Because PG production seems related to common clinical
problems, we evaluated the ability to produce PG of a number
of long-term metastatic breast cancer cell cultures. The
main questions asked were: Do metastatic breast cancer
cells produce PG? Can PG production be inhibited in vitro?
Does PG production by metastatic breast cancer correlate
with known prognostic factors?

METHODS

One of the authors (RC) has established 21 long term
cell cultures of metastatic breast cancer (5). These lines
came from 20 patients, the tumor of one patient giving rise
to two different cell lines. Eighteen cell lines were
established from malignant pleural effusions, while three
were established from solid metastasis. The cell lines were
grown in different culture media, depending on the particular needs of each cell line, as shown in Table 1. Cells

Table 1. PROSTAGLANDIN CONCENTRATIONS IN
CULTURE MEDIA

			PG Concentration (pg/ml)
I. Medium: L-15A			5.4
Cell lines:	MDA 309		140
	MDA 175		60
	MDA 415		480
II. Medium: L-15 10% FCS			27
Cell lines:	MDA 469		380
	MDA 461	P-38	3000
	MDA 461	P-43	100
	MDA 453		54
	MDA 436		9
	MDA 431		<1.25
	MDA 361		71
	MDA 330		120
	MDA 231		1100
III. Medium: L-15 10% REHA			52
Cell lines:	MDA 435		70
	MDA 331		140
	MDA 157		100
IV. Medium: CIGC			88
Cell lines:	MDA 470		520
	MDA 468		100
	MDA 416		470
	MDA 411		155
	MDA 390		170
	MDA 134		470

were grown in flasks until confluent growth was observed
(from three to seven days) and then were subcultured to
allow continued growth.

Thirteen of the 18 original pleural effusions from
which the long-term cell line cultures originated had been

stored and aliquots of these effusions were evaluated for PG concentrations.

Culture media samples were obtained at the time confluent growth of cells was observed. Fresh culture medium was used as control. A double antibody radioimmunoassay was used for PG determination (6). Duplicate samples were run for each cell line and pleural effusion.

The clinical characteristics of the patients from whom the original tumor samples were obtained were analyzed in an attempt to find correlations with the ability to produce PG.

RESULTS

PGE$_2$ concentrations in fresh media and each one of the media used to culture 21 cell lines are shown in Table 1. Analysis of the prognostic factors and the correlation with PG concentration were also performed. The numbers of patients are small; therefore, firm correlations are not possible. There is no significant difference in the ability to produce PG by age, menopausal status, race, family history, stage at diagnosis, disease-free interval, survival, alkaline phosphatase level, or distribution of metastatic sites. It is also of note that the four patients whose tumors did not produce PG in culture did have osseous metastasis.

However, there were minor trends suggesting that patients who were postmenopausal with positive family history of breast cancer, a disease-free interval longer than three years, an overall survival from diagnostic greater than five years, and normal alkaline phosphatase had a higher probability of having PG-producing tumors.

The PG concentrations in the original pleural effusions from which the cell lines were established are shown in Table 2. For comparative purposes, the PG concentrations of culture media of the corresponding cell line cultures are also shown in the same table. All 13 effusions examined contained a high concentration of PG. By contrast, two of the 12 corresponding cell lines analyzed failed to produce PG in culture.

Table 2: PG CONCENTRATIONS IN PLEURAL FLUID

Cell Line	PG Concentration (pg/ml)	
	Pleural Fluid	Culture Medium
MDA 134	2000	470
253	1240	ND
309	550	140
331	860	140
390	2000	170
411	640	155
415	2000	480
416	1480	470
431	500	<1.25
435	1260	70
436	270	9
468	2000	100
469	160	380

The next step was to inhibit PG synthesis in vitro by incubating the cell lines with either indomethacin or Ibuprofen. The five cell lines shown in Table 3 were chosen because of the rapid growth characteristics and not necessarily because of the high PG concentrations in the media. Three cell lines (231, 435, and 469) did have a significant PG concentration at the initiation of the experiment. The addition of 1 or 3 μg/ml of indomethacin substantially decreased the PG concentration for two of the three cell lines. Similarly, Ibuprofen inhibited PG production in two of three PG-producing cell lines. No clear dose response was observed.

Table 3. IN VITRO PG SYNTHESIS INHIBITION

Cell Line	PG Concentration (pg/ml)				
	Control Medium Without Inhibitor	Indomethacin 1 µg	3 µg	Ibuprofen 1 µg	3 µg
231	1100	605	275	1224	--
435	290	--	53	--	110
436	12	--	2.9	--	8.0
461	<1.25	<1.25	<1.25	1.8	3.2
469	380	380	167	101	101

COMMENT

Our results suggest that malignant cells found in malignant pleural effusions from breast cancer produce high amounts of PG. Since all 13 pleural effusions were from tumors that survived under in vitro conditions, this might represent a self-selected population. It remains to be established that their ability to produce PG is a universal property of metastatic breast cancer or a biologic characteristic of a small subgroup. It was of interest to note that not all cell lines produced the high concentrations of PG expected based on the PG concentrations of pleural fluid. This might be explained by different stimulatory or inhibitory factors in the pleural effusion and the culture medium, or the possibility that other cells contained in the pleural effusion might have contributed to PG production. The interesting trends in the clinical prognostic factor analysis suggest that breast cancer cells with a more benign biologic behavior are able to produce PG more often than tumors with a more malignant clinical course. One might hypothesize that the ability to produce PG is related to the degree of differentiation of tumors.

These preliminary experiments show that PG production by metastatic breast cancer cells can be inhibited in vitro by known PG synthetase inhibitors. More extensive studies need to be performed to establish the optimal dose as well as the drug of choice. Finally, in vivo measurement of PG production in patients with different stages of breast cancer is a logical next step. Correlations with known clinical factors might follow as well as therapeutic intervention if prostaglandin production is indeed positively correlated with poor prognosis, i.e., immunosuppression or osteolysis.

REFERENCES

1. Coombes RC, Neville AM, Gazet JC, et al (1979). Agents affecting osteolysis in patients with breast cancer. Cancer Chemother. Pharmacol. 3:41.
2. Tashjian AH, Voelkel EF, Levine L, et al (1972). Evidence that the bone resorbing stimulation factor produced by mouse fibrosarcoma is prostaglandin E_2. J. Exp. Med. 136:1329.
3. Plescia OJ, Smith AH, Grinwich K (1975). Subversion of immune system by tumor cells and role of prostaglandins. Proc. Natl. Acad. Sci. (USA) 72:1848.
4. Hortobagyi GN, Smith TL, Swenerton KD, et al (1981). Prognostic value of pre-chemotherapy skin tests in patients with metastatic breast carcinoma. Cancer 47:1369.
5. Cailleau R, Young R, Olive M, et al (1974). Breast tumor cell lines from pleural effusions. J. Natl. Cancer Inst. 53:661.
6. Levine L (1977). Levels of 13,14-dihydro-15-keto-PGE_2 in some biological fluids as measured by radioimmunoassay. Prostaglandins 14:1125–1139.

**Prostaglandins and Cancer: First
International Conference, pages 573-578
© 1982 Alan R. Liss, Inc., 150 Fifth Avenue, New York, NY 10011**

BONE RESORPTIVE ACTIVITY IN CONDITIONED MEDIUM FROM RAT
OSTEOSARCOMA CELL LINE

S.B. Rodan*, G.A. Rodan*, H.A. Simmons†, R.W. Walenga§,
M.B. Feinstein§ and L.G. Raisz†.
Departments of Medicine† , Oral Biology* & Pharmacology§
University of Connecticut Schools of Medicine and
Dental Medicine, Farmington, Connecticut 06032

Malignancy is frequently associated with hypercalcemia,
both in the presence and absence of bone metastases. In
most cases the hypercalcemia results from bone resorption, a
finely regulated process carried out by specialized cells,
the osteoclasts. Our understanding of the signals which
regulate osteoclastic activity is lagging due to the unavail-
ability of pure osteoclast cell populations. On the other
hand, cell populations highly enriched in osteoblasts are
shown to possess functional receptors for parathyroid hormone
(PTH) (Luben, et al., 1976; Peck et al., 1977), vitamin D
(Manolagas et al., 1980; Partridge et al., 1980) and the
response to these hormones among clonal cell lines derived
from the rat osteosarcoma, correlated with the presence of
osteoblastic features, such as elevated alkaline phosphatase
(Majeska et al., 1980) and synthesis of γ-carboxyglutamic
acid containing bone protein (Nishimoto and Price, 1980).
It was also found that the ability of various prostaglandin
analogues to stimulate cyclic AMP accumulation in the osteoblast-like osteosarcoma derived cells correlated with the
resorptive activity of these analogues in tissue culture
(Martin and Partridge, 1981). These findings suggested that
the osteoblasts may participate in the bone resorptive process
as signal transducing cells (Rodan and Martin, 1981), in a
way analogous to the participation of helper cells in the
immune process. To test this hypothesis we examined the resorptive activity in conditioned media from four osteosarcoma
derived clonal cell lines with different degrees of osteoblastic expression: (i) ROS 17/2·8, the osteoblastic cell
line, characterized by high alkaline phosphatase activity;
adenylate cyclase coupled PTH receptors; 1,25(OH)$_2$D$_3$

receptors; PTH and vitamin D inhibition of collagen and alkaline phosphatase synthesis; γ-carboxyglutamic acid containing
bone protein synthesis stimulated by 1,25(OH)$_2$D$_3$ (Price and
Baukol, 1980), and abundant osteogenesis in tumors formed by
s.c. injection of these cells; (ii) ROS 2/3, possessing all
of the above features to a lesser degree; (iii) ROS 24/1,
possessing lower alkaline phosphatase activity, no PTH stimulation of adenylate cyclase, undetectable receptors for
1,25(OH)$_2$D$_3$ and undetectable synthesis of bone γ-carboxyglutamic acid; (iv) ROS 25/1 has a fusiform fibroblastic morphology and no apparent osteoblastic features. The bone
resorption assay (Raisz and Niemann, 1969) was based on the
release of ^{45}Ca from 20 day old embryonic rat tibia, prelabeled in utero. We found that the conditioned medium from
ROS 17/2·8 had strong bone resorptive activity, equivalent
to that of saturating concentrations of PTH or PGE$_2$, 2.4-fold
over baseline (Table 1); resorptive activity in ROS 2/3 media
was 2-fold over baseline; ROS 24/1, 1.4-fold; and ROS 25/1
had none (Rodan, et al., 1981).

Table 1

BONE RESORBING ACTIVITY OF
CONDITIONED MEDIUM FROM DIFFERENT OSTEOSARCOMA CELL LINES

Cell Line	^{45}Ca Release (Experimental/Control)	
	2 Days	5 Days
ROS 17/2·8	1.60* ± 0.19	2.36* ± 0.10
ROS 2/3	1.35* ± 0.10	2.05* ± 0.18
ROS 24/1	1.22* ± 0.05	1.39* ± 0.06
ROS 25/1	0.95 ± 0.04	1.10 ± 0.05

*Significantly different than 1.0, $p < 0.05$, Student's t-
test. Values are means ±SE for 6 bones (Rodan et al., 1981).

We further proceeded to identify the resorptive factor produced by ROS 17/2·8 confluent cultures and found that the
activity was dialyzable through 3,500 M_r membranes and its
production was inhibited by the presence of 10 μM indomethacin or 10 μM flufenamic acid, inhibitors of cyclooxygenase.
The accumulation of resorptive activity in serum free BGJ
medium continued for at least 24 hours. Serial dilution of
24 hour medium showed that activity could be detected down to
a dilution of 1/128, which produced resorption levels

equivalent to 10^{-9} M PGE$_2$. With radioimmunoassay, about 100 picograms PGE in 0.2 ml were found in 24 hour conditioned media, a level consistent with the resorptive activity observed. Less than 10 picograms per 0.2 ml PGE was found in conditioned media from ROS 25/1.

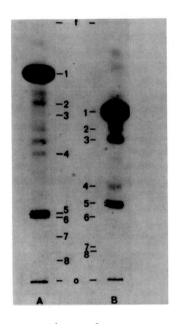

Figure la   Figure lb

Figure la: The products in conditioned medium of ROS 17/2·8: 1) Arachidonate 2) 12-Hydroxyeicosatetraenoic acid 3) PGA$_2$ and PGB$_2$ 4) PGD$_2$ 5) PGE$_2$ 6) Thromboxane B$_2$ 7) PGF$_{2\alpha}$ 8) 6-keto PGF$_{1\alpha}$ 0 - Origin. Lane A: Ethylacetate-acetic acid-iso-octane-water (90:20:50:100). Lane B: Chloroform-methanol-acetic acid-water (90:8:1:0.8). (Rodan et al., 1981)

Figure lb: TLC of ^{14}C-archidonate products in conditioned medium of ROS 17/2·8 (Lane A), of ROS 25/1 (Lane B) and of ROS 17/2·8 in the presence of indomethacin (Lane C).

To examine independently the identity of the resorptive factor, we incubated ROS 17/2·8 and ROS 25/1 cultures with 5 μM ^{14}C-arachidonate (54.6 mCi/mmole) for 24 hours, extracted the media with ethyl-acetate-acetic acid-iso-octane-water or chloroform-methanol-acetic acid-water and chromatographed the extract on thin-layer chromatography (Fig. 1b). PGE_2 was co-chromatographed with the samples while other standards ran on separate plates (Fig. 1a). The distribution of radio-activity was determined by autoradiography and the location of metabolites was determined by cupric acetate spray. The various metabolites were scraped off the plates and counted in liquid scintillation counter. We found that in ROS 17/2·8 (Fig. 1b, Lane A) about 70% of the recovered ^{14}C-arachidonate had been converted into PGE_2 to the extent of 180 pmoles per 24 hours, which was in good agreement with the radioimmuno-assay determination. On the other hand, virtually no PGE_2 was produced in ROS 25/1 (Fig. 1b, Lane B) under the same conditions. As expected, indomethacin at 10 µM completely inhibited the conversion of ^{14}C-arachidonate into PGE_2 in ROS 17/2·8 (Fig. 1b, Lane C).

Table 1

EFFECT OF CORTICOSTEROIDS ON PRODUCTION OF
BONE RESORBING ACTIVITY IN ROS CULTURES

Dexamethasone	Resorption (% ^{45}Ca released at 5 days)
None	85.3 ± 3
10^{-11} M	85.8 ± 8
10^{-10} M	76.4 ± 15
10^{-9} M	78.9 ± 10
10^{-8} M	75.3 ± 5
10^{-7} M	41.4 ± 6

Hydrocortisone	−indomet	+indomet (1µM)
None	87.05 ± 4	63.4 ± 6
10^{-8} M	75.4 ± 4	71.6 ± 12
10^{-7} M	49.0 ± 7	26.6 ± 3
10^{-6} M	52.2 ± 5	31.0 ± 3

Indomethacin (1 µM) (in resorption assay)	46.0 ± 10

Cells were cultured as described; media were changed to serum free BGJ containing dexamethasone or hydrocortisone ±indomethacin as indicated; media were diluted 1/8 and assayed for resorptive activity as described.

Corticosteroids inhibited the production of PGE in ROS 17/2·8 cultures. Thus, in the presence of dexamethasone at concentrations of 0, 10^{-10}, 10^{-9}, 10^{-8}, 10^{-7} M, the cultures (approx. 4×10^6 cells) produced 39.6, 45.0, 19.4, 13.5 and 11.7 ng PGE (by radioimmunoassay) in 24 hours, respectively. We also examined the resorptive activity of media from cells incubated with dexamethasone or hydrocortisone, and as can be seen in the above table (Table 2), corticosteroid concentrations between 10^{-8} and 10^{-7} M effectively inhibited the evolvement of resorptive activity. Indomethacin, present in the culture at 1 μM, was not as inhibitory as 1 μM hydrocortisone, whereas the two together had additive effects.

The findings summarized above show that osteosarcoma derived cells with osteoblastic properties release PGE_2 in sufficient amounts to produce bone resorption whereas other osteosarcoma cell lines which are equally tumorogenic, but lack osteoblastic features, produced almost none. PGE_2 was also produced by osteoblastic enriched cells from rat embryo calvaria and may represent a normal feature of osteoblastic cells. Since PGE_2 is a potent bone resorber, its production implicates the osteoblasts in the resorption process. The regulation of PGE_2 production by these cells has not been extensively studied, but it is possible that certain humoral factors promote bone resorption through this route. This system could be used to screen for the presence and potency of such factors. In the clinical context it is of interest that neither high concentrations of corticosteroids nor 1 μM indomethacin were as effective in inhibiting the release of resorptive activity into the cell culture media, as the two agents combined. Further studies of the control of prostaglandin synthesis in osteoblastic cells could offer insight into this and other questions related to intercellular communication involved in bone resorption.

REFERENCES

Chen TL, Feldman DJ (1981). Regulation of 1,25-Dihydroxyvitamin D_3 receptors in cultured mouse bone cells. J Biol Chem 256:5561.
Luben RA, Wong GL, Cohn DV (1976). Biochemical characterization with parathormone and calcitonin of isolated bone cells: provisional identification of osteoclasts and osteoblasts. Endocrinology 99:526.

Majeska RJ, Rodan SB, Rodan GA (1980). Parathyroid hormone-responsive clonal cell lines from rat osteosarcoma. Endocrinology 107:1494.

Manolagas SC, Haussler MR, Deftos LJ (1980). 1,25-Dihyroxy-vitamin D_3 receptor-like macromolecule in rat osteogenic sarcoma cell lines. J Biol Chem 255:4414.

Martin TJ, Partridge NC (1981). Initial events in the activation of bone cells by parathyroid hormone, prostaglandins, and calcitonin. In Cohn DV, Talmage RV, Matthews JL (eds): "Hormonal Control of Calcium Metabolism," Amsterdam: Excerpta Medica, p 147.

Nishimoto SK, Price, PA (1980). Secretion of the vitamin K-dependent protein of bone by rat osteosarcoma cells. J Biol Chem 255:6579.

Partridge NC, Frampton RJ, Eisman JA, Michelangeli VP, Elms E, Bradley RT, Martin TJ (1980). Receptors for 1,25(OH)$_2$ vitamin D_3 enriched in cloned osteoblast-like rat osteogenic sarcoma cells. FEBS Letters 115:139.

Peck WA, Burke JK, Wilkins J, Rodan SB, Rodan GA (1977). Evidence for preferential effects of parathyroid hormone, calcitonin, and adenosine on bone and periosteum. Endocrinology 100:1357.

Price, PA, Baukol, SA (1980). 1,25-Dihydroxyvitamin D_3 increases synthesis of the vitamin K-dependent bone protein by osteosarcoma cells. J Biol Chem 255:11660.

Raisz L, Niemann, I (1969). Effect of phosphate, calcium, and magnesium on bone resorption and hormone responses in tissue culture. Endocrinology 85:446.

Rodan GA, Martin TJ (1981). Role of osteoblasts in hormonal control of bone resorption--a hypothesis. Calcif Tissue Intl 33:349.

Rodan SB, Rodan GA, Simmons HA, Walenga RW, Feinstein MB, Raisz LG (1981). Bone resorptive factor produced by osteosarcoma cells with osteoblastic features is PGE$_2$. Biochem Biophys Res Commun 102:1358.

HOST TUMOR INTERACTION

Prostaglandins and Cancer: First
International Conference, pages 581-593

PROSTAGLANDINS IN RELATION TO TUMOUR-HOST INTERACTIONS

Peter Alexander

Division of Tumour Immunology
Institute of Cancer Research
Sutton, Surrey,
ENGLAND

INTRODUCTION

The role of the host in the growth and dissemination
of malignant tumours involves more than merely supplying
the neoplastic cells with oxygen and nutrition. Probably
the most important function of the host for the growth of
solid tumours is to provide the blood vessels and there are
also many instances where the supply of hormones by the
host is necessary for tumour growth. As yet, relatively
little is known of the role of PGs in tumour angiogenesis
or hormone dependence. In the metastasis of tumours
coagulation factors and particularly platelet aggregation
have been shown to play a role and if metastases are to
grow in bone osteolysis is required. PGs are clearly
involved in both these processes and if the manipulation of
PGs proves to be of therapeutic value, it may be in relation
to the control of metastases.

However, the aspect of host-interaction which has
until now attracted most attention involves immune mechanisms. A scenario to account for some of the contradictory
effects on tumours seen after manipulation of PGs (namely
that administration of PGs as well as inhibition of the
synthesis of PGs has been claimed to slow the growth of
some experimental tumours) is that PGs inhibit both the
division of tumour cells and also depress host immunity.
In vivo the net effect could depend on the magnitude of the
immune control of the tumour- if this is large, PGs
facilitate tumour growth, if small the cytostatic activity
predominates and the growth of tumour slowed. Failure to

detect an effect is then a reflection of fine balance. I
must admit that I am not attracted to a hypothesis which is
capable of explaining every conceivable outcome of an
experiment.

The body's first line of defence to infection and
foreign bodies of various kinds is innate immunity in which
phagocytic leukocytes are the principal effectors. These
processes are immediate and do not induce memory (i.e. no
secondary response); they are selective but do not show
the degree of specificity associated with lymphocyte-mediated immunity. The latter, as far as infection is concerned, is a second line of defence in that there is an induction period of several days but its eventual capacity for
elimination of infective organisms is greater. Specific
immunity, unlike innate immunity, has a potent memory leading to enhanced secondary responses. It is permissible to
consider lymphocyte-dependent (or specific) immunity as a
back-up mechanism in that survival is possible (just!) without it, whereas absence of phagocytes is incompatible with
life.

NON-SPECIFIC (BUT SELECTIVE) CYTOTOXICITY OF LEUKOCYTES

In vitro nucleated cells (including tumour cells) can
be destroyed in an immunologically non-specific way by
leukocytes. Phagocytic leukocytes may ingest the cells
after they have been killed but phagocytosis is a late
event and not the prime mover in these processes. The
best understood cytotoxic mechanism is that brought about
by potent oxidising species such as hydrogen peroxide and
oxidising radicals such as OH· or HO_2· (Ξ to O_2·⁻).
These are produced as part of the inflammatory process and
in vitro are responsible for the cytotoxicity of neutrophils
stimulated by Con A (Clark and Klebanoff, 1979) or of
macrophages treated with phorbol esters. These bursts of
extracellular oxidising activity from neutrophils and
macrophages are accompanied by the massive release of
unstable PGs, thromboxanes and leukotrienes (Goldstein et
al., 1978) but there is no indication that these products
of arachidonic acid or the more stable PGs derived from them
play a part in the cytotoxic process. In vitro the
susceptibility of target cells varies widely but killing
when it occurs is quick (i.e. within hours) and can be
protected against both by competitors for the active

oxidising species and by enzymes which catalyse their hydrolysis. The reasons for the wide variation in sensitivity of different target cells is not known nor is there any indication that the malignant phenotype predisposes to this type of cytotoxic process.

Another class of leukocytes capable of killing target cells in a selective - but not immunologically-specific - manner are referred to as NK cells (Herberman, 1980; Gidlund et al., 1981). They are non-phagocytic bone-marrow derived mononuclear cells (possibly larger than small lymphocytes), without the membrane markers characteristic for circulating B- and T-lymphocytes. Some investigators consider them to be monocyte progenitors, whereas others believe them to constitute a new class of myeloid cells. They cause lysis of susceptible target cells within a few hours but no evidence for the involvement of H_2O_2 or oxidising radicals has been reported. There is great variation in the susceptibility of different tumour cells to NK attack and cells after growth in tissue culture tend to be more responsive than those obtained directly from tumours. While tumour cells are the usual targets for studying NK activity, it is not known whether transformation to malignancy renders cells more susceptible to lysis by NK cells.

The third type of non-specific cytotoxic cells are macrophages and monocytes which have been activated by a variety of different substances of which the most potent are endotoxin, dsRNA (Alexander and Evans, 1971) and a lymphokine released by allergised T-cells (Evans and Alexander, 1971) called macrophage activating factor (MAF). The cytotoxicity of this class of macrophages differs markedly from that of peroxide-producing phagocytes (e.g. macrophages treated with phorbol esters) and NK cells (Alexander, 1976). Firstly, the initial effect is growth inhibition and lysis of the target cells may require 2 or 3 days. Secondly, transformed cells are much more susceptible than comparable (i.e. rapidly dividing) normal cells to this type of activated macrophage (Hibbs et al., 1972). Thus, in pairs of normal and virus-transformed fibroblasts and epithelial cells the cells of malignant phenotype sustain irreversible damage much more quickly than non-tumorigenic cells. Also, many transformed cells (e.g. sarcoma cells) which are resistant to NK cells and peroxide-producing cells are killed in vitro by these

activated macrophages. The reason for the increased susceptibility of transformed cells may be that these macrophages
induce cytostasis and that transformed cells cannot, like
normal cells, adapt to a period of quiescence and become
metabolically imbalanced and die after a day or so of growth
arrest. The growth inhibitory activity of the activated
macrophages has been attributed by one group of investigators to an increase in release following exposure to MAF
or endotoxin of the enzyme arginase (Currie, 1978) and by
Mannel et al., (1980) to the release of a direct acting
"cytotoxin" of 50,000 molecular weight. The release of
arginase causes rapid depletion of arginine from the medium
and a consequent inhibition of protein synthesis - the
effect of activated macrophages on the target cells can be
mimicked by transferring these to a medium without arginine.
The mode of action of the direct cytotoxin has not yet been
resolved. Activation with endotoxin causes increased
synthesis of PGs by macrophages and this has been claimed to
act as a feed-back control which limits the cytotoxicity of
these macrophages (Taffet and Russell, 1981).

ARE THE NON-SPECIFIC TUMORICIDAL ACTIONS OF LEUKOCYTES
RELEVANT IN VIVO?

    The most direct test to establish in vivo relevance of
macrophages and neutrophils in vivo would be to study tumour
development and growth in animals deprived of these cells.
While this type of experiment is possible for T-cells,
animals die in a few days if devoid of circulating phagocytic cells and there are, therefore, no mutants comparable
to the athymic nudes. The nearest example were strains of
rabbits which exhibited a high susceptibility to tuberculosis
which Lurie (1964) showed to be due to an inherited defect
in monocyte function. Interestingly, the strain of
rabbits which was susceptible to tuberculosis showed a
higher incidence of spontaneous cancers than the tuberculosis-
resistant strain. However, caution must be exercised not
to over-interpret this chance observation. Administration
of silica and carrageenan results in a partial depletion of
macrophages but this is transient and associated with major
and anatomically visible destruction of lymphoid tissue.
Changes in tumour resistance seen after giving these agents
could be due to a variety of factors. Equally inconclusive
are experiments in which agents, which both stimulate
macrophage proliferation and cause activation, are tested

as "immunotherapy" of cancer. In general, the therapeutic
activity of such agents when given systemically has been
rather small (especially in the very extensive clinical
trials for human cancer) and difficult to relate to
macrophages (Parr et al., 1977). When injected directly
into the tumour regressions confined to the injected lesions
are frequently seen. Since such local injection produces
inflammation within the tumour, it is not unreasonable to
attribute this local anti-tumour action to a tumoricidal
effect of one or more of the many components of an
inflammatory lesion.

The in vivo relevance of killing of tumour cells by
NK cells is in doubt. The NK activity of leukocytes varies
markedly with age (being maximal at 6 - 10 weeks), there is
a mutation ("beige") which is accompanied by a marked
defect in NK activity, and there are also a number of agents,
notably interferon, which raise NK activity. It is,
therefore, possible to compare both the genesis and growth
of cancers in backgrounds of widely varying NK activity.
While there are some experiments which indicate a correlation there are others where wide variation in NK activity
did not affect tumours (cf. Herberman, 1980). The claim
has been made that the rarity with which tumour xenografts
metastasize when grown in genetically immunosuppressed
nude mice is due to control of tumour dissemination by NK
cells. The possibility that antibody-dependent cell-
mediated immunity rather than NK cells is responsible has
not been excluded.

THE IN VIVO ROLE OF SPECIFIC IMMUNITY

The existence of macromolecules in the plasma membrane
of tumour cells which evoke a T-cell dependent immune
response in a syngeneic or autologous host has been clearly
shown for many chemically and virally induced rodent
tumours. The origin and chemical nature of these trans-
plantation-type tumour-specific antigens (TSTAs) in rodents
has not been .fully resolved but they may be related to the
gp70 coat proteins of oncorna viruses which are part of
the normal genome of rodents. There is no conclusive
evidence that a counterpart to the TSTAs is present in
many human cancer cells - perhaps because gp70-like
sequences form no part of the human genome. At this point

I must stress that a host response to some long-transplanted experimental tumours like the EL-4 leukaemia or the Lewis lung tumour cannot be attributed to TSTAs. When such tumours are transplanted into C57/Bl mice this is frequently referred to as a "syngeneic transplant" implying that any immunological difference between tumours and host can only be due to TSTAs. This is not true; while the tumours and the C57/Bl mouse share the same H-2 haplotype they can differ at many major histocompatibility loci because the mouse in which they arose is only vaguely related, because of genetic drift and other breeding factors, to the present day C57/Bl. Hence, such tumours are homografts and immunological manoeuvres which affect their growth may be relevant to a homograft reaction but are uninformative as far as true tumour immunity directed to TSTAs is concerned.

In relevant models, which can correctly be called "syngeneic" (i.e. tumours of recent origin transplanted into hosts which are genetically identical with the animal in which the tumour arose), the existence of a TSTA is demonstrated by the induction of T-cell dependent resistance to a tumour challenge by specific immunization. The biological significance of such a response is, however, unclear (cf. Alexander, 1977) in that the genesis (e.g. by administration of a carcinogen) of a TSTA containing tumour is the same in T-cell deprived as in normal hosts. Also, the local growth rate is not accelerated by immunosuppression. On the other hand, an important role for T-cell dependent immunity in the biological behaviour of some tumours is indicated (Alexander, 1976) by the findings that for tumours with TSTAs immunosuppression of the host causes

1) A marked increase in the incidence of distant metastases;*

Footnote: * The effect of T-cells on the distant dissemination of sarcomas and lymphomas of mice and rats can be striking. Tumours with a low incidence of spontaneous metastases will metastasize widely in immunosuppressed recipients and genetically athymic (i.e. "nude") hosts, so long as there is no xenograft barrier.

2) The tumours are less responsive to chemotherapy or local irradiation with X-rays;

3) A decrease in the number of macrophages present in the tumour.

Procedures which modulate T-cell activity will, therefore, affect these three properties of immunogenic experimental tumours, i.e. depressing T-cell activity will increase metastasis, decrease the macrophage content of tumours and make tumours less responsive to therapy; stimulating immunity can achieve the reverse. In our hands (Heckford et al., 1982) manipulation of PGs in vivo did not change such T-cell dependent biological properties of tumours. Thus administration of the potent cyclo-oxygenase inhibitor, flurbiprofen, did not increase response to chemotherapy, decrease incidence of metastases or alter the macrophage content of the rodent tumours studied.

EFFECTOR MECHANISMS OF SPECIFIC IMMUNITY

The effector mechanisms involved in the interaction of specific host immunity and tumours with TSTAs are likely to be various. We have evidence that distant metastatic spread when this is "immune-dependent" is controlled by antibodies directed against TSTAs (Proctor et al., 1973). A cytotoxic effect of antibodies can be caused by (1) lysis requiring complement; (2) lysis by Fc$^+$ leukocytes which combine with the antibody-coated target cells (i.e. ADCC) and then kill these by mechanisms which have not been elucidated, or (3) circulating antibody-coated target cells are phago-cytosed by the reticuloendothelial system. Immuno-phagocytosis is a highly efficient physiological process and is, for example, responsible for the rapid clearance of erythrocytes if mismatched blood is infused. We have evidence (Denham et al., 1980) that immunophagocytosis is responsible for protection against transplanted leukaemias by passive transfer of antibody. An in vivo role of complement-dependent or ADCC killing by antibodies has not so far been demonstrated in tumour immunology.

Cell-mediated cytotoxicity (not involving antibody)

is induced in animals immunized with a syngeneic TSTA-
positive tumour. These involve T-cells and the effector
mechanisms are of two types:-

(1) Allergized T_C (in the mouse defined by the surface
phenotype Ly 2,3$^+$; Ly 1^{-ve}) on meeting the specific
antigen proliferate and give rise to a population of cells
which has the capacity to lyse the specific target-
cytotoxic T-cells.

(2) Allergized T_H cells (in the mouse Ly$^+$; Ly 2,3^{-ve}) on
meeting the specific antigen release lymphokines with a
variety of physiological properties which include
a) MIF - with the capacity to attract macrophages;
b) macrophage arming factor (MAF) which renders macrophages
non-specifically cytotoxic (this has been discussed before);
c) lymphotoxin; glycoproteins which are in vitro cytotoxic
to some but not all nucleated cells.

    The effect of these various mechanisms in vivo remains
to be elucidated. The action of cytotoxic T-cells is
completely specific and these cells are, therefore, a good
candidate for the resistance to challenge induced by
immunization but whether they contribute to the other
manifestations of immunity to TSTA such as control of
metastatic spread or increased resistance to chemo- and
local radiotherapy is not clear. The cytotoxic mechanisms
initiated by lymphokines (i.e. macrophages exposed to MAF
or directly by lymphotoxins) are not specific but are
brought into being by the specific antigen to which the
host has been rendered immune. If these processes function
in vivo one would, therefore, expect an "innocent by-
stander" phenomenon, i.e. animals rendered immune to
tumour A should destroy an unrelated tumour B if B is
injected with A but not if B only is administered. This
phenomenon is rarely, if ever, encountered. The simplest
interpretation for the T-cell dependent accumulation of
macrophages within tumours is that this is caused by
lymphokines.

PRODUCTION OF PGs BY TUMOURS

That not all the cells present in malignant tumours
are cancer cells is self-evident but has often been for-
gotten when analyzing tumours and is a fact that has to be
borne in mind in reports on differences in PG production
by different tumours. For convenience, the normal cells
in a tumour can be referred to as "host cells" as this has
a precise meaning when dealing with transplanted tumours and
the concept is readily transferable to primary tumours.
The most obvious but frequently not the most numerous host
cells are those of the stroma and particularly the endothelial cells of the tumour blood supply without which a
tumour could not grow beyond a fraction of a millimeter in
diameter. In many tumours macrophages and leukocytes which
have entered via the blood constitute the major part of
the host cell component and occasionally outnumber the
cancer cells (Eccles and Alexander, 1974). In histological sections macrophages are, in general, only identified
as such if they have recently been involved in endocytosis
otherwise they are not picked out. In experimentally-
induced sarcomas of rodents the macrophage content was
found to range from 3 to 50% of the total cell number yet
histologically the sarcomas appeared very similar. In
human tumours up to 30% of the cells were found to be
macrophages (Gauci and Alexander, 1975). In general,
the proportion of macrophages within a tumour remains
reasonably constant during its growth but changes markedly
on treatment with radiotherapy or chemotherapy. The
macrophage content will be reduced if there is mono-
cytopaenia as a result of marrow damage by cytotoxic agents.
Immunosuppression also lowers the rate of entry of
macrophages (see above). On the other hand, during the
course of tumour regression the macrophage content increases
and this is very evident following local radiotherapy which
does not impair haemopoiesis. The progressive changes in
the cellular composition of tumours undergoing therapy
renders biochemical analysis of such tumours difficult to
interpret. Great caution must, therefore, be exercised
in the interpretation of PGs by tissue from tumours and
one might be led to conclude that there was a relationship
between immunogenicity of tumours and PG production by the

tumour cells when in reality the PG is largely synthesized
by the macrophages in the tumour.

IMPAIRMENT OF THE IMMUNE RESPONSE OF THE HOST BY TUMOURS

There have been many claims that the capacity of the
host to mount a general immune response is impaired by a
growing tumour and I note that there are reports that
manipulation of PGs can reverse the immunosuppression by
a tumour. This is unfortunately an area in which the
literature is very confusing not least because simplistic
deductions are made from in vitro tests about the immune
performance of the tumour-bearer. For example, there is
an extensive literature showing that the lymphocytes from
patients with advanced malignant disease - particularly
lymphoma - do not transform on exposure to PHA and frequently this was taken as evidence for immunosuppression caused
by the tumour. In those instances where a thorough study
has been made there was no lymphocyte lesion but it was the
presence in the patient's serum of acute phase proteins -
particularly the α-2M and α-1 protease inhibitors - which
interfere with the in vitro test but do not affect the
immune status of the patient (Hubbard et al., 1981).
Similarly, the magnitude of delayed hypersensitivity skin
reactions to antigens such as tuberculin can be reduced as
a result of tumour growth. In experimental animals we
(Eccles and Alexander, 1976) were able to show that this
could not be ascribed to a failure of specific immunity
since lymphocytes capable of transferring the delayed
hypersensitivity response were present. The reduced skin
reaction was due to the failure of monocytes to enter the
test area in sufficient numbers. There are instances where
true immune suppression has been documented in cancer
patients but frequently this has a metabolic basis as immune
reactions are clearly affected by malnutrition. In
animals a common artefact has been contamination of the
tumour with viruses, such as the LDH virus, which infect
the reticuloendothelial system and interfere with antigen
processing by macrophages which is essential for the
initiation of an immune response (Riley et al., 1978).
In my view, immunosuppression induced by tumours is not an

important phenomenon in the pathogenesis of cancer.

CONCLUSIONS

Where administration of PGs or inhibition of their synthesis has modulated tumour growth or dissemination at least five modes of action have to be considered:-

(1) Host immunity: The difficulties of facts and interpretation in this area are the subject of this paper. I must emphasize again that unless experimental tumours are truly syngeneic with the host in which they are grown, they are unsuitable for investigation of host-tumour interaction.

(2) Interference with dissemination via haemostatic mechanisms.

(3) Prevention of progressive growth of metastasis by preventing angiogenesis.

(4) Induction of differentiation: I consider that this is a most promising area in which to look for an interaction of PGs and the growth and spread of tumours. Of great clinical importance are "dormant" metastases. These are disseminated tumour cells which do not develop into clinically evident metastases until a triggering event occurs. One hypothesis (Eccles et al., 1980) is that for carcinomas this latency is due to differentiation of the cells shed from the growing tumour. PG production by the stroma surrounding the dormant tumour cells could determine whether they remain latent or grow progressively.

(5) Direct effect of PGs on growth of tumour cells: Some of the experiments claiming to show in vitro growth inhibition by PGs rely solely on changes in the rate of thymidine incorporation for a measure of DNA synthesis. There are many reasons why changes in thymidine incorporation need not reflect DNA synthesis or growth (e.g. an increase in thymidine phosphorylase activity (Perry and Marsh, 1964; Pauly, 1976) - will reduce thymidine incorporation even if DNA synthesis remains unaffected). Also, inhibition of cell growth in vitro by non-steroidal anti-inflammatory compounds has been reported but this was caused by non-PG related biochemical effects of these compounds (Bayer and Beaven, 1981).

Alexander P (1976). Dormant metastases which manifest on immunosuppression and the role of macrophages in tumours. IN Weiss L (ed). Fundamental aspects of metastasis. North-Holland Publishing Co. p 227.

Alexander P (1976). The functions of the macrophage in malignant disease. Annual Review of Medicine, 27:207.

Alexander P (1977). Innate host resistance to malignant cells not involving specific immunity. In Day SB et al. (ed). Cancer invasion and metastasis. Biologic mechanisms and therapy. Raven Press, New York.

Alexander P, Evans R (1971). Endotoxin and double stranded RNA render macrophages cytotoxic. Nature New Biol. 232:76.

Bayer BM, Beaven MA (1981). Cytostatic activity of pharmacological concentrations of indomethacin in cell cultures and inactivity of closely related compounds. Biochem. Pharmacol. 29: in the press.

Clark RA, Klebanoff SJ (1979). Role of the myeloperoxidase-H_2O_2-halide system in Concanavalin A-induced tumor cell killing by human neutrophils. J. Immunol. 122:2605.

Currie GA (1978). Activated macrophages kill tumour cells by releasing arginase. Nature (Lond.) 273:758.

Denham S, Hooton JWL, Barfoot RK, Alexander P, Mayol R, Wrathmell AB (1980). Mechanism by which antibodies to non-AgB antigens mediate rejection of rat leukaemia cells. Br. J. Cancer, 42:408.

Eccles SA, Alexander P (1974). Macrophage content of tumors in relation to metastatic spread and host immune reaction. Nature, 250:667.

Eccles SA, Alexander P (1974). Sequestration of macrophages in growing tumors and its effect on the immunological capacity of the limb. Br. J. Cancer, 30:42.

Eccles SA, Heckford SE, Alexander P (1980). Effect of Cyclosporin A on the growth and spontaneous metastasis of syngeneic animal tumours. Br. J. Cancer, 42:252.

Evans R, Alexander P (1971). Rendering macrophages specifically cytotoxic by a factor released from immune lymphoid cells. Transplantation, 12:227.

Gauci CL, Alexander P (1975). The macrophage content of some human tumors. Cancer Lett. 1:33.

Gidlund M, Orn A, Pattengale PK, Jansson M, Wigzell H, Nilsson K (1981). Natural killer cells kill tumour cells at a given stage of differentiation. Nature, 292:848.

Goldstein IM, Malmsten CL, Kindahl H, Kaplan HB, Radmark O, Samuelsson B, Weissmann G (1978). Thromboxane generation by human peripheral blood polymorphonuclear leukocytes. J. exp. Med. 148:787.

Heckford SE, Eccles SA, Powles TJ, Alexander P (1982).
Failure of Flurbiprofen to enhance the therapeutic effect
of Cyclophosphamide against rodent sarcomas and leukaemia.
Br. J. Cancer, in the press.
Herberman RB (ed). (1980). Natural cell-mediated immunity
against tumours. Academic, New York.
Hibbs JB, Lambert LH (1972). Macrophage-mediated non-
specific cytotoxicity - possible role in tumor resistance.
Nature New Biol. 235:48.
Hubbard WJ, Hess AD, Hsia S, Amos DB (1981). The effects
of electrophoretically "slow" and "fast" α-2 macro-
globulin on mixed lymphocyte cultures.
Johnston RB, Godzik CA, Cohn ZA (1978). Increased superoxide anion production by immunologically activated and
chemically elicited macrophages. J. Exp. Med. 148:115.
Lurie H (1964). In Resistance to Tuberculosis, experimental
studies in native and acquired defence mechanisms.
Cambridge: Harvard Univ. Press, p 330.
Mannel DN, Moore RN, Mergenhagen SE (1980). Macrophages
as a source of tumoricidal activity (tumor-necrotizing
factor). Infection and Immunity, 30:523.
Parr IB, Wheeler E, Alexander P (1977). Selective
mobilization of specifically cytotoxic T-lymphocytes at
sites of inflammation in relation to BCG-induced resistance to implants of syngeneic sarcoma in mice. J. Natl.
Cancer Inst. 59:1659.
Paulty JL (1976). Elaboration of pyrimidine specific
nucleosidases by human lymphoblastoid cells of established
cultures. Cancer Res., 36:2780.
Perry S, Marsh JC (1964). Uptake of tritiated thymidine
by leukaemic cells: Effects of various leukocyte
preparations. Proc. Soc. Exp. Biol. Med., 115:51.
Proctor JW, Rudenstam C-M, Alexander P (1973). A factor
preventing the development of lung metastases in rats
with sarcomas. Nature, 242:29.
Riley V, Spackman DH, Santisteban GA, Dalldorf G,
Hellstrom I, Hellstrom K-E, Lance EM, Rowson KEK,
Mahy BWJ, Alexander P, Chester Stock C, Sjögren HO,
Holland VP, Horzinek MC (1978). The LDH Virus: An
interfering biological contaminant. Science, 200:124.

**Prostaglandins and Cancer: First
International Conference, pages 595–607
© 1982 Alan R. Liss, Inc., 150 Fifth Avenue, New York, NY 10011**

ARACHIDONATE METABOLITES AND IMMUNITY

Charles W. Parker, M.D.
Howard Hughes Medical Institute Laboratory and
Dept. of Internal Medicine, Division of Allergy
and Immunology, Washington Univ. School.of Med.
St. Louis, Missouri 63110

INTRODUCTION

Prostaglandins (PGs) have been reported to exert a wide variety of regulatory effects on immune function affecting mitogenesis, cell mediated cytotoxicity, antibody biosynthesis, lymphokine formation, T and B cell differentiation, chemotaxis, anaphylactic mediator release, lysosomal enzyme release, interactions between cells, leukocyte colony formation, granuloma formation, allograft and tumor survival and immune complex mediated vasculitis (Stenson and Parker, 1980; Stenson and Parker, 1981; Goldyne and Stobo, 1981; Hume and Weidemann, 1980; Pelus and Strasser, 1977; Goodwin and Webb, 1980). Most of the experimental attention on the role of PGs in immunity has been focused on the E prostaglandins, probably in large measure because the available comparative studies have indicated that they are the most effective of the PGs on a molar basis. The overall predominant effect of PGs has been an inhibition of immunologic reactivity (Parker et al, 1974). However, in some situations enhancement rather than inhibition has been seen. Even where inhibition is consistantly seen, the magnitude of the inhibition may be markedly affected by the nature or dose of the mitogen or the time of addition of the PG. Moreover, in vivo some of the effects of PGs may partially counterbalance one another. These make it difficult to make a general statement for the role of PGs in immunity.

One of the questions that has recently received increasing attention is the possible involvement of arachidonate (AA) metabolites other than the PGs in immune function. Lymphoid cells produce a wide variety of AA

metabolites although there is still much more to be learned
about the level of their production under various conditions
of immunologic activation in vivo and even in some
circumstances the spectrum of products produced. Based on in
vitro studies macrophages (monocytes) appear to be a major
source of PGs (reviewed in Goldyne and Stobo, 1981).
Macrophages also produce very substantial amounts of
thromboxane A_2 (TxA_2). Macrophages also apparently make
prostacyclin (PC) although the level of PC production has
varied with the cell source, the purity of the macrophage
population and the state of cell activation. The role of
these metabolites is uncertain. In platelets cell
aggregation is stimulated by TxA_2 while PC is inhibitory.
TxA_2 also promotes aggregation in neutrophils. Indirect
evidence suggests that TxA_2 may be important in the control
of lymphocytic activation (Parker et al, 1979c). In human
lymphocytes a variety of inhibitors of thromboxane synthesis
very substantially inhibit lectin induced transformation and
stimulation of amino acid transport.

Several recent studies have expanded the variety of
lipids, both arachidonate metabolites and non-arachidonate
metabolites, which are known to act as intracellular or
intercellular mediators in the control of immunity (reviewed
in Stenson and Parker, 1981)). Two lymphokines originally
thought to be proteins have been shown to be biologically
active lipids bound to inactive proteins (Wolf and Merler,
1979). Platelets activating factor (1-O-alkyl-(primarily
C-16 or C-18)2-acetyl-sn-glyceryl-3 phosphorylcholine) has
been identified as an unusual group of closely related
phospholipids released by basophils or neutrophils depending
on the animal species. It causes a rapid release of granule
products from platelets and a variety of other acute
physiologic effects (Demopoulos et al, 1979). A lipoxygenase
product of neutrophils, mast cells, monocytes and probably
lymphocytes, 5-hydroxy-6,8,11,14-eicosatetraenoic acid
(5-HETE) has been shown to be chemotactic for neutrophils and
to promote inflammatory mediator release. 5-HETE is also an
effective inhibitor of lymphocyte transformation (Parker,
1981). 8, 9, 11 and 15 hydroxyeicosatetranoic acids have
recently been shown to be produced by mononuclear cells and
exert or may exert similar actions; 5,12
dihydroxyeicosatetraenoic acid (5,12, di HETE) which is
produced in these same cells under similar circumstances as
5-HETE, is a particularly potent inducer of neutrophile
aggregation and chemotaxis. Under certain circumstances 5,12

di HETE and other polyhydroxylated eicosatetraenoic acids may promote lymphocyte transformation although the effects are somewhat variable and their importance remains to be elucidated (Parker, unpublished data, 1981). The slow reacting substance (SRS) produced by a line of rat basophilic leukemia cells was reported several years ago by our laboratory to be an AA metabolite produced through the lipoxygenase pathway (Jakschik et al, 1977). More recently, SRS has been shown by ourselves (Parker et al, 1979a) and by Murphy et al, 1979 to be a family of oxygenated arachidonate metabolites with a sulfur containing side chain (glutathione, cysteinyl-glycine or cysteine) bound in thioether linkage. SRS is released by mast cells, neutrophils, and macrophages and causes smooth muscle contraction and alterations in vascular permeability. Studies in progress indicate that SRS promotes the uptake of Ca^{2+} by intestinal cells (in collaboration with S. Scheid and S. Findlay). Whether SRS has a broader role in the control of immune responses than its acute effects on immediate hypersensitivity remains to be elucidated.

Even this expanded list does not include all of the non phospholipid and triglyceride lipids which may be important in the control of immunity. For example, despite their chemical lability the endoperoxide products of the cyclooxygenase pathway, PGG_2 and PGH_2, and the fatty acid hydroperoxides produced by the lipoxygenase pathway have to be considered as possible intracellular mediators. These AA metabolites may exert different metabolic effects than the more stable end products of AA metabolism they give rise to. Even the prostaglandins themselves (PGEs, PGFs, and PGDs) are heterogeneous and may show similar or different actions depending on the tissue. In this connection it is of interest that mast cells and probably basophils make large amounts of PGD_2, (Stenson and Parker, 1981) in contrast to the other cells that participate in immune inflammation. Certainly the role of PGD_2 in immune modulation deserves more attention than it has previously received.

There is still much to be learned about how these various AA metabolites affect cellular function. In many cells PGs appear to affect intracellular metabolism by changing (usually raising) cAMP levels. However, this may not always be true and in any case PGs have the capability of lowering rather than raising cAMP in certain cells. PC also raises cAMP whereas the fatty

acid hydroperoxides have the capability of raising
intracellular cGMP levels, at least in some cell types.
Thymocyte and B lymphocyte maturation
      Despite extensive study the true role of the PGs in
the immune response is far from settled. It is
attractive to speculate that one of the physiologic roles
of PGs may be as mediators of lymphocyte maturation. The
addition of cAMP or PGE_2, but not $PGF_{2\alpha}$, to
thymocytes in vitro produces an increase in thymocyte
cAMP levels and ultimately leads to thymocyte
proliferation (Franks, et al, 1971). PGE_2 also induces
expression of early maturation antigens on both B and T
cells (Scheid, et al, 1975, 1978). Differentiating
murine T cells acquire the cell surface marker Thy-1
while B cells acquire complement receptors. PGE can also
increase the percentage of embryonic murine thymocytes
displaying the Thy-1 maturation antigen (Smith, et al,
1977). However, the extent to which PGE_2 is produced
locally in the thymus, in vivo is not clear. A variety
of hormones can produce similar effects on thymocytes in
vitro, apparently also acting through cAMP so it is
apparent that a number of alternative pathways exist for
the stimulation of thymocyte maturation.
T cell proliferative responses
      There are also ambiguities in regard to the
importance of some of the negative modulatory effects of
the PGs. In 1971 we reported that the PGEs and PGAs and
to a lesser extent the PGFs inhibited ^{3}H-thymidine
incorporation in PHA stimulated human peripheral blood
lymphocytes (Smith, et al, 1971). Other agents that
raised cAMP in these cells including isoproterenol and
theophylline, also inhibited the lymphocyte response to
mitogen. A variety of groups have also reported
inhibition of thymidine incorporation in mitogen
stimulated T cells by PGE. However, the minimal
inhibitory concentration of PG for 50% inhibition has
been as high as 1 X 10^{-4}M depending on the culture
conditions and the mitogen. Moreover, while Goodwin et
al (Goodwin, et al, 1978a) found that relatively low
concentrations of PGE_2 (3 X 10^{-8}M) inhibit PHA
induced thymidine incorporation this was only true when
suboptimal concentrations of PHA were used. In addition,
PG effects were more marked in partially purified T cells
than unpurified mononuclear cell mixtures (Goodwin, et
al, 1978: Novogrodsky, et al, 1979).
Finally, one group has isolated a human T lymphocyte

subpopulation in which mitogenesis was enhanced rather than inhibited by PGs and other cAMP agonists indicating that qualitatively different responses can occur depending on the T cell subpopulation (Goldyne and Stobo, 1981). These observations raise questions about the physiologic relevance and constancy of the PG inhibition. Nonetheless a number of laboratories have reported that indomethacin increases T cell proliferative responses in vitro indicating that at least under certain conditions in vitro enough PG is accumulating in the cultures to exert a suppressive effect. On the other hand, evidence for substantial enhancing effects of indomethacin in vivo where newly synthesized PGs may be excreted or more readily metabolized is very limited. With the present lack of information on PG levels in lymphoid tissues responding to antigen in vivo and the high concentrations of PG required for inhibition in vitro in most studies, it is difficult to be certain about the normal role of the PG inhibition of T cell proliferation.

B cell responses

The situation with regard to PGs and B cell proliferative responses is also subject to uncertainty. Stockman and Mumford (Stockman, et al, 1974) compared the effects of PGE_2 on mitogenesis by PHA, Con A and pokeweed mitogen (PWM) in human peripheral blood lymphocytes. They found that PGE_2 (1×10^{-5} to 1×10^{-7}M) inhibited PHA and Con A stimulated mitogenesis but had no effect on PWM induced mitogenesis. This supported the conclusion that PGs exert a more marked effect on T cells than on B cells. Nonetheless B cells also are susceptible to inhibition by PGs under appropriate circumstances as is demonstrated by the inhibition of antibody formation or induction of antibody producing cells in response to antigen by exogenous PGs that has been reported by a number of laboratories. For example, several groups have found that exogenous PGs inhibit the formation of plaque-forming (antibody-secreting) cells from mouse spleen lymphocytes in primary cultures (Melmon, et al, 1974; Webb and Nowowiejski, 1977; Zimecki and Webb, 1976). Other agents that raise cAMP levels (histamine, beta adrenergic agents) also were inhibitory.

In another study (Webb and Nowowiejski, 1977) spleen cell cultures incubated with indomethacin (1×10^{-7}M) and antigen (sheep red blood cells) produced more plaque forming colonies than did those without indomethacin,

whereas exogenous PGE restored the inhibition. Responses
to T-independent antigens such as DNP-Ficoll and
polyvinyl pyrolidone were also inhibited by exogenous
PGE_1 suggesting a direct action of the PGs on B cells.
Despite these interesting results the PG concentration
needed for effective inhibition has sometimes been as
high as $1 \times 10^{-4}M$ casting doubt on physiological
significance of the effect. Moreover, in contrast to
inhibitory effects of PGs the number of antibody
producing cells has been reported to be increased rather
than decreased when the cAMP agonist is only present in
the first 12 to 24 hours of the culture. Kishimoto and
Ishizaka (1976) have shown that PGE_1, and other agents
which increase intracellular cyclic AMP, initially
enhanced IgG and IgM responses to the hapten of DNP
conjugated antigen. However, an increase in the
intracellular cyclic AMP levels at later times in the
primed cells subsequently suppressed the antibody
response (Kishimoto and Ishizaka, 1976). This
enhancement of antibody synthesis could be due to
induction of differentiation in immature T (helper) or B
lymphocytes although there are a variety of alternative
possibilities such as an inhibition of T suppressor cells.
    Evidence for suppressive or enhancing effects of PGs
on B cell responses in man is very limited. Goodwin et
al (1978b) have investigated the effects of indomethacin
on the humoral immune response to bivalent influenza
vaccine in human subjects. Normal human subjects were
given indomethacin (100 mg/day) for 2 days before and 10
days after an injection with bivalent influenza vaccine
(A-New Jersey and A-Victoria). Compared to controls the
indomethacin treated group developed a significantly
increased antibody titer to A-Victoria, but showed no
difference in titer to A-New Jersey. Since almost all
the subjects had antibody to A-Victoria prior to
vaccination while none had antibody to A-New Jersey, this
indicated that indomethacin enhanced the secondary but
not the primary humoral response. Whether this
difference in the secondary antibody response would be
sustained at later times after boosting will require
further study. Certainly there is no really convincing
evidence at present for a major modulatory effect.

Mechanisms of the PG inhibition of T and B cell responses
    In view of the complexity of lymphocyte activation with
the existence of both helper and suppressor cells and the
accessory role of macrophages there are a variety of

possible mechanisms for PG induced inhibition of T and B cell responses. Studies by several groups have shown that lectin induced thymidine incorporation can be enhanced in human peripheral blood mononuclear cells or mouse spleen cells by depleting the cell population of glass-adherent cells (Goodwin and Webb, 1980). It was then found that the adherent cells were apparently acting as suppressor cells in these responses. The addition of prostaglandin synthetase inhibitors (PSIs) such as indomethacin enhanced the responses suggesting a possible role of PGs in the suppression. In the studies in human peripheral blood the suppresssor cell appeared to be a monocyte and these cells were shown to synthesize sufficient PGE$_2$ to account for the suppresssion (Goodwin et al, 1977). Goodwin and coworkers studied PHA-induced mitogenesis in normal individuals and patients with Hodgkin's disease where there is frequently anergy to delayed skin test antigens and impaired response in vitro to T cell mitogens like PHA (Goodwin, et al, 1977). When normal lymphocytes were exposed to indomethacin there was a 40 percent increase in the mitogenic response to PHA . In Hodgkin's disease the increase was 100 to 280 percent. In some instances the response was restored to normal levels. These investigators also demonstrated increased levels of PG production in mononuclear cell cultures from subjects with Hodgkin's disease and that the removal of adherent cells reversed the suppression. These observations suggested that the defect in cellular immunity might be secondary to increased PG production. In addition there is preliminary evidence that in certain disease states associated with decreased immune function including Hodgkins disease partial reversal may be achieved by indomethacin therapy, but much more study is needed (Goodwin, et al, 1978).

Other mechanisms for the suppressive effects of PGs have been suggested. Webb and his colleagues have identified a suppressor cell in mouse spleen that was activated by exogenous PG to make a 28,000 MW protein suppressor substance (Stenson and Parker, 1981). The suppressor cells were phenotypically Thy-1 and Ly-1$^+$2$^+$3$^+$ (Webb and Jamieson, 1976: Webb and Nowowiejski, 1978) indicating that they are probably relatively undifferentiated T cells. They have suggested a model in which activated lymphocytes synthesized by PG in turn induced suppressor cells to secrete a soluble suppressor protein. By contrast Goodwin and his colleagues have proposed that the inhibition of lectin-induced mitogenesis by PGs is a result of a direct effect of PGs on the lectin-stimulated lymphocytes. As far as B cell responses are concerned, Webb and Nowowiejski (1977) found that PGE_2 reduces the number of antibody producing cells in vitro only if it is added at the beginning or near the end of the culture. The late inhibition suggests a direct action on secretion of antibody by B cells, while the early effect of PGs is consistent with inhibition of the inductive phase either on helper T cells or B cell responsiveness to helper cells. As already indicated PGs may sometimes enhance instead of inhibit B cell responses if added early in the response. At present there is insufficient evidence to determine whether this effect is on B cell maturation, helper cell induction or suppressor cell inhibition.

In addition to the observations of Webb which indicate that PGs may promote the synthesis of a lymphokine, the work of Gordon, Bray and Morley (1976) suggests that PGs may suppress lymphokine production. They found that PGE_1 inhibited the production of an inhibition of macrophage migration by antigen stimulated sensitized guinea pig lymphocytes.

Attempts to determine the biochemical basis for PG inhibition at the intracellular level have been limited. We have found that several early activation events – protein phosphorylation, aminoisobutyric acid uptake, release of radiolabeled AA from prelabeled cells, and phosphatidyl inositol turnover are all inhibited by the PGEs (Chaplin et al, 1980, unpublished data, Parker et al, 1979b). Others have shown that PGE_1 and PGE_2 inhibit PHA and PPD-tuberculin induced inositol incorporation into phosphatidyl inositol (Offner and Clausen, 1974). Which, if any of these inhibitions is of primary importance in the inhibition of mitogenesis remains to be established. However, the inhibition of protein phosphorylation is of particular interest in that other cyclic AMP agonists are ineffective as inhibitors suggesting that a specialized pool of cAMP is involved or this agent is not acting through cAMP. Clearly, the biochemical mechanism of the PG inhibition deserves more study.   Cytotoxic T cell responses

The killing of target cells by cytotoxic T cells is modulated by intracellular cAMP and quite possibly cGMP levels. Agents that raise intracellular cAMP, including

PGs, inhibit the killing of target cells by sensitized T cells. In a mouse mastocytoma allogeneic system (Henney, et al, 1972; Lomnitzer, et al, 1976) PG was both the most effective cAMP agonist on a molar basis and the most efficient inhibitor of cytotoxicity in vitro or in vivo as evidenced by increased graft survival. PG analogs with long biologic half-lives in vivo considerably prolonged allograft survival in rats (Strom et al, 1977). Quagliata et al (1973) showed that PGs used in combination with procarbazine, a T cell depressent, considerably promoted survival of mouse skin allografts. On the other hand Louse and Diluzie reported that graft vs host responses in mice were enhanced by pretreatment of the splenocytes to be used for grafting with PGE_1; thus the timing of the exposure to PG was an important determinant in the response.

CONCLUDING REMARKS

One of the major problems in interpretation is the relative absence of in vivo studies. There is considerable uncertainity at this time as to the importance of PGs as physiological modulators of immune responsiveness in vivo. While there is no doubt that pharmacologic doses of PGs or PG analogues can markedly affect immune reactivity in vivo, the later may be acting in part by inducing endogenous steroid formation and both may be producing effects that would not occur under normal physiologic conditions. Certainly the changes in immune resistance to common pathogens during treatment of diseases such as rheumatoid arthritis, antiinflammatory agents such as aspirin or indomethacin have not been terribly impressive despite the use of maximally tolerated doses over an extended period of time. Thus while selected actions of PGs in modulatory interferon action or NK cell reactivity and in association with certain neoplasms as discussed elsewhere in this conference may be quite important, there is some doubt as to the overall importance of PGs in immune regulation. Nonetheless, it seems very possible that PGs do play a significant regulatory role. It should be kept in mind that conclusions as to effectiveness of prostaglandin synthetase inhibitors (PSI) such as aspirin in vivo are based primarily on studies of PG and PG metabolite excretion and may not be fully indicative of how effective the inhibition is in the relevant lymphoid organs which may account for only a small proportion of the total PG produced. Certainly some PG synthesis continues even at high PSI concentrations, particularly in nucleated cells since they can resynthesize their cyclooxygenase enzymes. Moreover, concomitant effects of PSI inhibitors on thromboxane and prostacyclin formation or less directly on the lipoxygenase pathway may alter the response to PG inhibition leading to a considerable underestimate as to the importance of the PGs. In addition, since PGs appear capable of acting at multiple control points in the immune response, it is possible that some of the effects may partially cancel one another.

REFERENCES

Demopoulos CA, Pinckard RN, Hanahan DJ, (1979) Platelet activating factor. J. Biol. Chem. 254:9355.

Franks DJ, Macmanus JP, Whitfield JF (1971) The effect of prostaglandins on cyclic AMP production and cell proliferation in thymic lymphocytes. Biochem. and Biophys. Res. Commun., 44:1177.

Goldyne ME, Stobo JD (1981) Immunoregulatory Role of Prostaglandins and Related Lipids. CRC Critical Reviews in Immunology, 2:189.

Goodwin JS, Messner RP, Bankhurst AD, Peake GT, Saiki JH, Williams RG Jr (1977) Prostaglandin producing suppressor cells in Hodgkin's diases. N. Engl. J. Med. 297:963.

Goodwin JS, Murphy S, Bankhurst AD, Selinger DS, Messner RP, Williams Jr., RC (1978) Partial reversal of the cellular immune defect in common variable immundeficiency with indomethacin. J. Clin. Lab. Immunol. 1:197.

Goodwin JS, Messner RP, Peake GT (1978a) Prostaglandin suppression of mitogen-stimulated lymphocytes in vitro changess with mitogen dose and preincubation. J. Clin. Invest. 62:753.

Goodwin JS, Selinger DS, Messner RP, Reed WP (1978b) Effect of indomethacin in vivo on humoral and cellular immunity in humans. Infec. Immun. 19:430.

Goodwin JS, Webb DR (1980) Regulation of the immune

Novogrodsky A, Rubin AL, Stenzel KH (1979) Selective suppressin by adherent cells, prostaglandin, and cyclic AMP analogues of blastogenesis induced by different mitogens. J. Immunol. 122:1.

Offner H, Clausen J (1974) Inhibition of lymphocyte responses to stimulus induced by unsaturated fatty acids and prostaglandins. Lancet 2:400.

Parker CW (1981) Arachidonic acid metabolism in activated lymphocytes in "Proceedings of the 14th International Leucocyte Culture Conference" Elsevier/North-Holland Biomedical Press B.V.

Parker CS, Sullivan TJ, Wedner HJ (1974) Cyclic AMP and the immune response. In "Advances in cyclic nucleotide research", Robison GA, Greengard P (eds) Raven Press, New York, Vol. IV, p. 1.

Parker CW, Huber MG, Hoffman MK, Falkenhein SF (1979a) Characterization of the two major species of slow reacting substance from rat basophilic leukemia cells as glutathionyl thioethers of eicosatetraenoic acids oxygenated at the 5 position. Evidence that peroxy groups are present and important for spasmogenic activity. Prostaglandins 18:673.

Parker CW, Kelly JP, Falkenhein SF, Huber MG (1979b) Release of arachidonic acid from human lymphocytes in response to mitogenic lectins. J. Exp. Med. 149:1487.

Parker CW, Stenson WF, Huber MG, Kelly JP (1979) Formation of thromboxane B_2 and hydroaxyarachidonic acids in purified human lymphocytes in the presence and absence of PHA. J. Immunol. 122:1572.

Pelus LM, Strasser HR (1977) Prostaglandins and the immune response. Life Sci. 20:903.

Quagliata F, Lawrence VJW, Phillips-Quagliata JM (1973) Prostaglandin D_1 as a regulator of lymphocyte function. Selective action of B lymphocytes and synergy with pro-carbazine in depression of immune responses. Cell. Immunol. 6:457.

Scheid MP, Goldstein G, Hammerling U, Byse EA (1975) Lymphocyte differentiation from precursor cells in vitro. Ann. N.Y. Acad. Sci. 249:531.

Scheid MP, Goldstein G, Byse EA (1978) The generation and regulation of lymphocyte populations. Evidence from differentiative induction systems in vitro. J. Exp. Med. 147:1727.

Smith JW, Steiner AL, Parker CW (1971) Human lymphocyte metabolism: Effects of cyclic and non-cyclic nucleosides on stimulation by phytohemagglutinin. J. Clin. Invest. 50:442.

Smith WL, Wilkin GP (1977) Immunochemistry of prostaglandin endoperoxide-cyclooxygenase: The detection of the cyclooxygenase in rat, rabbit and guinea pig kidneys by immunofluorescence. Prost. 13:873.

Strom TB, Carpenter CB, Cragoe DJ, Norris S, Devlin R, Perper RJ (1977) Suppression of in vivo and in vitro alloimmunity by prostaglandins. Trans. Proc. 9:1075.

Stenson WF, Parker CW (1980) Editorial: Prostaglandins, Macrophages and Immunity, J.I. 125:1.

Stenson WF, Parker CW (1981) Prostaglandins and the immune response. In "Comprehensive Endocrinology", Lee JB, (ed) Elsevier-North Holland, New York.

Stockman GD, Mumford DM (1974) The effect of prostaglandins on the in vitro blastogenic response of human peripheral blood lymphocytes. Exp. Hemat. 2:65.

Webb DR, Jamieson AT (1976) Control of mitogen-induced transformation: Characterization of a splenic suppressor cell and its mode of action. Cell. Immunol. 24:45.

Webb DR, Nowowiejski I (1977) The role of prostaglandins in the control of the primary 19S immune response to sRBC. Cell. Immunol., 33:1.

Webb DR, Nowowiejski I (1978) Mitogen-induced changes in lymphocyte prostaglandin levels: A signal for the induction of suppressor cell activity. Cell. Immunol. 41:72.

Wolf RI, Merler E (1979) Role of lipids of the immune response. I. ocalization to a lipid-containing fraction of the active moiety of an inhibitor (SIF) of lymphocyte proliferation. J. Immunol. 123:1169.

Zimecki M, Webb DR (1976) The regulation of the immune response to T-independent antigens by prostaglandins and B cells. J. Immunol. 117:2158.

Prostaglandins and Cancer: First
International Conference, pages 609-617
© 1982 Alan R. Liss, Inc., 150 Fifth Avenue, New York, NY 10011

THE ROLE OF ARACHIDONIC ACID PRODUCTS IN MACROPHAGE
FUNCTION

W. Dawson

Lilly Research Centre Limited

Erl Wood Manor, Windlesham, Surrey

INTRODUCTION

The macrophage plays a central role in the function of
the immune system and it follows therefore that its
regulation may have wide ramifications in many therapeutic
areas. It is interesting that whilst most of the early
studies on the immune system were conducted by
immunologists much of the work concerning macrophages
comes from laboratories concerned with pathology of
cells. However, accessory cells to the immune system have
been recognised to be of many types and have recently
received much attention. As the macrophage probably
plays a significant role in this area it has great
potential within the field of cancer immunology. This
short review will define various aspects of macrophage
function and look at the possibility that arachidonic acid
products may regulate these various functions with
particular regard to inflammation and cancer.

DISCUSSION

A simplistic view of the immune system suggests that
the presentation of an antigen to the T-lymphocyte is
performed by a monocytic type cell. This may be a
macrophage, spleen dendritic cell or a Langerhans cell in
the skin. There appear to be few, if any situations where
antigen is used by the lymphocyte without the
participation of an accessory cell. Subsequently
differentiation of the immune system occurs with the
development of either cellular immunity where the T-cell

becomes cytotoxic and also facilitates cytotoxicity by macrophages, or humoral immunity, where the T-cells interact with the B-lymphocytes, resulting in the formation of plasma cells and antibody synthesis. This leads to phagocytosis of opsonized particles by polymorphonuclear leucocytes (Figure 1).

Figure 1. Schematic representation of cellular and humoral immunity.

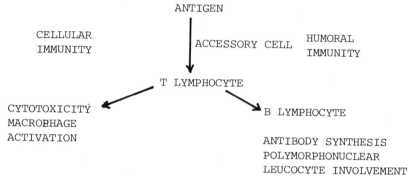

Whilst ultimately it may be possible to regulate sub-populations of lymphocytes as a therapeutic goal it does seem of more immediate interest to try to regulate the earliest stage in immune activation and so control antigen presentation by manipulating monocyte function (Spector & Willoughby, 1979).

The derivation of the monocyte from the pro-monocyte in the bone marrow is interesting. It allows the possibility of intervening in the early stage of differentiation of this cell type within the bone marrow or limiting its movement from bone marrow into blood or from blood into tissue. Clearly lymphocytes, monocytes and polymorphonuclear leucocytes derive differently from the bone marrow stem cells and this may give potential to modify selectively which cell types predominate.

The interaction between the cells involved in the immune system is important. Traditionally lymphokines have been considered to be important regulatory substances but a wider classification of cytokines as cellular messengers released by any cell type and having an effect on another cell seems to be more relevant and will include messengers produced by macrophages as well as those acting on these cells.

In addition, it has been demonstrated that the physical contact of the cells themselves may have particular relevance in the transfer of antigen from macrophage to lymphocyte (Clarke, Salisbury and Willoughby, 1970). The suggestion that prostaglandins may have a cytokine role is one of the more important aspects of their potential involvement in the immune system (Gordon, Bray and Morley, 1976). In any consideration of the action of chemicals on cells it is important to differentiate between pharmacology, where the action of specific compounds in specific biological systems is described and pathophysiology, where these substances are shown to have a role within a disease process. There is often a wide gap between the initial pharmacological characterisation of compounds and the subsequent demonstration of their release and function in a particular diseased state. Inherently, it seems better to consider products of the arachidonic acid cascade as regulatory substances rather than as mediators as this wide ranging family of compounds from both cyclooxygenase and lipoxygenase enzymes have members which have differing activities and in many instances opposite effects to each other. This is clearly so in the cyclooxygenase products and we do not yet have sufficient information on lipoxygenase products to know whether a similar situation pertains. To explore these concepts we can use the inflammatory process as an example.

The response of the mammalian system to injurious stimuli follows a set pathway. The initial response is the acute inflammatory reaction and involves in particular vascular change. The release of small molecular weight chemicals such as histamine, 5-hydroxytryptamine, kinins and arachidonic acid products causes an increased vascular permeability the end result of which is the appearance of symptoms of inflammation – heat, redness, pain and oedema. These chemicals seem to be released by both fixed tissue cells and also the initial wave of migrating cells which are predominantly of the polymorphonuclear leucocyte type. In many instances the stimulus producing the response will be controlled by the combined effects of vascular change and PMN migration with

subsequent phagocytosis. If the stimulus is more severe
then there is a later wave of monocytic infiltration with
the activation of monocytes within the tissue to
macrophages. Clearly at this stage there is no
involvement of the immune system.

However, in some situations, for example in rheumatoid
arthritis, for reasons yet unknown the inflammatory
reaction changes from an acute to a chronic state. The
presentation of an antigen within the inflammatory site
stimulates the T-lymphocytes, which in turn stimulate the
B-lymphocytes to develop into plasma cells, which are
responsible for antibody formation. Whilst
mechanistically this reaction is reasonably well
understood, causally it is not known whether the antigen
is bacterial, viral or is host tissue damaged by the early
phagocytic activity of both polymorphs and monocytes and
is thus recognised as "foreign". In pathological terms the
chronic inflammatory reaction such as occurs in rheumatoid
arthritis consists of accumulated polymorphs, lymphocytes
and macrophages. It would seem therefore to be a mixture
of both the acute and chronic inflammatory responses.

In addition to the cellular aspects of inflammation
the chemical aspects are also of interest. Arachidonic
acid is converted by the cyclooxygenase enzyme into
prostaglandin, thromboxane and prostacyclin products and
via the lipoxygenase enzyme to hydroxy acids (HETE) and
leukotrienes. (Figure 2)

Figure 2.   Schematic representation of the arachidonic
            acid cascade.

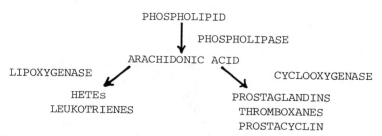

Are any of these compounds capable of influencing the
movement or function of cells involved within the immune
system? If we consider the migrating cells, the initial

phase of migration consists of margination of both PMN and monocytes within the blood vessel. The factors controlling this process are unclear but could in fact be chemotactic factors released at a site of inflammation or injury which by diffusing through the tissue, achieve a gradient from the site to the blood vessel. Having achieved margination the leucocytes then adhere to the inner wall of the vessel and this process may be dependent on the arachidonic acid cascade. Certainly the balance between thromboxane A_2 and prostacyclin (PGI_2) seem to be important as the thromboxanes increase adherence of both platelets and leucocytes whilst prostacyclin reduces adherence. More recently leukotriene B_4 has been shown to be a potent aggregatory substance (Ford-Hutchinson, Bray, Doig, Shipley & Smith, 1980 et al) but whether any or all of the substances are involved in the process of adherence is unknown. After adherence diapedesis of the leucocyte through the vessel wall occurs; this process is functionally uncharacterised in terms of chemicals. Finally the leucocytes arrive at the inflammatory site by moving up the chemotactic gradient towards the inflammatory or injurious stimulus. It is important to recognise that chemotaxis is only one of the events which occurs in the overall migratory process and it is probable that compounds may modify any part of migration to influence the number of cells arriving at the inflammatory site.

In practical terms the control of rheumatic diseases is achieved by two classes of pharmacological agents (Dawson, 1979). First, non-steroidal anti-inflammatory drugs work in the main by inhibiting prostaglandin synthetase and so limit the symptomology of the acute inflammatory response. There is no evidence that reduction or elimination of the cyclooxygenase products has any effect on the long term chronic condition. On the other hand, the suppresive drugs such as D-penicillamine and gold do seem to interfere with cellular functions, particularly of monocytes within the inflammatory cycle. It is encouraging to suppose, therefore, that modification of cellular movement or function may produce more lasting benefits to patients with inflammatory disease (Krane, 1981). It is interesting to note that whilst prostaglandins have been shown to influence some aspects of lymphocyte and macrophage function (Morley, 1981) experimentally, suppression of their formation for extended periods of time in patients undergoing chronic non-steroidal anti-inflammatory drug therapy does not appear to cause any impairment or increase in immune function. We must suppose therefore that whilst prostaglandin may have potent pharmacological activities their role in pathophysiology is much less clear cut, at least with respect to the immune system.

Various arachidonic acid products have been shown to have pharmacological effects on macrophages and their movement and function. PGE_2 (Higgs McCall & Youlten, 1975), thromboxane B_2 (Kitchen, Boot & Dawson, 1978), LTB_4 (Bray, Ford Hutchinson, Shipley and Smith, 1980) and some of the HETEs have been shown to increase chemokinetic movement of cells. Fewer of these compounds have been shown to increase chemotactic response, that is the directional movement of cells, but thromboxane B_2 (Kitchen et al, 1978), LTB_4 (Smith, Ford Hutchinson and Bray, 1980; Goetzl, 1981) and 15-HETE are possible contenders. There has been some speculation that LTB_4 (Smith, 1981) may modify phagocytosis of both polymorphs and monocytes. However, these have been pharmacological studies and whether these properties are functional within disease states remains to be determined. There are many other biological activities, notably of the macrophage in which the actions of these prostanoids have not been studied. In addition to chemokinesis, chemotaxis and phagocytosis the cells can secrete enzymes, have an accessory function to the immune system and can become cytotoxic. Little is known of the activity of arachidonic acid products in these systems. As has already been discussed, to these functions should be added the initial phase of margination, adherence and diapedesis and a complete analysis is probably necessary before roles may be assigned for the arachidonic acid compounds in pathophysiological processes.

One other facet is important. Whilst the arachidonic acid products may or may not modify many of these cellular functions they are not the only potential cytokines. The ultimate expression of activity of these cells will depend on a balance between both positive and negative cytokinens in the tissue in vivo during the disease state (Figure 3).

Within the field of oncology, the evidence that inhibition of the cyclooxygenase enzyme provides

Figure 3. Schematic representation of function and its regulation within macrophages.

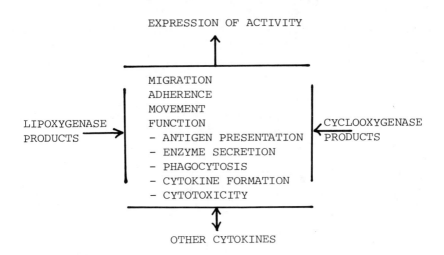

EXPRESSION OF ACTIVITY

LIPOXYGENASE PRODUCTS

MIGRATION
ADHERENCE
MOVEMENT
FUNCTION
- ANTIGEN PRESENTATION
- ENZYME SECRETION
- PHAGOCYTOSIS
- CYTOKINE FORMATION
- CYTOTOXICITY

CYCLOOXYGENASE PRODUCTS

OTHER CYTOKINES

therapeutic advantage is not clear. The experimental and clinical data has been reviewed recently (Honn, Bockman and Marnett, 1981) in the context of the rationale for the therapeutic use of these compounds. Selective inhibitors of the lipoxygenase pathway are not available, although the ability of benoxaprofen to inhibit the lipoxygenase pathway (Walker & Dawson, 1979) with relatively modest inhibition of the cyclooxygenase enzyme is of interest. Clearly the biological data is not yet available to allow a reasoned assessment of the potential therapeutic benefit of lipoxygenase inhibitors.

The involvement of macrophages in surveillance and in tumor growth is of particular interest. Evans and Alexander (1972), Alexander (1976), and Keller (1974) have explored the cytotoxic properties of macrophages in tumour systems and the regulation of these mechanisms by prostanoids seems a fruitful avenue of exploration. It is probable that factors other than those deriving from the arachidonic acid cascade will be involved and the resolution of these questions can only come from a concerted multidisciplinary research programme.

References

Alexander PA, (1976). The function of the macrophage in malignant disease. Ann Rev Med 27: 207.

Bray MA, Ford-Hutchinson AW, Shipley ME, Smith MJH. (1980). Calcium ionophore A23187 induces release of chemokinetic and aggregating factors from polymorphonuclear leucocytes. Br J Pharmac 71: 507

Clarke JA, Salisbury AJ and Willoughby DA, (1970). Application of electron probe microanalysis and electron microscopy to the transfer of antigenic material. Nature 227: 69.

Dawson W, (1979). Mechanisms of action of antiinflammatory drugs. In Samuelsson B, Ramwell PW, Paoletti R (eds): "Adv in Prost and Thromb Res". New York: Raven Press 8: 1741.

Evans R, Alexander P. (1972). Mechanism of immunologically specific killing of tumour cells by macrophages. Nature 236: 168.

Ford-Hutchinson AW, Bray MA, Doig MV, Shipley ME, Smith MJH, (1980). Leukotriene B, a potent chemokinetic and aggregating substance released from polymorphonuclear leukocytes. Nature 286: 264.

Goetzl EJ, (1981). Oxygenation products of arachidonic acid as mediators of hypersensitivity and inflammation. Med Clin N Amer 65: 809.

Gordon D, Bray MA, Morley J, (1976). Control of lymphokine secretion by prostaglandins. Nature 262: 401.

Honn KV, Bockman RS, Marnett LJ, (1981). Prostaglandins and cancer: a review of tumor initiation through tumor metastasis. Prostaglandins 21: 833.

Higgs GA, McCall E, Youlten LJF, (1975). A chemotactic role for postaglandins released from polymorphonuclear leucocytes during phagocytosis. Br J Pharmac 53: 539.

Keller R, (1974). Mechanisms by which activated normal macrophages destroy syngeneic rat tumour cells in vitro. Immunol 27: 285.

Kitchen EA, Boot JR, Dawson W, (1978). Chemotactic activity of thromboxane B_2, prostaglandins and their metabolites for polymorphonuclear leucocytes. Prostaglandins, 16: 239.

Krane SM, (1981). Aspects of the cell biology of the rheumatoid synovial lesion. Ann Rheum Dis 40: 433.

Morley J. (1981). Lymphokine reports 3: in press.

Smith MJH, (1981). Leukotriene B_4. Gen Pharmac 12: 211.

Smith MJH, Ford-Hutchinson AW, Bray MA, (1980). Leukotriene B: a potential mediator of inflammation. J Pharm Pharmacol 32: 517.

Spector WG, Willoughby DA, (1979). The cell of the inflammatory response. Eur J Rheumatol 3: 3.

Walker JR, Dawson W, (1979). Inhibition of rabbit PMN lipoxygenase activity by benoxaprofen. J Pharm Pharmacol 31: 11.

**Prostaglandins and Cancer: First
International Conference, pages 619-631
© 1982 Alan R. Liss, Inc., 150 Fifth Avenue, New York, NY 10011**

DOES PROSTAGLANDIN SYNTHESIS EFFECT *IN VIVO* TUMOUR GROWTH
BY ALTERING TUMOUR/HOST BALANCE?

OTTO J. PLESCIA

Waksman Institute of Microbiology, Rutgers-The
State University of New Jersey, New Brunswick,
New Jersey 08903

INTRODUCTION

The title of this paper is unique among the others
presented in this Conference in that it is in the form of
a question. This title was assigned to me by the organizers
of this Conference, and I suspect that they are intrigued by
the possibility that prostaglandin synthesis by tumour cells
may alter tumour/host balance, and thus affect tumour growth,
but that they are not quite convinced by the results published thus far. I regard this a challenge to answer the
question posed in the title, and try in the process to make
believers among those who may have reservations.

My approach will be to rephrase the question by asking
several implicit subsidiary questions. These are: (1) Are
prostaglandins physiological immunoregulatory agents? 2)
Do malignant tumours produce excess prostaglandins? 3) Are
malignant tumours immunosuppressive? 4) Is tumour-mediated
immunosuppression linked to prostaglandin synthesis? 5) Do
drugs that regulate prostaglandin synthesis affect tumour
growth?

Answers to the above questions will be based primarily
on the results of our study, and those of others, of experimental animal model systems comprising inbred strains of
mice and several syngeneic tumour lines, including cell lines
induced by chemical carcinogens and oncogenic viruses.

IMMUNOREGULATORY ROLE OF PROSTAGLANDINS

Antigenic stimulation of immunocompetent mice by sheep red blood cells (SRBC) results in the induction of antibody-forming cells in a matter of days. These antibody-forming cells are plasma cells derived from B lymphocytes that are activated by the specific concerted action of antigen, macrophages, and T helper and suppressor lymphocytes. This action depends, among other factors, on cellular interactions that are regulated by mediators derived from antigen-reactive cells in response to antigen. Lymphokines and monokines have clearly been identified as mediators in antibody formation, and evidence is accumulating that prostaglandins also play a physiological role (Quagliata, Lawrence, Quagliata, 1972; Loose, DiLuzio, 1973; Bach, Bach, 1973; Ferraris, DeRobertis, 1974; Pelus, Strausser, 1977; Strom, et al., 1977; Webb, Nowowiejski, 1977; Goldyne, Stobo, 1980; Goodwin, Webb, 1980; Leung, Mihich, 1980).

Our own study of prostaglandins began with an investigation of the role of carrier determinants of an immunogen in the activation of helper T lymphocytes (Plescia, 1969; Plescia, Hirsch, 1973) and of the possible role of cyclic AMP (cAMP) in this activation (Plescia, Yamamoto, Shimamura, 1975). Within two minutes, after injection of SRBC into mice, the splenic level of cAMP increases three to five-fold. This is followed about four hours later by the appearance of antigen-specific helper T lymphocytes.

The cAMP response can be elicited only in immunocompetent mice and by T lymphocyte-dependent immunogens. Also, this response is antigen-specific, but paradoxically it is not additive when mixtures of unrelated antigens, each in an amount that elicits a maximal cAMP increase, are used. To resolve this apparent paradox, we postulated that a common mediator is released by certain antigen-specific lymphocytes in response to antigen and subsequently, in a second step, stimulates cAMP biosynthesis in a larger population of spleen cells with receptors for the postulated mediator (Skelly, Plescia, 1976).

Histamine and prostaglandins (PGE and PGF2α) were tested as possible mediators of the cAMP response to antigen. Both histamine and PGE were active, but not PGF2α. The kinetics and the magnitude of the cAMP response to these agents were equivalent to the response to antigen. Histamine antagonists and indomethacin, an inhibitor of prostaglandin synthetases, were next tested for their ability to inhibit the cAMP response to antigen. Only indomethacin proved to be active, clearly implicating prostaglandins as the common mediator system responsible for the relatively large and quick increase in the splenic level of cAMP in mice after being immunized. This conclusion was confirmed by Webb and Osheroff (1976), who quantitated the splenic level of prostaglandins directly in mice immunized with SRBC.

Having identified prostaglandins as physiological mediators of the cAMP response to antigen, we next considered the possible role of prostaglandins in the activation and function of helper and suppressor T lymphocytes. Mice, immunized with SRBC, develop peak levels of helper and suppressor T lymphocytes in their spleen four and eight hours, respectively, after the injection of SRBC. These helper and suppressor cells can be quantitated, using *in vitro* assay systems recently developed by us, so that we are able to assess the role of prostaglandins in the generation of these cells *in vivo* and their function *in vitro*.

Pretreatment of mice with indomethacin, not only abrogates the cAMP response to antigen as found previously, but also interferes with the generation of helper and suppressor T lymphocytes. This suggests that the cAMP response mediated by prostaglandins is somehow associated with the activation of both helper and suppressor cells. Confirmation is based on the finding that PGE, added exogenously to cultures of normal spleen cells in the absence of antigen, results in the generation of helper cells, and also suppressor cells. Larger amounts of PGE are required to generate suppressor cells (Racis, Griffiths, Plescia, unpublished results).

Helper and suppressor cells, generated *in vivo* by mice in response to antigen, have been identified as the Lyt 1^+ and Lyt $2,3^+$ subsets of T lymphocytes, respectively. Their functional activity, *in vitro,* requires intact cells that presumably react with antigen activated B lymphocytes and macrophages subject to genetic restriction at the H2 locus. Pretreatment of these functional cells with indomethacin reduces significantly their activity *in vitro* in stimulating or suppressing induction of anti-SRBC antibody-forming cells. Thus, prostaglandin synthesis seems to

be required not only for the generation of helper and
suppressor cells but also for their functional activity.

PROSTAGLANDIN SYNTHESIS BY TUMOURS

Several speakers at this Conference have addressed the
question of prostaglandin synthesis and the role of
prostaglandins in the initiation and promotion of carcinogenesis. The evidence indicates that transformation of
animal cells by carcinogens and viruses is generally
accompanied by an increased capacity of the transformed
cells to synthesize prostaglandins. Lines of transformed
tumorigenic cells may differ quantitatively in their
synthetic capacity, but most show increased activity
(Grinwich, Plescia, Pelus, Strausser, unpublished results),
and equally important, synthesis of PGE is preferentially
stimulated so that tumours produce excess PGE which we, and
others, have shown to be a physiological immunoregulatory
agent. Whether or not increased synthesis of prostaglandins
is an essential phenotypic trait of transformed cells is not
certain, but whatever the reason for the increased synthesis
generally associated with transformation, tumours should,
through the excess of PGE they produce, offset the immunological balance between host and tumour.

TUMOUR-MEDIATED IMMUNOSUPPRESSION

Suppression of Antibody Response

Groups of C57B1/6J mice were inoculated with MC16
tumour cells (a syngeneic fibrosarcoma induced by methylcholanthrene), and BALB/cJ mice were inoculated with
MCDV-12 ascites tumour cells (induced by Rauscher leukemia
virus). At different times thereafter, these tumour-bearing
mice and normal control mice were immunized with SRBC, and
their antibody response was monitored. Depression of the
antibody response was noted in the tumour-bearing mice, and
the extent increased with time of tumour growth prior to
challenge with SRBC (Plescia, Smith, Grinwich, 1975). The
MCDV-12 line grew faster in syngeneic recipients than the
MC16 line, and its growth resulted in a more rapid decline
in antibody response to SRBC. Since the tumours and SRBC
were antigenically unrelated, it was evident that the

immunosuppression associated with tumour growth was general
in nature and not antigen-specific, and also independent of
the etiology of the tumours. Chemical and virus-induced
tumour lines were used.

The same kind of results were noted with other
syngeneic tumour lines, indicating the generality of immunosuppression associated with progressive tumour growth. They
did not indicate, however, that the tumour was the direct
cause of the immunosuppression although a direct relationship
between rates of tumour growth and immunosuppression
suggested it. Induction of antibody response to SRBC was
therefore carried out in vitro, co-culturing a fixed number
of normal spleen cells, a variable number of syngeneic tumour
cells and SRBC. The tumour proved very active in suppressing the antibody response (Plescia, Smith, Grinwich, Feit,
1975). Complete suppression occurred in cultures with tumour
to spleen cells in a ratio of 1:100, providing direct
evidence of the immunosuppressive activity of syngeneic
tumour cells. Pretreatment of the tumour cells with mitomycin C abrogated their immunosuppressive activity, as did X-
irradiation. Viability is therefore essential for immunosuppressive activity, and suggests a positive action by the
tumour cells against host spleen cells. This is further
suggested by the observed increase in immunosuppressive
activity when tumour and spleen cells are allowed to interact prior to the addition of SRBC to initiate the antibody
response.

Suppression of Cell-Mediated Immunity

The finding of a generalized depression of the antibody response in tumour-bearing mice was considered to be,
not a fortuitous event, but a reflection of a mechanism that
tumours might use to escape from immunological rejection by
subverting the immune system. This hypothesis prompted a
study of the effect of a syngeneic tumour on the development of cellular immunity since specific tumour immunity is
largely dependent on cell-mediated immunity rather than on
antibody-mediated immunity.

For this purpose, the cellular immune response to a
tumour allograft was studied in a histoincompatible strain
of mice bearing a transplanted syngeneic tumour. Tumour
cells of the MC16 line were inoculated subcutaneously in

syngeneic C57B1/6J mice, and at different times thereafter
groups of these mice, and a control group that received
diluent, were inoculated in a contralateral site with allogeneic DBA/2J mastocytoma cells.

The objective of this type of experiment was to assess
the effect of a growing viable syngeneic tumour on the
capacity of its host to reject a tumor allograft. From the
growth profile of the DBA/2J tumor allograft in C57B1/6J
mice as a function of the interval of time between inoculation
of the syngeneic tumour and challenge with tumor allograft,
it was clear that the tumour allograft grew faster and more
extensively in these mice, and more important it was not
rejected by mice bearing a syngeneic tumour for as few as 5
days at the time the tumour allograft was inoculated (Plescia,
Grinwich, Plescia, 1976). These results may be summarized
by saying that a syngeneic tumour can so depress the cellular
immune capability of its host that proliferating tumour cells,
even strongly antigenic allogeneic tumour cells, can and do
escape immunological rejection.

Targets of Immunosuppressive Tumour Cells

Suppression of cell-mediated immunity in tumour-bearing
mice implicated T lymphocytes as targets of immunosuppressive tumours. The antibody response to SRBC is dependent on
both T and B lymphocytes, so that its suppression might have
been due to the action of tumours against either T or B
lymphocytes, or both. T and B lymphocyte-specific mitogens
were used to probe the functional activity of T and B
lymphocytes in spleens of tumour-bearing mice. Compared
with spleens of normal mice, the mitogen response (measured
in terms of DNA synthesis) to phytohemagglutinin (a T cell
mitogen) was depressed, the extent increasing with time of
tumour growth. In contrast, the response to LPS (a B cell
mitogen) remained stable. Suppression of spleen cells
(responsive to T cell mitogen) in tumour-bearing mice
occurred at a rate equal to suppression of the antibody
response to SRBC and suppression of the cell-mediated
response to a tumour allograft. These results point to T
lymphocytes as the chief target of immunosuppressive tumours.
Further support for this conclusion is based on our finding
that normal spleen cells become unresponsive to phytohemagglutinin, but not to LPS, on culturing them *in vitro*
with syngeneic tumour cells.

The antibody response to SRBC, as noted above, is T and B cell dependent, but it is also dependent on macrophages. Moreover, macrophages may well be critically important in tumour immunity. Accordingly, macrophages from tumour-bearing animals, and also macrophages cultured *in vitro* with syngeneic tumour cells, were tested for phagocytic and bactericidal activity. No significant change in macrophage function was evident as a result of their interaction with known immunosuppressive tumours both *in vivo* and *in vitro* (Plescia, Grinwich, Sheridan, Plescia, 1978). This was surprising in view of reports of tumour-derived factors that repulse macrophages (Fauve, Hevin, Jacob, Gaillard, Jacob, 1974), and the apparent inactivity of macrophages that infiltrate tumours (Evans, 1972). Nevertheless, it is a fact that syngeneic tumours we tested did not suppress phagocytic activity of macrophages under the same conditions and in the same test systems in which they clearly suppressed T lymphocytes.

Natural killer cells (NK) have recently been recognized as a family of cytotoxic cells that are active against a broad spectrum of tumour cells. These NK cells may constitute a critical first line of host defense in tumour immunosurveillance, and are therefore the object of intense investigation. We have tested spleen cells of mice, bearing immunosuppressive syngeneic tumours, for possible change in NK activity associated with tumour growth, and could find none in an *in vitro* assay using the same tumour cells as targets. This was unexpected because others had reported some effect by prostaglandins on NK activity (Droller, Schneider, Perlmann, 1978; Brunda, Herberman, Holden, 1980), and we had shown prostaglandins to be mediators of tumour immunosuppression.

PROSTAGLANDINS AS MEDIATORS OF TUMOUR IMMUNOSUPPRESSION

Prostaglandins were first considered and tested as possible mediators of immunosuppression by syngeneic tumours because several tumour lines had been reported to synthesize and release abnormal amounts of prostaglandins (Humes, Strausser, 1974; Sykes, Maddox, 1972; Tashjian, et al., 1972), which we were investigating as mediators of immunological responses.

Indeed, the addition of prostaglandins of the E series (PGE1 and PGE2) to cultures of normal spleen cells mimicked syngeneic tumour cells in suppressing the antibody response of the spleen cells to SRBC (Plescia, Smith, Grinwich, 1975). More importantly, the addition of indomethacin, an inhibitor of prostaglandin synthetases, to cultures of tumour and spleen cells reduced significantly the suppression of the antibody response to SRBC. These results were regarded as an important first clue to the role of prostaglandins in the subversion of the immune system by syngeneic tumours, and this study was extended to include the effect of prostaglandins on the mitogenic response of normal spleen cells and also the effect of inhibitors of prostaglandin synthetases on tumour-mediated suppression of the mitogenic response.

To cultures of spleen cells were added either PGE2 or PGF2α, in different amounts. Five min later, mitogen (PHA-M or LPS) was added, and mitogenic stimulation was assessed as before. Only PGE2, which is the series of prostaglandins produced in greatest amount by tumour cells, showed a suppressive effect, and like tumour cells it suppressed preferentially the T cell response to PHA-M (Plescia, Grinwich, Plescia, 1976).

The fact that prostaglandins could induce the same kind of immunosuppression as tumours suggested, but did not prove, that they were the mediators of tumour immunosuppression. Decisive evidence was obtained through the use of inhibitors of prostaglandin synthetases; namely, indomethacin, aspirin and flufenamic acid. Immunosuppressive tumour cells were pretreated with these inhibitors prior to culturing them with normal syngeneic spleen cells and testing the response of the spleen cells to SRBC or T cell mitogen. Inhibition of prostaglandin biosynthesis by the tumour cells resulted in a significant decrease in suppression of both the antibody and mitogen response (Plescia, Smith, Grinwich, 1975; Plescia, Grinwich, Plescia, 1976). Also, treatment of tumour-bearing mice with inhibitors of prostaglandin synthesis prevented completely tumour-mediated suppression of their antibody response to SRBC (Grinwich, Plescia, 1977).

EFFECT OF PROSTAGLANDIN SYNTHESIS INHIBITORS ON TUMOUR GROWTH

Treatment of tumour-bearing mice with inhibitors of prostaglandin synthesis not only prevents suppression of their antibody response, as noted above, but also affects tumour growth. This effect on tumour growth varies with the antigenicity of the tumour. The MC16 tumour is weakly antigenic, and its growth in syngeneic mice is significantly reduced by indomethacin but not prevented (Plescia, Smith, Grinwich, 1975). In contrast, the Moloney sarcoma virus-induced tumor is highly antigenic in syngeneic BALB/c mice, and its growth is completely prevented by indomethacin provided the tumour-bearing mice are immunocompetent at the time the virus is inoculated (Strausser, Humes, 1975).

DISCUSSION

The answer to the question whether or not prostaglandin synthesis can affect tumour growth is yes. The reasons, based on the results of our study of prostaglandins over the past several years and reviewed in this report, are that: (1) Prostaglandins are now recognized as essential physiological immunoregulatory agents, and any abnormal change in their concentration in lymphoid tissue during the course of an active immune response is apt to affect that response. Excess of PGE tends to be immunosuppressive at the level of T lymphocytes so that tumours which produce excess PGE can, and do, suppress T cell-dependent immune responses. (2) Treatment of mice, bearing syngeneic immunosuppressive tumours, with inhibitors of prostaglandin synthesis retards, and in some instances prevents, tumour growth.

If one asks the question does, rather than can, prostaglandin synthesis affect tumour growth, the answer is a qualified yes. Yes, if two conditions are satisfied. The host must be immunocompetent at the time tumour is inoculated or develops spontaneously, and the tumour must be sufficiently antigenic rendering it subject to rejection by tumour-specific activated cytotoxic T lymphocytes.

The reason for the first requirement is obvious. It matters little if tumours produce an excess of prostaglandins capable of subverting their host's immune system if it is initially inadequate. The requirement that tumours be antigenic is based on the fact that excess prostaglandins suppress largely T lymphocytes, including precursors of antigen-specific cytotoxic T cells, and not B lymphocytes, phagocytic monocytes and NK cells. Therefore, only if host rejection of a tumour is significantly dependent on tumour-specific cytotoxic T lymphocytes will prostaglandin synthesis affect tumour growth. This should be the case if the tumour is sufficiently antigenic.

The fact that immunosuppressive tumours, that produce excess prostaglandins, do not seem to suppress macrophages or NK cells is reason for optimism. These cells constitute the non-specific arm of tumour immunity. Thus, if they are insensitive to suppression by tumours, one can hope to develop a form of immunotherapy designed to activate macrophages and NK cells. This strategy is essential if the tumour is not antigenic and thus not subject to rejection by antigen-specific cell-mediated immunity. In the case of those tumours that are both antigenic and produce excess prostaglandins which can subvert T lymphocytes, one should also include as part of the immunotherapeutic regimen inhibitors of prostaglandin synthesis, which we have found to be effective, and perhaps even prostaglandin antagonists.

SUMMARY

Prostaglandins are physiologically released by lymphocytes on stimulation by antigen, and function as important mediators of immune responses, especially those that are dependent on T lymphocytes. Excess PGE suppresses T cell function, and interferes with the normal development of antigen-specific cell-mediated immunity and antibody response to T cell-dependent antigens. Macrophages and natural killer cells are relatively unaffected by excess PGE.

Tumour cells, compared with normal cells, generally produce large amounts of PGE and are therefore immunosuppressive in syngeneic hosts. This tumour-mediated suppression of T cell-dependent immune responses can affect host/tumour balance, and therefore tumour growth. Tumour growth is affected provided that the tumour is sufficiently antigenic to be rejected by antigen-specific cytotoxic T lymphocytes, that are suppressed by PGE produced by the tumour. In such cases the host/tumour balance can be shifted in the host's favor by treating the host with inhibitors of prostaglandin synthesis, such as indomethacin. This treatment is particularly effective if the immune system of the host is normal and has not been subverted by the tumour by the time treatment is started.

REFERENCES

Bach MA, Bach JF (1973). Studies on thymus products IV. The effects of cyclic nucleotides and prostaglandins on rosette-forming cells. Interactions with thymic factor. Eur J Immunol 3: 778.

Brunda M, Herberman R, Holden H (1980). Inhibition of murine natural killer cell activity by prostaglandins. J Immunol 124: 2682.

Droller M, Schneider M, Perlmann P (1978). A possible role of prostaglandins in the inhibition of natural and antibody-dependent cell-mediated cytotoxicity against tumor cells. Cell Immunol 39: 166.

Evans R (1972). Macrophages in syngeneic tumors. Transplantation 14: 468.

Fauve R, Hevin B, Jacob H, Gaillard J, Jacob F (1974). Anti-inflammatory effects of murine malignant cells. Proc Natl Acad Sci 71: 4052.

Ferraris J, DeRobertis F (1974). Release of prostaglandins by mitogen- and antigen-stimulated leukocytes in culture. J Clin Invest 54: 378.

Goldyne M, Stobo J (1980). Prostaglandin E2 as a modulator of macrophage-T lymphocyte interaction. J Invest Dermat 74: 297.

Goodwin J, Webb D (1980). Regulation of the immune response by prostaglandins. Clin Immunol Immunopathol 15: 106.

Grinwich K, Plescia OJ (1977). Tumor-mediated immunosuppression: prevention by inhibitors of prostaglandin synthesis. Prostaglandins 14: 1175.

Humes J, Strausser H (1974). Prostaglandins and cyclic nucleotides in Moloney sarcoma tumors. Prostaglandins 5: 183.

Leung K, Mihich E (1980). Prostaglandin modulation of development of cell-mediated immunity in culture. Nature 288: 597.

Loose L, DiLuzio N (1973). Effect of prostaglandin E1 on cellular and humoral immune responses. J R E S 13: 70.

Pelus L, Strausser H (1977). Prostaglandins and the immune response. Life Science 20: 903.

Plescia OJ   (1969).   Role of the carrier in antibody formation.   Adv Immunol 50: 78.

Plescia OJ, Grinwich K, Plescia AM   (1976)   Subversive
activity of syngeneic tumor cells as an escape
mechanism from immune surveillance and the role of
prostaglandins.   Ann NY Acad Sci 276: 455.

Plescia OJ, Grinwich K, Sheridan J, Plescia AM   (1978).
Subversion of the immune system by tumors as a mechanism
of their escape from immune rejection.   Prog Biochem
Pharmacol 14: 123.

Plescia OJ, Hirsch J   (1973).   Isolation and characterization
of functional antigen-carrying T cells.   Ann NY Acad
Sci 207: 49.

Plescia OJ, Smith A, Grinwich K, Feit C   (1975).   The
problem of cancer immunotherapy in perspective.   In
Gottlieb A, Plescia OJ, Bishop D (eds):   "Fundamental
Aspects of Neoplasia,"   New York: Springer Verlag, p
139.

Plescia OJ, Smith A, Grinwich K   (1975).   Subversion of
immune system by tumor cells and role of prostaglandins.
Proc Natl Acad Sci 72: 1848.

Plescia OJ, Yamamoto I, Shimamura T   (1975).   Cyclic AMP and
immune responses: changes in the splenic level of cyclic
AMP during the response of mice to antigen.   Proc Natl
Acad Sci 72: 888.

Quagliata F, Lawrence V, Quagliata J   (1972).   Prostaglandin
El as a regulator of lymphocyte function.   Cell Immunol
6: 457.

Skelly R, Plescia OJ   (1976).   Specificity and control of
the cyclic AMP response of mice to antigen.   Fed Proc
35: 532.

Strausser H, Humes J   (1975).   Prostaglandin synthesis
inhibition: effect on bone changes and sarcoma tumor
induction in Balb/c mice.   Int J Cancer 15: 724.

Strom T, Carpenter C, Crague E, Norris S, Devolin R,
Perper R   (1977).   Suppression of the in vivo and in
vitro alloimmunity by prostaglandins.   Trans Proc 9:
1075.

Sykes J, Maddox J   (1972).   Prostaglandin production by
experimental tumors and effects of antiinflammatory
compounds.   Nature New Biol 237: 59.

Tashjian A Jr, Voelkel E, Levine L. Goldhaber P   (1972).
Evidence that the bone resorption-stimulating factor
produced by mouse fibrosarcoma cells is prostaglandin
E2.   J Exp Med 136: 1329.

Webb D, Nowowiejski I (1977). The role of prostaglandins in the control of the primary 19S immune response to SRBC. Cell Immunol 33: 1.

Webb D, Osheroff P (1976). Antigen stimulation of prostaglandin synthesis and control of immune responses. Proc Natl Acad Sci 73: 1300.

ACKNOWLEDGEMENTS

The studies reported here were carried out by the following graduate students and associates of mine: K. Grinwich, A. Smith, R. Skelly, S. Racis, A. Plescia, J. Sheridan, J. Brown, E. Griffiths, T. Shimamura, C. Feit, and I. Yamamoto. Financial support was provided by the Charles and Johanna Busch Fund, USPHS Grant AI-11006, and USPHS Contract NCI-NO1-CM-67106.

**Prostaglandins and Cancer: First
International Conference, pages 633-649**
© 1982 Alan R. Liss, Inc., 150 Fifth Avenue, New York, NY 10011

INTERRELATIONSHIP OF ENDOGENOUS MACROPHAGES, PROSTAGLANDIN
SYNTHESIS AND TUMOR CELL CLONOGENICITY IN HUMAN TUMOR
BIOPSIES

Sydney E. Salmon, M.D.

University of Arizona Cancer Center and
Department of Internal Medicine, Hematology/
Oncology, Tucson, Arizona 85724

INTRODUCTION

Macrophages are thought to play a regulatory or "mana-
gerial" role in normal hemopoiesis and in the immune response (Kurland and Bockman, 1978; Bockman and Rothschild,
1979). Some evidence also suggests that in sufficiently
high concentrations, activated macrophages may also have
antitumor properties in transplantable animal tumor systems
(Hibbs, 1974). Since 1975, my laboratory has pursued detailed studies of in vitro clonogenicity of tumor cells in
fresh biopsies from spontaneous human cancers in an effort
to better define biological and clinical correlates of putative human "tumor stem cells" (Hamburger and Salmon,
1977; Salmon, 1980). The primary technique which we have
used has been in vitro colony formation in semi-solid
medium. Morphological, cytogenetic and biomarker studies
have provided excellent evidence that the assay system promotes the growth of human tumor colonies as opposed to normal fibroblasts, lymphocytes, myeloid precursors or other
cellular elements in the biopsy specimen. For some tumor
types, self-renewal studies (replating experiments) or formation of tumors from colonies transplanted into nude mice
have provided support for the contention that some of the
tumor colony-forming cells which proliferate in vitro in
this assay system bear a close relationship to tumor stem
cells in vivo. Tumor cell cloning efficiency is usually
low (circa 1:1000 nucleated cells), and similar to that of
normal bone marrow progenitors (Salmon, 1980). Chemosensitivity testing of cytotoxic agents in the tumor stem cell
assay has proven to be predictive of clinical response in

cancer patients to specific anticancer drugs (Salmon et al., 1978; Salmon, 1980), hormones, and biological response modifiers such as the interferons (Salmon, 1981). Thus, the assay system appears to have relevance to biological events relevant to tumor growth in vivo. In the course of this work, we have observed that endogenous macrophages within the tumor cell population appear to modulate in vitro clonogenicity with differing effects observed in multiple myeloma and in malignant effusions from epithelial neoplasms such as ovarian or breast cancer. I will summarize prior observations from my laboratory relating to modulation of in vitro tumor cell clonogenicity and provide additional data relevant to the relationship between the macrophages and prostaglandin synthesis inhibitors and prostaglandin synthesis in culture in relation to tumor cell clonogenicity. Our observations and other data are then viewed from the perspective of a hypothesis relating to macrophage promotion of tumor growth.

METHODS

The human tumor stem cell assay procedure was carried out with only minor modifications of the method of Hamburger and Salmon (1977; Salmon, 1980). Balb-C spleen-conditioned medium was used to stimulate myeloma colony growth but not required for studies involving carcinomas. In selected experiments, using techniques detailed by Buick et al. (1980; Buick and Salmon, 1980), cell suspensions prepared from malignant effusions were subjected to procedures for separating adherent cells from the non-adherent non-phagocytic (NA/NP) cells prior to plating. The NA/NP cell fraction is macrophage depleted, and enriched for tumor cells, whereas the adherent cell fraction is enriched for monocytes and macrophages (Buick et al, 1980; Buick and Salmon, 1980). "Reconstitution studies" and prostaglandin radioimmunoassays for PGE_2 and $PGF_{2\alpha}$ were performed as delineated by Buick et al. (1980). The 13',13' dimethyl PGE_2 analog, which is stable in tissue culture, was utilized in specific experiments designed to test growth stimulation effects in the presence of indomethacin. When utilized, indomethacin and PGE_2 were added to the agar in the Petri dishes to permit continuous exposure to the cell populations present during the entire duration of culture.

MULTIPLE MYELOMA

Our studies of multiple myeloma suggest that macrophage derived factors played a modulating role on clonogenicity of myeloma stem cells in soft agar culture. Conditioned medium derived from adherent mononuclear cells
from the spleen of mineral oil-treated Balb-C mice is required to obtain myeloma colony growth in at least 80% of
patients whose cells could be grown in vitro in the agar
culture system (Hamburger and Salmon, 1977). The condi-
tioning factor is non-dialyzable, heat labile and susceptible to proteolytic enzymes (Hamburger et al., 1979).
Morphologically, Giemsa stained plates of the adherent
spleen cells had the appearance of macrophages. Despite
this requirement for a macrophage-conditioned medium, endogenous adherent phagocytic mononuclear cells within the
myeloma patients' marrow were not required for clonogenicity (Hamburger and Salmon, 1977). On the contrary, clonogenicity of myeloma colony-forming cells was improved when
adherent and/or phagocytic mononuclear cells were removed
prior to plating (Hamburger and Salmon, 1977), suggesting
that endogenous macrophages in the myeloma patients' marrow
cells inhibit clonogenicity. Observations on the effect of
depletion of adherent and/or phagocytic cells are summarized in Table 1.

TABLE 1

Effect of Population Depletion on Myeloma Colony Formation*

Population depleted	Experiment No.	Number of M-CFU-c per 5×10^5 cells plated[a]	
		Before depletion	After depletion
Adherent	1	11± 7.2	92± 8.3
	2	52± 8.7	83± 6.8
	3	65± 8.6	101±11.2
	4	28± 5.6	123± 9.8
	5	44± 4.8	220±28.5
Adherent phagocytic	5	48± 8.1	80±22.0
Phagocytic	6	70±14.5	200±37.4

*Reproduced from J Clin Invest (Hamburger and Salmon, 1977)
with permission of the publishers.
[a]Mean ± SEM of four plates.

Optimal myeloma colony growth has thus been obtained by
plating just the NA/NP cell population which is enriched
for myeloma cells. Reconstitution studies were carried
out wherein adherent mononuclear cells from the patients'
marrow were plated below the agar feeder layer and the
overlying tumor cell plating layer. The clonogenic myeloma
cells were rendered NA/NP prior to plating. In these experiments, increasing inhibition of myeloma colony formation occurred with increasing numbers of adherent mononuclear cells plated on the bottom of the dish (data not
shown). This suggested a dose-dependent inhibition of
myeloma cell clonogenicity resulting from diffusable
factors released by the adherent cells.

    Figure 1 summarizes fractionation and prostaglandin
modulation experiments on cells from two myeloma patients.

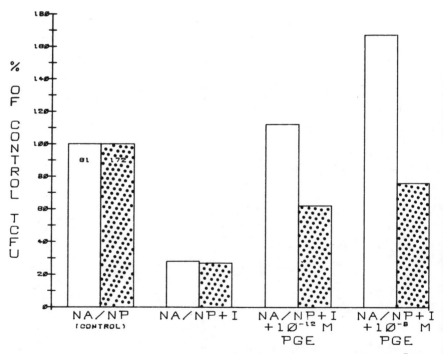

Fig. 1 Effects of cell fractionation, indomethacin (10^{-5}M),
and PGE_2 on myeloma colony formation. The number of
colonies in the controls appears in the bars. I=Indometha-
cin.

One patient's myeloma cells were harvested from the marrow while the second patient's cells were from a malignant pleural effusion. Both myeloma samples were depleted of endogenous adherent and phagocytic macrophages prior to culture. Effects of added 10^{-5}M indomethacin alone or with added PGE_2 were tested to assess the modulating effects of these agents on clonogenicity of NA/NP myeloma cells. As can be appreciated from figure 1, addition of indomethacin markedly reduced myeloma colony formation. The indomethacin effect appears to be specifically mediated via inhibition of prostaglandin production by the myeloma cells as the effect of indomethacin could largely be reversed with the addition of physiological quantities (10^{-12}-10^{-8}M) of PGE_2. Thus, in myeloma, colony formation does not require endogenous tumor macrophages as long as a non-dialyzable growth factor from Balb-C mouse macrophage-conditioned medium is provided. PGE synthesis intrinsic in the myeloma cell population appears to be linked to myeloma colony formation. As evidenced by the PGE_2 effects of physiological amounts of PGE_2 in the presence of indomethacin and macrophage depletion, prostaglandin biosynthesis appears to be constitutive in enriched myeloma cell progenitors which give rise to myeloma colonies in vitro. Effects of higher concentrations of PGE_2 (e.g., 10^{-6}M) have not yet been tested to determine whether the proliferative response continues to increase (or is inhibited) at pharmacological concentrations of PGE_2.

STUDIES OF EFFUSIONS FROM OVARIAN CANCER AND OTHER EPITHELIAL NEOPLASMS

Morphological assessment of the cell population present in carcinomatous effusions which gave rise to tumor colonies established that they contained an admixture of normal host cells (including macrophages, lymphocytes and mesothelial cells) as well as tumor cells (Buick et al., 1980). In our initial studies (Table 2) of ovarian cancer, we questioned the role of macrophages in such effusions and found that phagocytic depletion of macrophages in ovarian effusions markedly reduced ovarian tumor colony formation (Hamburger et al., 1978). Recently, using cell separation procedures, Buick et al. (1980) established that the adherent mononuclear cells present in the effusions provided the predominant source of PGE_2 production in such effusions.

Effect of Depletion of Macrophages
on Ovarian Tumor Cell Growth*

		No. of colonies/500,000 cells
Trial	Control	Macrophages
1	157±30[a]	31± 6
2	146±35	17± 8
3	99± 9	5± 3
	147±20	58±10

*Modified from Cancer Res (Hamburger et al., 1978)
with permission of the publishers.
[a]Mean±SE.
Cell populations in malignant effusions from patients
with ovarian cancer were depleted of phagocytic macrophages by ingestion of carbonyl iron prior to plating.

Recently, Berens et al. have confirmed and extended this
observation with a larger group of fractionated malignant
effusions (Berens and Salmon, 1981). Overall, PGE synthesis by adherent cells was 30-fold greater than that of the
NA/NP cells (Berens and Salmon, 1981). The low synthetic
rate of PGE observed in macrophage depleted cells in the
NA/NP fraction not only contrasts sharply with the high
levels synthesized in the adherent layer, but also with the
high levels of PGE that have been observed with long term
established tumor cell lines. As depicted in figure 2, we
recently observed that indomethacin addition to unfractionated effusions or depletion of the adherent phagocytic
cells generally results in significantly reduced ovarian
or breast tumor colony formation. However, colony formation per se in unfractionated effusions correlated positively with the number of tumor cells present and not with
the macrophage or lymphocyte content (Buick et al., 1980).
Reconstitution studies wherein separated NA/NP cells were
added back over varying numbers of adherent cells but
separated by a layer of agar usually did reconstitute
growth of tumor colonies in a dose-dependent fashion, with
optimum stimulation usually attained when the number of adherent cells was similar to that present in the unfractionated effusion. This result contrasts with our findings in
myeloma wherein reconstitution with adherent cells inhibited myeloma colony formation.

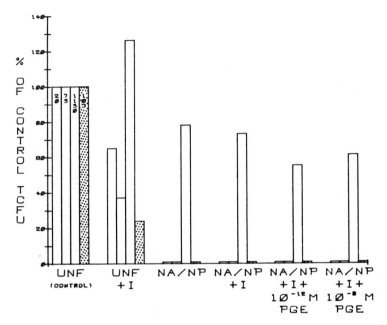

Fig. 2 Effect of cell fractionation, indomethacin (10^{-5}M), and PGE_2 on ovarian and breast tumor colony formation. UNF=Unfractionated cells. Other abbreviations in Fig. 1 and the text.

Data on a series of reconstitution experiments in various carcinomas are depicted in figure 3. These experiments indicate that growth stimulation of human tumor colony forming cells by adherent cells is mediated by diffusable factors released by them, and in a dose-dependent fashion. Furthermore, plating numbers of adherent cells that were significantly higher than were present in the original effusion usually resulted in inhibition of colony formation suggesting that optimal ratios of macrophages to tumor cells to promote chemosensitivity may be present in malignant effusions. Thus, we had established that tumor colony growth of unfractionated effusions could frequently be inhibited with pharmacological doses of indomethacin that inhibited PGE synthesis, and that prostaglandins such as PGE were produced by the primarily adherent cells present in malignant effusions. Furthermore, we found that the cells in the adherent fraction also promoted tumor colony formation by release of diffusable factors.

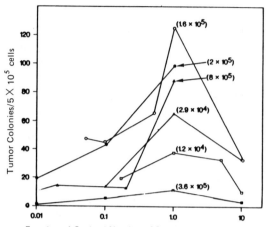

Fraction of Optimal Number of Stimulating Adherent Cells

Fig. 3   Ability of autologous adherent cells to reconstitute tumor colony formation by enriched tumor cells in six
patients with carcinoma.   Inasmuch as the absolute tumor
colony modulating activity of adherent cells varied from
patient to patient, the reconstitution data have been normalized with respect to the concentration of adherent cells
beneath the feeder layer that produced peak stimulation of
tumor colony formation.   Results are mean of duplicate
plates.   Reproduced from Cloning of Human Tumor Stem Cells
(Salmon, 1980), with permission of the publisher.

These experiments indicate that growth stimulation of
human tumor colony forming cells by adherent cells is
mediated by diffusable factors released by them, and in
a dose-dependent fashion.   Furthermore, plating numbers
of adherent cells that were significantly higher than
were present in the original effusion usually resulted in
inhibition of colony formation suggesting that optimal
ratios of macrophages to tumor cells to promote clonogenicity may be present in malignant effusions.   Thus, we
had established that tumor colony growth of unfractionated
effusions could frequently be inhibited with pharmacological doses of indomethacin that inhibited PGE synthesis,
and that prostaglandins such as PGE were produced by the
primarily adherent cells present in malignant effusions.

Furthermore, we found that the cells in the adherent fraction also promoted tumor colony formation by release of diffusable factors. Nonetheless, these experiments did not prove that the diffusable growth stimulants produced by the adherent cells were prostaglandins. In order to test that possibility directly, we recently began a series of experiments wherein NA/NP tumor cells were plated in the absence of adherent cells and with the addition of indomethacin alone or with physiological concentrations of PGE_2 (figure 2). As is apparent from figure 2, physiological concentrations of PGE_2 (10^{-12}-10^{-8}M) did not restore growth. This indicates that, in the absence of PGE secreting adherent cells, PGE per se was not a sufficient stimulus for breast or ovarian carcinoma growth in vitro. Whether higher concentrations of PGE_2 or other prostaglandins secreted by macrophages (e.g., $PGF_{2\alpha}$) would support growth remains to be tested. Alternatively, growth promoters other than prostaglandins but also secreted by adherent cells may enhance in vitro clonogenicity of the tumor cells.

DISCUSSION

The cell separation and reconstitution studies we have carried out with spontaneous human tumors provide clear evidence that endogenous adherent and phagocytic host macrophages within the growing tumor can significantly modulate in vitro clonogenicity of tumor cells. In myeloma, endogenous macrophages appear to inhibit clonogenicity. After inhibition of the cyclooxygenase system with indomethacin, phagocyte-depleted myeloma cells have their clonogenic growth stimulated when exogenous PGE_2 is added to replace endogenous prostaglandin synthesis. On the other hand, in carcinoma cells from effusions, the endogenous macrophages generally stimulate growth in vitro unless very low or much higher than normal numbers of macrophages are recombined in the reconstitution studies. However, great biological variability in the stoichiometry of this growth modulation is observed from tumor to tumor, suggesting a complex interaction of stimulatory and inhibitory factors. Although endogenous macrophages in carcinomatous effusions appear to be the primary source of prostaglandin synthesis, our results thus far do not suggest that prostaglandins are the primary stimulus for colony formation by carcinomas.

During the past few decades, studies of cell lines
and transplantable tumor models have predominated as the
major approaches for study of human tumor biology. These
approaches have been quite valuable for studies of inherent
mechanisms of proliferation of relatively autonomous and
homogenous tumors (Buick et al., 1980). As evidenced by
data summarized in this chapter, in vitro tumor growth of
spontaneous tumors, as assessed in clonogenic assay, is no-
where near as autonomous or homogenous as would be implied
from long term cell lines. Some of the biological differences between spontaneous human tumors and long term
cell lines of transplanted tumors are summarized in Table 3.

TABLE 3

Differences Between Spontaneous Human Tumors
and Established Tumor Cell Lines

Characteristic	Spontaneous Tumor Biopsies	Tumor Cell Lines
1. Prolonged in vitro growth in tissue culture	Not without adaptation or selection	Yes
2. Cloning efficiency	Low	High
3. Host cell modulation by macrophages	Significant	Not significant after repeated passages
4. In vivo metastatic potential	Present	Often reduced or lost on serial in vitro passage
5. Prostaglandin production by tumor cells	Low	High

These differences may at least, in part, account for the
differences that we have observed in our growth modulating
studies as compared to investigations with cell lines or
transplantable animal tumors. Interactions between host
and neoplastic cells in the agar culture system are in

many ways analogous to those observed in studies of in
vitro hemopoiesis. In both hemopoiesis and lymphopoiesis,
macrophages can exert either stimulatory or inhibitory effects on clonogenic proliferation of progenitor cells.
With respect to cancer, the observation that adherent and
phagocytic macrophages can potentiate in vitro growth of
a wide variety of carcinomas has provided the basis for developing a hypothesis on the growth-promoting interaction
between macrophages and clonogenic tumor cells in human
cancer and on the relation of this interaction to the cellular immune response. Based on other evidence, Prehn
(1977) had previously suggested that there is a "lymphodependent" phase of tumor growth (in which the immune
system supports the growth of a cancer). On the basis of
our initial macrophage depletion studies in carcinomas and
macrophage-conditioned medium stimulation of clonal growth
of myeloma and other evidence, we proposed an initial
"macrophage hypothesis" in 1978 (Salmon and Hamburger,
1978). We suggested that one or more macrophage-derived
promoter substances facilitated clonal growth of human
cancers in vivo, as well as having a stimulatory effect on
B-lymphocyte proliferation. We also proposed that such
macrophage effects were critical in the promotional step
in the two-step model of skin carcinogenesis (Boutwell,
1974) and in the induction of myeloma in the Balb-C mouse
(Potter et al., 1978). Of interest, tumor promoters are
now known to exert potent effects on macrophages and to
stimulate their production of prostaglandins (Humes et al.,
1978, 1980). Additional data supportive for the concept
that autologous macrophages can potentiate tumor growth
include the observation in an in vivo tumor model by Evans
(1978).

The cell separation and reconstitution studies reviewed in this chapter further define the host cell requirements for in vitro clonal growth of human neoplasms,
and indicate that growth promotion or inhibition was con-
veyed by soluble factors from the adherent cells which
diffused through the agar. Furthermore, we found that
elaboration of prostaglandins by host macrophages occurred
concomitantly with this process. These findings, and the
knowledge that macrophage-derived prostaglandins can potently inhibit the proliferation of T cells (Kurland and
Bockman, 1978; Bockman and Rothschild, 1979) as well as
modulate fetal development, led me recently to propose an
even broader hypothesis: that the macrophage is a promoter

of both fetal and cancer growth as well as immunological
tolerance to both of these growth processes (Salmon, 1980).
This more general hypothesis is depicted in figure 4.

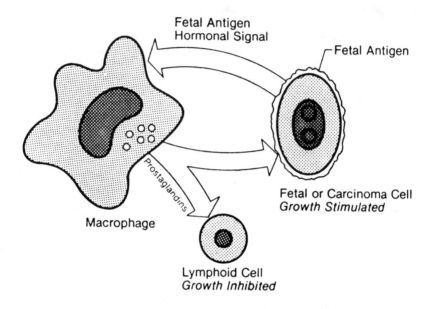

Fig. 4 Hypothetical relationship of the macrophage as a
promoter of fetal and cancer growth and immunological
tolerance, including possible roles for fetal antigens or
hormones and prostaglandins. Factors secreted by the responding activated macrophage stimulate fetal (or carcinoma) growth. The secretion of prostaglandin E also
initiates immunological tolerance by inhibiting the
T-lymphocyte response to histocompatibility or tumor antigens. Thus, in cancer, the macrophage is "tricked into
thinking" that a fetus is present. Reproduced from Cloning
of Human Tumor Stem Cells (Salmon, 1980) with permission of
the publisher.

It is well recognized that there are similarities
between maternal tolerance to the fetus and the immunological tolerance of a patient's immune system to a progressively growing cancer (Uriel, 1975). In both circumstances, progressive growth of the immature cells occurs

while the local cellular immune response to histocompatibility or tumor antigens appears to be inhibited. With respect to cancer, a central question has been to identify the mechanism by which cancers can grow progressively despite the presence of demonstrable tumor immunity in the host lymphoid cells. Certain biological markers also appear to be expressed in both fetal and tumor issues: these include embryonic antigens and prostaglandins.

The central postulate upon which the new hypothesis is based is that a normal function of macrophages is to respond to the presence of fetal antigens or hormones by secretion of prostaglandins and/or other growth factors which normally stimulate the proliferation of immature cells (expressing fetal properties) while simultaneously inhibiting the immune response. Macrophage-derived prostaglandins could potentially inhibit allogenic immunoproliferative responses in both mother and fetus, thus contributing directly to maternal-fetal tolerance. While the specific fetal biological signals which we postulate remain to be directly identified, they might well be some of the already recognized "oncofetal antigens" (e.g., α-fetoprotein, AFP; human chorionic gonadotropin, HCG; and carcinoembryonic antigen CEA). HCG (Lange et al., 1976) and AFP (Gershwin et al., 1978) have been reported to suppress cellular immunity in vitro; these effects might be macrophage mediated. Activated macrophages secrete high levels of prostaglandin E which, in turn, potently suppresses the proliferation of normal T-lymphocytes (Pelus and Strausser, 1977), as well as modulating other aspects of immunity.

This hypothesis on the role of macrophages in fetal growth would be quite relevant to the cancer problem as the expression of fetal antigens and other features of "immaturity" are characteristic abnormalities associated with neoplastic clones. Retention of the ability to recognize a fetal antigenic or hormonal signal and respond by secreting immunosuppressive as well as growth factors would provide the environment which would allow an evolving carcinoma arising from a transformed cell to have a growth advantage. Recent investigations support the concept that fetal antigens can stimulate tumor growth. The induction of myeloma in the Balb-C mouse can be facilitated by the administration of AFP (Gershwin et al., 1980). Administration of irradiated normal fetal liver cells has been shown to enhance the growth of a rat fibrosarcoma while blocking the expression of immune cytotoxicity (Keller, 1979). If the various fetal signals and macrophage responses which we hypothesize to occur in the fetus also occur in patients harboring neoplastic cells, then both growth of the carcinoma and inhibition of the immune response to tumor antigens would be anticipated. Thus, this hypothesis could provide simultaneous explanations for two long-standing biological enigmas: (1) maternal-fetal tolerance, and (2) the mechanism by which a carcinoma can "slip through" the immune response.

With respect to cancer growth, we proposed that the early growth of a carcinoma requires both a transformed clonogenic cell expressing one or more fetal antigens and an appropriate microinductive environment. Plescia et al. (1975) have observed that small numbers of tumor cells can induce immunosuppression in association with PGE_2 production. Tumors are known to be rich in prostaglandins and the studies by Buick et al. (1980; Buick and Salmon, 1980) would suggest that these are secreted primarily by functional macrophages which have migrated into spontaneous human tumors. The use of compounds which block either the elaboration of or the response to prostaglandins and other growth factors secreted by macrophages could have an anti-promotional effect, either before or after the neoplastic transforming event has occurred. In the two-step model of carcinogenesis in the mouse skin, prostaglandin synthesis inhibitors block the promotional step (Verma et al., 1977). Tumor promotion in this model is known to require a mono-nuclear inflammatory response to the tumor promoter. Clinically, macrophages present in the lymph node, liver or lungs of a patient might provide an important component of the local environment for colonization by circulating clonogenic tumor cells. How might this vicious circle be reversed? A two-pronged approach to cancer treatment might be considered. Inhibitors of macrophage function and growth factor secretion or effect would be used to block the promotional step, while conventional cytotoxic or hormonal agents would be used to directly attach the neoplastic cells. The clinician may have already discovered the two-pronged approach to cancer treatment empirically by combining biological response modifiers or hormones (e.g., corticosteroids and PG synthesis inhibitors) along with conventional cytotoxic drugs. Since macrophages in high concentrations may have suppressive effects on tumor growth (Hibbs, 1974), the possibility remains that macrophage subpopulations could be identified which could be induced to suppress tumor growth at clinically achievable macrophage-tumor cell ratios.

The proof of any given hypothesis is, of course, in the testing, and a variety of relevant biological experiments can be designed which may either support, refute or lead to modification of the macrophage-oncofetal tolerance hypothesis.

ACKNOWLEDGEMENTS

The author thanks Drs. Anne Hamburger and Ronald Buick and Mr. Michael Berens for their scientific collaborations and Ms. Barbara Soehnlen for skilled technical assistance. These studies were supported by grants CA-21839 and CA-17094 from the U.S. Public Health Service, Bethesda, Maryland 20205.

REFERENCES

Berens ME, Salmon SE (1981). Prostaglandin and prostaglandin synthesis inhibitor effects on tumor colony formation in agar: evidence for modulation of host-tumor cell interactions in primary human tumor biopsies. In Proc International Conf on Prostaglandins and Cancer, August 30-September 2, Georgetown, Maryland, #42, p 48.

Bockman RJ, Rothschild M (1979). Prostaglandin E inhibition of T-lymphocyte colony formation. J Clin Invest 64:812-819.

Boutwell RK (1974). The function and mechanism of promoters of carcinogenesis. CRC Crit Rev Toxicol 2:419-443.

Buick RN, Fry SE, Salmon SE (1980). Effect of host-cell interactions on clonogenic carcinoma cells in human malignant effusions. Br J Cancer 41:695-704.

Buick RN, Salmon SE (1980). Variables in the demonstration of human tumor clonogenicity: cell interactions and semi-solid support. In Salmon SE (ed): "Cloning of Human Tumor Stem Cells," New York: Alan R. Liss, p 127-134.

Evans R (1978). Macrophage requirement for growth of a murine fibrosarcoma. Br J Cancer 37:1086-1089.

Gershwin ME, Castles JJ, Makishima AA (1978). The influence of α-fetoprotein on Maloney sarcoma virus oncogenesis: evidence for generation of antigen nonspecific suppressor T cells. J Immunol 121:978-985.

Gershwin ME, Castles JJ, Makishima R (1980). Accelerated plasmacytoma formation in mice treated with α-fetoprotein. J Natl Cancer Inst 64:145-150.

Hamburger AW, Salmon SE (1977). Primary bioassay of human tumor stem cells. Science 197:461-463.

Hamburger AW, Salmon SE, Kim MB, Trent JM, Soehnlen B, Alberts DS, Schmidt HJ (1978). Direct cloning of human ovarian carcinoma cells in agar. Cancer Res 38:3438-3443.

Hamburger AW, Kim MB, Salmon SE (1979). The nature of cells generating human myeloma colonies in vitro. J Cell Phys 98:371-376.

Hibbs JB (1974). Discrimination between neoplastic and non-neoplastic cells in vitro by activated macrophages. J Natl Cancer Inst 53:1487-1492.

Humes JL, Davies P, Bonney RJ, Kuehl FA Jr (1978). Phorbol myristate acetate stimulates the release of arachidonic acid and cyclo-oxygenase products by macrophages. Fed Proc 37:1318.

Humes JL, Burger S, Galavage M, Kuehl FA Jr, et al (1980). The diminished production of arachidonic acid oxygenation products by elicited mouse peritoneal macrophages: possible mechanisms. J Immunol 124:2110-2116.

Keller R (1979). Competition between foetal tissue and macrophage-dependent natural tumor resistance. Br J Cancer 40:417-423.

Kurland JI, Bockman RJ (1978). Prostaglandin E production by human blood monocytes and mouse peritoneal macrophages. J Exp Med 147:952-957.

Lange PT, Hakala TR, Fraley EE (1976). Suppression of antitumor lymphocytic mediated cytotoxicity by human gonadotropins. J Urol 115:95-98.

Pelus L, Strausser H (1977). Prostaglandins and the immune
response. Life Sci 20:903-913.

Plescia OJ, Smith AH, Grinwich K (1975). Subversion of the
immune system by tumor cells and the role of prostaglandins. Proc Natl Acad Sci, USA, 72:1848-1851.

Potter M, Cancro M (1978). In Saunders GF (ed): "Plasma-
cytogenesis and the differentiation of immunoglobulin-
producing cells in cell differentiation and neoplasia."
New York, Raven Press, p 145-161.

Prehn RT (1977). Immunostimulation of the lymphodependent
phase of neoplastic growth. J Natl Cancer Inst 59:1043.

Salmon SE, Hamburger AW, Soehnlen B, Durie BGM, Alberts DS,
Moon TE (1978). Quantitation of differential sensiti-
vity of human tumor stem cells to anticancer drugs. New
Engl J Med 298:1321-1327.

Salmon SE, Hamburger AW (1978). Immunoproliferation and
cancer: a common macrophage-derived promoter substance.
Lancet 1:1289-1290.

Salmon SE (1980). "Cloning of Human Tumor Stem Cells."
New York: Alan R. Liss.

Salmon SE, Young L, Stebbing N (1981). Antitumor activity
of natural and cloned human interferons in the human
tumor stem cell assay. Proc Amer Soc Clin Oncol, Washington DC, April 30-May 2, #1152, p 290.

Uriel J (1975). Fetal characteristics of cancer. In
Becker FF (ed): "Cancer, a Comprehensive Treatise."
Vol. 3, New York: Plenum Press, p 21-49.

Verma AK, Rice HM, Boutwell RK (1977). Prostaglandins and
skin tumor promotion: inhibition of tumor promoter-
induced ornithine decarboxylase activity in epidermis
by inhibitors of prostaglandin synthesis. Biochem
Biophys Res Commun 79:1160-1166.

**Prostaglandins and Cancer: First
International Conference, pages 651-655
© 1982 Alan R. Liss, Inc., 150 Fifth Avenue, New York, NY 10011**

DIFFERENTIAL EFFECTS OF INDOMETHACIN AND PGE_2 ON THE DEPRESSED
RESPONSES OF CANCER PATIENTS

Tilden, A.B., Dougherty, P.A. and Balch, C.M.

University of Alabama in Birmingham

University Station, Birmingham, Alabama   35294

Cancer patients exhibit decreased immunocompetence as
measured by a variety of in vitro and in vivo immunological
responses (1, 2, 3). These depressed immune responses have
been attributed to increased suppressor cell activity in
patients with osteogenic sarcoma (4), bladder cell carcinoma
(5), Hodgkin's lymphoma (6, 7), multiple myeloma (8), and
acute leukemia (9). Abnormalities in prostaglandin mediated-
suppression have been demonstrated in a number of tumors in
animals and humans (10, 11, 7). We examined the influence of
PG-producing suppressor cells on depressed mitogen respones
in head and neck (H & N) cancer and in melanoma patients.
    Proliferative responses of Ficoll-Hypaque purified
peripheral blood mononuclear cells (PBMC) to Concanavalin A
(Con A) (5 µg/ml) and photohemagglutinin (PHA) (20 µg/ml)
were determined by the uptake of ^{3}H-thymidine (12). The
effect of indomethacin (1 µg/ml) on mitogen response was
studied in 42 patients with H & N cancer and 57 melanoma
patients. Indomethacin caused a significant increase (P <
.01) in the proliferative responses of PBMC from H & N
cancer and melanoma patients whereas it caused significantly
less change in the responses of PBMC from normal subjects
(Table I).
    We suspected the indomethacin enhancement of lymphocyte
proliferation was due to inhibition of excessive prostaglandin
production by suppressor monocytes. Goodwin and colleagues
(7) first demonstrated such an abnormality in the depressed
mitogen responses of Hodgkin's lymphoma patients. We therefore compared the amount of PGE_2 produced by cultured PBMC
of cancer patients and normal individuals. PGE_2 production
was measured by testing 48 hour PBMC culture supernatants in

TABLE I
Effect of Indomethacin on Mitogen Responses
Indomethacin Induced Mean Percent Increase in Mitogen
Responses Above Control Levels

	PHA	ConA
H & N Cancer (36)[a]	45%[b]	71%[b]
Melanoma (33)	38%[b]	70%[b]

(a) Number of patients studied
(b) Significantly greater than normal controls, $P < .01$

a competitive inhibition radioimmunoassay (RIA) for PGE_2 (13). Cultured PBMC from 24 H & N cancer patients produced significantly more PGE_2 than PBMC for 45 normal controls (8.97 ± 0.85 ng/ml vs. 4.72 ± 0.44 ng/ml, respectively, $P < .001$). Suprisingly, PGE_2 production by PBMC from 16 melanoma patients was similar to control values (4.89 ± 0.78 ng/ml) (Table II).

Table II
Amount of PGE_2 Produced by Cultured PBMC

	H & N Cancer (24)[a]	Melanoma (16)	Normal (45)
Mean ng/ml PGE_2 ± ISE	8.97 ± 0.85[b]	4.89 ± 0.78	4.72 ± 0.44

(a) Number of individuals studied
(b) Significantly greater than normals $P < .001$

Since melanoma patients did not exhibit elevated PGE production, we tested whether lymphocyte hypersensitivity to PGE_2 might result in depressed mitogen response. We thus compared the suppressive effects of exogenous PGE_2 on PBMC from melanoma patients and normal individuals. We examined the magnitude of PHA and Con A responses in the presence of a range of PGE_2 doses to determine whether lymphocyte function in melanoma patients might be more easily suppressed than normal lymphocytes by equivalent concentrations of PGE_2. The results showed that PGE_2 dose response curves for PBMC from melanoma patients did not differ significantly from those obtained for normal subjects (Table III).

TABLE III
SUPPRESSION OF MITOGEN RESPONSE BY EXOGENOUS PGE_2

PGE$_2$ Dose (Molarity)	Con A (1 µg/ml)		PHA (20 µg/ml)	
	Melanoma Patients (10)[a]	Normal Controls (7)	Melanoma Patients (10)	Normal Controls (7)
3×10^{-9}	19 ± 7[b]	26 ± 5	11 ± 6	18 ± 4
3×10^{-8}	29 ± 5	46 ± 3	42 ± 6	43 ± 5
3×10^{-7}	52 ± 4	57 ± 2	57 ± 5	60 ± 4
3×10^{-6}	59 ± 4	65 ± 3	65 ± 5	65 ± 4

(a) Number of individuals studied
(b) % Inhibition of the mitogen response ± on SE.

Since indomethancin is known to have multiple effects on cellular metabolism (14), we then examined whether lymphocyte proliferation could be altered by a structurally unrelated inhibitor of PG synthesis, RO-205720, (Roche). We found that RO-205720 (at 20 µg/ml) did not significantly enhance the mitogen response of PBMC from either 13 melanoma patients or 17 normal controls. In contrast, the responses of PBMC from 25 H & N cancer patients were significantly enhanced by this drug (Table IV).

TABLE IV
Effect of RO-205720 on Mitogen Response
Mean Percent Increase in Mitogen Response
in the Presence of RO-20-5720 (20 µg/ml)

	PHA	ConA
H & N Cancer (25)[a]	64%[b]	46%[b]
Melanoma (13)	24%	-8%
Controls (17)	38%	10%

(a) Number of individuals studied
(b) Significantly greater than controls, P < .05

In summary, indomethacin enhances mitogen responses in both H & N cancer patients and melanoma patients. In H & N cancer patients the mechanism of action appears to be blockage of excessive PGE_2. Melanoma patients, on the other hand, exhibit normal levels of PGE_2 production and normal sensitivity to the suppressive effects of PGE_2. Thus indomethacin appears to enhance mitogen responses in melanoma patients by a mechanism unrelated to prostaglandin.

References

1. Golub, S.H., O'Connell, T.X. and Morton, D.L. 1974. Correlation of In Vivo and In Vitro Assays of Immunocompetence in Cancer Patients. Cancer Research, 34;1833-1840.

2. Eilber, F.R., Nizze, J.A. and Morton, D.L. 1975. Sequential Evaluation of General Immune Competence in Cancer Patients Correlation with Clinical Course. Cancer, 35;660-666.

3. Zembala, M., Mytar, B., Popiela, T. and Asherson, G.L. 1977. Depressed In Vitro Peripheral Blood Lymphocyte Response to Mitogens in Cancer Patients: The Role of Suppressor Cells. Int. J. Cancer, 19;605-610.

4. Yu, A., Watts, H., Jaffe, N. and Parkman, R. 1977. Concomitant Presence of Tumor-Specific Cytotoxic and Inhibitor Lymphocytes in Patients with Osteogenic Sarcoma. N. Engl. J. Med., 297;121-126.

5. Bean, M.A., Kodera, Y., Cummings, K.B. and Bloom, B.R. 1977. Occurrence of Restricted Suppressor T-Cell Activity in Man. J. of Exp. Med., 146:1455-1461.

6. Twomey, J.J., Laughter, A.J., Farrow, S. and Douglas, C.C. 1975. Hodgkin's Disease: An Immunodepleting and Immunosuppressive Disorder. J. Clin. Invest., 56;467-471.

7. Goodwin, J.S., Messner, R.P., Bankhurst, A.D., Peake, G.T., Saiki, J.H. and Williams, R.C., Jr. 1977. Prostaglandin-Producing Suppressor Cells in Hodgkin's Disease. N. Engl. J. Med., 297(18);963-968.

8. Broder, S., Humphrey, R., Durm, M., Blackman, M., Meade, B., Goldman, C., Strober, W. and Waldmann, T. 1975. Impaired Synthesis of Polyclonal (Non-Paraprotein) Immunoglobulins by Circulating Lymphocytes from Patients with Multiple Myeloma: Role of Suppressor Cells. N. Engl. J. Med., 293;887-892.

9. Broder, S., Poplck, D., Whang-Peng, J., et. al. 1978. Characterization of a Suppressor-Cell Leukemia: Evidence for the Requirement of an Interaction of Two T Cells in the Development of Human Suppressor Effector Cells. N. Engl. J. Med., 298;66-71.

10. Plescia, O.J., Smith, A.H. and Grinwich, K. 1975. Subversion of Immune System by Tumor Cells and Role of Prostaglandins. Proc. Nat. Acad. Sci. USA, 72(5);1848-1850.

11. Pelus, L.M. and Bockman, R.S. 1979. Increased Prostaglandin Synthesis by Marcrophages from Tumor-Bearing Mice. J. Immunol., 123;2118-2122.

12. Tilden, A.B. and Balch, C.M. 1981. Indomethacin Enhancement of Immunocompetence in Melanoma Patients. Surgery, 90(1);77-84.

13. Toffet, S.M. and Russell, S.W. 1981. Macrophage Mediated Tumor Cell Killing: Regulation of Expression of Cytolytic Activity by Prostaglandin E$_2$. J. Immunol., 126;424-427.

14. Shen, T-Y. and Winter, C.A. 1977. Chemical and Biological Studies on Indomethacin, Sulindae and Their Analogs. Adv. Drug Res., 12;89.

**Prostaglandins and Cancer: First
International Conference, pages 657–662**
© 1982 Alan R. Liss, Inc., 150 Fifth Avenue, New York, NY 10011

MODULATION OF PROSTAGLANDINS IN HORMONE DEPENDENT MAMMARY
CARCINOMA

M.K. Foecking, R.V. Panganamala, H. Abou-Issa
and J.P. Minton
Depts. Physiological Chemistry and Surgery, The
Ohio State University
Columbus, Ohio   43210

Prostaglandins production in DMBA-induced mammary carcinoma may be hormonally modulated. The DMBA-induced
mammary tumor is a hormone dependent tumor. Prolactin and
estrogen are thought to be of primary importance in the
control of growth of this tumor. Prostaglandin synthesis in
the murine mammary gland varies with the stage of the estrus
cycle (Krazek 1980), suggesting that mammary prostaglandin
production is sensitive to fluctuations in ovarian hormones.
This paper reports the measurement of prostaglandin production in mammary tumors by the modification of a method
recently reported for rat aorta, (Panganamala 1981). The
relationship between tumor prostaglandin production and
in vivo hormonal minipulation was investigated.

METHODS

Animals

Mammary tumors were induced in female Sprague-Dawley
rats by gastric intubation of 10 mg of 7,12-dimethylbenz(a)
anthracene (DMBA) at 50 days of age, followed by 3 weekly
doses of 5 mg DMBA. Bilateral ovariectomy was performed in
tumor-bearing rats to induce tumor regression. Growth of
the tumors, as recorded by measurement with vernier calipers
was observed over a period of 10-14 days. Growing tumors
showed an increase of greater than 20% in the sum of two
diameters compared to the measurement taken at the beginning of the treatment period; regressing tumors showed a
greater than 20% decrease. If the change in tumor size
was less than 20%, the tumor was considered stable.

Assay of Prostaglandins

The production of prostaglandins by tumor tissue was determined by measuring the rate of release of prostaglandins
into an aqueous incubation medium. The method used was a
modification of a method used in rat aortic tissue (Panganamala). Tumors were sliced to a thickness of 0.35 mm to
ensure adequate diffusion of oxygen into all parts of the
tissue as well as release of exported metabolites to the
extracellular medium. All measurements were made in freshly
excised tumor tissue, since PGE_2 production in frozen tumors
(-196°C) was found to be elevated compared to fresh tumors
(unpublished observations).

The tumors were rapidly excised from decapitated rats,
weighed, and then sliced to a thickness of 0.35 mm using
a McIlwain Tissue Chopper. The sliced tumors were washed
in 0.5 ml of cold (4°C) incubation buffer (50mM Tris, 150
mM NaCl, pH 8.0) for 5 minutes. The cold buffer was discarded, and the samples were incubated in 1 ml of incubation
buffer at 20°C with gentle agitation for 1 hour. Aliquots
of 40-60 μl were removed at 6 time points throughout the
incubation. These aliquots were stored in 50 mM Tris buffer
(pH 8.0) containing 0.1% albumin at 4°C until radioimmunoassay. An ethanol extract of the tumor tissue at the final
time point showed that 90% ± 3% of the PGE_2 was released
from the tissue into the medium, for all the tissues measured. Thus, most of the synthesized prostaglandin is released
into the medium and not bound to the tissue.

Each aliquot was diluted to a known volume with Tris-
albumin buffer to permit measurement of several different
prostaglandin species by radioimmunoassay. We measured
PGE_2, 6-keto-$PGF_{1\alpha}$, and $PGF_{2\alpha}$ release from tumor tissue
using this method.

Prostaglandin E_2 was measured by radioimmunoassay
(Caldwell 1972) using an antibody donated by Dr. Thomas
Ferris, Dept. of Medicine, Ohio State University. The
antibody to 6-keto-$PGF_{1\alpha}$ was purchased from Seragen (Boston
Mass.). ^3H-PGE_2 and ^3H-6-ketoprostaglandin $F_{1\alpha}$ were
purchased from New England Nuclear (Boston, Mass.). The

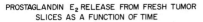

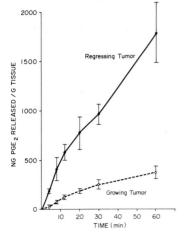

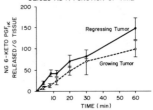

Figure 1 (left) Representative time course for PGE_2 release from a growing tumor and from a regressing tumor. The error bars represent standard deviation. Each curve is the mean of triplicate analysis from a single tumor. Figure 2 (above right) Representative time course for 6-keto-$PGF_{1\alpha}$ release from a growing and from a regressing tumor. The error bars represent standard deviation. Each curve is the mean of triplicate analysis from a single tumor.

determination of ng of prostaglandin released per gram of tissue at 10 minutes was used for comparisons between tumors. Comparisons between means were computed using Student's t test.

RESULTS

The amount of PGE_2 and 6-keto-$PGF_{1\alpha}$ released from tumor slices incubated at 20°C increased with time. Representative time courses showing release of PGE_2 and 6-keto-$PGF_{1\alpha}$ are shown in Figures 1 and 2. No PGE_2 or 6-keto-$PGF_{1\alpha}$ release was detected from tissue slices incubated in the presence of 300 µM indomethacin. Furthermore, extraction of these tumors at the final time point showed that PGE_2 and 6-keto-$PGF_{1\alpha}$ levels were undetectable, implying that inhibition was at the level of synthesis and not release.

Tumors appeared in the rats 6-12 weeks after administration of DMBA. Ovariectomy resulted in regression of mammary tumors in 70% of the cases in this study.

The results in Table 1 show that there is an inverse relationship between tumor growth and the production of PGE_2 and 6-keto-$PGF_{1\alpha}$ as measured by release from tumor slices.

Table 1

Inverse Relationship Between Prostaglandin
Production and Growth in DMBA-induced Rat
Mammary Tumors

	PGE_2[1]	6-Keto-PGF 1α
GROWING	48 ± 10	27 ± 8
STABLE	86 ± 15	---
REGRESSING	206 ± 62	57 ± 11

[1]ng Prostaglandin released/g tissue/10 minutes: mean±S.E.

The differences between the groups were statistically significant at the following levels: PGE_2- growing vs. regressing, $p < 0.025$, growing vs. stable, $p < 0.05$, stable vs regressing $p < 0.025$. The same inverse relationship was also seen in 6-keto-$PGF_{1\alpha}$ release (growing vs. regressing, $p < 0.025$). Non-regressing tumors from ovariectomozed rats released 102±26 ng PGE_2/g tissue/10 minutes, which is half the level of PGE_2 production found in regressing tumors.

DISCUSSION

The measurement of the release of prostaglandins into an aqueous medium has been reported as a method for determining prostaglandin synthesis in rat aortic tissue(Pangamala) This paper reports a modification of this method to mammary tumor slices. This method has the advantage of allowing for kinetic studies, since sampling is non-destructive, and organic extractions are no longer necessary. The method allows for the determination of several different prostaglandin species by different radioimmunoassay. PGE_2, 6-keto -$PGF_{1\alpha}$ and $PGF_{2\alpha}$ release from tumor tissue have been measured in our laboratory.

An inverse relationship between tumor growth and prosta glandin production (PGE_2 and $6\text{-keto-PGF}_{1\alpha}$) was observed. The inverse relationship between prostaglandin production and tumor growth suggests that prostaglandins may be functionally involved in the control of tumor growth and regression. It remains to be determined whether any or all of the prostaglandins are directly modulated by the hormones estrogen and/or prolactin. Since estrogen stimulates prolactin release, ovariectomy results in a decrease in prolactin along with the depletion of estrogen. The interaction of both of these hormones with prostaglandin synthesis is being studied. The responses of PGE_2 and prostacyclin (as measured by $6\text{-keto-PGF}_{1\alpha}$) in regressing tumors are qualitatively similar, suggesting that the difference between growing and regressing tumors is at the level of cyclooxygenase, or availability of substrate fatty acid.

If prostaglandins are modulated by hormones in this mammary tumor model, then changes in prostaglandin production should correlate with alterations in endogenous hormone levels, as well as with the resulting growth response. Tumors from ovariectomized rats which are non-regressing are of particular interest since the alteration in the endogenous hormone environment is separated from the usual tumor response, which is regression. The level of prostaglandin production in non-regressing tumors was lower than the level from regressing tumors, and not different from the value seen in stable tumors. Since the non-regressing tumors fell under the classification of stable (as described in Methods), PGE_2 levels seem to correlate more closely with the growth response of the tumor than with the estrogen levels. Further investigation is underway to more clearly define the relationship between the hormones, estrogen and prolactin, and prostaglandin production and tumor growth.

Knazek R A , Watson K C , Lim M F , Cannizzaro A M , Christy R J , Liu S C (1980) Prostaglandin synthesis by murine mammary gland is modified by the state of the estrus cycle. Prostaglandins 19:891.

Panganamala R V , Gillespie A C , Merola A J (1981). Assay of prostacyclin synthesis in intact aorta by aqueous sampling. Prostaglandins 21:1.

Caldwell B V , Speroff L , Brock W A , Auletta J F ,

Gordon JW, Anderson CG, Hobbins JC (1972).
Development and application of a radioimmunoassay for
F prostaglandins. In Southern EM (ed.): "The
Prostaglandins: Clinicap Applications in Human Repro-
duction", Mount Kisco: Futura Publishing Co., p. 257.

Prostaglandins and Cancer: First
International Conference, pages 663-666
© 1982 Alan R. Liss, Inc., 150 Fifth Avenue, New York, NY 10011

INTERFERON-INDUCED RESISTANCE OF HUMAN NATURAL KILLER CELLS TO PGE$_2$-MEDIATED SUPPRESSION

Kam H. Leung and Hillel S. Koren,
Division of Immunology,
Duke Medical Center,
Durham, NC., U.S.A.

Natural killer (NK) cells display spontaneous cytotoxicity against a variety of tumor cells and may play a role in immunosurveillance to cancer (Roder and Haliotis, 1980). Although first discovered as a potent anti-viral (Friedman, 1977) and antitumor (Gresser and Tovey, 1978) protein, interferon (IFN) has been shown to be a major biological response modifier of NK activity (Bloom, 1980). In contrast prostaglandin E$_2$ (PGE$_2$) suppresses NK activity (Droller, et al, 1978). The purpose of this study was to examine the effect of PGE$_2$ on IFN and polyinosinic-polycytidylic acid (poly I:C) (an IFN inducer) activated NK cells. The data suggest that IFN and Poly I:C induce a partial resistance of NK cells to suppression by PGE$_2$.

Human mononuclear cells isolated from peripheral blood were cultured in RPMI-1640 medium supplemented with 10% FCS for 18 hr. Their NK activity against K-562 target cells was measured in a 2 hr ^{51}Cr release assay. To examine if PGE$_2$ can inhibit cytolytic activity of IFN-activated NK cells, the cytotoxicity of nonadherent cells cultured with IFN or poly I:C for 18 hr was assessed in the presence or absence of PGE$_2$ in the NK assay.

Table I shows that PGE$_2$ (30-3,000nM) inhibited the control endogenous NK cytolytic activity in a dose-dependent manner when added to the NK assay. Fifty % inhibition of endogenous activity was obtained by 300nM PGE$_2$. Human fibroblast interferon (IFNβ) caused an augmentation of NK activity and a concommittant loss of sensitivity to PGE$_2$-mediated suppression; PGE$_2$ at 3,000nM caused less than 50% inhibition of IFN-activated cells. PGE$_2$ at 30nM was no longer suppressive to IFN-activated cells. Similarly, poly I:C also caused a partial loss of sensitivity to PGE_2-mediated suppression. The loss of sensitivity to PGE_2-mediated suppression was shown to be dependent on the dose of IFN (α and β) or poly I:C used (data not shown). Doses of IFN or poly I:C that did not augment NK activity had little effect on the loss of sensitivity to PGE_2-mediated suppression.

Using large granular lymphocytes (LGL) obtained by Percoll gradient sedimentation (Timonen, et al, 1981) highly enriched for NK activity, we showed that similar results to those obtained with nonadherent cells were obtained, suggesting that the activation by IFN and the subsequent loss of sensitivity to suppression did not involve other cell types. Although we could not detect any appreciable amounts of PGE_2 in the medium of nonadherent cell culture by radiomunoassay (level of sensitivity $>3x10^{-10}$ M), indomethacin was added to the nonadherent cell culture to ensure the complete absence of PGE_2 synthesis in the local environment of the cells. Overnight pretreatment of nonadherent cells with 3,000nM of indomethacin did not affect their sensitivity to PGE_2-mediated suppression (Table 1). Furthermore, the presence of indomethacin during an overnight pretreatment with poly I:C or IFN did not substantially affect the acquired resistance to PGE_2-mediated suppression. Hence, enodgenous PGE_2 does not seem to be responsible for the loss of susceptibility to PGE_2-mediated suppression.

Previous reports have shown that desensitization induced by exposure of cells to agonists results in specific loss of responsiveness to those agonists (Raff, 1976). Therefore, we investigated the possibility that PGE_2 may induce a specific loss of sensitivity to PGE_2-mediated suppression of NK cells. Table 1 shows that pretreatment of nonadherent cells with 3,000nM of PGE_2 for 18 hr indeed resulted in a loss of susceptibility to PGE_2-mediated suppression. In separate experiments, treatment of nonadherent cells with $PGF_{2\alpha}$ and isoproterenol caused little loss of that susceptibility indicating that the effect is specific to PGE_2.

In this study, we have demonstrated that IFN-activated NK cells become resistant to PGE_2-mediated suppression; moreover, that PGE_2 also causes a specific desensitization. Within the local environment of a tumor, PGE_2 could be produced by intratumoral macrophages (Pelus and Bockman, 1979) and/or tumor cells (Goodwin, et al, 1980). IFN or other yet unidentified factors primarily produced by tumor-infiltrating or tumor-associated lymphoid cells (Mantovani, et al, 1980) could provide the required signal(s) necessary for the activation of

Table I

THE EFFECT OF PGE$_2$ on Poly I:C and INTERFERON-
ACTIVATED NK CELLS

% Specific ^{51}Cr Release $\pm$ S.E.M.

PGE$_2$ (nM) in the Assay

Treatment	0	30	300	3,000
Control	28+2	22+1(32)	15+1(46)	11+1(61)
IFN(10^{3}u/ml)	47+3	49+3(-4)	39+3(17)	32+2(32)
Poly I:C(100ug/ml)	46+4	47+3(-2)	41+3(11)	35+5(24)
Indomethacin (3,000nM)	28+3	19+2(32)	15+2(46)	9+1(68)

Nonadherent cells were cultured in the presence or absence of IFN, polyI:C, PGE$_2$ or indomethacin for 18 hr at 37°C. The effector cells were then washed and assayed for NK activity in the presence or absence of PGE$_2$. The E:T was 10:1 in a 2 hr assay against K562 target cells. The numbers in parentheses represent percent of inhibition by PGE$_2$.

NK cells. The final outcome of an immune response depends on the balance between positive and negative influences. Our results offer an explanation as to how NK cells may protect themselves from suppression by PGE$_2$. The possible mechanisms for I F N induction of resistance to suppression by PGE$_2$ may be due to alteration of effector cell surface characteristics (Gresser, 1979) and/or to change in the cellular metabolism such as cyclic nucleotides (Tovey, et al, 1979).

Acknowledgements. We thank Ms. Connie Hayes for her secretarial assistance. This work was supported in part by USPHS grants CA23354 and CA29589. H.S.K. is a recipient of Research Career Development Award CA00581 from the NCI.

References

1 Bloom, B. R. 1980. Nature, 284: 593.
2 Droller, J. J., Schneider, M. U. and Perlmann, P. 1978. Cell Immunol. 39:165.
3 Friedman, R. M. 1977. Bacteriol. Rev. 41:543.
4 Goodwin, J.S., Husby, G. and Williams, R.C., Jr. 1980. Cancer Immunol. Immunother. 8:3.
5 Gresser, I. 1977. Cell. Immunol. 34:406.
6 Gresser, I. and Tovey, M. G. 1978. Biochim. Biophys Acta 516:231.
7 Mantovani, A., Allavena, P., Sessa, C., Bolis, G. and Mangioni, C. 1980. Int. J. Cancer 25:573.
8 Pelus, L. M. and Bockman, R. S. 1979. J. Immunol. 123:2118.
9 Raff, M. 1976. Nature 259:265.
10 Roder, J.C., and Haliotis, T. 1980. Immunol. Today 1:96.
11 Timonen, T., Ortaldo, J. R. and Herberman, R. B. 1981. J. Exp. Med. 153:569.
12 Tovey, M. G., Rochette - Egly, C. and Castagna, M. 1979. Proc. Natl. Acad. Sci. 76:3890.

Prostaglandins and Cancer: First
International Conference, pages 667–672
© 1982 Alan R. Liss, Inc., 150 Fifth Avenue, New York, NY 10011

LEUKOTRIENES RELEASED BY HUMAN MONOCYTES MEDIATE TUMOR
ANTIGEN INDUCED LEUKOCYTE ADHERENCE INHIBITION (LAI).

D. M. P. Thomson,* Kerry Phelan* and
M. K. Bach†
*The Montreal General Hospital Research
Institute Montreal, Quebec, Canada. †The UpJohn
Company, Kalamazoo, Michigan, USA

The phenomenon of antigen-induced leukocyte adherence
inhibition (LAI) is a method for demonstrating human antitumor immunity (Halliday and Miller, 1972). The assay is
based on the fact that leukocytes from a tumor-bearing
host, after in vitro incubation with the sensitizing tumor
extracts, lose their ability to adher to glass surfaces.
We adapted and modified (Grosser and Thomson, 1975) a tube
method from Holan et al. (1974) to demonstrate human antitumor immunity.

Holt et al. (1975) and Maluish and Halliday (1975)
found that the LAI-reactive cell, when it bound a sensitizing antigen, released mediators causing other leuko-cytes
to be nonadherent. The cells that reacted with tumor
antigen and released mediators were T cells. Holan et al.
(1974) in his original studies in an animal model found
that macrophages binding tumor antigen were directly
inhibited from adhering to the glass tubes. No mediators
were detected.

We, too, studied the cells involved in the tube LAI
assay (Grosser and Thomson, 1975). By two different
experimental approaches, we failed to detect mediators in
the tube assay (Grosser and Thomson, 1975).Later, we enriched the reactive peripheral blood leukocytes (PBL) for
T and B or T lymphocytes and combined them with PBL from
control subjects, but still the admixture did not mediate
LAI (Marti et al., 1976). When deleted and/or enriched
subpopulations of PBL were put into the assay, only leukocytes enriched for monocytes reacted (Grosser et al.,

1976). Serum or IgG from patients whose leukocytes exhibited a positive LAI response was able to arm normal leukocytes to respond positively in the assay (Marti et al., 1976; Marti and Thomson, 1976).

In early cancer, seldom absent is the measureable antitumor response. In late cancer, seldom present is the measureable antitumor response because excess circulating tumor antigen in vivo triggers armed monocytes to express their programmed cell functions (Grosser and Thomson, 1976). We discovered that prostaglandin E_2 and other substances that were able to raise intracellular cyclic AMP, briefly incubated with leukocytes in vitro, reversed to positive the negative assay results of advanced cancer patients (Kaneti et al., 1981; Thomson et al., 1981). The studies with PGE_2 suggested that more PBL were participating in the response than could be accounted for by the number of monocytes, recognized morphologically, in the peripheral blood.

So experiments were undertaken with different drugs that block various pathways of arachidonic acid metabolism to determine whether arachidonate metabolites were responsible for LAI. In initial studies we found that drugs which inhibited the lipoxygenase pathway of arachidonic acid metabolism inhibited the LAI response (Thomson et al., 1981). These studies seemed to suggest that leukotrienes mediated LAI.

As described in this paper, armed human monocytes challenged with the sensitizing tumor antigen release a mediator that induces LAI and appears physiologically to act in a manner identical to LTC_4 and LTD_4.

RESULTS AND DISCUSSION

Armed Monocytes Release Mediators Upon Immunologic Challenge

Normal human monocytes were purified by adherence to microexudates or to plastic in the presence of 20% FCS, armed with serum from LAI^+-breast cancer patients or LAI^- control subjects, and after washing away all unbound IgG challenged with the sensitizing and control tumor extracts, simultaneously and separately. Twenty to 120 minutes later, the resultant supernatants were collected

TABLE 1.

Armed Human Monocytes Challenged with the Sensitizing Tumor Antigen Release a Mediator Inducing Leukocyte Adherence Inhibition of Normal Leukocytes

Armed Monocytes†	Drug**	NAI*
Normal Serum		2±4
Breast Cancer Serum		54±2
Breast Cancer Serum	No Drug	44±6
Breast Cancer Serum	Indomethacin (10^{-6})	43±15
Breast Cancer Serum	No Drug	34±15
Breast Cancer Serum	ETYA (10^{-6}M)	12±7
Breast Cancer Serum	No Drug	52±20
Breast Cancer Serum	NDGA (10^{-6}M)	12±16
Breast Cancer Serum	No Drug	46±20
Breast Cancer Serum	FPL 55712 (10^{-13}M)	−10±7
Breast Cancer Serum	No Drug	100±7
Breast Cancer Serum	Arylsulfatase	24±15

†Monocytes armed with serum were challenged simultaneously and separately with the specific and nonspecific cancer extract; the supernatants were added to normal leukocytes and the difference in nonadherent leukocytes was determined by computer-driven image analysis.

* $NAI = \dfrac{A-B}{B} \, 100$ A = a sample of no. of nonadherent cells incubated with the supernatant from the monocytes incubated with the breast cancer extract.

  B = a sample of no. of nonadherent cells incubated with the supernatant from the monocytes incubated with the stomach cancer extract.

NAI >30 are positive. The difference in mean NAIs are statistically significant ($p<0.001$).

**Drugs were preincubated with the monocytes for 30 minutes before challenge with antigen with the exception of FPL 55712 which was added to the supernatant.

and examined for their ability to inhibit the glass adherence of normal leukocytes. Only monocytes armed with LAI[+] serum and exposed to the sensitizing antigen released a mediator that was able to inhibit the glass adherence of normal leukocytes (Table 1). This effect was enhanced by adding either PGE_2 (5×10^{-6}M) or aminophylline (10^{-5}M) to the supernatant. By contrast, the nonadherent cells (T and B cells) from controls, incubated with LAI[+] serum, produced no detectable mediators upon challenge with tumor antigen.

The monocyte mediator was detected at 20 and 40 minutes after challenge, occasionally at 60 minutes after, but never at 120 minutes after challenge. A human macrophage cell line, U-937, when armed with specific antibody and challenged with the sensitizing antigen also released a mediator that inhibited the adherence of normal PBL.

Inhibition of the Monocyte's Mediators

Table 1 shows that the synthesis of the monocyte mediator was not inhibited by Indomethacin but was inhibited by ETYA and NDGA. Arylsulfatase destroyed the mediator activity. And FPL 55712 blocked the effect of the mediator. In addition, both the synthesis and action of the mediator were calcium dependent since La^{3+}, Intal, Nifedipine, and Trifluoroperazine inhibited the release of the mediator by the monocytes and blocked the mediator's actions on the normal PBL.

Effect of Pure LTC and LTD on Leukocyte Adherence Inhibition

Pure LTC or LTD, supplied by Bach et al., (1980), when added to normal leukocytes inhibits their glass adherence properties: pure populations of PMN and mononuclear cells are affected about equally. Consequently, it was not surprising to find that LTC or LTD also inhibited an LAI[+] response. Furthermore, PGE_2 and leukotrienes show synergism in their action on leukocytes. About 46 nM of LTD induces significant leukocyte nonadherence, but if the leukocytes are briefly exposed to PGE_2 before LTD, only 46 pM of LTD is needed. FPL 55712 blocked the effect of the leukotrienes inducing leukocyte adherence inhibition. About 10^{-15}M FPL 55712 was able to completely inhibit 10^{-6}M LTC. Intal (10^{-8}M) also blocked the action of the leukotrienes inducing leukocyte adherence.

Armed Monocytes Release ^{3}H-Arachidonic Acid Metabolites Upon Immunologic Challenge

Purified and armed monocytes were prelabelled with ^{3}H-arachidonic acid and then challenged with specific and nonspecific tumor extracts. The release of ^{3}H-arachidonic acid metabolites by the monocytes was measured over 2 hrs. The armed monocytes challenged with specific tumor antigen released at least 50% more ^{3}H-arachidonic acid metabolites than when challenged with the nonspecific tumor extract. This difference was maintained over 2 hours. The armed U-937 macrophage cell line behaved similarly. Monocytes from cancer patients were purified by adherence to plastic dishes, prelabelled with ^{3}H-arachidonic acid and then challenged with specific and nonspecific cancer extracts. Somewhat suprisingly, we discovered that the monocytes responded by releasing ^{3}H-arachidonic acid metabolites when challenged with the specific cancer extract, indicating that they were still armed. Monocytes from control subjects released equal amounts of ^{3}H-arachidonic acid metabolites when challenged with specific and nonspecific cancer extracts.

SUMMARY

Arming of monocytes seems to be biologically important because infinitesimal amounts of cytophilic antibody bestow on the immunologically nonspecific yet phagocytic cell exquisite specificity to recognize an antigen. And when the cytophilic antitumor IgG is cross-linked, the human monocytes synthesize and release measureable amounts of a biologically active factor having properties consistent with the action of leukotrienes. The physiologic significance of leukotriene release is unanswered; nonetheless, leukotrienes have chemotactic and chemokinetic effects on leukocytes which may be important in the migration of leukocytes to sites of inflammation, and increase the permeability of microvessels which in conjunction with the vasodilatation induced by prostaglandins E_2 and I_2 might be important in the development of edema.

REFERENCES

Bach MK, Brashler JR, Hammarstrom S, Samuelsson B. (1980). identification of leukotriene C-1 as a major component of slow reacting substance from rat mononuclear cells. J. Immun. 125:115.

Grosser N, Marti JH, Proctor JW, Thomson DMP. (1976). Tube leukocyte adherence inhibition assay for the detection of anti-tumor immunity. I. Monocyte is the reactive cell. Int. J. Cancer 18:39.

Grosser N, Thomson DMP. (1975). Cell-mediated immunity in breast cancer patients evaluated by antigen-induced leukocyte adherence inhibition in test tubes. Cancer Res. 35:2571.

Halliday WJ, Miller S. (1972). Leukocyte adherence inhibition: A simple test for cell-mediated tumor immunity and serum blocking factors. Int. J. Cancer 9:477.

Holan V, Hasek M, Rubenik J, Jitka CH. (1974). Antigen-mediated macrophage adherence inhibition. Cell.-Immunol. 13:107.

Holt PG, Robert LM, Fimmel PJ, Keast D. (1975). The LAI microtest: A rapid and sensitive procedure for the demonstration of cell-mediated immunity in vitro. J. Immunol. Methods. 8:277.

Kaneti J, Thomson DMP, Reid EC. (1981). Prostaglandin E_2 affects the tumor immune response in prostatic carcinoma. J. Urology (in press).

Maluish AE, Halliday WJ. (1975). Quantitation of anti-tumor cell-mediated immunity by a lymphokine-dependent reaction using small volumes of blood. Cell.Immunol.17:131.

Marti JH, Grosser N, Thomson, DMP. (1976). Tube leukocyte adherence inhibition assay for the detection of anti-tumour immunity.: II. Monocyte reacts with tumour antigen via cytophilic anti-tumour antibody. Int. J. Cancer 18:48.

Marti J, Thomson DMP. (1976). Anti-tumour immunity in malignant melanoma assay by tube leucocyte-adherence inhibition. Br. J. Cancer 34:116.

Thomson DMP, Phelan K, Scanzano R, Fink A. (1981). The regulation of the human antitumor immune response to organ-specific neoantigens. Transplant. Proceed. (in press).

Thomson DMP, Phelan K, Schwartz Scanzano R. (1981). A dye-extraction methods to quantitate the standard and PGE_2 stimulation tube adherence inhibition assay. Tumor Diagnostik 2:68.

Prostaglandins and Cancer: First
International Conference, pages 673-677
© 1982 Alan R. Liss, Inc., 150 Fifth Avenue, New York, NY 10011

Inhibition of Tumor Cell Adherence By Prostaglandins

J. Fantone, S. Kunkel, and J. Varani
Dept. of Pathology, Univ. of Michigan School of Medicine
Ann Arbor, Michigan 48109
This work was supported in part by NIH
Grants CA29550, CA29551, and HL-00905

Introduction:
The precise mechanism by which circulating tumor cells metastasise to a specific site is not fully understood. Current evidence suggests that the initiation of a metastatic focus is dependent on the biologic characteristics of both circulating tumor cells and the vascular or lymphatic walls. Recent studies have suggested that the adherence of platelets to tumor cell surfaces could initiate a metastatic focus by the generation of tumor cell emboli. Several authors have demonstrated anti-metastatic effects of prostaglandins (PGs) which inhibit, platelet aggregation and suggest that these effects are a result of the inhibition of platelet adherence to circulating tumor cells (1,2). The data presented here show that treatment of Walker 256 carcinosarcoma cells (WCC) in vitro with PGI_2, 15-S-15-methyl PGE_1, and $PGF_{2\alpha}$ can directly inhibit tumor cell adherence to plastic plates and nylon fibers induced by the tumor promotor, phorbol myristate acetate, (PMA) and the chemotactic peptide, N-formyl-methionyl-leucyl-phenylalanine (f Met-Leu-Phe). This study suggests that endogenous prostaglandin synthesis especially by endothelial cells may play an important role in modulating tumor cell adherence and metastasis in vivo by their <u>direct</u> effects on tumor cells.

Methods and Materials: (WCC) were used in all studies and were grown in suspension culture in RPMI-1640 medium supplemented with 10% fetal calf serum, (FCS) as previously described (3). Tissue culture reagents were purchased from

Grand Island Biological Co. (Grand Island, N.Y.) and FCS
from Kansas City Biological Co. (Kenexa, Kansas).
15-S-15-M-PGE$_1$, PGI$_2$, and PGF$_{2\alpha}$ were the generous gift of
Dr. John Pike (Upjohn, Co., Kalamazoo, Mich.). All other
reagents were obtained from Sigma Chemical Co. (St. Louis,
MO.). Adherence assays to nylon fibers and plastic culture
dishes were performed as previously described (3,4). In
specific experiments cells were pre-incubated in theophylline (2.5x10^{-4}M) for 10 min., 37°C, 5% CO$_2$ and then
incubated with prostaglandins for 15 min. at 37°C prior to
the addition of the stimulants, f-Met-Leu-Phe and PMA. All
samples were run in duplicate or triplicate, the number of
adherent cells determined and the percent inhibition of
adherence calculated. Mean values and standard errors of
the mean were determined and the students t-test was
employed in comparing treated and non-treated cell groups.

Results: The effect of pre-treatment of tumor cells with
theophylline and prostaglandins (PGI$_2$, PGF$_{2\alpha}$, 15-S-15-
M-PGE$_1$) on PMA induced tumor cell adherence to plastic
plates is shown in Table 1. In three separate experiments,
there was significant inhibition of tumor cell adherence by
all three prostaglandins at a concentration of 10^{-4}M both
in the presence and absence of theophylline. 15-S-15-
M-PGE$_1$ (without theophylline) showed greater than 50%
inhibition of tumor cell adherence to plastic plates at
concentrations ranging between 10^{-6} to 10^{-4} (exp. #2).
This response was dose dependent with 27.4% inhibition
observed at a concentration of 10^{-8}M and 88.9% inhibition
at 10^{-4}M. Theophylline appeared to increase the 15-S-15-M
PGE$_1$ mediated inhibition at 10^{-5}M (exp. #3) from 55.6% to
89.1%.
    PGI$_2$ had inhibitory effects on tumor cell adherence to
plastic plates similar to the PGE$_1$ analogue. At 10^{-4}M
concentration there was greater than 50% inhibition observed in 2 experiments (exp. #1 & #3) in the presence of
theophylline. The inhibition of tumor cell adherence by
PGI$_2$ was dose dependent with less inhibition observed at
concentrations of 10^{-5}M and 10^{-6}. At low doses of PGI$_2$
theophylline had a potentiating effect increasing the
inhibition at 10^{-5}M PGI$_2$ from 26.8% to 43.3%. Variability
in the effects of PGI$_2$ on different tumor cell preparations
similar to the PGE$_1$ analogue was also seen. PGF$_{2\alpha}$ also
exhibited inhibitory effects on tumor cell adherence to
plastic plates. However, the response of the tumor cells
to PGF$_{2\alpha}$ was much more variable than PGI$_2$ and 15-S-15-M

Table 1: Inhibition of Tumor Cell Adherence to Plastic Plates by Prostaglandins

	% Inhibition ± S.E.M.			
Experiment	#1	#2	#3	
Concentration (M)	+Theophylline	-Theophylline	-Theophylline	+Theophylline
15-S-15- methyl PGE$_1$ 10^{-4}	63.9±2.7	88.9±10.9	107.0±5.2	93.7±0.0
10^{-5}	56.8±4.9	-	55.6±3.4	89.1±5.1
10^{-6}	-	51.3±3.4	-	-
10^{-8}	-	27.4±8.2	-	-
PGI$_2$ 10^{-4}	50.4±4.2	38.4±9.2	71.1±4.8	73.1±22.9
10^{-5}	30.4±3.4	-	26.8±14.7	43.3±3.4
10^{-6}	-	-7.1±14.0	-	-
PGF$_{2\alpha}$ 10^{-4}	44.5±2.3	-5.8±0.0	54.6±23.0	35.7±8.1
10^{-5}	52.0±1.2	-	32.7±1.8	-
10^{-6}	-	-29.2±0.1	-	-
Control	29.1±1.7	-	-	7.8±2.5

PGE$_1$ with no inhibition seen in exp. #2 even at high concentrations. In additional studies pre-treatment of WCC with each of the three PGs significantly inhibited f Met-Leu-Phe stimulated tumor cell adherence to nylon fibers by greater than 75% at a concentration of 10^{-4}M in the absence of theophylline (data not shown).

The effect of 4 agents, histamine, cholera toxin, L-epinephrine, and dibutyryl cAMP on tumor cell adherence to plastic plates was determined. These agents are known to alter neutrophil functions in vitro and increase intracellular cAMP. When tumor cells were pre-incubated with each of these reagents and subsequently stimulated with PMA, there was significant inhibition of tumor cell adherence at concentrations between 10^{-4} to 10^{-6}M. Theophylline also potentiated the inhibition of adherence at 2.5×10^{-6}M dibutyryl cAMP. Preliminary data (not shown) demonstrates that pretreatment of WCC cells with the PGE$_1$ analogue, PGI$_2$, and PGF$_{2\alpha}$ at concentrations of 10^{-4}M will increase intracellular cAMP levels in WCC by approximately 3-fold. The data suggests that inhibition of tumor cell adherence may be mediated through alteration of tumor cell cAMP levels.

Discussion: Previous authors (1,2) have suggested that PGs and thromboxanes (Txs) may modulate platelet adherence to tumor cells and alter the size of circulating aggregates and their potential for embolization and metastasis. The data presented here demonstrates that PGs can modulate tumor cell adherence in vitro by their <u>direct</u> action on the tumor cell. This suggests that in certain systems, the local production of PGs (especially PGI_2 by endothelial cells) may play an important role in vivo by directly modulating tumor cell adherence to endothelium and/or basement membranes.

Since the localization of tumor cells is the initial event in the establishment of a metastatic site it is reasonable to postulate that the metastatic potential of certain tumors is intimately related to their responsiveness or lack there of to PGI_2. Under normal conditions the local production of PGI_2 by vascular endothelium could function to inhibit tumor cell adherence and metastasis. However, when the endothelial cells are injured and the production of PGI_2 decreased, the homeostatic balance may be altered in favor of increased tumor cell adherence and metastasis formation. Under these conditions, the exogenous administration of PGs that would inhibit tumor cell adherence may offer an effective therapeutic option. In addition, one could postulate that in certain circumstances the evolution of highly metastatic tumor cell lines from

Table 2: Effect of Agents Which Increase cAMP Levels on Tumor Cell Adherence

Drug	Concentration	% Inhibition $\pm$ S.E.M.
Histamine	10^{-4}M	92.3 ± 27.5
	10^{-5}M	65.9 ± 14.1
Cholera Toxin	10^{-5}M	90.7 ± 20.0
	10^{-6}M	61.6 ± 4.7
L-Epinephrine	10^{-5}M	63.6 ± 8.8
Dibutyryl cAMP	2.5×10^{-5}M	107.0 ± 3.8
	2.5×10^{-6}M	2.5 ± 5.7
	2.5×10^{-6}M + Theo-phylline (5×10^{-4}M)	44.7 ± 2.8

relatively dormant parent lines may be the result of a lack
of responsiveness of adherent tumor cells to PGs.

1. Stringfellow, D.A., and Fitzpatrick, F.A. Prosta-
    glandin D_2 controls pulmonary metastasis of malignant
    melonoma cells. Nature, 282:76–78, 1979.
2. Honn, K.V., Cicone, B., and Skoff, A. Prostacyclin: A
    potent antimetastatic agent. Science 212:1270–1272, 1981.
3. Varani, J., Wass, J., Piontek, G., and Ward, P.A.
    Chemotactic factor induced adherence of tumor cells.
    Cell Biol. Int. Rep., 5:525–530, 1981.
4. Varani, J. and Fantone, J.C. Phorbol myristate acetate
    induced adherence of tumor cells (submitted).

**Prostaglandins and Cancer: First
International Conference, pages 679-684**
© 1982 Alan R. Liss, Inc., 150 Fifth Avenue, New York, NY 10011

TUMOR ANTIGEN INDUCED CHANGES IN TRANSMEMBRANE POTENTIAL OF
LEUKOCYTES OF CANCER PATIENTS AND MODULATION BY LEUKOTRIENES
AND PROSTAGLANDINS.

George Shenouda,* D. M. P. Thomson* M. K. Bach†

*The   Montreal   General   Hospital   Research
Institute, Montreal, Quebec, Canada
†The UpJohn Company, Kalamazoo, Michigan, U.S.A.

INTRODUCTION

Human anti-tumor immunity has been studied in our
laboratory by the tube leukocyte adherence inhibition assay
(Grosser and Thomson, 1975). The LAI phenomenon is mediated
by human monocytes armed with cytophilic antitumor antibody
(Grosser et al., 1976; Marti et al., 1976). In this study we
describe a basic physiologic change in the transmembrane
potential (TMP) of peripheral blood leukocytes (PBL) from
patients with different types of cancer following challenge
by their sensitizing tumor antigen (TA).

TMP changes associated with receptor-ligand interaction
have been demonstrated in other cell types (Zierler, 1959;
Mathews et al., 1973; Gallin and Gallin, 1977). PBL are too
small for the direct measurements of TMP by microelectrodes.
We have, therefore, measured TMP indirectly by use of the
lipophilic-cation ^{3}H-tetraphenylphosphonium (TPP$^+$). This
ion equilibrates rapidly across biological membranes and the
measurements of its distribution reflect the magnitude and
direction of TMP changes. The use of 'lipophilic ions' to
measure TMP changes across biological membranes was introduced by Skulachev (1971). This technique has been applied
to monitor TMP changes in PMN (Korchak and Weissmann, 1978)
and neuroblastoma-glioma hybrid cell suspensions
(Lichtshtein et al., 1979).

MATERIALS & METHODS

(1) Donor of leukocytes

Venous blood from patients with breast, malignant melanoma, colon cancer and from normal control patients was drawn into heparinized Vacutainer® tubes. Buffy-coat PBL were isolated as described by Grosser and Thomson (1975) and suspended at a concentration of 0.5×10^7 cells/ml in Medium 199. Either PGE_2 or aminophylline stimulation was carried out by incubating 10^7 PBL with 0.5 ml of PGE_2 ($10^{-5.5}$M) or aminophylline (10^{-5}M) for 5 min at room temperature before reconstituting to the final PBL concentration. Mononuclear and polymorphnuclear cells (PMN) were prepared by Ficoll/Hypaque gradient from heparinized venous blood of control patients.

(2) Tumor extracts

Preparation of tumor extracts from metastases to the liver has been described in detail (Grosser and Thomson, 1975). PBL were challenged, simultaneously and separately, with a pair of tumor extracts one being specific to the type of cancer the patient has, the other being used as a control.

(3) Arming of monocytes

Adherent monocytes were armed with serum (1:4 dilution) from breast cancer patients for 30 min at 37°C in a 5% CO_2, humidified atmosphere. Then, they were challenged with breast cancer extract as the specific antigen and malignant melanoma as the non-specific antigen. The mediator released was tested in the TPP^+ uptake experiment using control PBL as indicator cells. In some experiments ETYA 10^{-5}M was added to the monocytes during the 0.5h. arming, and in other experiments FPL 55712 (10^{-6}M) was added to the generated mediator. Besides, the human non-adherent macrophage cell line, U937, was armed and challenged with the TA extracts to determine TPP^+ uptake.

(4) TPP^+ uptake measurements

1.5×10^6 PBLs in 300 μl were incubated at 37°C for 30 min with 10 μM ^3H-TPP^+ (NEN) to reach equilibrium. Then, they were challenged, separately and simultaneously, with the sensitizing and control TA, and at appropriate times the uptake was stopped by the addition of 3 ml of ice-cold saline followed by rapid filtration on a 0.5 µM pore-diameter Celotate® filter (Millipore). This was followed by a further 3 ml ice cold saline rinse. The filters were then placed in 10 ml of Ready-Solv H.P. liquid scintillation fluid (Beckman) and the radioactivity counted.

RESULTS AND DISCUSSION

Expression of Results

The direction and magnitude of TMP changes of PBL is reflected by the cellular level of TPP^+. We compared the TPP^+ uptake of PBL from cancer patients (e.g. breast cancer) when incubated with their specific antigen (e.g. breast cancer antigen) to the TPP^+ uptake of the same cells when challenged with the nonspecific antigen (e.g. malignant melanoma antigen). The results are expressed as an Index of TPP^+ uptake:

$$\frac{\text{cpm in presence of specific TA} - \text{cpm in presence of nonspecific TA}}{\text{cpm in presence of nonspecific TA}} / 10^6 \text{ cells} \times 100$$

PBL from cancer patients exhibited a triphasic re-sponse:- early hyperpolarization, depolarization and late hyperpolarization over a period of 15 min. In order to compare different TPP^+ indices of different patients we used the RATE of TPP^+ uptake:

$$\frac{\text{index of } TPP^+ \text{ uptake at the point of depolarization} - \text{at the point of hyperpolarization}}{\text{time elapsed between these 2 points}}$$

TMP Changes of PBL from Cancer Patients

The rate of TPP^+ uptake of breast cancer patients' PBL when challenged with the breast cancer antigen was 28 ± 5 as compared to 6.6 ± 4.6 for controls' PBL ($p<0.001$). $PGE_{2\alpha}$ or aminophylline stimulated PBL from breast cancer patients show a rate of TPP^+ uptake of 27 ± 3.3 when chal-lenged with specific TA, whereas PBL from controls had an TPP^+ uptake of 6.6 ($p<0.001$). Similarly, PGE_2 stimulated

PBL from melanoma patients showed a rate of TPP$^+$ uptake of 32 ± 7.5 when stimulated with malignant melanoma TA in comparison to a TPP$^+$ uptake of 8 ± 2.3 when stimulated with breast cancer antigen. PBL of breast cancer patients did not show any TMP changes when stimulated with the normal breast tissue antigen as reflected by a rate of TPP$^+$ uptake of 3.2 ± 0.2.

The results show that PBL from cancer patients possess receptors for their sensitizing TA and this receptor-TA interaction induces TMP changes.

Further confirmation of this specificity is demonstrated by the rate of TPP$^+$ uptake of 6.4 ± 1.3 for PBL from breast cancer patients preincubated for 15 min. with their specific breast cancer antigen while the same PBL not preincubated show a rate of uptake of 32 ± 11 ($p<0.05$). The same PBL preincubated with an unrelated TA show TMP changes similar to the nonpreincubated PBL when challenged with the specific TA.

PBL from advanced breast cancer patients showed no TMP changes since the rate of TPP$^+$ uptake was 5.5 ± 0.8, but if they were preincubated with PGE$_2$ $10^{-5.5}$M their rate of TPP uptake increased to 11 ± 1.3 ($p<0.01$).

The results correlated perfectly with those of the tube LAI assay where fewer patients responded as the stage of cancer increased, and most advanced cancer patients respond positively if they were stimulated with either PGE$_2$, or aminophylline (Grosser and Thomson, 1975; Kaneti et al., 1981). We demonstrate here that the primary defect is refractoriness of TMP changes of advanced cancer patients' PBL after receptor-TA interaction, and PGE$_2$ or aminophylline stimulation of the cells, by affecting the intracellular level of cAMP, reverses the refractory state.

The armed non-adherent macrophage cell line, U937, shows identical TMP changes (rate of TPP$^+$ 15 ± 1.2) when challenged with TA similar to the arming serum (e.g. breast cancer extract and serum from a breast cancer patient), but they show no TMP changes (3.2 ± 1.2) if armed with serum of normal control subjects ($p<0.001$).

Monocyte Mediators Induce TMP Changes

Purified monocytes armed with serum from breast cancer patients and challenged with the breast cancer extract release a mediator which cause TMP changes when added to PBL from control patients; rate of TPP^+ uptake was 32 ± 12. In comparison, when the mediator was obtained from monocytes armed with serum from normal patients challenged with breast cancer extract the rate of TPP^+ uptake was 13 ± 1.8. ETYA, an inhibitor of the lipoxygenase pathway of arachidonic acid metabolism, abrogated the release of the mediator that induced TMP changes, rate of TPP^+ uptake was 12 ± 2 ($p<0.025$).FPL 55712, a competitive inhibitor of leukotrienes, inhibited the mediator induced rate of TPP^+ uptake of normal PBL to 7 ± 3.5 ($p<0.005$).

Pure LTC and LTD enhanced the rate of TPP^+ uptake when added to control PBL (17 ± 6.5) compared to zero rate of TPP^+ uptake without LTC or LTD. Both mononuclear cells and PMNs respond equally to the leukotrienes, 17.3 ± 3.5 and 14.3 ± 4.1. The TPP^+ uptake by PBL was inhibited by FPL 55712.

Armed human monocytes challenged with the sensitizing tumor antigen release a mediator that induces TMP changes, and the mediator is similar in its actions to pure LTC and LTD.

REFERENCES

Gallin EK, Gallin JI (1977). Interaction of chemotactic factors with human macrophages: Induction of transmembrane potential changes. J Cell Biology 75:277.

Grosser N, Marti JH, Proctor JW, Thomson DMP (1976). Tube leukocyte adherence inhibition assay for the detection of anti-tumor immunity. I. Monocyte is the reactive cell. Int J Cancer 18:39.

Grosser N, Thomson DMP (1975). Cell-mediated anti-tumour immunity in breast cancer patients evaluated by antigen-induced leukocyte adherence inhibition in test tubes. Cancer Res. 35:257.

Kaneti J, Thomson DMP, Reid EC (1981). Prostaglandin E_2 affects the tumor immune response in prostatic carcinoma. J. Urology (in press).

Korchack HM, Weissmann G (1978). Changes in membrane potential of human gramulocytes antecede the metabolic responses to surface stimulation. Proc Natl Acad Sci USA 75:3818.

Lichtshtein D, Kaback HR, Blume AJ (1979). Use of a lipophilic cation for determination of membrane potential in neuroblastoma-glioma hybrid cell Suspensions. Proc Natl Acad Sci USA. 76:650.

Marti JH, Grosser N, Thomson DMP (1976). Tube leukocyte adherence inhibition assay for the detection of anti-tumour immunity.: II. Monocyte reacts with tumour antigen via cytophilic anti-tumour antibody. Int J Cancer 18:48.

Marti J, Thomson DMP (1976). Anti-tumour immunity in malignant melanoma assay by tube leucocyte-adherence inhibition. Br J Cancer 34:116.

Mathews EK, Petersen OH, Williams JA (1973). Pancreatic acinar cells acetylcholine-induced membrane depolarization, calcium efflux and amylase release. J Physiol (Lond) 231:283.

Skulachev VP (1971). Energy transformations in the respiratory chain. In Sanadi, DR (ed): Curr Top Bioenergy Vol 4, Academic Press, p. 127.

Zierler KL (1959). Effect of insulin on membrane potential and potassium content of rat muscle. Am J Physiology 197:515.

Prostaglandins and Cancer: First
International Conference, pages 685-689
© 1982 Alan R. Liss, Inc., 150 Fifth Avenue, New York, NY 10011

PGE$_2$-INDUCED ANGIOGENESIS

David M. Form, Younan A. Sidky, Louis Kubai and
Robert Auerbach
Dept. of Zoology, Univ. of Wisconsin, Madison,
WI 53706

Tumor-induced angiogenesis, i.e. the eliciting of new
blood vessels, is believed to be essential for the successful growth of solid tumors (Sidky and Auerbach, 1975;
Auerbach and Sidky, 1979). In addition to tumor cells,
lymphocytes (Folkman and Cotran, 1976; Folkman, 1976), and
macrophages (Polverini et al., 1977) have also been shown to
be capable of inducing neovascular reactions. Recent
attempts to isolate angiogenesis-inducing factors have led
to the description of numerous factors obtained from a broad
spectrum of cellular sources (Auerbach, 1981).

In an attempt to provide some unifying concept that
might consolidate the diverse studies on angiogenesis, the
idea that prostaglandins of the E series might play a significant role in many of the angiogenesis-inducing systems has
been proposed (Ben Ezra, 1978a; cf. Auerbach, 1981),
although experimental data in support of the concept has
been quite limited (Ben Ezra, 1978b; Cooper et al., 1980).
Reports of the association of PGE$_2$ with tumors, activated
macrophages and inflammataory exudates (cf. Auerbach, 1981)
has made this an attractive theory. Our experiments were
designed to determine to what extent prostaglandin-E$_2$ could
induce angiogenesis.

The primary assay system for neovascularization was the
chorio-allantoic membrane (CAM) of explanted chick embryos
grown in petri dishes (Auerbach et al., 1974). The method
permits the continued observation of induced neovascular
reactions including sequential measurements and photographic
documentation of the vascular response. To obtain a

controlled release of PGE_2, thin sheets of Elvax (ethylene vinyl acetate), containing PGE_2 at different concentrations, were prepared according to published procedures (11). Disc-shaped pellets, 1 mm in diameter, each containing approximately 1 mg of this slow-release polymer were used as implants on the CAM of 8-day old chick embryos. Uniformity and release kinetics were monitored using $^3HPGE_2$. As shown in Fig. la pellets containing 10^{-5} mg PGE_2 released their labelled prostaglandin into saline slowly over a 6-day period. Comparable release rates were found for pellets containing higher concentrations of PGE_2. The release kinetics was similar to that reported by Rhine et al (1980) for the release of bovine serum albumin from Elvax. Since release rates were more uniform after the first 24 hours, pellets were kept in saline for 24 hours before use. The kinetics of PGE_2 release into the CAM is shown in Fig. 1b, in which the value of PGE_2 release on day 0 represents the amount of prostaglandin released into saline prior to placement of the pellet on the CAM.

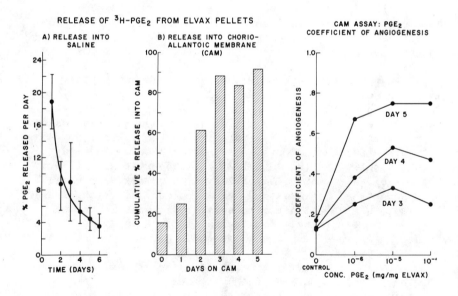

RELEASE OF $^3H\text{-}PGE_2$ FROM ELVAX PELLETS

CAM ASSAY: PGE_2
COEFFICIENT OF ANGIOGENESIS

A) RELEASE INTO SALINE

B) RELEASE INTO CHORIO-ALLANTOIC MEMBRANE (CAM)

Figure 1

PGE$_2$-containing pellets induced two distinct types of vascular activity on the CAM. The first involved the appearance of a reticulated network of capillaries near positive pellets, apparent within 24-48 hours and declining after the 4th day. The second response, a more typical neovascular reaction (Folkman, 1976), marked by oriented blood vessels, bends and loops, first became noticeable 3 days after implantation of the pellet, becoming more fully developed on days 4 and 5 (Fig. 1c). This angiogenic response was seen associated with an opaqueness under or near the pellet which appeared to act as a focus for the angiogenic response.

Using a scoring method for angiogenesis developed by Folkman (1976) pellets were seen to be either negative (o), weakly positive (+) or clearly positive (++). The extreme responses observed by Folkman for some tumor extracts (+++. ++++) were not seen in our tests. Scoring was carried out on coded embryos. After uncoding, the scores for all pellets from each group were added together and divided by the maximum possible score (2 x # pellets) to give a coefficient of angiogenesis. Pellets containing 10^{-4}, 10^{-5} and 10^{-6} mg PGE$_2$ releasing approximately 0.2 ng, 2.0 ng or 20 ng per day into thee CAM were tested. By day 4 a definite angiogenic response (P<.05) was obtained with pellets containing 10^{-4} or 10^{-5} mg PGE$_2$ while by day 5 all three concentrations of PGE$_2$ were significantly (P<.025) more angiogenic than the control pellets. Similar results were obtained using PGE$_1$-containing pellets.

The amount of PGE found by us to be optimal for inducing angiogenesis is similar to that reported for a variety of tumors (Owen et al., 1980; cf. Auerbach, 1981), for activated macrophages (Stenson and Parker, 1980), for inflammatory exudates (Vane, 1976) and for synovium (Dayer et al., 1976). The relation of PGE production incident to the release of lymphokines has been discussed previously (Auerbach and Sidky, 1979; Auerbach, 1981). A variety of angiogenesis induced factors have been isolated and partially characterized (cf. Auerbach, 1981). They appear to fall into two classes: low molecular weight factors that could well turn out to be in the prostaglandin family, and larger, non-dialyzable ones some of which may in fact be comprised of a small active component attached to a heavier carrier molecule.

Angiogenesis is a complex biological process that can be
regulated at various points. Dissolution of vascular continuity, induction of cell migration, triggering of endothelial cell replication, induction of capillary sprouting
and extension of vascular continuity all must occur in an
orderly fashion (Auerbach, 1981; Form et al., 1981). There
is no reason to expect, therefore, that the prostaglandins
should be the only mediators of neovascularization. On the
other hand, the fact that prostaglandin-E$_2$, in amounts
equivalent to those accompanying inflammatory lesions, synovial swelling and some tumor nodules, can by itself be adequate to elicit neovascularization suggests that the array
of angiogenesis factors may be at least partially reduced to
a few key elements.

References

Auerbach R. (1981). Angiogenesis-inducing factors: A
review. in Lymphokines, vol. 4, ed. E. Pick (in press).

Auerbach R. and Sidky Y.A. (1979). Nature of the stimulus
leading to lymphocyte-induced angiogenesis. J. Immunol.
123: 751.

Auerbach R., Kubai L., Knighton D. and Folkman J. (1974). A
simple procedure for the long-term cultivation of chicken
embryos. Dev. Biol. 41: 391.

Ben Ezra D. (1978a). Neovasculogenesis. Triggering factors
and possible mechanisms. Surv. Ophthalmol. 24: 167.

Ben Ezra D. (1978b). Neovasculogenic ability of prostaglandins, growth factors and synthetic chemoattractants.
Am. J. Ophthalmol. 86: 455.

Cooper C.A., Bergamini M.V.W. and Leopold I.H. (1980). Use
of flurbiprofen to inhibit corneal neovascularization.
Arch. Ophthalmol. 98: 1102.

Dayer J.-M., Krane S.M., Russell G.G. and Robinson D.R.
(1976). Production of collagenase and prostaglandins by
isolated adherent rheumatoid synovial cells. Proc. Natl.
Acad. Sci. 73: 945.

Folkman J. (1976) "Tumor angiogenesis" in Cancer, vol. 3, ed. F.F. Becker, Plenum Press, NY, pp. 355.

Folkman J. and Cotran R. (1976). Relation of vascular proliferation to tumor growth. Int. Rev. Exp. Pathol. 16: 207.

Form D.M., Sidky Y.A., Kubai L. and Auerbach R. (1981). PGE$_2$ and angiogenesis. (submitted for publication).

Owen K., Gomolka D. and Droller M.J. (1980). Production of prostaglandin E$_2$ by tumor cells in vitro. Cancer Res. 40: 3167.

Polverini P.J., Cotran R.S., Gimbrone M.A. Jr. and Unanue E.R. (1977). Activated macrophages induce vascular proliferation. Nature 269: 804.

Rhine W.D., Hsieh D.S.T. and Langer R. (1980). Polymers for sustained macromolecule release: Procedures to fabricate reproducible delivery systems and control release kinetics. J. Pharmaceut. Sci. 69: 265.

Sidky Y.A. and Auerbach R. (1975). Lymphocyte-induced angiogenesis (LIA): a quantitative and sensitive assay of the graft-vs.-host reaction. J. Exp. Med. 141: 1084.

Stenson W.F. and Parker C.W. (1980). Prostaglandins, macrophages and immunity. J. Immunol. 125: 1.

Vane J.R. 1976). Prostaglandins as mediators of inflammation. Adv. Prostaglandin and Thromboxane Res. 2: 71.

This research has been supported by grants EY-3243, AI-14607 and CA-28626 from the National Institutes of Health. DWF is a postdoctoral trainee supported by a training grant (CA-9106) from the National Cancer Institute.

**Prostaglandins and Cancer: First
International Conference, pages 691-695
© 1982 Alan R. Liss, Inc., 150 Fifth Avenue, New York, NY 10011**

HUMAN LUNG CANCER AND PROSTAGLANDINS

IF Stamford, A Bennett, MA Carroll, CN Hensby,
WF Whimster and F Williams.
Departments of Surgery and Morbid Anatomy, King's
College Hospital Medical School, London SE5 8RX,UK
and Department of Clinical Pharmacology, Royal
Postgraduate Medical School, London W12 DH5, UK.

The amounts of prostaglandin-like material (PG-lm)
extracted from human mammary carcinomas correlate. with local
tumor invasiveness, spread to bone and early death (Bennett
et al 1977, 1979; Rolland et al 1980). We have now studied
human lung tumors which also metastasize to bone and soft
tissues, and are the most common malignancy.

PATIENTS AND METHODS

Of the 171 patients initially suitable for operation 134
are evaluable (108 men, 26 women); 37 patients were excluded
due to other primary or secondary cancers or other lung
disease. None had been treated previously for lung cancer
or had received radiotherapy or chemotherapy.

Fresh surgically resected tumor and lung tissue were
obtained at pneumonectomy and lobectomy and samples were
taken for histology. The remainder of each tissue was cut
finely and washed several times in Krebs solution. Weighed
samples were homogenised either in ethanol:Krebs solution (1:1)
acidified to approximately pH3 with formic acid (to indicate
basal amounts of tissue PG-lm), or in Krebs alone (which
allows new prostaglandin synthesis from endogenous precursors
released during homogenisation). The extract of this latter
homogenate yields "total PG-lm" since it reflects newly synthesised + basal PG-lm. Individual samples were extracted
(Unger, Stamford and Bennett 1971) and bioassayed against
PGE_2 using the rat gastric fundus preparation (Gilmore, Vane

and Wyllie 1968). Tumor samples from 4 patients were also purified by column and thin layer chromatography prior to analysis by gas chromotography-mass spectrometry.

Tumor types were classified according to their degree of differentiation (ie squamous and adenocarcinomas - well and poorly differentiated - and undifferentiated large and small cell carcinomas). Measurements of tumor size and histological assessments of tissue macrophages, lymphocytes, neutrophils, necrosis and mitotic figures were made, without prior knowledge of PG-1m results.

RESULTS AND DISCUSSION

The "total" and "basal" amounts of PG-1m extracted from the tumors were usually greater than amounts from normal tissue (P<0.0001 for both). Amounts of PG-1m extracted from different tumor types varied widely (Table 1), with well differentiated adenocarcinomas yielding the highest amounts, and undifferentiated cancers yielding the least. Table 1 also relates these values to the expected prognosis, which tends to be better with the higher amounts of PG-1m, except for squamous carcinomas which show a reverse trend. With squamous carcinomas less than 3cm diameter the difference in PG-1m between well differentiated and poorly differentiated tumors was particularly marked (median amounts of 22 and 435ng PGE_2 equivalents/g, P=0.002). Amounts of PG-1m extracted from normal lung resected with the tumor did not vary significantly between different tumor types.

Histological examination showed that mitotic figures tended to correlate inversely with PG-1m; the slower growing adenocarcinomas had few mitotic figures and high amounts of PG-1m, whereas the fast growing undifferentiated small cell carcinomas had many mitotic figures and low amounts of PG-1m. Moderate necrosis or neutrophil content tended to be associated with highest amounts of tumor PG-1m. There was no correlation between PG-1m and fibrosis, the numbers of lymphocytes, or tumor size (divided into 4 groups, Soorae and Abbey Smith 1977). Macrophages were present in normal tissue and their numbers correlated with PG-1m (total, P<0.0001; basal, P<0.05).

Analysis by gas chromatography-mass spectrometry of extracts from squamous carcinomas (2 well-differentiated and

Table 1. Tumors of different types in relation to prognosis and yield of prostaglandin-like material

Carcinoma Type	Prognosis	N	Basal PG-lm	Total PG-lm
Squamous WD	Best	48	21(12-47))c	47(22-110))c
Squamous PD	Moderate	28	48(19-190))	145(55-460))
Adenocarcinoma WD	Best	13	100(49-830))b	170(88-1800))a
Adenocarcinoma PD	Moderate	7	41(34-62))	86(59-110))
Adenosquamous		3	32-55	120-300
Large cell UD (mostly squamous)	Poor	30	15(5-39)	37(17-145)
Small cell UD	Bad	4	0.8-14	3-44
Overall tumor values		133	28(11-79))d	70(24-190))d
Normal tissue		132	16(6-38))	33(14-63))

WD, PD and UD are respectively well, poorly or undifferentiated tumors. The results are median values with semiquartile ranges in parentheses. a, $P<0.1$; b, $P<0.05$; c, $P<0.01$; d, $P<0.0001$.

1 poorly differentiated) and 1 undifferentiated large-cell carcinoma, showed the presence of arachidonic acid and several metabolites including thromboxane B_2, 6-keto-PGF$_{1\alpha}$ and 12 hydroxy-eicosatetraenoic acid (12-HETE). Three metabolites (15-keto-13,14-dihydro TXB$_2$, 6,15-diketo-13,14 dihydro PGF$_{1\alpha}$ and 6,15-diketo PGF$_{1\alpha}$), not previously described in lung tumors were also found. No primary prostaglandins or metabolites of eicosatrienoic acid or eicosapentaenoic acid were found; if they were present their recovered amounts were less than 80ng/g tissue. No search was made for leukotrienes. The contribution of the various constituents to the biological activity is not known. Many of the metabolites tested on the rat stomach are only weakly active, 6-keto-PGF$_{1\alpha}$, 6,15-diketo-PGF$_{1\alpha}$ and thromboxane B_2 being at least 300 times less potent than PGE$_2$ (Bennett et al 1980).

Since all the tumor homogenates contained the lipoxygenase product 12-HETE, and all originally contained PGI$_2$ and thromboxane A_2 as indicated by complete spectra of their degradation products 6-keto-PGF$_{1\alpha}$ and thromboxane B_2, these eicosanoids may be the major substances formed. However, we do not know how much the tumor blood vessels and constituents contribute to the amounts present in extracts. The relevance of these findings to the tumor biology and patient prognosis remains to be determined.

REFERENCES

Bennett A, Berstock DA, Raja B, Stamford IF (1979). Survival time after surgery is inversely related to the amounts of prostaglandins extracted from human breast cancers. Br J Pharmac 66:451P.

Bennett A, Charlier EM, McDonald AM, Simpson JS, Stamford IF, Zebro T (1977). Prostaglandins and breast cancer. Lancet ii:624.

Bennett A, Jarosik C, Sanger GJ, Wilson DE (1980). Antagonism of prostanoid-induced contractions of rat gastric fundus muscle by SC19220, sodium meclofenamate, indomethacin or trimethoquinol. Br J Pharmac 71:169.

Gilmore N, Vane JR, Wyllie JH (1968). Prostaglandin released by the spleen. Nature 218:1135.

Rolland PH, Martin PM, Jacquemier J, Rolland AM, Toga M (1980). Prostaglandin in human breast cancer: evidence suggesting that an elevated prostaglandin production is a marker of high metastatic potential for neoplastic cells. J Nat Cancer

Inst 64:1061.
Soorae AS, Abbey Smith R (1977).   Tumor size as a prognostic
factor after resection of lung carcinoma.   Thorax 32:19.
Unger WG, Stamford IF, Bennett A (1971).   Extraction of
prostaglandins from human blood.   Nature 233:336.

**Prostaglandins and Cancer: First
International Conference, pages 697-700**
© 1982 Alan R. Liss, Inc., 150 Fifth Avenue, New York, NY 10011

PROSTAGLANDIN PRODUCTION BY SQUAMOUS CELL CARCINOMA OF
HUMAN UTERINE CERVIX IN VITRO

Tsuneki Nagasaka[1], Wendell D. Winters[2], Olive M.
Soriero[1] and Michael J.K. Harper[1]
Departments of Obstetrics and Gynecology[1] and
Microbiology[2], The University of Texas Health
Science Center at San Antonio, 7703 Floyd Curl
Drive, San Antonio, Texas 78284, U.S.A.

There have been numerous reports describing the production of prostaglandins (PGs) by some human and experimental animal tumors. PGs have been found to be associated
with a number of cellular activities including proliferation, differentiation, malignant transformation, metastatic
characteristics, hypercalcaemia, immunity and platelet
aggregation, but their exact role is yet unclear. The aims
of the present study were to measure the production of PGs
by newly established cultures of squamous cell carcinoma of
human uterine cervical origin and to determine the source of
the PGs produced.

Squamous cell carcinomas of human uterine cervix from
18 patients were used in this study. Sterile specimens of
tumor tissue were obtained at the time of surgery and maintained in monolayers by serial subpassages. The cells (ca.
1.2×10^6) were cultured in 10ml Dulbecco's modified essentia
medium with 10% heat-inactivated fetal bovine serum, 50µg/ml
gentamycin and 5µg/ml fungizone added, in 75cm^2 plastic
flasks at 37°C in a humidified atmosphere of 5% CO_2 and 95%
air (Winters et al., 1974). The medium was changed approximately every 48 hours, and 1ml aliquots of media from the
same passage stage were collected, acidified to pH 4.5 with
acetate buffer, extracted twice with 4 ml ethyl acetate and
chromatographed on silicic acid columns before radioimmunoassay of PGE and PGF (Harper et al., 1978; Harper et al.,
1981).

During the initial passage, concentrations (mean ± S.
E.M., in ng/ml) of both PGE and PGF were relatively high

(PGE: 18.59 ± 8.17; PGF: 5.17 ± 1.24). However, after this time, levels of PGs were significantly decreased (PGE: 0.70 ± 0.18; PGF: 1.51 ± 0.18) in all cultures tested (p < 0.05) as shown in Fig. 1. The decrease of PGE was more dramatic than that of PGF.

Similar patterns of the production of PGE or PGF were observed in all three tumor cell cultures following the addition of arachidonic acid (AA) into the culture medium during the dose-response and time-course experiments conducted at three subpassage intervals (passage 9,10 and 11). Therefore, the data from these experiments were pooled and expressed as means ± S.E.M. for different cell cultures combined (Fig. 2). Incubation for periods of 2, 4 or 6 days did not produce any significant differences in the concentrations of PGE and PGF. The results for dose-response studies of cultures at 6 days after AA treatment revealed that PGs production was dose dependent. When incubated with 10.0 μg/ml of AA, the cancer cells produced significantly higher (p < 0.001) amounts of PGs (PGE: 3.44 ± 0.23; PGF: 1.83 ± 0.13) than control cancer cells without AA treatment (PGE: 0.33 ± 0.017; PGF: 1.27 ± 0.041). Neither PGE nor PGF concentrations were significantly increased over control values by AA treatment at levels of 0.1 or 1.0 μg/ml.

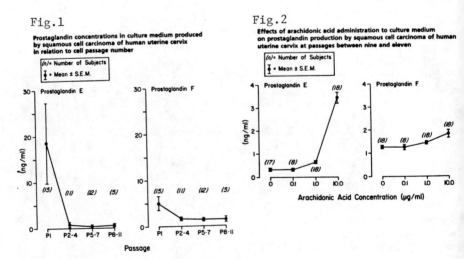

Fig.1

Prostaglandin concentrations in culture medium produced by squamous cell carcinoma of human uterine cervix in relation to cell passage number

Fig.2

Effects of arachidonic acid administration to culture medium on prostaglandin production by squamous cell carcinoma of human uterine cervix at passages between nine and eleven

This appears to be the first report on the production
of PGs by squamous cell carcinomas of human uterine cervix
during serial in vitro subpassage. These cancer cells produced high amounts of PGE and PGF at initial passage. However, the production of both PGE and PGF decreased after
the second passage in all cases. These decreases may be
explained due to any or all of the following: (1) at the
initial passage level, tumor cells mixed with macrophages,
monocytes, lymphocytes and platelets may exist. These
mixed cell populations could produce considerable amounts of
prostanoids; (2) during serial subpassages, metabolic pathways or enzyme activities have changed in the tumor cell populations; (3) after the second subpassage, the substrate for
PG production, namely arachidonic acid, is depleted. The
first explanation is probable, but the tissue separation
and cell preparation methods applied destroy and/or separate
the leukocyte cell populations from the tumor cells well. The
second explanation is undeniable. The pattern and sequence
of PGs synthesized by monocytes and macrophages are in part
a function of in vitro culture conditions, time in culture
and the species studied (Bockman, 1981). The alterations of
metabolic pathways in the cancer cells may occur during
serial subpassages. However, in our studies in the presence
of AA, the human tumor cells showed significant increases of
PG production at subpassages nine through eleven. Moreover,
the production of PGs did not show any significant increase
as the incubation period was increased from 2 to 6 days,
despite continued cell growth. The most likely explanation
for our findings is that AA is rapidly depleted during serial
subculture of human squamous cell carcinomas of the uterine
cervix. The present results of the effects of AA on the
production of PGs in cultured cells are in agreement with
the generally similar results on the established cell lines,
e.g., HeLa, L and HEp-2 (Cohen and Jaffe, 1973), on the
primary cultures from mouse mammary tumors (Burstein et al.,
1977) and on the mouse neuroblastoma cells (Tansik and White,
1979). We suggest that the depletion of substrate plays a
major role in the decreased production of PGs during serial
subpassage of cells.

In summary, cells from 18 human squamous cell carcinomas of the uterine cervix had the capacity to produce PGs
after long-term serial subpassage in vitro, if the substrate,
arachidonic acid, was added. These human cancer cells may
provide a useful model system for future studies on the
relationships between PGs and cancer.

Acknowledgments

This work was supported by the Ford Foundation
(Postdoctoral Fellowship to Tsuneki Nagasaka) and the
Spuelin J. Burress Research Fund (Wendell D. Winters).

Bockman RS (1981). Prostaglandin production by human blood
monocytes and mouse peritoneal macrophages: Synthesis
dependent on in vitro culture conditions. Prostaglandins
21:9.
Burstein S, Gagnon G, Hunter SA and Maudsley DV (1977).
Elevation of prostaglandin and cyclic AMP levels by
arachidonic acid in primary epithelial cell cultures of
C3H mouse mammary tumors. Prostaglandins 13:41.
Cohen F and Jaffe BM (1973). Production of prostaglandins
by cells in vitro: Radioimmunoassay measurement of the
conversion of arachidonic acid to PGE$_2$ and PGF$_2\alpha$. Biochem
Biophys Res Comm 55:724.
Harper MJK, Norris CJ, Friedrichs WE and Moreno A (1981).
Poly I:C accelerates ovum transport in the rabbit by a
prostaglandin-mediated mechanism. J Reprod Fert 63
(in press).
Harper MJH, Valenzuela G and Hodgson BJ (1978). Accelerated
ovum transport in rabbits induced by endotoxin. 1. Changes
in prostaglandin levels and reversal of endotoxin effect.
Prostaglandins 15:43.
Tansik RL and White HL (1979). Prostaglandin synthesis in
homogenates of cultured neuroblastoma cells. Prostaglandins and Medicine 2:225.
Winters WD, Neri A and Morton DL (1974). New cell line
derived from a human chondrosarcoma. In Vitro 10:70.

Prostaglandins and Cancer: First
International Conference, pages 701–703
© 1982 Alan R. Liss, Inc., 150 Fifth Avenue, New York, NY 10011

PROSTAGLANDINS IN TUMOR-ASSOCIATED CELLS

A. Fulton, A. Rios, S. Loveless and G. Heppner

Michigan Cancer Foundation, Detroit, MI

Many human and experimental tumors synthesize high levels of prostaglandins. Several studies have suggested that high prostaglandin levels, particularly of the E class, serve as markers of malignant potential for human breast tumors (Powles, et al., 1976, Bennett, et al., 1977, Rolland, et al., 1980). Fitzpatrick and Stringfellow (1979) have shown, in contrast, that high levels of prostagland D_2 are inversely related to the metastatic potential of the B_{16} murine melanoma sublines. We have examined a series of mouse mammary lesions ranging from pre-neoplastic HANs (hyperplastic alveolar nodules) to neoplastic lesions of both low and high metastatic potential to determine the levels and cellular sources of prostaglandin E_2 (PGE_2).

Two of the tumors used for these studies (68H and 410) are subpopulations isolated from a single spontaneous mammary carcinoma arising in a BALB/cfC_3H mouse. The 410.4 tumor is a transplantable tumor originally isolated from the lung of a mouse bearing the 410 tumor. The 4501 and 4526 tumors are sublines derived by dilution cloning of the 410.4 tumor. The C_4 HAN, originally obtained from Dr. D. Medina, and the C_4 tumor which spontaneously arises from it were also studied. The characteristics of these tumors are described in Table 1 and by Miller, et al. (1979).

As shown in Table 1, the lowest levels of PGE_2 are seen in the pre-neoplastic HANs (9 ng/g) while higher levels are seen in the spontaneously occurring tumors which arise from these lesions (37 ng/g). The poorly metastasizing 68H and 410 tumors contain levels of PGE_2 of 27 ng/g and 75 ng/g, respectively, while the highly metastatic variants of 410 (410.4, 4501 and 4526) produce much higher levels of PGE_2. Lung metastases isolated from mice bearing subcutaneously growing 4526 tumors maintain the high PGE_2 level.

Table 1. PGE_2 Levels in Mouse Mammary Neoplasms

Sample	Characteristics	PGE_2 (ng/g)
C_4 HAN	Pre-neoplastic Benign	9+5
C_4 Tumor	Neoplastic Non-metastasizing	37+10
68H Tumor	Neoplastic Low-metastasizing	27+5
410 Tumor	Neoplastic Low-metastasizing	75+22
410.4 Tumor	Neoplastic High-metastasizing	135+30
4501 Tumor	Neoplastic High-metastasizing	429+163
4526 Tumor	Neoplastic High-metastasizing	543+94
4526 Lung metastases		432+100

To determine the PGE_2 activity of tumor cells freed of host infiltrative cells, tumor cells are grown in in vitro culture for 10-12 passages. Cells are trypsinized, harvested and split. After replating, cells are allowed to grow for 24h at which time the tissue culture media is replaced by fresh media. Incubation continues for a further 24h, at which time cells and supernatant fluids are harvested and PGE_2 activity determined. While cultured tumor cells release PGE_2 into the culture fluid, the relative PGE_2 levels correspond to neither the levels seen in tumors freshly isolated from mice nor to malignant potential.

The contribution of host infiltrative cells to tumor-associated prostaglandin levels is determined by isolating

these cells from tumor nodules. Tumors are enzyme dissociated, plastic-adherent cells removed and the remaining
cells separated by the isokinetic gradient technique of
Pretlow (1969). PGE_2 activity is associated with both the
tumor parenchymal cells and the tumor-associated macrophage population but little activity is seen in the lymphocyte fractions.

Parallel studies of primary human breast tumors have
shown that most contain measurable quantities of PGE_2 and
PGF_{2a}. Further studies will determine whether the prostaglandins levels are related to disease-free interval or
site of recurrence.

(Supported by NIH Grants CA·16175, CA 27437, the
E. Walter Albachten Fund and the United Foundation of
Greater Detroit).

References

Bennett A, McDonald AM, Stamford IF, Charlier EM, Simpson JJ
and Zebro T (1977). Prostaglandins and breast cancer.
Lancet II:624.

Fitzpatrick FA and Stringfellow DA (1979). Prostaglandin
D_2 formation by malignant melanoma cells correlates inversely with cellular metastatic potential. Proc. Natl.
Acad. Sci. 76:1765.

Miller FR and Heppner GH (1979). Immunologic heterogeneity
of tumor cell subpopulations from a single mouse mammary
tumor. J.N.C.I. 63:1457.

Powles TJ, Dowsett M, Easty GC, Easty DM and Neville AM
(1976). Breast cancer osteolysis, bone metastases, and
anti-osteolytic effect of aspirin. Lancet I:608.

Pretlow TG, Boone CW (1969). Separation of mammalian cells
using programmed gradient sedimentation. Exp. Mol.
Pathol. 11:139.

Rolland PH, Martin PM, Jacquemier J, Rolland AM, and
Toga M (1980). Prostaglandin in human breast cancer:
Evidence suggesting that an elevated prostaglandin production is a marker of high metastatic potential for
neoplastic cells. J.N.C.I. 64:1061.

Prostaglandins and Cancer: First
International Conference, pages 705-711
© 1982 Alan R. Liss, Inc., 150 Fifth Avenue, New York, NY 10011

PROSTAGLANDIN SYNTHESIS AND BINDING BY GROWING AND
REGRESSING MAMMARY CARCINOMA

Sue C. Liu and Richard A. Knazek

National Institutes of Health, National Cancer
Institute, Laboratory of Pathophysiology
Bethesda, MD 20205

Prostaglandins have been found in virtually every
mammalian tissue. Thought to act near their sites of synthesis, the effects are protean with opposing actions being
observed within a tissue when the concentrations of the
same prostaglandin are changed or when different prostaglandins are elaborated (Manku, 1979). Changes in cell
differentiation, growth, and function have been induced by
exogenous prostaglandins while the abilities of cells to
synthesize prostaglandins have been modified by exposure
to a variety of extrinsic stimuli in vitro (Karmali, 1980;
Salz, 1978; Thomas, 1974). The role prostaglandins play in
tumor pathophysiology is less clear, having been indicated
in the hypercalcemia of malignancy (Tashjian, 1978), blood
flow (Rankin, 1977), neovascularization (Gullino, Private
Communication), and metastasis (Rolland, 1980). Similarly,
a review of inhibitors of prostaglandin synthesis shows
both stimulation and inhibition of cell growth (Hail, 1977;
Karmali et al, 1979; Tashjian et al, 1977). These seeming-
ly contradictory observations are likely due to the complex
interactions and feedback loops in the cascade of arachidonate metabolism. In addition, different tissues may vary
in their ability to respond to a given prostaglandin held at
a fixed concentration. Just as the effects of a hormone are
modified by its circulating concentrations, they are also
mediated by changes in affinity or quantity of the specific
hormone receptor on or within the target cells (Kahn et al,
1979). In like manner, the protean effects of prostaglandins are mediated by means of specific receptors within the
target cells (Powell et al, 1975; Rao, 1975, 1976; Schafer,
1978). The studies reported herein describe the prosta-

glandin receptor in the hormone-dependent NMU rat mammary tumor and correlate its characteristics with the growing and regressing states.

MATERIALS

Tumors

Female Buffalo rats were treated with nitrosomethyl urea (Gullino et al, 1975) and were fed Purina rat chow and water ad libitum, while being maintained 3-4 per cage in an animal room kept between 75-78°F having a 6 am to 6 pm light-dark cycle.

Prostaglandins

Tritium-labeled prostaglandins E_2 (New England Nuclear, NET-428, [5,6,8,9,11,12,15-^{3}H(N)]-PGE$_2$, 75-165 Ci/mmole) and $F_{2\alpha}$ (Nuclear, NET-433, [5,6,8,9,11,12, 14,15-^{3}H(N)]-PGF$_{2\alpha}$ 150 Ci/mmole) had a radio chemical purity greater than 99% by high performance liquid chromatography. The non-labeled prostaglandins PGE$_2$, PGF$_{2\alpha}$ were purchased from Sigma Chemical Co.

Membrane Preparations

When the tumors reached 1-2 gm the hosts were oophorectomized or sham-operated before decapitation 0-9 days later. When the tumors were to be used for prostaglandin receptor studies, they were excised, immediately minced in an ice-water bath, and homogenized in 10 volumes of buffer, composed of 250 mM sucrose, 10 mM Tris-HCl pH 7.4, 0.1% sodium azide, 1mM dithiothreitol, and 1 mM Ca Cl$_2$. After preliminary 120g centrifugation at 4°C for 15 min, the supernatant was centrifuged for 20 min at 15,000g. The pellet was then resuspended in 10 volumes Tris-Sucrose and recentrifuged at 15,000g. These pellets were resuspended in assay buffer composed of 50 mM Tris-HCl and 15 mM MgCl$_2$ at pH 7.4 to yield a concentration of 2 to 5 mg protein/ml immediately prior to the binding assay.

Tumor membranes were prepared in a slightly different manner for investigation of prostaglandin synthesis. A portion of each tumor was frozen in liquid N_2 immediately after excision, pulverized and then homogenized in 300 mM Sucrose/25mM Tris-HCl pH 7.6. After centrifuging the homogenate at 120 xg, the supernatant was centrifuged at 100,000 xg for 1 hour at 4°C. The pellet was resuspended in the homogenization buffer to provide 2 mg protein/ml.

PG Binding Assay

Membrane fractions were incubated at 23°C for 45 min with concentrations of [^{3}H]PGF$_2\alpha$ as indicated. Incubations were carried out in a total volume of 250 ul which included 100 ul of membrane suspension. After incubation, a 125 ul aliquot of the suspension was rapidly filtered through a Whatman GF/C glass microfiber filter and washed with two 3 ml portions of ice-cold 50 mM Tris-HCl, buffer pH 7.4. The number of CPM bound to the air-dried filters were then determined by counting in Beckman Ready-Solv HP liquid scintillation fluid.

Except where noted, additional tubes containing 10^{-5}M non-radioactive PG were also included in each experiment to provide the value for "non-specific" binding. The difference between the values for total and non-specific binding was the specific binding and amounted to 50% to 80% of total radioactivity bound.

PG Synthesis Assays

One-half ml of the membrane suspensions were placed in six glass tubes containing 0.5 ml buffer composed of 4 mM GSH, 0.34 mM hydroquinone, 10 mM glucose, 1.2 mM MgCl$_2$, 1.3 mM CaCl$_2$, 115 mM NaCl, and 25 mM Tris at pH 8.1, three with and three without 10^{-3}M indomethacin. After incubating at 37° for 2 hours, the tubes were plunged into an ice water bath and were vortexed with 20 ml ice cold petroleum ether., Subsequently, the aqueous phase was acidified with 10 ul concentrated formic acid and approximately 1000 CPM of ^{3}H-PGF$_2\alpha$ and ^{3}H-PGE$_2$ were added to permit individual estimates of recovery. The prostaglandins were then extracted from the aqueous suspensions into chloroform and dried under nitrogen. The samples were dissolved in 0.2 ml of a benzene-ethylacetate-methanol (B-EA-M) solution mixed in a ratio of 60:40:2 by volume and applied to a 1 gm silicic acid column (Sigma, Sil-A-200) that had been pre-washed with 60:40:0 B-EA-M and benzene. Compounds eluted with an initial volume of 18 ml 60:40:0 B-EA-M were discarded. Subsequent elution with 20 ml 60:40:20 B-EA-M yielded the PGE and $PGF_{2\alpha}$ fraction which, after drying, was incubated with 1 ml of 0.1M KOH in absolute methanol for 45 minutes to convert PGE to PGB. This permitted separation of PGE (as PGB) from $PGF_{2\alpha}$ by repeating the above chromatography with fresh columns (Alexander et al, 1975).

The partially purified prostaglandins PGE (as PGB) and $PGF_{2\alpha}$ were thus separated prior to the quantitation which was accomplished by dextran-charcoal RIA using anti-PGB antibody (provided by Dr. John Pisano, NIH) and anti-$PGF_{2\alpha}$ antibody (New England Nuclear, NEA-057B). The amounts of PG synthesized were determined by correcting for recovery and then subtracting the corrected quantities present in the indomethacin-containing tubes from the corrected quantities present in the tubes without indomethacin. The amounts were normalized for the amounts of protein present.

RESULTS

Binding of both PGE_2 and $PGF_{2\alpha}$ to tumor membranes reached equilibrium after 30 min incubation. The binding was saturable and 44-58% reversible within 15 min of adding excess unlabeled PGE_2 or $F_{2\alpha}$, respectively. Sudden 2-3 fold increases in specific binding of both types of PG were observed ~ 4 days after oophorectomy (Table 1). Scatchard

Table 1

Specific Binding of Prostaglandins to Growing and
Regressing NMU Mammary Carcinoma Membranes

Ligand	Days following Oophorectomy			
	0	3	4	8
^3H-$PGF_{2\alpha}$	1600 ± 300	1100 ± 400	4700 ± 500	6400 ± 2000
^3H-PGE_2	2500 ± 200	1350 ± 250	3550 ± 850	3400 ± 700

Values are CPM ± S.D.

analysis of $PGF_{2\alpha}$ binding to growing tumor membranes revealed K_d = 2.9 nM and binding capacity = 25 fmole/ mg protein. The same analyses of binding data obtained with regressing membranes showed K_d = 2.2 nM and binding capacity = 38 fmole/mg. Only a very low affinity PGE_2 receptor was detectable in both growing and regressing tumor membranes.

The amounts of PGE_2 and $F_{2\alpha}$ synthesized during the 2 hour incubation rose from 0.13 and 10.5 ng/mg protein in the growing tumors to 1.2 and 26.5 ng/mg protein in the regressing tumors 5 days after ovariectomy, respectively (Table 2).

Table 2

Prostaglandin Synthesis by Growing and Regressing
NMU Mammary Carcinoma Membranes

Indome-thacin	Days following oophorectomy				
	0	1	4	5	7
$PGF_{2\alpha}$ +	1.5 ±.5	2.0 ±.4	7.6 ±.4	15.6 ±1.5	9.0 ±.6
−	12.0 ±1.0	15.6 ±.6	26.0 ±2.0	42.0 ±5.4	29.2 ±4.5
PGE +	0.5 ± .1	0.4 ± .2	.5 ± .2	.4 ± .1	.5 ± .1
−	0.6 ± .1	1.2 ± .2	1.3 ± .2	1.6 ± .2	1.1 ± .5

PG values are expressed as ng /mg protein · 2 hours ± S.D.

DISCUSSION

The data reported herein demonstrate specific binding sites for prostaglandin E_2 and $F_{2\alpha}$ within the NMU mammary carcinoma. While binding of PGE_2 to tumor membranes was of low affinity and, therefore, of uncertain significance, those same membranes possessed a high affinity for $PGF_{2\alpha}$ suggesting a purposeful role in tumor pathophysiology. The suggestion that $PGF_{2\alpha}$ plays an important role in tumor

regression is strengthened by the simultaneous demonstration of both increased numbers of receptors and
PGF$_{2\alpha}$ synthesis after regression has been induced by
ovariectomy.

Other investigators have induced regression in the
hormone-dependent MTW9 tumor by injections of PGF$_{2\alpha}$, a
response thought to be a result of luteolysis since
regression was reversed by the addition of exogenous
progesterone (Jubiz et al, 1979). However, the fact
that progesterone has also been shown to decrease PGF$_{2\alpha}$
binding in the ovary in vitro (Rao, 1976) suggests a more
direct interaction may exist between these hormones, with
progesterone suppressing the ability of PGF$_{2\alpha}$ to alter tumor
growth in vitro. Clearly the contractile effects of PGF$_{2\alpha}$
upon the uterus and fallopian tubes are well known (Kuehl,
1973) as are the opposing effects of progesterone on the
same tissues. Progesterone may, therefore, act as a
permissive hormone, modifying the ability of PGF2α to modulate the growth of the NMU tumor. The evidence
presented thus far suggests that PGF$_{2\alpha}$ plays a significant
role in this hormone-dependent regression process.

Alexander RW, Kent RW, Pisano J, Keiser HR, Cooper T (1975).
  Regulation of post-occlusive hyperemia by endogenously
  synthesized prostaglandins in the dog heart. J Clin
  Invest 55:1174.
Gullino PM, Pettigrew HM, Grantham FH, (1975). N-Nitroso-
  methylurea as mammary gland carcinogen in rats. J Natl
  Cancer Inst 54:401.
Gullino PM, Ziche M. Private Communication.
Hail V, Mello MCF, Horakova Z, Beaver MA. Antiprolifera-
  tion activity of anti-inflammatory drugs in two mammalian
  cell culture lines. J Pharm Extl Therap 202:446.
Jubitz W, Frailey J, Smith JB, (1979). Inhibitory effect of
  prostaglandin F$_{2\alpha}$ on the growth of a hormone-dependent rat
  mammary tumor. Cancer Res 39:998.
Kahn CR, Neville DM, Roth J (1973). J Biol Chem 248:244.
Karmali RA, (1980). Review: Prostaglandins and cancer.
  Prostaglandins and Medicine 5:11.
Karmali RA, Horrobin DF, Menezes J, Patel P. Relationship
  between concentrations of PGA$_1$, E$_1$, E$_2$ and F$_{2\alpha}$ and rates
  of cell proliferation. Pharm Res Comm 11:69.

Kuehl FA Jr, Cirrilo VJ, Ham EA, Humes JL (1973). In Bergstrom S, Berhard S (eds): "Advances in Biosciences, Internat Conf on Prostaglandins," Vol 9, New York, Pergammon, p 155.

Manku MS, Horrobin DF, Karmazyn M, Cunnane SC (1979). Prolactin and zinc effects on rat vascular reactivity: Possible relationship to dihomo-γ-linolenic acid and to prostaglandin synthesis. Endocrinology 104:774.

Powell WS, Hammarstrom S, Samuelsson B (1975) Occurence and properties of a prostaglandin F_{2a} receptor in bovine corpora lutea. European J Biochem 56:73.

Rankin JHG, Jirtle R, Phernetton TM (1977). Anomalous responses of tumor vasculature to norepinepherine and PGE_2 in rabbit. Circ Res 41:496.

Rao Ch V (1975). Steroid hormone modulation of ^{3}H-prostaglandin E, binding to bovine corpus luteum cell membranes. Prostaglandins 9:567.

Rao Ch V (1976). Inhibition of prostaglandin $F_{2\alpha}$ binding to its receptors by progesterone. Steroids 27:831

Rolland PH, Martin PM, Jacquemier J, Rolland AM, Toga M (1980). Prostaglandin in Human Breast Cancer: Evidence suggesting that an elevated prostaglandin production is a marker of high metastatic potential for neoplastic cells. JNCI 64:1061.

Salz JM, Evan D, Gallet D. (1978). Role of cAMP and protein kinase on the steroidogenic action of ACTH, PGE, and dibutryl cAMP in normal adrenal cells and adrenal tumor cells from human. J Cyclic Nucl Res 4:311.

Schafer AI, Cooper B, O'hara D, Handin, RI (1978) Identification of platlet receptors for PGI_2 and PGD_2, J Biol Chem 254:2914.

Tashjian AH Jr (1978). Role of Prostaglandins in the production of hypercalcemia by tumors. Cancer Res 38:4138.

Tashjian AH Jr, Voekel EF, Levine L (1977). Plasma concentrations of 13,14-dihydro -15-keto-prostaglandin E_2 in rabbits bearing the VX_2 carcinoma: Effects of hydrocortisone and indomethacin. Prostaglandins 14: 309.

Thomas DR, Philpott GW, Jaffe BM (1974). The Relationship between concentration of prostaglandin E and rates of cell replication. Exptl Cell Res 84:40.

**Prostaglandins and Cancer: First
International Conference, pages 713-718**
© **1982 Alan R. Liss, Inc., 150 Fifth Avenue, New York, NY 10011**

PROSTAGLANDIN MODULATION OF ADCC IN HUMAN MALIGNANT
MELANOMA.

J. Lee Murray, M.D.
Cancer Research Program
Oklahoma Medical Research Foundation
825 N. E. 13th Street
Oklahoma City, OK   73104

Monocytes and activated macrophages are important in
host defense, as demonstrated by their ability to kill
antibody coated target cells following binding via Fc receptors (antibody dependent cellular cytotoxicity - ADCC)
(Holm 1972). Since monocytes release PGE_2 following
activation (Humes et al 1977), and since preliminary
observations suggest that exogenously added PGE_2 inhibits
interferon induced macrophage tumoricidal activity
(Schultz et al 1978) we examined whether a similar feedback mechanism was responsible for controlling
cytotoxicity toward antibody coated erythrocyte targets.
Our results suggested that in vitro human monocyte but not
lymphocyte ADCC could be augmented by inhibitors of PGE_2
synthesis following in vivo preactivation by
immunostimulant.

RESULTS

Monocyte (MØ) and lymphocyte (L) ADCC in 12
controls, as well as 17 malignant melanoma patients
receiving adjuvant immunotherapy with subcutaneous C.
parvum, were compared. Monocytes and lymphocytes were
separated using adherence techniques (Koller et al 1973)
and tested against anti-D coated human O+ RBC targets as
reported previously (Koller, LoBuglio 1981). Percent
monocyte ADCC was markedly higher in patients than
controls, (25 ± 2 S.D. vs 8 ± 1; p < .0001) whereas percent
lymphocyte ADCC was similar in both groups at E:T ratios of
1:2 (8 ± 2 vs 9 ± 2).

As demonstrated in Table 1, a 20 percent increase in monocyte ADCC occurred in patients with the addition of indomethacin at 10^{-6}M concentration. A similar yet smaller increase was observed following addition of PGE_2 antibody, suggesting that PGE_2 was acting as a feedback inhibitor of further cytotoxicity. There was no significant increase in spontaneous ^{51}CR released with the addition of either indomethacin or PGE_2, suggesting that the increase seen was not due to a direct action of these reagents on the target (data not shown). Monocytes alone are responsible for PGE_2 production since lymphocyte ADCC was not augmented. Moreover, monocyte preactivation precedes augmentation of ADCC by indomethacin in that control non-activated monocytes did not show a similar increase. The addition of PGE_2 at 10^{-6}M neutralized the effect of PGE_2-AB; in fact, a greater suppression from baseline occurred.

TABLE 1

COMPARISON OF MØ AND L-ADCC IN CONTROLS VS PATIENTS WITH THE ADDITION OF INHIBITORS OF PGE_2

	CONTROLS (9)		PATIENT (7)	
	MØ	L	MØ	L
O	3 ± 3	2 ± 1.6	18 ± 8	7 ± 6
+I 10^{-6}M°	3 ± 4	2 ± 2	22 ± 10¶	9 ± 9
O	5 ± 4	2 ± 1	21 ± 7	10 ± 7
+ PGE_2-AB* (1:100)	4 ± 1	2 ± 2	24 ± 8¶	12 ± 13
+PGE_2-AB** +PGE_2(10^{-6}M)	3 ± 1	$1.4 \pm .7$	19 ± 3	11 ± 5

° Percent ADCC with addition of indomethacin (10^{-6}M)
¶ Significant increase in patient MØ ADCC with addition of indomethacin (p = .02; trend with PGE_2-AB at 1:100 dilution:p = .15; paired t analysis)
* Antibody to PGE_2 at 1:100 dilution.
** Addition of PGE_2 (10^{-6}M) neutralized effect of PGE_2-AB

To determine whether the lack of augmentation of monocyte ADCC was masked by a low E:T ratio, the number of effector cells was increased. Figure 1 shows the effect of adding effector cells to the assay at E:T ratios of 5:1.

As previously demonstrated, a significant increase in monocyte ADCC occurred only in patients despite the higher ratio, implying that monocyte preactivation was a critical factor.

A series of experiments was performed whereby peripheral blood mononuclear cells were preincubated with PGE_2-AB prior to separation into monocyte and lymphocyte enriched fractions. (Table 2) Interestingly, slight augmentation of patient monocyte ADCC still occurred, implying that PGE_2 secretion is an early event. The increase was not as great as that seen with continuous presence of inhibitor. Actual inhibition of patient lymphocyte ADCC occurred, suggesting that early PGE_2 secretion by activated monocytes may serve to enhance lymphocyte function. Controls were unaffected. In two experiments the presence of PGE_2-AB throughout the four hour assay did not alter the kinetics of the ADCC reaction (data not shown). These studies suggest that PG_2-AB acts by binding to PGE_2 as it is produced throughout the duration of the assay and does not irreversibly shut off PGE_2 synthesis.

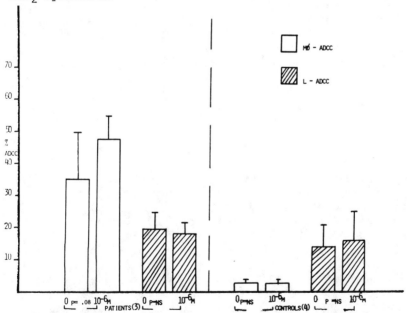

Figure 1: The effect of indomethacin on monocyte (MØ) and lymphocyte (L) ADCC at E:T ratio of 5:1. An increase in ADCC was seen only in the patient monocyte fraction.

TABLE 2
EFFECT OF PREINCUBATING CELLS WITH
ANTI-PGE$_2$ PRIOR TO CYTOTOXICITY

		MØ;1:2°	+Preinc.† PGE$_2$-AB	L;1:2°	+Preinc. PGE$_2$-AB
Controls	(3)	10 ± 3	12 ± 4	19 ± 1	18 ± 10
Patients	(4)	29 ± 4	33 ± 7*	25 ± 8	18 ± 4
		MØ;10:1	+Preinc. PGE$_2$_AB	L;10:1	+Preinc. PGE$_2$-AB
Controls	(3)	N.T.**	N.T.	36 ± 2	23 ± 3
Patients	(3)	N.T.	N.T.	50 ± 18	38 ± 7

° Effector:target ratio = 1:2
† Mononuclear preincubated for 30' with PGE$_2$-AB (1:200
Dil), washed, separated into L and MØ fractions and
used in cytotoxicity assay.
* Slight increase in percent ADCC in patient monocyte
fraction only (p = N.S.)
** N.T. = Not tested

DISCUSSION

The above data suggest that PGE$_2$ acts as a feedback
mechanism to limit monocyte ADCC. The inhibition follows
an early triggering event of monocyte activation which can
be reversed by adding inhibitors such as indomethacin and
PGE$_2$-AB to the assay.
Studies using other in vitro systems have
demonstrated similar results. For example, PGE$_2$ acts to
limit hematopoietic colony stimulating factor (CSF)
production and thereby reduce myeloid colony growth.
(Kurland et al 1977) A similar mechanism is responsible
for limiting T cell proliferation in vitro. (Bockman,
Rothschild 1979)
It appears that PGE$_2$ secretion by macrophages is
initiated by immunoglobulin binding to the Fc receptor.
(Rouzer et al 1980). Droller et al. (1978) studied the
effect of prostaglandin inhibitors on natural as well as
antibody dependent lymphocyte cytotoxicity against tumor
cell lines. Addition of inhibitors increased both natural

and antibody dependent lymphocyte cytotoxicity from 3 to
15%. Preincubation of targets but not effector cells with
inhibitors resulted in augmented activity, suggesting an
inhibitor effect of tumor cell production of PGE_2 rather
than a stimulatory effect on effector cells. Unlike our
study, monocytes and lymphocytes were not tested
separately; hence, it is difficult to determine whether
monocyte ADCC alone was affected.

Macrophages must be stimulated to become cytotoxic
and in the absence of a continuous antigen or endotoxin
stimulus they rapidly lose tumoricidal activity (Hibbs
1975). Taffet and Russell (1981) noted that the loss of
tumoricidal activity by peritoneal macrophages was due to
feedback inhibition by PGE_2 following stimulation by
lipopolysaccharide (LPS). Despite inhibitory
concentrations of PGE_2 after one hour, cytolytic activity
gradually developed, and 12 to 16 hours incubation was
necessary for full inhibition of cytolysis. Hence, PGE_2
did not block the development of activity. Treatment with
indomethacin abrogated PGE_2 synthesis and the shutdown of
cytotoxicity. The following events occurred only in the
continuous presence of activator (LPS).

Our data are quite similar to the above in that higher
augmentation in preactivated macrophages occurred only with
the continuous presence of inhibitor rather than with
preincubation; furthermore, the kinetics of cytotoxicity
were not changed.

Our results may have important clinical implications
in view of studies suggesting a relevant role for ADCC in
vivo. (Haskil, Felt 1976). The data suggest that PGE_2
inhibitors may act synergistically with non-specific
immunostimulants to augment cytotoxicity, and hence may be
useful in a clinical trial setting.

References
Bockman RS, Rothschild M (1979) Prostaglandin E
    inhibition of T lymphocyte colony formation. J. Clin.
    Invest., 64:812-819
Droller MJ, Perlman P, Schneider MV (1978) Enhancement of
    natural and antibody-dependent lymphocyte cytotoxicity by
    drugs which inhibit prostaglandin production by tumor-
    target cells. Cell. Immunol., 39:154-164
Haskill JS, Felt JW (1976) Possible incidence of antibody-
    dependent macrophage-mediated cytotoxicity directed
    against murine adenocarcinoma cells in vivo. J.
    Immunol., 117:1992-1998

Hibbs JB, Jr. (1975). Activated macrophages as cytotoxic
effector cells. II. Requirement for local persistence
of inducing antigens. Transplantation, 19:81-87

Holm G (1972) Lysis of antibody-treated human erythrocytes
by human leukocytes and macrophages in tissue culture.
Int. Arch. Allergy Appl. Immunol., 43:671-682

Humes JL, Bonney RJ, Pelus L, Dahlgren ME, Sadowski SJ,
Kuehl FA, Jr., Davies P (1977). Macrophages synthesize
and release prostaglandins in response to inflammatory
stimuli. Nature (Lond.), 269:149-151

Koller CA, King, GW, Hurtubise PE, Sagone AL,LoBuglio AF
(1973) Charterization of glass adherent mononuclear
cells. J. Immunol, 111:1610-1615

Koller CA, LoBuglio AF (1981) Monocyte mediated antibody
dependent cell-mediated cytotoxicity: The role of the
metabolic burst. Blood, 58:293-299

Kurland JI, Bockman, RS, Broxmeyer HE, Moore MAS (1978)
Limitation of excessive myelopoiesis by the intrinsic
modulation of macrophage-derived prostaglandin E.
Science, 199:552-555

Rouzer CA, Scott WA, Kempe J, Cohn ZA (1980) Prostaglandin
synthesis by macrophages requires a specific receptor-
ligand interaction. Proc. Natl. Acad. Sci, USA,
77:4279-4282

Schultz RM, Pavlidis NA, Stylos WA, Chirigos MA (1978)
Regulation of macrophage tumoricidal function: A role by
prostaglandins of the E series. Science, 202:320-321

Taffet SM, Russell SW (1981) Macrophage-mediated tumor
cell killing: Regulation of expression of cytolytic
activity by prostaglandin E. J. Immunol., 126:424-427

**Prostaglandins and Cancer: First
International Conference, pages 719-723**
© **1982 Alan R. Liss, Inc., 150 Fifth Avenue, New York, NY 10011**

RENAL CELL CARCINOMA & URINARY PROSTAGLANDIN: CASE REPORT

M. Lee Beckman, Francis Deture, P.W. Ramwell

Georgetown University
Departments of Medicine, Division of Nephrology
and Physiology & Biophysics
Washington, D.C. 20007

Renal cell carcinoma (RCC) has been associated with
the production of prolactin, gonadotropins, cortisol, erythropoietin, parathyroid hormone, renin and also arachidonic acid metabolites. (Cronin, 1976). High concentrations
of prostaglandins have been found in both the primary tumor
and distant metastases, but attempts to correlate PG production with plasma PG levels have been inconclusive (Cummings, 1975; Robertson, 1972; Zusman, 1974; Brereton, 1974).
All such studies have included only patients with advanced,
metastatic disease with multiple clinical and chemical abnormalities. This case report provides an important new
perspective on the potential diagnostic and descriptive significance of urinary PGs in a mildly hypertensive man with
only localized non-metastatic RCC and normal plasma $PGF_{2\alpha}$.

CASE REPORT

The patient was a 64 year old white man with newly
diagnosed hypertension of 160/100 mmHg and asymptomatic microscopic hematuria. An intravenous pyelogram (IVP) showed
a 4.5 cm mass in the lower pole of the right kidney, confirmed by renal arteriography. The metastatic workup revealed no evidence of tumor spread; he underwent a right
radical nephrectomy which revealed a 5.2 by 2.4 by 4.1 cm
gray-white encapsulated tumor. This was a well-differentia-
ated, papillary, renal cell carcinoma. He has remained
normotensive since 3 days post-operative; with no evidence
of tumor recurrence after more than 18 months.

METHODS

Blood and urine were studied 48 hours pre-operatively and 18 days post-operatively. He received no drugs known to affect arachidonic acid metabolism. Blood was drawn from the antecubital vein and assayed for blood urea nitrogen, creatinine, sodium, chloride, CO_2, potassium, total protein, albumin, calcium, and phosphorus by a standard SMA-12 autoanalyzer. 24 hour urine collections were fast-frozen for PGE and PGF (iPGE, iPGF) according to a previously described method (Granstrom,1976). All prostaglandin analyses were done in duplicate and the variation between paired samples did not exceed 10%. Statistical significance was determined by the student's "t" test at 95% confidence limits. All samples were analyzed as a group in two separate assays. Interassay variability in our laboratory is less than 10%.

RESULTS

Pre-operative and post-operative blood chemistry were normal (Table 1). The post-operative creatinine clearance fell by 26%; serum electrolytes remained normal. These data were considered normal for the post-nephrectomy patient. The remaining left kidney did not increase appreciably in size as estimated from the post-operative IVP. Plasma $i\text{-}PGF_{2\alpha}$ was normal, both pre- and post-operatively was less than 150 ng/ml, $p<0.05$.

TABLE 1

Status Units	BP mmHg	BUN mg/dl	Creatine mg/dl	Creatinine Clearence ml/min	$i\text{-}PGF_{2\alpha}$ ng/ml
Pre-OP	160/100	24	1.2	90	85*
Post-OP	130/76	18	1.6	69	116*

Table 1 - Results of pre-operative and post-operative blood chemistry and blood pressure (BP).

Figure 1 shows the total daily excretion of i-PGE and i-PGF for the patient and nine normal men (ages 23 to 39). Pre-operatively the patient excreted 787 ng/24h i-PGE and 1142 ng/24h $i\text{-}PGF_{2\alpha}$ both values significantly above normal values $p<0.05$. Post-operatively his daily excretion fell to 329 ng/24h i-PGE and 625 ng/24h i-PGF$_{2\alpha}$, values not significantly different from the normal. The normal mean for i-PGE is 390+55 (SE) ng/24h (range 212 to 560 ng/24h) and the normal for i-PGF$_{2\alpha}$ is 494+66 (SE) (range 229 - 722 ng/24h).

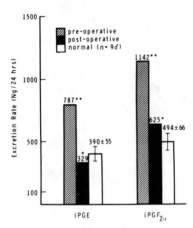

Figure 1. - Total daily excretion of i-PGE and i-PGF$_{2\alpha}$ for the patient and for nine normal men, mean $\pm$ SEM. *Not significant, ** p<0.05.

DISCUSSION

Several studies clearly demonstrate the ability of RCC tumors and their metastases to produce PGs (Cummings, 1975; Robertson, 1976; Zusman, 1974). Such studies involve only patients with advanced metastatic disease and measurable clinical abnormalities, i.e., hypercalcemia. However, a definite relationship between plasma PGs and RCC is not evident and plasma PGs do not reliably reflect the clinical disease state. One notes that blood samples from peripheral venous sites are reflective of tumor PG production only if the amounts released by the tumor are so large as to escape single-passage pulmonary degradation. However, urinary i-PGE and i-PGF$_{2\alpha}$ do reflect intrarenal synthesis and not glomerular filtration of plasma PGs (Frolich, 1975). Therefore, their levels may be elevated with early RCC before excessive tumor PG production allows elevated plasma levels.

Increases in urinary prostaglandins are already associated with different disease entities. Papanicolaou describes an inverse relationship between urinary i-PGE and i-PGF$_{2\alpha}$ and the time course of essential hypertension (Papanicolaou, 1975). Other investigators implicate over-production of i-PGE in the pathogenesis of Bartter's syndrome (Bartter, et al.-1976; Gill, et al.-1976; Flickman, et al.-1976; Verbeckmoes, et al.-1976, Norby, et al.-1976). The latter reports such a patient whose clinical course was accurately reflected in urinary, but not plasma, i-PGE and i-PGF$_{2\alpha}$ values.

Recently, in our laboratory we found that an increase in urine i-TXB$_2$ was associated with kidney allograft rejection. Furthermore an increase in urine i-TXB$_2$ was seen in deep venous thrombosis (Foegh, et al.-1981).

We suggest that urinary PGs may reflect locally confined renal pathology, thus providing an early indication of renal disease, before the plasma levels are elevated. This theory is supported by the statistical significance of our case report where striking elevations of urinary PGs are associated with early RCC and mild hypertension in the face of normal plasma i-PGF$_{2\alpha}$. Similarly, elevated urinary PGs may prove of diagnostic and/or prognostic benefit for other types of localized renal pathology.

Bartter FC, Gill J, Frolich J, Bowden R, Hollenfield J, Keiser H, Oates J, Seyberth H, Taylor A (1976). Prostaglandins are over-produced by the kidney and mediate hyperreninemia in Bartter's Syndrome. Clin Res 24:490A.

Brereton HD, Haluska PV, Alexander RW, Mason DH, Keiser HR, DeVita Jr. VT (1974). Indomethacin responsive hypercalcemia in a patient with renal cell adenocarcinoma. NEJM 291:83.

Cronin RE, Kaeling WD, Miller PD, Stables DP, Gaboro PA, Ostray PR, Schrier RW (1976). Renal cell carcinoma unusual systemic manifestations. Medicine 55:291-311.

Cummings KB, Whels RF, Robertson RP (1975). Prostaglandins: increased production by renal cell carcinoma. Surgical Forum 26:572.

Fickman M, Telfer N, Zia P, Speckart P, Golub M, Rude R (1976). Role of prostaglandins in the pathogenesis of Bartter's Syndrome. Am J Med 60:785.

Foegh M, Winchester JF, Zmudka M, Helfrich GB, Cooley C, Ramwell PW, Schreiner GE. (1981) Urine i-TXB$_2$ in renal allograft rejection. Lancet 2:431

Granstrom E, Kindahl H (1976). Radioimmunoassays for prostaglandin metabolites. Adv. Prost Thromb Res. 1:81.

Frolich JD, Wilson TW, Sweetman BJ, Smigel M, Niess A, Carr K, Watson JT, Oates JA (1975). Urinary prostaglandins: their identification and origin. J Clin Invest 55:763.

Gill JR, Frolich JC, Bowden RE, Taylor EA, Keiser HR, Seyberth HW, Oates JA, Bartter FC (1976). Bartter's syndrome: a disorder characterized by high urinary prostaglandins and a dependence of hyperreninemia on prostaglandin synthesis. Am J Med 61:43.

Norby L, Flammenbaum W, Lentz R and Ramwell PW (1976). Prostaglandins and aspirin therapy in Bartter's syndrome. Lancet 2:604.

Papanicolaou N, Mountokalakis T, Safar M, Bariety J, Milliez P (1976). Deficiency in renomedullary prostaglandin synthesis related to the evaluation of essential hypertension. Experientia 32:1015.

Robertson RP, Baylink DJ, Marini JJ, Adkinson HW (1972). Elevated prostaglandins and suppressed parathyroid hormone associated with hypercalcemia and renal cell carcinoma. J. Clin Endo Met 41:164.

Verkerckmoes R, Van Damme B, Clement J, Amery A, Michielson P (1976). Bartter's syndrome with hyperplasia of renomedullary interstitial cells: Successful treatment with indomethacin. Kidney Int 9:302.

Zusman R, Snider JJ, Cline AC, Caldwell BJ, Speroff L (1974). Antihypertensive function of a renal cell carcinoma. NEJM 290:843.

Supported by the Office of Naval Research and the National Institute of Health.

Prostaglandins and Cancer: First International Conference, pages 725-730
© 1982 Alan R. Liss, Inc., 150 Fifth Avenue, New York, NY 10011

AGE RELATED IMMUNOSUPPRESSION:
PUTATIVE ROLE OF PROSTAGLANDINS

Anna Bartocci*, Franco M. Maggi†,
Roy D. WelkerΔ, and Fulvia Veronese*
*NCI - NIH - Bethesda, MD
†Georgetown Univ. Wash., D.C.
ΔLitton Bionetics, Inc. Kensington, MD

INTRODUCTION

Aging is associated with depressed humoral and cellular immunity in man and experimental animals (Weksler, 1980; Pahwa, 1981; Piguet, 1980; Delfraissy, 1980; Nakano, 1980). The suppression of immunofunctions may contribute to the pathogenesis of diseases that show a peak of incidence late in life, like cancer and autoimmune disorders. Immunosuppression is not always associated with an increased incidence of spontaneous tumors, since immunosurveillance is not the only factor modulating the expression of neoplastic disease. Nevertheless the increasing incidence of cancer and the decline in cell-mediated immunity with age present an interesting association.

Many of the earlier studies on the mechanism of reduction of immunocompetence with age were focused on macrophages (Mφ). The Mφ has a major role in the immune response both as an essential accessory cell and as a regulatory cell that can either enhance or suppress immune reactions. The suppressor activity is manifested mainly by activated Mφ through the release of several mediators including prostaglandins, interferon, thymidine and oxygen-derived radicals (Metzger, 1980). Inhibitory effects of prostaglandins of the E series on the immune response have been described and related to the presence of an adherent prostaglandin producer suppressor cell (Metzger, 1980; Goodwin, 1977 and 1979; Droller, 1987; Grimm, 1978).

In this study, we investigated the relationship between Mφ and prostaglandins (PGs) in the aging related immune suppression. We present evidence of an increased prosta-

glandins production by Mφ with aging and an inhibition of
tumor growth after multiple aspirin treatments in tumor-
bearing old mice.

MATERIALS AND METHODS

Peritoneal and Spleen Cell Preparations
Peritoneal exudate cells (PEC) were collected from
old or young mice by i.p. injection of 10 ml complete RPMI
1640 medium. The number of viable cells was determined and
differential counts were made on Giemsa stained preparation.
Peritoneal Mφ cultures were prepared and purified by adherence (Schultz, 1977). Supernatants were obtained after
24 hours of incubation and assayed for prostaglandins.
Animals were sacrificed and the spleen aseptically
removed and mashed. Single cell suspensions were divided
in two parts and incubated in 6 well Costar Plates. After
two hours of incubation at 37°C in CO_2, non-adherent spleen
cells were removed by repeated washing.

Radioimmunoassay (RIA) of PGE_2 and 6 KETO $PGF_{1\alpha}$
The RIA was performed as originally designed by Granstrom (1976) and modified in our laboratory (Pomerantz,
1980). The PGE_2 antibody was purchased from Steranti.
The 6 KETO $PGF_{1\alpha}$ antibody was provided by Dr. P.W. Ramwell,
^{3}H-labelled PGE_2^α and 6 KETO $PGF_{1\alpha}$ were purchased from New
England Nuclear, and the unlabelled products were a gift
of Dr. E. Pike (Upjohn, Kalamazoo, MI). Statistical analysis of the results were performed using the Students t-test
for unpaired data.

Tumor Cell Line
WM-7 were derived from spontaneous fibrosarcoma of
old, untreated BALB/c Cr mice. A standard strain of Rauscher
Murine Leukemia Virus (R-MuLV) propagated in vivo was used to
infect WM-7 tumor cell line. These cells were then designated R-WM-7. Infection center assays (Rowe, 1970) indicated
that 95 to 100% of R-WM-7 cells were shedding the virus.

RESULTS

Adherent cells from old mice release more PGE_2 and
Prostacyclin (PGI_2) than the young matched controls.
Table 1 shows the prostaglandin release by peritoneal
macrophages from old (18-24 months) and young (8 weeks)
male BALB/c mice. Supernatants of 24 hour cultured cells
from old animals contain significantly higher amounts of
both PGE_2 and 6 keto $PGF_{1\alpha}$ (breakdown product of prostacyclin) with a peak of PG release in the "18-months old" group.

A similar age-dependent pattern was observed in female animals. Results of RIA measurements of PGE_2 and 6 keto PGF_1 in supernatant of macrophages from 8 weeks and 17 months old female BALB/c mice are summarized in Table 1.

TABLE 1

RELEASE OF 6 KETO $PGF_1\alpha$ and PGE_2 BY PERITONEAL Mɸ FROM FEMALE (♀) AND MALE (♂) BALB/c CR MICE

AGE	SEX	6 KETO $PGF_1\alpha$	PGE_2
7 weeks	♀	1.605 ± 0.251	0.673 ± 0.067
7 weeks	♂	1.309 ± 0.407	0.520 ± 0.076
17-18 months	♀	2.855 ± 0.282*	1.472 ± 0.129**
17-18 months	♂	4.911 ± 1.403*	2.079 ± 0.570*
24 months	♂	3.661 ± 0.393***	1.407 ± 0.278**

The levels are expressed as ng per 10^6 cells ± S.E.
*p<0.05   **p<0.02   ***p<0.005

Associated with the increased prostaglandin synthetase activity, an absolute higher number of peritoneal macrophages was observed in old animals. Differential counts of PEC (peritoneal exudate cells) are shown in Figure 1. The higher number of peritoneal macrophages correlates with an increased total count of PEC.

The PG synthetase activity was also tested in splenic adherent cells. The levels of PGE_2 and 6 keto $PGF_1\alpha$ in supernatant of 24-hour cultured cells are summarized in Table 2. Results are expressed as release of prostaglan-

TABLE 2

RELEASE OF $PGF_1\alpha$ and PGE_2 BY SPLENIC ADHERENT CELLS FROM ♂ BALB/c Cr MICE

AGE	SEX	6 KETO $PGF_1\alpha$	PGE_2
7 weeks	♂	0.790 ± 0.05	0.810 ± 0.1
24 months	♂	2.347 ± 0.471*	3.550 ± 0.320**

The levels are expressed as ng per incubation well ± S.E.   *p<0.02   **p<0.001

dins per spleen. Adherent splenic cells from 18-months-old animals release twice as much PGE_2 and prostacyclin when compared to cells from young animals.

In order to investigate the possible role of PG release in tumor growth in aging mice, different cell doses of R-WM7 were inoculated in groups of young and old BALB/c mice (Table 3). The tumor is a syngeneic fibrosarcoma chronically infected with R-MuLV. The increased immunogenicity

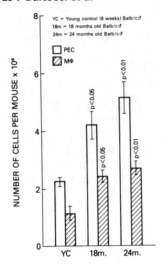

has been shown to result in the regression of the tumor in young but not in old mice (Al Ghazzouli). Multiple treatments of old mice with Aspirin (10 µg/mouse) not only increased the survival time (from 43 to 56 days) but led in a few animals to the regression of the tumor (Table 3).

FIGURE 1

TABLE 3
TUMOR INCIDENCE IN MICE CHALLENGED WITH:[a]

Cells Dose	R-WM-7 Cells[b] 8 Weeks	R-WM-7 Cells 18-24 Months	MST[d]	R-WM-7 Cells + Aspirin[c] 18-24 Months	MST
10^7	0/10	10/10	43	8/10	57
10^6	0/10	8/10	--	NT	--
10^5	0/10	5/10	--	NT	--
10^4	0/10	2/10	--	NT	--

[a] Mice were inoculated s.c.
[b] WM-7 = Spontaneous Fibrosarcoma of Balb/C Cr Mice.
R-WM-7 = WM-7 Infected with Rauscher-Murine Leukemia Virus (R-MuLV)
[c] Aspirin = 10µg/Mouse
[d] Median Survival Time

DISCUSSION

Our findings support the hypothesis that prostaglandins production by macrophages may constitute a mechanism of immunosuppression in vivo. A number of subsequent studies demonstrated suppression of lymphoproliferative response by MΦ from mice, rats, and humans (Oehler, 1978; Herberman, 1980 and 1981) via their production of PGEs. The inhibitory effect of PGEs seems to be mediated by a direct effect on lymphocytes increasing intracellular cyclic AMP (C-AMP) (Droller, 1978).

The results show different patterns of prostaglandin production by peritoneal Mϕ and splenic adherent cells. Peritoneal Mϕ from old mice release considerable amounts of prostacyclin (PGI$_2$), and show a potent suppressor activity on the lymphoproliferative response in mice (data in progress).

However, splenic adherent cells from these old mice release equivalent or higher amounts of PGE$_2$ but less PGI$_2$, and show less suppressor activity. Since PGI$_2$ is reported to be a potent stimulator of C-AMP formation (Best, 1977; Tateson, 1977), we can speculate a contribution of both PGE$_2$ and PGI$_1$ in the macrophage mediated immunosuppression.

Further investigation will be necessary to obtained direct evidence of the relative importance of these two compounds and their interaction in macrophage mediated suppression in aging.

REFERENCES

Al-Ghazzouli, J.K., Donahoe, R.M., Huang, K.Y., Sass, B., Peters, R.L. and Keloff, G.J.: J. of Immunol., 117:2239, 1976.

Best, L.C., Martin, T.J., Russell, R.G. and Preston, F.E.: Nature, 267:859, 1977.

Delfraissy, J.F., Galanaud, G., Dormont, J. and Wallon, C.: Clin. Exp. Immunol. 39:208, 1980.

Droller, H.J., Schneider, M. and Perlmann, P.: Cell Immunol., 39:165, 1978.

Goodwin, J.S., Bankhurst, A.D. and Messner, R.P.: J. Exp. Med. 146:1719, 1977.

Goodwin, J.S. and Messner, R.P.: J. Clin. Invest., 64:434, 1979.

Granstrom, E. and Kindahl, H.: Prost. Thromb. Res., I:81, 1976.

Grimm, W., Seitz, M., Kirchner, H. and Gemsa, D.: Cell Immunol. 40:419, 1978.

Herberman, R.B., Holden, H.T., Djeu, J.Y., Jerrells, T.R., Varesio, L., Tagliabue, A., White, S.O., Oehler, J.R. and Dean, J.H. In Macrophage and Lymphocytes, Part B. M.R. Escober and H. Friedman (Eds.), Plenum Publishing Corporation, New York, 1980.

Herberman, R.B. In Human Suppressor Cell. B. Serrou (Ed), North Holland Publishing Co., Amsterdam, 1981.

Metzger, Z., Hoffeld, J.T. and Oppenheim, J.J.: J. of Immunol. 124:983, 1980.

Nakano, K. and Cinader, B.: Eur. J. Immunol.: 10:309, 1980.
Oehler, J.R., Herberman, R.B. and Holden, H.T.: Pharm. Ther.
A, 2:551, 1978.
Pahwa, S.G., Pahwa, R.N. and Good, R.A.: J. Clin. Invest.,
67:1094, 1981.
Piguet, P.F.: Scand. J. Immunol., 12:233, 1980.
Pomerantz, K., Maddox, Y., Maggi, F., Ramey, E. and Ramwell,
P.: Life Sciences, 27:1233, 1980.
Rowe, W.P., Pugh, W.E., and Hartley, J.W.: Virology,
42:1136, 1970.
Schultz, R.M., Papamatheakis, J.D., Luetzeler, J., Ruiz, P.
and Chirigos, M.A.: Cancer Res. 37:358, 1977.
Tateson, J.E., Moncada, S. and Vane J.R.: Prostaglandins,
13:389, 1977.
Weksler, M.E.: Proc. Soc. Exp. Biol. Med., 165:200, 1980.

PHARMACOLOGICAL MANIPULATION OF PROSTAGLANDIN SYNTHESIS ON TUMOR GROWTH AND METASTASES IN VIVO

**Prostaglandins and Cancer: First
International Conference, pages 733-752
© 1982 Alan R. Liss, Inc., 150 Fifth Avenue, New York, NY 10011**

PROSTACYCLIN/THROMBOXANE RATIOS IN TUMOR GROWTH AND
METASTASIS

Kenneth V. Honn
Departments of Radiation Oncology, Radiology
and Biological Sciences
Wayne State University, Detroit, MI 48202

INTRODUCTION

The ability of a primary neoplasm to metastasize
represents one of the major obstacles in the search for a
cure for human cancers. A metastatic lesion represents the
result of an intricate series of sequential events in which
malignant cells, released from a primary tumor, disseminate
to distant sites. A complex array of factors may influence
the metastatic potential of a tumor, e.g., the growth
potential of the tumor, the degree of vascularization,
host/tumor immunologic interactions, etc. These are
discussed in several excellent reviews of the metastatic
process (Weiss, 1977; Sugarbaker and Ketcham, 1977; Roos
and Dingmans, 1979; Clark, 1979; Donati et al., 1981). One
aspect of this process which has received considerable
attention is the interaction of the metastasizing tumor
cells with the hemostatic system of the host (Donati et
al., 1981). The association of circulating tumor cells
with host platelets has been reported by numerous
investigators and the ability of a wide spectrum of tumor
cell types to aggregate platelets in vitro has been
reported (Gasic et al., 1973, 1976). Morphological
evidence for a close association of hematogenously
disseminating cancer cells with thrombotic material had
suggested that anticoagulant therapy could be useful in
preventing or reducing the secondary spread of tumor cells.
Numerous anticoagulants such as heparin (Elias et al.,
1973), warfarin (Lione and Bosman, 1978), aspirin (Gasic et
al., 1973), indomethacin (Giraldi et al., 1980), and dipyri-
damole (Gastpar, 1977) have been investigated as possible

antimetastatic agents with both positive and negative results. The role of arachidonic acid (20:4) metabolites, notably thromboxane A_2 (TXA_2) and prostacyclin (PGI_2), (Figure 1) in the modulation of platelet aggregation has been firmly established (Moncada and Vane, 1979). TXA_2 produced by platelets is a potent large vessel vasoconstrictor and induces platelet aggregation, whereas PGI_2 is a strong vasodilator and the most potent inhibitor of platelet aggregation known (Moncada and Vane, 1979). Each substance has an opposing action on platelet aggregability resulting in a balanced control mechanism (Moncada and Vane, 1979). An imbalance between PGI_2 formation and TXA_2 formation could be a dramatic consequence. The platelet anti-aggregation effects of non-steroidal antiinflammatory agents (NSAIA), such as aspirin or indomethacin, are mediated via differential inhibition of platelet and vascular wall cyclooxygenase, the former being more sensitive to inhibition (Baenziger et al., 1977). If the association of the metastasizing tumor cell with platelets is of critical importance, then manipulation of PGI_2/TXA_2 ratios may alter the metastatic cascade.

Thromboxane A_2 and PGI_2 exert antagonistic effects on platelet aggregation mediated by opposing effects on platelet cyclic AMP (cAMP). TXA_2 prevents a rise in platelet cAMP levels in response to an external stimulus (Marcus, 1978) whereas PGI_2 inhibits aggregation by increasing platelet cAMP levels (Gorman et al., 1977). The rapid synthesis and short half-lives of PGI_2 and TXA_2 these compounds make them ideal bioregulators (Hamberg et al., 1975; Salmon et al., 1978).

Cyclic AMP, a nucleotide present in a wide variety of organisms ranging from bacteria to man, is considered to be a major regulator of numerous cellular activities (Sutherland, 1972). It has been shown that cAMP, either endogenously generated or exogenously supplied, inhibits proliferation both in vivo and in vitro of normal as well as transformed cells. In many cases there is an inverse relationship between the amount of intracellular cAMP and the rate of cell growth (Heidrick and Ryan, 1971). Recent evidence indicates that TXA_2 and PGI_2 are produced by a wide variety of tissues (Gorman et al., 1979; Ali et al., 1980; Sun et al., 1977). Consideration of their opposing effects on cAMP production suggest their possible role in normal and/or abnormal cellular proliferation.

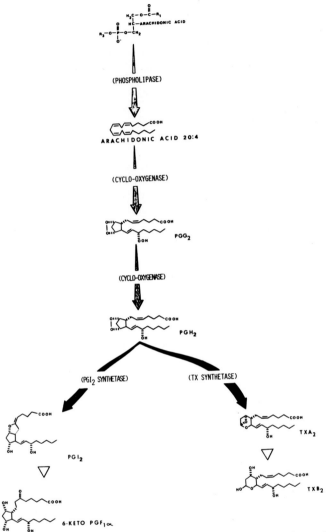

Figure 1. Biosynthesis of prostacyclin (PGI$_2$) and thromboxane A$_2$ (TXA$_2$) by the oxidative cyclization of the polyunsaturated fatty acid (20:4). The endoperoxide intermediate PGH$_2$, serves as a pivotal point in the biosynthesis of prostaglandins and related compounds. PGH$_2$ can serve as substrate for prostacyclin synthetase and thromboxane (TX) synthetase. PGI$_2$ and TXA$_2$ can be nonenzymatically converted to their stable metabolites 6-keto-PGF$_1\alpha$ and TXB$_2$, respectively.

HYPOTHESES

We propose the hypothesis that the primary tumor, tumor cell shed vesicles and/or circulating tumor cells disrupt the balance between PGI_2 and TXA_2 in favor of platelet aggregation. If this hypothesis is correct then the following criteria should be substantiated by experimental fact: 1) the exogenous adminstration of PGI_2 should reduce lung colony formation by tail vein injected tumor cells, 2) a therapeutic synergism should result from the use of PGI_2 with a phosphodiesterase inhibitor, [since the effect of PGI_2 is mediated by increasing concentrations of adenosine $3',5'$-monophosphate (cAMP) in platelets it follows that phosphodiesterase inhibitors by slowing the breakdown of cAMP should potentiate the antithrombogenic action of PGI_2 and thus the anti-metastatic effect.], 3) an inhibitor of endogenous PGI_2 synthesis should enhance metastasis, 4) thromboxane synthetase inhibitors should also function as antimetastatic agents, and 5) agents that augment in vivo PGI_2 synthesis or activity should function as anti-metastatic agents.

Consideration of the mechanism of action of PGI_2 and TXA_2 in the regulation of platelet cAMP levels has led us to propose the following additional hypothesis. Prostacyclin increases cAMP levels in the platelet while TXA_2 prevents a rise in cAMP levels in response to external stimuli (Gorman et al., 1977). Considering that increased cAMP levels are believed to inhibit cell division (Kreider et al., 1975; Friedmann et al., 1976), we therefore propose that thromboxane synthetase inhibitors, PGI_2 and agents which may increase PGI_2 production could have an effect on inhibition of tumor growth. If this hypothesis is correct, then the following criteria should be substantiated by experimental fact: 1) thromboxane synthetase inhibitors should decrease tumor cell replication, 2) thromboxane A_2 or its stable metabolite thromboxane B_2 should enhance tumor cell proliferation, 3) the TXA_2 mimicking agent (Smith, 1980) (15S)-Hydroxy-$11\alpha,9\alpha$-(epoxymethano) prosta-5Z,13E-dienoic acid, should enhance tumor cell proliferation, 4) exogenous PGI_2 should decrease tumor cell proliferation, and 5) agents that stimulate PGI_2 production should decrease tumor cell proliferation.

Role of Prostacyclin in the prevention of metastasis

Prostacyclin and its major degradatory product, 6 keto-PGF$_1$ were tested for their effect on lung colony formation by B16 amelanotic melanoma (B16a) cells. Experimental methods for tumor cell isolation and injection were as described previously (Honn et al., 1981; Sloane et al., 1981).

Prostacyclin produces a dose related decrease in experimental metastasis of the B16a melanoma (Table 1). A significant decrease was observed with as little as 25 μg/animal. At the highest dose tested (200 μg) lung metastatic colonies were reduced to 14% of controls. Metastasis to the liver and spleen were also reduced with PGI$_2$ suggesting that the decrease in lung metastasis does not merely reflect a redistribution of tumor cells (Table 1). The byproduct of PGI$_2$ hydrolysis, 6-keto PGF$_1$α was ineffective at a dose of 50 μg/animal; however, at 200 μg/animal a slight reduction in lung metastasis was noted, probably due to the pulmonary vasodilator effect of this compound (Hyman and Kadowitz, 1979). However, it should be noted that although PGI$_2$ is a potent pulmonary vasodilator, such vasodilation is not principally responsible for the antimetastatic effects which have been observed. Honn et al. (1981) have demonstrated that prostaglandin E$_2$ (PGE$_2$), which is an approximately equipotent vasodilator but does not inhibit platelet aggregation, was ineffective in reducing B16a melanoma tumor cell metastasis. Theophylline, a platelet phosphodiesterase inhibitor (Moncada and Vane, 1979), at 100 μg/animal produced a slight but insignificant decrease in pulmonary metastasis. However, the combination of theophylline plus PGI$_2$ (100 μg/animal) resulted in a four fold reduction in pulmonary metastasis over PGI$_2$ alone at the same dose (Table 1).

Heparin and warfarin anticoagulation have been demonstrated to decrease the incidence of metastasis from small numbers ($<10^5$) of i.v. injected tumor cells. However, metastasis from large numbers ($>10^6$) of injected tumor cells was not prevented (Gralnick, 1981).

In order to assess the effect of a single PGI$_2$ injection on a large circulating tumor burden, mice were pretreated with theophylline (100 μg, i.p.) + PGI$_2$ (150 μg, i.v.) before the injection of 3 x 10^6 B16a melanoma cells. A tumor burden of 3 x 10^6 cells resulted in > 500 tumor colonies in the control, while theophylline + PGI$_2$ treated mice exhibited 37±10 colonies (Fig. 2).

If PGI$_2$ is efficacious in preventing metastatic tumor colony formation, then an inhibitor of endogenous PGI$_2$ synthesis should enhance metastasis. To test this hypothesis we synthesized 15-hydroperoxy arachidonic acid 15-(HPETE) from arachidonic acid utilizing soybean lipoxygenase. Hydroperoxy fatty acids are in general very potent and specific inhibitors of prostacyclin synthetase (Salmon et al., 1978; Siegel et al., 1979).

Compared to controls, 100 μg of 15-HPETE increased lung tumor colony formation almost 200% (Table 2). A dose of 200 μg nearly quadrupled that number (Table 2). Liver metastasis increased 667% and 944% with 100 μg and 200 μg of 15-HPETE respectively (Table 2). There was also an increase in metastasis to the spleen (Table 2). In order to ascertain if exogenous PGI$_2$ could reverse the effects of 15-HPETE, animals were injected with 100 μg 15-HPETE followed by an i.p. injection of 100 μg theophylline. Thirty minutes later 100 μg PGI$_2$ was administered. The results in Table 2 indicate that PGI$_2$ significantly reversed the effect of 15-HPETE in lung, liver and spleen, reducing metastatic colony formation to below control levels.

Collectively these results indicate that a vital role may be played by in vivo PGI$_2$ synthesis in preventing the spread of metastatic disease. Furthermore, exogenous PGI$_2$ may be efficacious as an adjuvant chemotherapeutic agent to reduce the total tumor burden prior to and immediately following therapies aimed at the the removal or destruction (surgery/radiotherapy) of the primary neoplasm.

Thromboxane Synthetase Inhibitors and Metastasis

We have presented data in the preceeding section to indicate that PGI$_2$ may function as a potent antimetastatic agent. According to the hypothesis which we presented earlier, it follows that TX synthetase inhibitors should

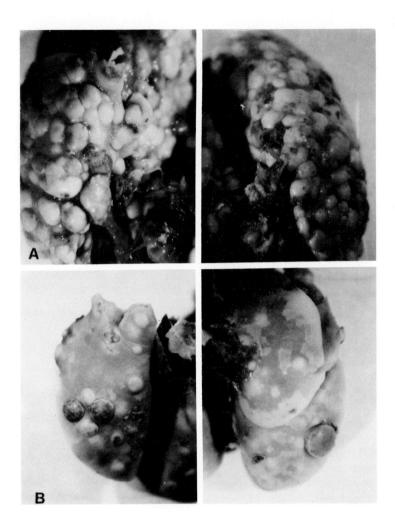

Figure 2. Inhibition of lung colony formation from tail vein injected B16a cells (3 x 10^6) by PGI_2 pretreatment. A. Representative lungs from untreated controls. B. Representative lungs from animals pretreated with PGI_2 prior to tumor cell injection.

Table 1: Effects of PGI_2 on pulmonary and extrapulmonary metastasis following injection of 3×10^5 viable B16a melanoma cells

Treatment	Lungs	Liver	Kidney	Spleen	Brain
MEM control	144 ± 18^a	13 ± 5	0	1 ± 0.5	0
TRIS control	130 ± 9	8 ± 3	0	3 ± 1	0
PGI_2 25 µg	95 ± 10	2 ± 0.5	0	0	0
PGI_2 50 µg	77 ± 5	0	0	0	0
PGI_2 100 µg	43 ± 13	0	0	0	0
PGI_2 200 µg	15 ± 7	0	0	0	0
6-keto $PGF_1\alpha$ 50 µg	138 ± 15	0	0	0	0
6-keto $PGF_1\alpha$ 200 µg	100 ± 14	3 ± 1	0	0	0
Theophylline 100 µg+PGI_2 100 µg	10 ± 5	0	0	0	0
Theophylline 100 µg	119 ± 8	7 ± 3	0	0	0

[a] Mean ± SEM; n = 7

also function as antimetastatic agents. We have screened three compounds which are endoperoxide analogues. These compounds and their actions are as follows: 1) 9,11-diazo-prosta-5,13-dienoic acid (U51605), a TX synthetase and PGI_2 synthetase inhibitor (Fitzpatrick and Gorman, 1978); 2) 9,11-iminoepoxy-prosta-5,13-dienoic acid (U54701), an inhibitor of TX synthetase and stimulator of PGI_2 synthetase (Fitzpatrick et al., 1979); 3) 9,11-epoxy-imino-prosta5,13-dienoic acid (U54874), a TXA_2 receptor antagonist (Fitzpatrick et al., 1978). It is evident from the data present in Table # that all of these compounds significantly reduced pulmonary metastasis from tail vein injected B16a melanoma cells.

Table 2. Effect of 15-hydroperoxyarachidonic acid (15-HPETE) and PGI$_2$ on pulmonary and extrapulmonary metastasis following injection of 3 x 10^5 viable B16a melanoma cells[a].

Treatment	Lung	Liver	Kidney	Spleen	Brain
MEM control	144±18[c]	13± 5	0	1±0.5	0
TRIS control	130± 9	8± 3	0	3±1	0
Ethanol control	127±14	9± 5	0	0	0
15-HPETE 100 µg[b]	380±40	60±21	0	17±6	0
15-HPETE 200 µg	500	85±33	0	22±8	0
15-HPETE 100 µg + theophylline 100µg + PGI$_2$ 100 µg	39±16	3±2	0	0	0

[a] 25 µl i.v. (tail vein)
[b] Injected in 25 µl ethanol i.v. (tail vein)
[c] Mean ± SEM; n = 7

However, the most effective drug tested was 9,11-iminoepoxy-prosta-5,13-dienoic acid, the agent which is reported to inhibit TX synthetase and stimulate PGI$_2$ synthetase. At an injected dose of 200 µg this compound reduced tumor colony formation from 102±26 in the controls to 6±1.3 in the treated group.

Considering the complexity of events leading to the eventual establishment and growth of a secondary metastatic lesion, there is little doubt that experimental metastasis via tail vein injection of dissociated tumor cells is an artificial and partial model. Nevertheless, it has its usefulness when standardization of experimental conditions is critical. However, in order to assess the effects of TX synthetase inhibitors on spontaneous metastasis, animals bearing subcutaneous B16a melanoma and Lewis lung carcinoma tumors were treated with the TX synthetase inhibitor 1-(7-carboxyheptyl) imidazole (Yoshimoto et al., 1978). Treatment (2mg/animal/day/i.p.) began with the appearance of a palpable tumor. The data in Table 4 clearly indicates the antimetastatic effects of this TX synthetase inhibitor in the complete metastasis model. Spontaneous metastasis was inhibited 60% for the B16a tumor and 66% for the 3LL tumor.

Table 3. Effect of thromboxane synthetase inhibitors and receptor antagonist on pulmonary metastasis from subcutaneous B16a melanoma cells.

Treatment	Tumor Colonies
Control[a]	$\underline{102 \pm 26}$[b]
U51605	
100 μg	75 ± 23
200 μg	56 ± 13
U54701	
100 μg	21 ± 7
200 μg	6 ± 1.3
U54874	
100 μg	47 ± 17
200 μg	35 ± 9

[a]3×10^5 B16a cells injected in 50 μl.
[b]Number of metastatic colonies on lung surface (bilateral), mean ± SEM; n = 10

Table 4. Effect of 1-(7-carboxyheptyl) imidazole on pulmonary metastasis from subcutaneous B16a melanoma and Lewis lung carcinoma tumors

	Control	1-(7-carboxyheptyl)imidazole
B16a melanoma	48 ± 10[a]	19 ± 9
Lewis lung carcinoma	89 ± 17	30 ± 11

[a]No. of metastatic colonies on lung surface (bilateral), mean ± SEM; n = 12.

Nafazatrom (Bay g 6575) a New, Potent Antimetastatic Agent.

Nafazatrom (Fig. 3) has been reported to possess significant antithrombotic activity in model systems of experimental thrombosis (Seuter et al., 1979). Thrombus formation in the femoral arteries of rabbits was inhibited at a minimal effective dose of 1 mg/kg p.o. Nafazatrom also possesses significant thrombolytic properties similar to urokinase (Seuter et al., 1979). The mechanism of action for these antithrombotic effects appears related to the ability of the drug to stimulate PGI_2 production by the vascular wall (Vermylen et al., 1979). Nafazatrom significantly increased bioassayable PGI_2 release from aortic rings obtained from normal and diabetic rats (Carreras et al., 1980). In addition, plasma, obtained from human volunteers after ingestion of a single dose (1.2g) of Nafazatrom, stimulated PGI_2 release from slices of rat aorta (Vermylen et al., 1979). The reported action of this new drug on PGI_2 production and its low toxicity in vivo (Seuter et al., 1979; Vermylen et al., 1979) suggested its possible use as an antimetastatic agent.

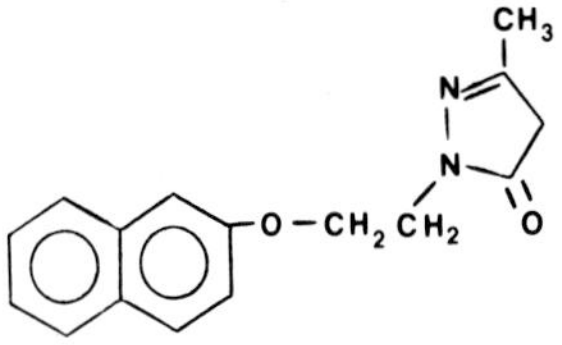

1-[2-(β-napthyloxy)ethyl]-
3-methyl-2-pyrazolin-5-one
(Bay g 6575, Bayer Pharm-
aceutical)

Figure 3. Chemical structure of Nafazatrom (BAY g 6575).

Mice were pretreated (3 days) with 0.02 and 0.08 mg (s.c.) Nafazatrom prior to tail vein injection of 5×10^4 B16a melanoma cells. Both doses produced significant reduction (90% and 99% respectively) in lung tumor colony formation (Table 5). Representative lungs from control and 0.08 mg Nafazatrom treated animals are shown in Fig. 4. This compound was also effective when injected 1 hr prior to tumor cell injection, an effect which was potentiated by theophylline (Table 5). Theophylline alone (200 μg i.p.) was ineffective.

Table 5. Effect of Nafazatrom on metastasis from tail vein injected B16a melanoma cells[a]

Treatment	Lung Tumor Colonies
Control	181 ± 45[b]
0.02 mg Nafazatrom[c]	19.3 ± 7.5
0.08 mg Nafazatrom[c]	2.7 ± 1.3
Theophylline 200 µg[d]	165 ± 38
Theophylline 200 µg + 0.08 mg Nafazatrom[d]	33.6 ± 18
0.08 mg Nafazatrom[d]	65 ± 36

a. 5 x 10[4] cells injected intravenously in 50 µl.
b. x̄ ± SEM; n = 6.
c. Animals pretreated daily (3 days) before tumor cell injection.
d. Injected 1 hour prior to tumor cells.

Nafazatrom was also evaluated in spontaneous metastasis models. Mice bearing subcutaneous B16a melanoma and Lewis lung carcinoma tumors were injected (s.c.) daily with 0.01 to 0.08 mg Nafazatrom. All doses tested significantly reduced spontaneous metastasis to the lungs of tumor bearing mice (Table 6). In addition, the number of mice positive for metastasis was also reduced from 12/12 in the controls to 5/12 in B16a and 2/12 in Lewis lung with 0.08 mg of Nafazatrom (Table 6). Collectively, these results point to significant antimetastatic properties of Nafazatrom, an effect which may be mediated by the ability of this drug to stimulate endogenous PGI_2 production.

Table 6. Effect of Nafazatrom on spontaneous metastasis from subcutaneous B16a melanoma[a] and Lewis lung carcinoma[b] tumors.

Treatment	B16a	3LL
Control	14.1 ± 3.1[c] (12/12)[d]	34.5 ± 6.4[c] (12/12)[d]
Nafazatrom[e]		
0.01 mg	1.7 ± 0.7 (7/12)	--
0.02 mg	2.5 ± 0.9 (7/12)	--
0.04 mg	3.1 ± 0.8 (8/12)	--
0.08 mg	1.4 ± 0.8 (5/12)	2 ± 0.5 (2/12)

a. 1.8 x 10[5] cells injected subcutaneously.
b. 1 x 10[5] cells injected subcutaneously.
c. No. of metastatic tumor colonies on bilateral lung surface; X̄ ± SEM; n = 12.
d. No. of animals positive for metastasis
e. Injected daily subcutaneously in 0.2 ml.

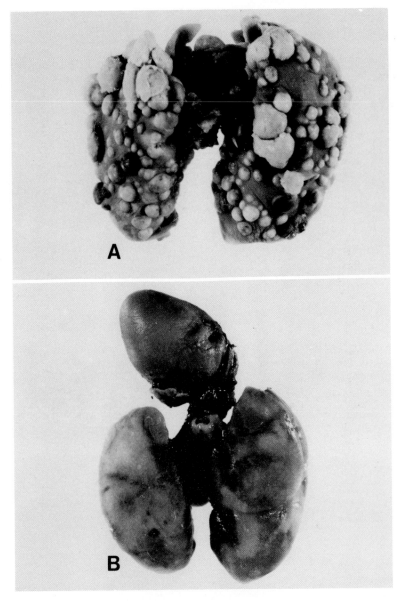

Figure 4. Inhibition of lung colony formation from tail vein injected B16a cells by pretreatment (0.08 mg x 3 days, s.c.) with Nafazatrom. A. Representative lungs from untreated control animal. B. Representative lungs from animals receiving Nafazatrom pretreatment.

Thromboxane A_2 and Prostacyclin Control of Tumor Cell Growth.

Considering the bidirectional control of platelet cAMP levels by TXA_2 and PGI_2, we proposed the hypothesis that these compounds may play a role in tumor cell proliferation. To test this hypothesis we examined the effects of the endoperoxide analogues (U51605, U54701, U54874) on DNA synthesis by B16a (Honn et al., in press) and 3LL cells in vitro. All three compounds significantly reduced DNA synthesis by these tumor cells at non-cytotoxic doses (Table 7). U54701 was slightly more efficacious than U51605 or U54874 in 3LL cells (Table 7). Similar inhibition of DNA synthesis by B16a and 3LL cells has been obtained with two additional, structurally unrelated, TX synthetase inhibitors (data not shown) indicating that such inhibition was not peculiar to the endoperoxide structure.

Cultured B16a cells exposed to U51605 and U54701 (5-25 μg/ml) for 7 days demonstrated a dose dependent inhibition of proliferation. At 25 μg/ml inhibition of proliferation by U51605 and U54701 was 85% and 70% respectively.

Table 7. Inhibition of DNA synthesis in Lewis lung carcinoma cells with thromboxane synthetase inhibitors and a thromboxane A_2 receptor antagonist.

Test Compound	Dose (μg/ml)	3LL 4 hr	3LL 18 hr
U51605	1	88.8±7.4	77.3±11.8
	10	35.5±2.9	44.3± 2.3
	25	18.6±1.9	30.2± 2.4
U54701	1	88.0±7.4	58.9± 3.4
	10	53.9±1.7	44.7± 8.1
	25	28.8±2.1	36.1± 3.7
U54874	1	107.2±1.8	84.8±22.4
	10	66.8±1.3	75.8± 6.2
	25	38.5±1.6	33.0± 1.5

[a] % control ± SEM

The above results would suggest that endogenous TXA_2 production by the tumor cells is a necessary positive signal for proliferation. The mechanism of action of thromboxanes in the stimulation of tumor cell proliferation is unknown. However, we have observed that B16a melanoma cells pretreated (48 hrs) with TXB_2 (20 μg/ml) and subsequently challenged with PGE_1 (1 μg/ml) have diminished release (87% decrease) of cAMP into the media when compared to PGE_1 stimulated control cultures (Honn et al., in press). Whether this reflects decreased cyclic nucleotide synthesis or increased catabolism is unknown at present. However, if the mechanism of action of these compounds centers around the downward modulation of cAMP levels, agents such as PGI_2, known to increase cAMP levels, should inhibit proliferation. Treatment of B16a melanoma cells in culture for 7 days with PGI_2 produced a dose dependent decrease in cell proliferation with a 50% inhibition at 10 μg/ml. Collectively these results suggest the possibility of bidirectional control of tumor cell proliferation by the balance between endogenous and/or exogenous PGI_2/TXA_2.

As stated earlier, the antithrombogenic and antimetastatic effects of Nafazatrom are believed to be mediated in part by an increase in PGI_2 levels. Considering the effects of exogenous PGI_2 on tumor cell replication we examined the effects of Nafazatrom on DNA synthesis by B16a cells in culture. Exposure of B16a cells to Nafazatrom for 4 hr produced a dose dependent decrease in DNA synthesis with an ED_{50} of 0.6 μg/ml (Fig. 5). Similar inhibition by Nafazatrom has been observed with the Lewis lung carcinoma,

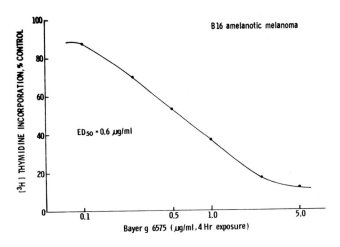

Figure 5. Nafazatrom inhibition of DNA synthesis by B16a melanoma cells.

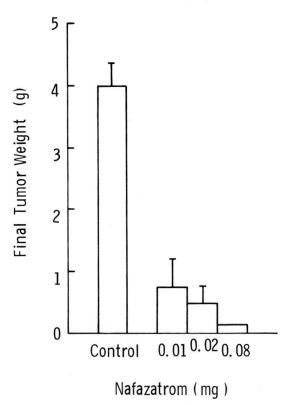

Figure 6.   Inhibition of tumor growth by Nafazatrom.

Friend erythroleukemia cells, a reticular cell sarcoma and neuroblastoma   N-2   cells   (unpublished   observations). Animals   bearing   subcutaneous   Lewis   lung   tumors   were injected (s.c.) with Nafazatrom (0.01 - 0.08 mg/animal/da x 22 da).   A significant reduction in final tumor weight was observed in all treated groups (Figure 6).

ACKNOWLEDGEMENT

Work in the authors' laboratory has been supported by research grants from the National Institutes of Health,

CA29405, CA29997, the American Cancer Society, BC-356, the Milheim Foundation for Cancer Research and the Comprehensive Cancer Center of Metropolitan Detroit. The work with Nafazatrom has been supported by the Miles Institute for PreClinical Pharmacology. The authors also wish to thank Drs. T.T. Tchen and J.D. Taylor for advice and encouragement. We thank Dr. J. Pike for the generous supply of eicosanoids. The use of Dept. of Chemistry laboratory facilities is gratefully acknowledged. The expert typing of M. Patricia Hensler is also gratefully appreciated.

REFERENCES

Ali, AE, Barrett, JC and Eling, TE (1980) Prostaglandin and thromboxane production by fibroblasts and vascular endothelial cells. In: Advances in Prostaglandin and Thromboxane Research (B. Samuelsson, P.W. Ramwell and R. Paoletti, eds), Raven Press, NY 6, 533.

Baenziger, NL, Dillender, MJ, Majerus, PW (1977) Cultured human skin fibroblasts and arterial cells produce a labile platelet-inhibitory prostaglandin. Biochem. Biophys. Res. Commun. 78, 294.

Carreras, LO, DAF Chamone, P Klercky and J Vermylen (1980) Decreased vascular prostaglandin (PGI$_2$) in diabetic rats. Stimulation of PGI$_2$ release in normal and diabetic rats by the antithrombotic compound Bay g 6575. Thromb. Res. 19, 663.

Clark, R, (1979) Systemic cancer and the metastatic process. Cancer 43, 790.

Donati, MB, JF Davidson and S Garattini (1981) Malignancy and the hemostatic system. Raven Press, New York, 138 p.

Elias, EG, Sepulveda, F and Mink, IB (1973) Increasing the efficacy of cancer chemotherapy with heparin: "Clinical Study". J. Surg. Oncol. 59, 189.

Fitzpatrick, FA and RR Gorman (1978) A comparison of imidazole and 9,11-azoprosta-5,13-dienoic acid, two selective thromboxane synthetase inhibitors. Biochim. et Biophys. Acta 539, 162.

Fitzpatrick, FA, GL Bundy, RR Gorman and T Honohan (1978) 9,11-Epoxyiminoprosta-5,13-dienoic acid is a thromboxane A$_2$ antagonist in human platelets. Nature 275, 764.

Fitzpatrick, FA, GL Bundy, RR Gorman and T Honohan, J McGuire and F Sun (1979) 9,11-iminoepoxyprosta-5,13-dienoic acid is a selective thromboxane A_2 synthetase inhibitor. Biochim. et Biophys. Acta 573, 238.

Friedman, DL, RA Johnson and LE Zeilig (1976) The role of cyclic nucleotides in the cell cycle. Adv. Cyclic Nucleotide Res. 7, 69.

Gasic, GJ, TB Gasic, N Galanti, T Johnson and S Murphy (1973) Platelet-tumor cell interactions in mice. The role of platelets in the spread of malignant disease. Int. J. Cancer 11, 704.

Gasic, GJ, PAG Koch, B Hsu, TB Gasic and S Niewiarowski (1976) Thrombogenic activity of mouse and human tumors: effects on platelets, coagulation, and fibrinolysis, and possible significance for metastasis. Z. Krebsforsch 86, 263.

Gastpar, H (1977) Platelet-cancer cell interaction in metastasis formation: a possible therapeutic approach to metastasis prophylaxis. J. Med. 8, 103.

Giraldi, T, G Sava, M Kopitar, J Brzin and V Turk (1980) Neutral proteinase inhibitors and antimetastatic effects in mice. Eur. J. Cancer 16, 449.

Gorman, R, S Bunting and O Miller (1977) Modulation of human platelet adenylate cyclase by prostacyclin (PGX). Prostaglandins 13, 377.

Gorman, R, R Hamilton and NK Hopkins. (1979) Prostacyclin and thromboxane A_2 biosynthesis and regulation of adenylate cyclase in human diploid cell lines. In: J.R. Sane and S. Bergstrom (eds.) Prostacyclin, NY, Raven Press, p. 85.

Gralnick, HR (1981) Cancer cell procoagulant activity. In: "Malignancy and the Hemostatic System" (MB Donati, JF Davidson and S Garattini eds.) Raven Press, New York. p. 57.

Hamberg, M, M Svensson and B Samuelsson (1975) Thromboxanes: a new group of biologically active compounds derived from prostaglandin endoperoxides. Proc. Nat. Acad. Sci. USA 72, 2994.

Heidrick, M, and W Ryan (1971) Adenosine 3',5'-cyclic monophosphate and contact inhibition. Cancer Res. 31, 1313.

Honn, KV, B Cicone and A Skoff (1981) Prostacyclin: a potent antimetastatic agent. Science 212, 1270.

Honn, KV, JR Dunn and J Meyer Thromboxanes and
prostacyclin: positive and negative modulators of
tumor cell proliferation. In: Prostaglandins and
Cancer (Powles, J, Bockman, R, Honn, KV, Ramwell, P
eds) New York, Alan Liss (in press).

Hyman, A and P Kadowitz (1979) Pulmonary vasodilator
activity of prostacyclin (PGI_2) in the cat. Cir Res.
45, 404.

Kreider, J, D Wade, M Rosenthal and T Densley (1975)
Maturation and differentiation of B16 melanoma cells
induced by theophylline treatment. J. Nat. Cancer
Inst. 54, 1457.

Lione, A and HB Bosman (1978) The inhibitory effect
of heparin and warfarin treatments on the
intravascular survival of B16 melanoma cells in
syngeneic C57 mice. Cell Biol. Int. Rep. 2, 81.

Marcus, A (1978) The role of lipids in platelet
function: with particular reference to the
arachidonic acid pathway. J. Lipid Res. 19, 793.

Moncada, S and J Vane (1979) The role of prostacyclin
in vascular tissue. Fed. Proc. 38, 66.

Roos, E and KP Dingmans (1979) Mechanisms of metastasis.
Biochim. Biophys. Acta. 560, 135.

Salmon, J, D Smith, R Flower, S Moncada and J Vane. (1978)
Further studies on the enzymatic conversion of
prostaglandin endoperoxide into prostaglandin by
porcine aorta microsomes. Biochim. Biophys. Acta.
523, 250.

Seuter, F, W Busse, K Meng, F Hoffmeister, E Moeller and H
Horstmann (1979) The antithrombotic activity of Bay g
6575. Arzneim-Forsch/Drug Research 29, 54.

Siegel, M, R McConnell, S Abrahams, N Porter and P
Cuatrecasas (1979) Regulation of arachidoniate
metabolism via lipoxygenase and cyclooxygenase by
12-hpete, the product of human platelet lipoxygenase.
Biochem. Biophys. Res. Comm. 89, 1273.

Sloane, B, J Dunn and K Honn (1981) Lysosomal cathepsin B:
correlation with metastatic potential. Science 212,
1151.

Smith, JB (1980) The prostanoids in hemostasis and
thrombosis. Am. J. Path. 99, 743.

Sugarbaker, EV and AS Ketcham (1977) Mechanisms and
prevention of cancer dissemination: an overview.
Sem. Oncol. 4, 19.

Sun, F, J Chapman and J McGuire (1977) Metabolism of prostaglandin endoperoxide in animal tissues. Prostaglandins 14, 1055.

Sutherland, E (1972) Studies on the mechanism of hormone action. Science 177, 401.

Vermylen, J, DA Chamone and M Verstraete (1979) Stimulation of prostacyclin release from vessel wall by Bay g 6575. An antithrombotic compound. Lancet 1, 518.

Weiss, L (1977) A pathobiologic overview of metastasis. Sem. in Oncology 4, 5.

Yoshimoto, T, S Yamamoto and D Hayarshi (1978) Selective inhibition of prostaglandin endoperoxide thromboxane isomerase by 1-carboxyalkylimidazoles. Prostaglandins 16, 529.

**Prostaglandins and Cancer: First
International Conference, pages 753-757**
© 1982 Alan R. Liss, Inc., 150 Fifth Avenue, New York, NY 10011

PROSTAGLANDINS AND CELL PROLIFERATION IN INTESTINAL TUMORS
IN VIVO

P.J.M. TUTTON, FRANCES M. PETRY, AND D.H. BARKLA

DEPARTMENT OF ANATOMY, MONASH UNIVERSITY, CLAYTON

VICTORIA 3168, AUSTRALIA

In a series of earlier reports from this laboratory
the effects of several biogenic amines and their
antagonists on cell proliferation in the crypt epithelium
of both the small and the large intestine and in dimethyl-
hydrazine(DMH)-induced adenocarcinomas of the large
intestine of rat have been detailed. For reviews, see
Tutton (1977) and Tutton & Barkla (1980a; 1981a). Cyclic
nucleotide derivatives have also been shown to influence
cell proliferation in these three tissues (Tutton &
Barkla, 1980b,c; 1981b). Factors inhibiting cell
proliferation in DMH-induced tumors of rat colon have, in
most instances, also inhibited the growth of human
colonic tumors propagated as xenografts in immune-deprived
mice (Tutton & Steel, 1979; Barkla & Tutton, 1981). The
present report concerns the effects of prostaglandin
precursors, inhibitors of prostaglandin synthesis and some
synthetic prostaglandin analogues on epithelial cell
proliferation in the intestine and in intestinal tumors.
    Throughout the following experiments a Vinblastine
based, stathmokinetic technique was used to estimate the
mitotic rate (that is, the cell proliferation rate) in the
jejunal crypt epithelium, the colonic crypt epithelium
and in DMH-induced colonic tumors in male Sprague-Dawley rats.
Details of this stathmokinetic technique and the induction
of tumors has previously been described (Tutton & Barkla,
1976). The following procedures were then used to
manipulate prostaglandin metabolism. First, rats were
injected with arachidonic acid - a precursor of the
2-series prostaglandins. Secondly, rats were subjected
to bilateral surgical adrenalectomy, thus depriving them

of various hormones including cortisol, a hormone that,
amongst other things, reduces the availability of
prostaglandin precursors, possibly by inhibiting the
enzyme phospholipase A_2 (Lewis, Piper & Vigo, 1979).
Thirdly, adrenalectomised rats were treated with either
the steroidal anti-inflammatory drug, Dexamethasone or the
non-steroidal, cyclooxygenase inhibitor, Flurbiprofen.
Fourthly, to distinguish between prostaglandin-mediated
and other effects of arachidonic acid administration,
rats were treated with a combination of Flurbiprofen and
arachidonic acid. Finally, animals were treated with
16,16-dimethyl analogs of PGE_2 and $PGF_2\alpha$.

RESPONSE TO ARACHIDONIC ACID

Intraperitoneal injection of arachidonic acid at a
dose of 100mg/kg resulted in significant suppression of
cell proliferation in the jejunal crypts, the colonic
crypts and in colonic tumors (see Table 1). Administration
of the cyclooxygenase inhibitor, Flurbiprofen at a dose of
1mg/kg with the arachidonic acid prevented the suppression
of cell proliferation in both jejunal crypts and the colonic
tumors, but in colonic crypts cell proliferation was still
suppressed, suggesting the participation of a non-
prostaglandin arachidonic acid metabolite - possibly via
a lipoxygenase pathway.

TABLE 1. Response to arachidonic acid.

Treatment	Mitotic rate - mean ± SE - Mitoses/cell/hr.		
	Jejunal Crypts	Colonic Crypts	Colonic Tumors
Nil (Control)	0.048±0.002	0.024±0.003	0.018±0.003
Arachidonic acid	0.031±0.006	0.008±0.001	0.00 ±0.002
Arachidonic acid + Flurbiprofen	0.046±0.005	0.007±0.004	0.024±0.005

RESPONSE TO ADRENALECTOMY

Following bilateral adrenalectomy, cell proliferation
was significantly suppressed in both the jejunal crypt
epithelium and in the colonic tumors but not in the colonic

crypts (see Table 2). This suppression of cell proliferation was, in both tissues, reversed by administration of a
glucocorticoid agent (i.e. a non-steroidal anti-inflammatory drug) Dexamethasone but not by a mineralocorticoid
hormone, aldosterone acetate. In adrenalectomised rats,
Flurbiprofen on the other hand returned cell proliferation
rates to the control value in the jejunal crypt epithelium,
but failed to influence the effect on adrenalectomy in
colonic tumors.

TABLE 2.   Response to adrenalectomy.

Treatment	Mitotic rate - mean ± SE - Mitoses/cell/hr.		
	Jejunal Crypts	Colonic Crypts	Colonic Tumors
Nil (Control)	0.048±0.002	0.024±0.003	0.018±0.003
Adrenalectomy	0.025±0.002	0.015±0.005	0.000+0.002
Adrenalectomy + aldosterone	0.027±0.003	–	0.00±0.007
Adrenalectomy + dexamethasone	0.044+0.003	–	0.029±0.009
Adrenalectomy + Flurbiprofen	0.039±0.005	0.018±0.004	0.003±0.008

RESPONSE TO PROSTAGLANDIN ANALOGS

Rats were treated with 16,16-dimethyl PGE_2 or
16,16-dimethyl $PGF_{2\alpha}$ (Upjohn Ltd.) at doses ranging from
0.025 to 250µg/kg (see Table 3). The PGE_2 analog failed
to significantly influence cell proliferation in any of
the tissues examined. The $PGF_{2\alpha}$ analog, on the other
hand, significantly promoted cell proliferation in the
jejunal crypt epithelium but yet strongly suppressed cell
proliferation in colonic tumors.

TABLE 3.   Response to prostaglandin analog.

Treatment	Mitotic rate - mean ± SE - Mitoses/cell/hr.		
	Jejunal Crypts	Colonic Crypts	Colonic Tumors
Nil (Control)	0.048±0.002	0.024±0.003	0.018±0.003
16,16-dimethyl PGE₂ 250µg/kg	0.044±0.009	0.021±0.008	0.018±0.002
2.5µg/kg	–	–	0.033±0.008
0.025µg/kg	–	–	0.022±0.001
16,16-dimethyl PGF₂α 250µg/kg	0.081 ±0.016	0.017±0.008	0.00±0.001
2.5µg/kg	0.073 ±0.005	–	0.00±0.008
0.025µg/kg	0.051 ±0.003	–	0.015±0.006

DISCUSSION

The obvious question arising from such *in vivo* studies
is - to what extent are the observed effects of prosta-
glandin-related agents direct or indirect? In the case
of glucocorticoid hormones acting on colonic tumor cells
the effect appears to be a direct one since suitable
hormone receptors are present (Alford, Do, Geelhoed, Tsangaris
& Lippman, 1979), and growth of colonic tumor cells in
serum free medium *in vitro* is also promoted by these
hormones (Murakami & Masui, 1980). However, the effect of
glucocorticoid hormone withdrawal on colonic tumors does
not appear to involve prostaglandins since it is not
opposed by a dose of Flurbiprofen that is adequate to
oppose the effect of injected arachidonic acid. With the
sole exception of the effect of glucocorticoids on tumor
cell proliferation, it must be acknowledged that it is
currently not possible to distinguish between direct and
indirect effects of agents used in the present study.

Despite the above mentioned reservations, the
present results do raise the serious possibility that
prostaglandins may have an important role in the biology
of colonic tumors. Much remains to be surveyed even
within the present framework of *in vivo* experiments.
Results with arachidonic acid treated and adrenalectomised
rats must be analysed after treatment with lipoxygenase
inhibitors such as Benoxaprofen, as a means of establishing a *prima facie* case for the involvement of leukotrienes.
It is also important to assess the role of analogs of
other cyclooxygenase metabolites, such as Prostacyclin
and Thomboxane A_2. Experiments along these lines are
currently being conducted in our laboratory.

Acknowledgements.

This work was done during the tenure of a research
grant awarded by the Anti-Cancer Council of Victoria to
P.J.M. Tutton and D.H. Barkla, whilst F.M. Petry was the
recipient of a National Health & Medical Research Council
of Australia Scholarship. Prostaglandin analogs used in
these experiments were generously supplied by the Upjohn
Company, Kalamazoo, Michigan, U.S.A., and Flurbiprofen was
generously supplied by the Boots Company Pty. Ltd.,
Sydney, Australia.

REFERENCES

Alford TC, Do HM, Geelhoed GW, Tsangaris WT, Lippman ME (1979). Steroid hormone receptors in human colon cancers. Cancer 43:980.

Barkla DH, Tutton PJM (1981). The influence of histamine and serotonin antagonists on the growth of xenografted human colorectal tumors. J Natl Cancer Inst in press

Lewis GP, Piper PJ, Vigo C (1979) The effects of glucocorticoids on the distribution and mobilisation of arachidonic acid in fat cell ghosts. Brit J Pharmacol 67:393.

Murakami H, Masui H (1980) Hormonal control of human colon carcinoma cell growth in serum-free medium. Proc Nat Acad Sci USA 77:3464.

Tutton PJM (1977). Neural and endocrine control systems acting on the population kinetics of the intestinal epithelium. Med Biol 55:201.

Tutton PJM, Barkla DH (1976) Cell proliferation in the descending colon of dimethylhydrazine-treated rats and in dimethylhydrazine-induced adenocarcinomata. Virchows Arch Abt B Cell Path 21: 147.

Tutton PJM, Barkla DH (1980a) Neural control of colonic cell proliferation. Cancer 45:1172.

Tutton PJM, Barkla DH (1980b) A final common pathway promoting cell proliferation in normal and in neoplastic intestinal epithelia. In Appleton DR (ed): "Cell Proliferation in the Gastrointestinal Tract," London: Pitman Medical, p 298.

Tutton PJM, Barkla DH (1980c) The influence of dibutyryl adenosine cyclic monophosphate on cell proliferation in the epithelium of the jejunal crypts, the colonic crypts and in colonic carcinomata of rat. Clin exp. Pharmacol Physiol 7:275.

Tutton PJM, Barkla DH (1981d) Neural control of cell proliferation in colonic carcinogenesis. In Malt RA (ed): "Colonic Carcinogenesis," MTP Press.

Tutton PJM, Barkla DH (1981b) The effects of cyclic nucleotide derivatives on the growth rate of human colonic carcinomata propagated in immune-deprived mice and on the cell production rate in the colonic crypt epithelium. Br J Cancer in press.

Tutton PJM, Steel GG (1979) Influence of biogenic amines on the growth of xenografted human colorectal carcinomas. Br J Cancer 40:743.

**Prostaglandins and Cancer: First
International Conference, pages 759-766
© 1982 Alan R. Liss, Inc., 150 Fifth Avenue, New York, NY 10011**

EFFECT OF PROSTAGLANDIN SYNTHESIS INHIBITORS ON TUMOR GROWTH
IN VIVO

Alan Bennett

Department of Surgery, King's College Hospital
Medical School,
London SE5 8RX, UK

TUMOR GROWTH

Prostaglandins and related substances can be formed by
malignant cells and by the host cells within tumors (see
Bennett 1979, 1981). Because of the different types of
cancers and species, and the wide varieties of cells and
prostanoids involved, it would be surprising if studies revealed a uniform picture. Indeed, even with just PGE_1 or
PGE_2, some cell types in culture show growth inhibition and
others show stimulation (see Bennett 1979, 1981). Despite
this variability, and the fact that anti-inflammatory drugs
may have a mixture of properties, drugs which inhibit prostaglandin synthesis usually inhibit tumor growth in vivo, although occasionally they have no effect. Those that demonstrate an inhibition include studies by Tashjian et al (1973),
Humes et al (1974), Plescia et al (1975), Hial et al (1976),
Lynch et al (1978), and several from our own group (see
Bennett 1981). Those that show only a small inhibition or
no effect include Sykes and Maddox (1972), Feher and Gidali
(1974), Pollard et al (1977), Favalli et al (1980) and Hofer
et al (1980). No papers report an increase in tumor size
with non-steroidal anti-inflammatory drugs, although Favalli
et al (1980) found that indomethacin hastened the development of mouse B-16 melanomas; nevertheless, all the mice
had palpable tumors at day 8. What is the significance of
a reduction in tumor size? Local growth of a primary cancer
is rarely a cause of death. More important is metastatic
spread, so does the effect on the primary tumor reflect the
effect on metastases? This aspect will be discussed subsequently.

How do inhibitors of prostaglandin synthesis reduce
primary tumor size? In some cases, at least part of the
effect might be due to reduction of inflammation and swelling,
but in others this explanation seems untenable. Indomethacin
caused complete regression of some tumors (Lynch et al 1978);
flurbiprofen given to mice from time of tumor transplanation
halved the tumor size, but had no significant effect when
given to mice after their tumors had grown substantially
(Bennett et al 1979). Indomethacin can overcome a prosta-
glandin-induced inhibition of the immune system, but this
too may not be its anti-tumor mechanism: Lynch et al (1978)
thought that their tumor was non-immunogenic, and this may
be the case with the NC carcinoma used by Bennett et al (1979).

Do anti-inflammatory drugs affect tumor cell numbers?
Here again the results are variable. Clearly there is a
reduction in those tumors that disappear. One group has
claimed that B-16 melanomas from indomethacin-treated mice
had more viable cells. However, whereas in their first
paper (Favalli et al 1980) the cell numbers were almost
double those in control tumors, in their second paper (Hofer
et al 1980) the difference was only about 8% taking into
account the smaller tumors from indomethacin-treated mice.
Besides malignant cells, viable lymphocytes were also present,
so that it is not possible to ascertain from their data which
cell type was affected. If, as Hofer et al (1980) assume,
indomethacin decreases the numbers of lymphocytes in the
tumor, their results could indicate a dramatic increase in
malignant cells. But the reverse might be true if, for
example, indomethacin diverted metabolism of prostaglandin
precursors into chemotactic leukotrienes. More convincing
is the finding by Tutton and Barkla (1980) that flurbiprofen
speeded cell division in dimethylhydrazine-induced rat
colonic tumors.

TUMOR METASTASIS

The results with non-steroidal anti-inflammatory drugs is
less variable than with the topics discussed so far. Aspirin
or indomethacin have been found either to inhibit metastasis
or to have no effect. No study shows a statistically significant increase in metastasis. An anti-metastatic effect
has been found with various tumors in mice (Kolenich et al
1972; Gasic et al 1973), and rats (Pollard et al 1977);
other data on survival can be interpreted similarly. How-

ever, in rats injected intravascularly with Walker tumor cells
(Powles et al 1973), or in rabbits given VX2 tumors (Galasko et al
1979), the development of soft tissue metastases was not
reduced, although bone destruction by the tumors was inhibited.

SURVIVAL

As with metastasis, some studies with non-steroidal anti-
inflammatory drugs on their own show benefit, and some have
no effect. None shows a worse survival. Work demonstrating
a beneficial effect includes that of Lynch et al (1978),
Bennett et al (1979, 1981) and Trevisani et al (1980). Those
showing little or no effect include papers by Strausser and
Humes (1975), Hial et al (1976), Galasko and Bennett (1976),
Powles et al (1978) and Powles and Millar (1979).

INTERACTION WITH CONVENTIONAL ANTI-CANCER TREATMENTS

Mice with NC carcinomas were given two low doses of
local radiotherapy which did not affect the weight of the
tumor removed 4 days after the second irradiation. However,
concurrent administration of flurbiprofen resulted in substantially smaller tumors. The extent to which this may
indicate an increased response to radiotherapy has not been
evaluated; flurbiprofen may have merely reduced an inflammatory response to the radiation.

An increased response with chemotherapeutic drugs seems
better established, since the effect has been demonstrated
as an increase in survival time. With rat tumors made
resistant to chlorambucil, tumor sensitivity was often restored by giving flurbiprofen or indomethacin (Powles et al
1978; Powles and Millar 1979). Furthermore, 3 patients
had tumors resistant to chemotherapy which became sensitive
when treatment with flurbiprofen was also given (Powles et
al 1978).

Our results with NC carcinomas in mice may be somewhat
analogous to these findings. Melphalan and methotrexate
had little effect on tumor size (Bennett et al 1979) or on
survival of mice following tumor excision (Bennett et al 1979;
Berstock et al 1979; Bennett et al 1981). However, when
flurbiprofen was given with the chemotherapeutic drugs to
mice with resected primary tumors, survival time increased

significantly (Berstock et al 1979; Bennett et al 1981).
Figure 1 shows this effect in female mice.   Similar results
have been obtained with indomethacin (A Bennett, D A Berstock
and M A Carroll, unpublished).

FIG 1. EFFECTS OF TREATMENTS ON MOUSE SURVIVAL

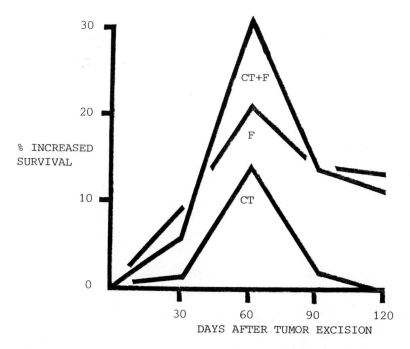

Survival is shown as % difference from control, the
horizontal line at 0.   Mice received chemotherapy with
melphalan and methotrexate (CT, N=72), flurbiprofen
(F, N=56), CT+F (N=71) or vehicle (N=51 controls).
Control vs: CT, P=0.37; F, P=0.038; CT+F, P=0.003.
CT+F   vs: CT, P=0.02; F vs CT, P=0.19.

Since the mice die of metastatic spread, mainly to the lungs
and mediastinum, the prolongation of survival may be due to
an inhibition of processes involved in metastatic spread and/
or to the development of established metastases. Possible
mechanisms by which the non-steroidal anti-inflammatory drugs
act, in addition to those discussed previously, involve
interference with platelet aggregation (Gasic et al 1973),
interference with tumor blood supply which may be modulated
by prostaglandins, inhibition of calcium binding by cell
membranes (Northover 1973), or possibly removal of prosta-
glandin-induced "cytoprotection"; prostaglandins protect
the gastric mucosa from damage (Robert 1977) but this may
involve stimulation of blood flow, mucus secretion etc.

In addition to an increase in survival, flurbiprofen
given with chemotherapy reduced the local recurrence of tumor
at the excision site, whereas the separate therapies had
little effect (Berstock et al 1979; Bennett et al 1981).
This reduction of recurrence did not seem to involve the
trapping of malignant cells in the sutured wound, since no
tumor developed in mice given a contralateral sutured cut
at the time of tumor excision (Bennett et al 1981). Nor
did flurbiprofen seem likely to act by displacing methotrexate from binding sites on plasma proteins, as can occur
with some drugs (Schiffman et al 1978). As indicated by
toxicity studies in normal mice, flurbiprofen did not increase
the bioavailability of the chemotherapeutic drugs, or it
simultaneously protected against their toxic effects. Powles
et al (1978) and Powles and Millar (1979) found that indomethacin reduced the toxic effects of methotrexate on gut and
bone in rats.

Indomethacin may not interact favourably with all chemotherapeutic agents in all types of tumor and all species,
but this point needs further investigation. Hofer et al
(1980), studying mouse B-16 melanoma, reported that indomethacin had no effect on the tumor response to various chemotherapeutic agents, or was deleterious. However, the data
on tumor size, weight and cell numbers are somewhat variable,
and there are problems of interpretation such as the numbers
of viable cells discussed earlier.

It is important to determine the extent to which inhibitors of prostaglandin synthesis interact with cancer in man.
Patients with cancer may take such drugs for relief of pain
which may or may not be related to the malignancy, or for

the relief of symptoms due to cancer therapy (Mennie et al 1975; Tanner et al 1981). Non-steroidal anti-inflammatory drugs cannot yet be recommended for adjuvant therapy in cancer, because their efficacy and safety have yet to be determined in man. Benorylate, a relatively weak inhibitor of prostaglandin synthesis, seems to be safe but not efficacious in breast cancer (Powles et al 1980), and corticosteroids which inhibit the release of prostaglandin precursors, are included in some cancer treatments. The evidence from animal experiments suggest that other nonsteroidal inhibitors of prostaglandin synthesis should be tried in human cancer subjects and studies with flurbiprofen are now in progress (unpublished).

REFERENCES

Bennett A (1979). Prostaglandins and cancer. In Karim SMM (Ed): "Practical Applications of Prostaglandins and their Synthesis Inhibitors", Lancaster: MTP Press, P149.
Bennett A (1981). Prostaglandins and inhibitors of their synthesis in cancer growth and spread. In Rose DP (ed): "Endocrinology of Cancer. Vol III", Florida: CRC Press, in press.
Bennett A, Berstock DA, Carroll MA (1981). Enhanced anticancer effect by combining cytotoxic drugs with the prostaglandin synthesis inhibitor flurbiprofen. Br J Pharmac, in press.
Bennett A, Houghton J, Leaper DJ, Stamford IF (1979). Cancer growth, response to treatment and survival time in mice: beneficial effect of the prostaglandin synthesis inhibitor flurbiprofen. Prostaglandins 17:179.
Berstock DA, Houghton J, Bennett A (1979). Improved anticancer effect by combining cytotoxic drugs with an inhibitor of prostaglandin synthesis. Cancer Treatment Reviews 6:69.
Favalli C, Garaci E, Etheredge E, Santoro MG, Jaffe BM (1980). Influence of PGE on the immune response in melanoma-bearing mice. J Immunol 125:897.
Feher I, Gidali J (1974). Prostaglandin E_2 as a stimulator of haemopoietic stem cell proliferation. Nature 247:550.
Galasko CSB, Bennett A (1976). Relationship of bone destruction in skeletal metastases to osteoclast activation and prostaglandins. Nature 263:508.
Galasko CSB, Rawlins R, Bennett A (1979). Timing of indomethacin in the control of prostaglandins, osteoclasts and bone destruction produced by VX2 carcinoma in rabbits.

Br J Cancer 40:360.
Gasic GJ, Gasic TB, Galanti N, Johnson T, Murphy S (1973).
Platelet tumor-cell interactions in mice.   The role of plate-
lets in the spread of malignant desease.   Int J Cancer 11:704.
Hial V, Horakova Z, Shaff RE, Beavan MA (1976).   Alteration
of tumor growth by aspirin and indomethacin: studies with
two transplantable tumors in mouse.   Eur J Pharmacol 37:367.
Hofer D, Dubitsky AM, Reilly P, Santoro MG, Jaffe BM (1980).
The interactions between indomethacin and cytotoxic drugs
in mice bearing B-16 melanomas.   Prostaglandins 20:1033.
Kolenich JJ, Mansour EG, Flynn A (1972).   Haematological
aspects of aspirin.   Lancet 2:714.
Lynch NR, Castes M, Astoin M, Salomon JC.(1978).   Mechanism
of inhibition of tumour growth by aspirin and indomethacin.
Br J Cancer 38:503.
Mennie SAT, Dalley V, Dinneen LC, Collier HOJ (1975).   Treat-
ment of radiation-induced gastrointestinal distress with
acetylsalicylate.   Lancet 2:942.
Northover BJ (1973).   The effect of anti-inflammatory drugs
on the binding of calcium to cellular membranes in various
human and guinea-pig tissues.   Br J Pharmacol 48:496.
Pollard M, Burleson GR, Luckert PH (1977).   In Day SB (ed):
"Cancer Invasion and Metastasis: Biologic Mechanisms and
Therapy".   New York: Raven Press, P357.
Plescia OJ, Smith AH, Grinwich K (1975).   Subversion of
immune system by tumor cells and role of prostaglandins.
Proc Nat Acad Sci 72:1848.
Powles TJ, Alexander P, Millar JL (1978).   Enhancement of
anti-cancer activity of cytotoxic chemotherapy with production of normal tissues by inhibition of prostaglandin
synthesis.   Biochem Pharmacol 27:1389.
Powles TJ, Clark SA, Easty DM, Easty GC, Neville AM (1973).   The
inhibition by aspirin and indomethacin of osteolytic tumour
deposits and hypercalcaemia in rats with Walker tumour, and
its possible application to human breast cancer.   Br J Cancer
28:316.
Powles TJ, Dady PJ, Williams J, Easty GC, Coombes RC (1980).
Use of inhibitors of prostaglandin synthesis in patients
with breast cancer.   In Samuelsson B, Ramwell PW, Paoletti
R (eds):   "Advances in Prostaglandin and Thromboxane Research",
Vol 6, New York: Raven Press p511.
Powles TJ, Millar JL (1979).   Non-steroidal anti-inflamma-
tory drugs and cytotoxics.   Cancer Treat Rev 6(Suppl):63.
Schiffman FJ, Uehara Y, Fisher JM, Rabinovitz M (1978).
Potentiation of chlorambucil activity by phenylbutazone.
Cancer Lett 4:211.

Strausser H, Humes J (1975). Prostaglandin synthesis inhibition: Effect on bone changes and sarcoma tumour induction in BALB/c mice. Int J Cancer 15:724.

Sykes JAC, Maddox IS (1972). Prostaglandin production by experimental tumours and effects of anti-inflammatory compounds. Nature (New Biology) 237:59.

Tanner NSB, Stamford IF, Bennett A (1981). Plasma prostaglandins in mucositis due to radiotherapy and chemotherapy. Br J Cancer 43:767.

Tashjian AH, Voelkel EF, Goldhaber P, Levine L (1973). Successful treatment of hypercalcemia by indomethacin in mice bearing a prostaglandin-producing tumor. Prostaglandins 3:515.

Trevisani A, Farretti E, Capuzzo A, Tomasi V (1980). Elevated levels of prostaglandin E_2 in yoshida hepatoma and the inhibition of tumour growth by non-steroidal anti-inflammatory drugs. Br J Cancer 41:341.

Tutton PJM, Barkla DH (1980). Influence of prostaglandin analogues on epithelial cell proliferation and xenograft growth. Br J Cancer 41:47.

Prostaglandins and Cancer: First
International Conference, pages 767–774
© 1982 Alan R. Liss, Inc., 150 Fifth Avenue, New York, NY 10011

ANTITUMOUR ACTIVITY OF FLURBIPROFEN $\underline{IN}$ $\underline{VIVO}$ AND $\underline{IN}$ $\underline{VITRO}$

Kurt Hellmann and Barbara A. Pym

Cancer Chemotherapy Department
Imperial Cancer Research Fund,
London, WC2, England.

INTRODUCTION

Sykes (1974) first demonstrated the occurrence of prostaglandins in animal tumours. Of special interest were her findings of substantial concentrations of PGE_2 in the Lewis lung carcinoma, only surpassed by those found in sheep seminal fluid. Sykes speculated that there might be special significance in the occurrence of such large amounts in a tumour which metastasized spontaneously, regularly and predictably in all inoculated animals and that the prostaglandins were involved in a fundamental way in the metastatic process.

This theme was later taken up by others (Bennett et al. 1977), but in view of the lack of influence of prostaglandin synthesis inhibitors on the appearance of metastases (Sykes 1974) the general applicability of this hypothesis to the clarification of the mechanism of metastasis formation seemed and still seems highly unlikely, even if one or more tumours are found to have mechanisms of dissemination involving prostaglandins.

Recently a closer investigation of the anti-tumour actions of one prostaglandin inhibitor,

Flurbiprofen (FLPR), was undertaken in this laboratory and this paper will concern itself only
with this potent agent.

FLPR AND METASTASIS

Most of our experiments designed to unravel
the role of prostaglandins and prostaglandin
inhibitors in the metastatic process were done
with the Lewis lung carcinoma. At maximum
tolerated doses, FLPR given either subcutaneously
or by the oral route had no effect on the development of metastases nor did it influence the growth
of the primary subcutaneous tumour implant.

Experiments were then done in which the
primary Lewis lung implant was irradiated with or
without subsequent treatment by FLPR and this too
had no evident effect on the outcome of the growth
of the primary or the development of the secondary
tumours. Similar experiments with radiation were
therefore done with the sarcoma 180 which dissem-
inates, but does not metastasize and with this
tumour there was a very evident potentiation of
the effects of radiation by FLPR (Table 1). FLPR
alone however seems to have some slight, but
consistent activity in this tumour.

In several experiments with the S180 in which
a single radiation dose of 800 rads was given 10
days following the inoculation of the tumour together with FLPR before and after the radiation
and the animals followed for a further 3 weeks,
there was a significant increase in the number of
animals who were tumour free as compared with those
who had radiation or FLPR alone. Although the
FLPR given alone had only a slight effect on the
growth of sarcoma 180, the combination with
radiation showed a considerable increase in the
inhibitory activity of the radiation. The

FLURBIPROFEN & RADIATION
S180 (solid)

Drug	Dose (mg/kg) s.c.	No. Doses/ Day		Rads d.10	Mean (g)	T/C %
Control					4.46	
FLPR	2	3	d.2-14	–	3.04	68
FLPR	2	3	d.2-14	800	1.17	26
				800	2.32	52
Control					5.9	
FLPR	2	3	d.4-14		5.0	84
		2	d.15-16			
FLPR	2	3	d.4-14	800	2.14	36
			d.15-16	800	3.67	62
Control					4.5	
FLPR	2	3	d.10-14		3.68	81
		2	d.9-16			
FLPR	2	3	d.10-14	800	2.29	50
			d.9-16	800	2.74	60
Control					5.57	
FLPR	2	3	d.3-14		4.3	77
		2	d.13-16			
FLPR	2	3	d.3-14	800	2.08	37
		2	d.13-16	800	3.48	62

No./Gp.11   FLPR/RTX/180 1-4

TABLE 1

mechanism of this radiotherapeutic potentiation is not yet clear.

It was considered possible that prostaglandins might play some part in the implantation of circulating metastatic cells and therefore lungs of mice which were subsequently inoculated with Lewis lung tumour were irradiated with a single dose of radiation of between 2-3,000 rads several days before implantation of the tumour to increase the chances of circulating tumour cell implantation. Following tumour implantation 4mg/kg FLPR was given twice daily subcutaneously until the end of the experiment.

It seemed possible that if prostaglandins played a part in the active promotion of adherence or implantation of circulating tumour cells that prostaglandin inhibitors might prevent this process. In the event it can be seen from Table 2 that only where the tumour was implanted 6 days after irradiation were the number of additional metastases significantly higher than in the un-irradiated controls and in these animals additional treatment with FLPR resulted in a significant reduction of metastases. It may be that further exploration of this effect may yield even more decisive differences.

RTX OF LUNGS PRIOR TO 3LL IMPLANT
Mice C57 ♀ No./Gp. 10

Group	Rad.dose to lungs day 0	Day post x-ray tumour implanted	FLPR.4mg/kg s.c. x2/d. on d.post RTX	2° Mean
1	nil	0	nil	32
2	2360	0	nil	48
3	2360	0	5 - 21	44.7
4	nil	4	nil	59
5	2670	4	nil	91
6	2670	4	5 - 23	83
7	nil	6	nil	59.7
8	2670	6	nil	104
9	2670	6	7 - 26	69

t.test groups 1,2,3 - not significant
gp.4 v gp.5 = $p0.01$ gp.7 v gp.8 = $p<0.001$
gp.4 v gp.6 = $p>0.05$ gp.7 v gp.9 = $p>0.1$
gp.5 v gp.6 = $p>>0.1$ gp.8 v gp.9 = $p<<0.01$
TABLE 2

Similar experiments with the spontaneously metastasizing melanoma B16 did not reveal any significant differences between the irradiated groups and those that were treated additionally with FLPR. However the conditions were not identical with those employed in the Lewis lung experiments since the growth rate of the B16 secondary tumours is much slower than that of the Lewis lung metastases. It is necessary therefore to excise the primary B16 tumour implants by day 12 in order to allow the animals 40-50 days for the secondaries to become visible. The B16 tumours were also treated with a somewhat different fractionation scheme. Doses of 250 rads daily were used on days 7-10 post implantation and a dose of 2.5mg/kg of FLPR given subcutaneously 3 times a day from day 4 after implantation to day 13. The animals were then followed until they died and extensive post-mortem examination made to ascertain what effect had been obtained on B16 metastases formation. There were no significant differences either in the number or distribution of the metastases when the controls were compared with the FLPR treated animals.

IN VITRO ANTITUMOUR ACTIVITY OF FLPR

At the same time tissue culture experiments were undertaken to see if FLPR had a direct effect on B16 melanoma cells grown in vitro. Surprisingly it was found that there was a direct correlation between concentrations of FLPR and cytotoxicity of B16 cells. The assays were done by colony count so as to enable the effect of FLPR to be measured directly on the proliferative capacity of the B16 cells. As can be seen from Table 3 which shows the results of one experiment, a 50% inhibition of colony growth (ID_{50}) was reached at 8μg/ml. Similar results were obtained in two further experiments with the ID_{50} varying between 8 and 12μg/ml.

FLURBIPROFEN ON B16 CELLS TISSUE CULTURE (COLONY COUNT)

Expt. 1 DOSE	CONTROL	$4\mu gcm^{-3}$	$8\mu gcm^{-3}$	$10\mu gcm^{-3}$	$12\mu gcm^{-3}$
Mean Colony Count	129	94	66	46.2	39.8
S.E.	4.37	5.8	6.3	1.56	2.94
% Survival (T/C)	100	72	51	35	30

Cells set up as normal 200 cells/plate. Cells dosed day 1 drug left in culture medium for duration of experiment. Cells were stained and colonies counted day 10.

TABLE 3

In view of these results, the lack of activity of FLPR on the growth rate of primary B16 is surprising.

Further studies on the direct cytotoxicity of FLPR used the Lewis lung cells grown in suspension, but here there were no significant effects even at 16µg/ml (Table 4).

FLURBIPROFEN ON 3LL CELL COUNT (Coulter Counter) $(X10^6)$

	Day 1	Day 2	Day 3
Control	.551	1.39	6.76
16µg/ml	.592	1.70	6.86
8µg/ml	.609	1.67	6.87
4µg/ml	.569	1.91	6.41
2µg/ml	.583	1.74	6.62

Each value is mean of 3 readings

TABLE 4

Tests were also carried out with FLPR on L1210 leukaemia which did not however reveal any activity on this cell line nor did FLPR potentiate or antagonise the actions of other drugs such as 5-fluorouracil, cyclophosphamide, razoxane, methotrexate or chlorambucil in either L1210 leukaemia or the lymphoma TLX5.

IN SUMMARY

1. Prostaglandin synthesis inhibition does not appear to interfere with metastases formation in the Lewis lung carcinoma or the B16 melanoma.
2. FLPR has a direct cytotoxic or proliferative inhibitive activity in some tumours such as the B16 melanoma.
3. There is a seeming contradiction which may relate to pharmacokinetics and cell cycle kinetics between the findings in 1 and 2 since circulating

B16 cells should be at risk of destruction or inhibition of proliferation by FLPR.
4.   FLPR does not appear to be active against transplantable tumours such as the TLX5 and Lewis lung carcinoma, but there is some small and consistent activity against the S180.
5.   FLPR does not appear to antagonise or potentiate the activity of a number of anticancer drugs.
6.   FLPR appears to increase the effectiveness of radiotherapy against the S180.
7.   FLPR does not appear to increase the effect of radiotherapy against the Lewis lung carcinoma.

CONCLUSION

FLPR may be of some value in conjunction with radiotherapy in the treatment of human cancer and should have a clinical trial, particularly in association with radiotherapy for the treatment of malignant melanoma.

REFERENCES

Bennett A, Charlier EM, McDonald AM, Simpson JS, Stamford IF, Zebro T (1977). Prostaglandins and Breast Cancer. Lancet 2: 624-626
Sykes JAC (1974) Ph.D. Thesis. University of London

**Prostaglandins and Cancer: First
International Conference, pages 775–781
© 1982 Alan R. Liss, Inc., 150 Fifth Avenue, New York, NY 10011**

EFFECTS OF INDOMETHACIN ON MURINE FIBROSARCOMAS

Neil R. Lynch* and J.C. Salomon

Institut de Recherches Scientifiques sur le Cancer, CNRS, Villejuif, France

SUMMARY.

In this communication we consider the possibility that anaphylactic (allergic) reactions can complement antitumour mechanisms, and also evaluate the influence of tumour-bearing mice. Both indomethacin and *C. parvum* demonstrate anti-tumour activity in the tumour models studied, while exerting opposing effects on intratumour PGE2 concentrations. The influence of these agents on tumour histamine concentrations and mononuclear cell infiltration was also examined, and the possibility that the latter contributed to intratumour prostaglandin levels considered. Using the natural killer cell-deficient beige (bg/bg) mouse mutant, we obtained results that might be interpreted as indicating an involvement of these cells in the indomethacin effect. That, however, caution should be taken in the analysis of this model is suggested by our finding that these mice also have a defect in anaphylactic reactivity.

In previous publications we have described various aspects of the relationship between a transplantable 3 methylcholanthrene-induced fibrosarcoma of C3H mice (McC3-1) and the host response (1-5), and have reviewed the possible association between allergic-type reactions and antitumour mechanisms (6). A summary of our results is:

(1) Passive local anaphylactic reactions had an accessory activity in the rejection of this solid tumour; the effect being dependent upon vasoactive amines.

(2) The tumour, however, inhibited allergic-type reactivity in its host, due at least in part to the elaboration of a soluble (dialyzable*) factor. This inhibition was exerted at the mast cell — vasoactive amine level.

(3) The tumour contained high levels of both "PGE2-like" material, and histamine, that generally increased with tumour size. For histamine, this increase was not limited to the tumour tissue.

(4) Continuous oral indomethacin or aspirin administration decreased the tumour prostaglandin concentrations (this effect not being evident with theophylline or hydro-

*Present address: CEPIALET-IND (PAHO-WHO), Aptdo. 4043, Caracas, Venezuela.
*Unpublished observations.

cortisone treatment*).

(5) Indomethacin or aspirin (but not theophylline, hydrocortisone or heparin) administration significantly slowed the growth of established tumours.

While this effect was generally reversed after drug withdrawal, in some cases complete elimination of the tumour occurred. No prophylactic effects were observed.

The sensitivity of the tumour to these drugs diminished with successive serial transplant passages.

(6) Oral indomethacin potentiated the therapeutic effects of immunomodulators such as BCG and *C. parvum,* particularly when their activity was sub-optimal; e.g. with large tumour burden, or systemic (rather than intratumoural) injection.

The duration of the "tumour-free" interval depended, however, upon the continued administration of the drug in many cases.

(7) No *specific* anti-tumour immunity was detected in the animals that had completely eliminated their tumours under indomethacin administration alone; in marked contrast to after *C-parvum*-induced cure. A relatively short-lived non-specific tumour resistance was, however, observed in the former animals.

(8) The tumours could cause bone resorption, and augmented plasma calcium levels; these effects being diminished by indomethacin.

(9) *In vitro* studies revealed that indomethacin had no direct effect on tumour cell proliferation.

(10) The splenic PHA responsiveness of tumour-bearing animals was drastically depressed, probably due to non-specific suppressor cell (macrophage-like*) activity.

Short-term indomethacin treatment (either *in vivo* or *in vitro*) did not augment the PHA response, although long-term administration (at equivalent tumour burden) caused a slight elevation, and induced a small decrease in suppressor activity.

Tumour cell culture supernatants were in fact stimulatory for the PHA responsiveness of normal spleen cells, and indomethacin reduced this effect.

(11) The tumour enhanced, rather than depressed, splenic Jerne PFC responses, although it decreased the adjuvant effect exerted by indomethacin administered prior to antigen injection.

We have, therefore, suggested that at least part of the therapeutic effect of indomethacin is due to a reactivation of prostaglandin-depressed anaphylactic reactivity in the tumour-bearing animals (3, 4).

Using previously described methods we have subsequently obtained more direct data supporting this possibility. We used the 72 hr latent period passive cutaneous anaphylactic (IgE PCA) titres of a DBA/1 antiovalbumin serum, determined in the skin of the test animals, as a partial evaluation (2) of the anaphylactic reactivity of the host. It can be seen in Table 1 that although short-term oral indomethacin administration (4 days, ~ 100 μg/mouse/day) neither augmented the PCA titres determined in the skin of these mice, nor restored the depressed titres in tumour-bearers, a longer period of treatment

---

*Unpublished observations.

TABLE 1. EFFECT OF McC3-1 AND INDOMETHACIN ON PCA TITRE OF DBA/1
ANTI-OA ANTISERUM

Animal	Tumour cell dose	Day after graft	Indo. days	Tumour* diameter, mm	PCA* titre
Normal	–	–	–	–	640
Indo.	–	–	4	–	640
McC3-1	trocar	38	–	23.8±3.9	80
McC3-1 + Indo	trocar	38	4	24.3±4.1	80
Indo	–	–	33	–	1280
McC3-1	2×10^4	41	–	18.3±2.6	160
McC3-1 + Indo	10^5	41	33	16.2±3.8	640

*Mean ± SD tumour diameters determined in groups of 12 mice, and PCA titres in groups of 3 animals (see ref.2).

TABLE 2. EFFECT OF INDOMETHACIN AND I.T.*C.PARVUM* ON McC57-2 GROWTH, AND
HISTAMINE PGE2 AND MONONUCLEAR CELL CONTENT

Treatment	Days after graft	Indo. days	Tumour* diam. mm	Histamine* ng/mg	PGE2* ng/mg	MNC
Control	40	–	19.4 ±6.3	9.1 ±3.4	0.310 ±0.069	+
Indo.	68	58	16.7 ±5.5	3.2 ±2.4	0.028 ±0.011	++
C. parvum	40	–	8.8 ±4.1	4.7 ±3.1	0.906 ±0.312	+++
C. parvum + Indo.	46	36	6.8 ±4.0	5.6 ±3.6	0.131 ±0.098	+++

*Mean ± SD in groups of 12 mice.

(day 8 to 41 after grafting) increased the titres in the latter animals. It should be noted that in order to compensate for the antitumour effect of the prolonged indomethacin treatment, the control tumour-bearers were initially grafted with lower tumour cell numbers. This reactivation of depressed anaphylactic reactivity in the tumour-bearing animals might be considered to be a direct consequence of the indomethacin-mediated inhibition of PGE2 synthesis (see later), as this prostaglandin is capable of inhibiting mast cell degranulation (7). It might also be proposed that the effect on anaphylactic reactivity is a secondary phenomenon, related for example to diminished histamine levels (see later) causing reduced thachyphylactic or negative feedback auto-inhibition (7). This latter possibility is difficult to dismiss considering the variable effects of vaso-active amine antagonists on tumour growth (1). This variability might now be explained by the conflicting activities of these drugs; inhibition of both tachyphylactic-type effects, and allergic reactivity.

It is also important to remark here that the twice-daily IP injection of 1.5 μg PGE2 into otherwise normal mice for a week caused no consistent change in PCA titres determined in their skin (unpublished results). This lack of effect of PGE2 may, however, be due to the technical difficulties inherent in this type of experiment; PGE2 continuously produced within a tumour would probably be more effective than when injected at widely spaced, though regular, intervals.

As we have previously reported for McC3-1 fibrosarcomas (3), a 3 methylcholanthrene induced transplantable tumour of C57B1/6 mice (McC57-2) was found to contain high levels of "PGE2-like" material (Table 2), as measured by bio-assay (based essentially on the technique described in ref. 3). Tumour histamine concentrations (assayed by instrumental modifications of the method previously employed in ref. 5) were also high. We also attempted to quantitate mononuclear cell (MNC) infiltration into non-necrotic regions of these tumours, but adopted a qualitative assessment based on comparison with the scanty infiltrate into control tumours. As further presented in Table 2, long-term indomethacin administration (day 10 to 68 after grafting) caused a significant slowing of the growth of these tumours; sufficient time was allowed to elapse for the indomethacin group so that the tumours were roughly comparable in size to those of the control animals. In the drug-treated tumours a significant decrease in histamine concentration was observed. One possible explanation for this is that the inhibition of prostaglandin (PGE2?) synthesis reversed the "anaphylactic deficit" (2, 5) experienced by the tumour-bearers, thus diminishing the stimulus for the accumulation of histamine (5). Although we were unable to evaluate changes in mast cell concentrations, MNC infiltration was noted to be somewhat elevated in indomethacin-treated, compared to control, tumours. It is not, however, possible to determine from our results whether the augmented MNC infiltration was the cause, or a consequence, of the anti-tumour effect of this drug.

We also found (Table 2) that the intratumour injection of C. parvum (1, 4) caused a marked antitumour effect, that was accompanied by a substantial elevation in PGE2-like concentrations, and MNC infiltration. This observation might indicate that the high prostaglandin levels are due, at least in part, to the MNC response. Indomethacin treatment augmented the antitumour effect of *C. parvum,* thus reaffirming our impression that changes in PGE2 levels bear little relation to the anti-tumour mechanism; indomethacin and *C. parvum* both demonstrated therapeutic effects, but exerted opposing influences on the levels of this prostaglandin. In the present studies, we have not examined changes in the levels of other members of the prostaglandin series, and so cannot comment on their possible participation.

While our previous results indicated no specific antitumour immunity in mice that had eliminated their tumours under indomethacin administration, a short-lived non-specific resistance was observed (3). We wished to further evaluate the apparent lack of T-cell-dependent immune involvement in the indomethacin effect, by using fibrosarcomas growing in congenitally thymusless nude (nu/nu) mice. However, as we have previously noted for *C. parvum*-treated C3H tumour-bearers (4), toxicity became evident during the drug administration. In the nude system this could not even be satisfactorily overcome by starting with very low doses of oral indomethacin (1–5 µg/ mouse/day). We then tested the effect of indomethacin on a 3 methylcholanthrene-induced fibrosarcoma (McBg-1; see ref. 8 for methods) of beige (bg/bg) mice, which have been reported to be deficient in natural killer (although, significantly, not natural cytotoxic) cells (9, 10). We were only able to test one tumour in relatively small numbers of recipient mice, that had been bred from two pairs that were originally obtained from Jackson Laboratories (Bar Harbour, Maine, U.S.A.). Problems with toxicity during oral indomethacin administration to tumour-bearers were also encountered, although this was substantially overcome by starting at ~ 5 µg/mouse/day and gradually increasing to ~ 100 µg/mouse/day). From our results, such as those presented in Table 3, we concluded that the McBg-2 tumour in bg/bg mice was relatively resistant to indomethacin, under the conditions of the test.

This tumour, however, when growing in the phenotypically normal bg/+ heterozygote appeared to be sensitive to the drug treatment, although interestingly, in most experiments it grew less vigorously in the control animals. These results could be interpreted to suggest that the effect of indomethacin is dependent upon the activity of NK cells. Before this possibility can be accepted, however, various beige tumours should be tested. Also, as indicated in Table 4, a deficiency in NK activity is not the only defect demonstrable in these animals. Thus bg/bg mice, as compared to their bg/+ counterparts, were found to be virtually incapable of expressing anaphylactic-type reactivity. This was not due to an incapacity in the synthesis of anaphylactic antibody, whether IgE or IgG_1 (PCA titres determined in the skin of Fischer rats or Swiss mice respectively). Despite the presence of circulating anaphylactic antibody, the homozygotes did not, however, undergo significant active systemic anaphylaxis (ASA) as measured by % haemoconcentration (2) 20 min after intravenous antigen challenge. Passive cutaneous anaphylaxis (PCA) induced by skin sensitization with DBA/1 antiovalbumin serum was also of considerably lower intensity in bg/bg compared to bg/+, for both IgE and IgG_1 antibody activity. That the defect in bg/bg was localized at the level of the mast cell was suggested by the finding that these animals were at least as, if not more, sensitive to histamine plus serotonin challenge (2) than their heterozygotic counterparts. Considering, therefore, our previously demonstrated association between antitumour mechanisms and

TABLE 3. EFFECT OF CONTINUOUS ORAL INDOMETHACIN ON McBg-1
GROWTH IN bg/bg AND bg/+ MICE

Treatment	Tumour* diameter (day 31) mm	Tumour regression	Survival* days
bg/bg Control	25.8 ± 10.1	0/23	44.3 ± 8.7
bg/bg Indo.	19.2 ± 6.4	0/19	49.6 ± 10.3
bg/+ Control	16.9 ± 4.4	3/15	N.D.
bg/+ Indo.	8.3 ± 3.1	5/13	N.D.

*Mean ± S.D. in groups of 10 mice.
N.D. = not determined.

TABLE 4. ANAPHYLACTIC REACTIVITY IN bg/bg AND bg/+ MICE

Mouse	Anaphyl. Ab titre		ASA* % Hb conc.	PCA titre		Hist. + Sero.* % Hb conc.
	IgG$_1$	IgE		IgG$_1$	IgE	
bg/bg	640	320	13 ± 1	<40	<40	63 ± 5
bg/+	640	160	52 ± 9	640	320	36 ± 7

*Mean ± SD in groups of 5 mice.

anaphylactic activity, the deficit in the latter exhibited by beige mice must be taken into consideration when attempting to use these animals as models lacking effective NK activity.

In conclusion, therefore, although we do not consider anaphylactic-type reactions to exert primary antitumour activity, they may play an accessory role, and part of the therapeutic effect of indomethacin in the fibrosarcoma models examined might be related to a potentiation of these reactions.

BIBLIOGRAPHY

1. LYNCH, N.R. & SALOMON, J.C. (1977). Passive local anaphylaxis; demonstration of antitumour activity and complementation of intratumor BCG. J. Natl. Cancer Inst. *58*, 1093.
2. LYNCH, N.R. & SALOMON, J.C. (1977). Tumour-associated inhibition of immediate hyper-sensitivity reactions in mice. Immunology *32*, 645.
3. LYNCH, N.R., CASTES, M., ASTOIN, M. & SALOMON, J.C. (1978). Mechanism of inhibition of tumour growth by aspirin and indomethacin. Brit. J. Cancer *38*, 503.
4. LYNCH, N.R. & SALOMON, J.C. (1979). Tumour growth inhibition and potentiation of immunotherapy by indomethacin. J. Natl. Cancer Inst. *62*, 117.
5. SCHIENMANN, P., LEBEL, B., LYNCH, N.R., SALOMON, J,C., PAUPE, J.R. & BURTIN, C.J. (1979). Histamine levels in the blood and other tissues of male and female mice. II. Mice carrying a 3-methylcholanthrene induced tumour. Agents & Actions *9*, 95.
6. LYNCH, N.R., SALOMON, J.C. & TURNER, K.J. (1978). Evolutionary development of IgE and the role of anaphylactic-type reactions in resistance to solid tumours. Cancer Immunol. Immunoth. *4*, 223.
7. BOURNE, H.R., LICHTENSTEIN, L.M., MELMON, K.L. *et al* (1974). Modulation of inflam-mation and immunity by cyclic AMP. Science (Wash.) *184*, 19.
8. SALOMON, J.C., CREAU-GOLDBERG, N. & LYNCH, N.R. (1980). Cancer induction by methylcholanthrene and metastatic spread of transplantable tumors in Chediak Higashi (Beige) mice. Canc. Immunol. Immunoth. *8*, 67.
9. KARRE, K., KLEIN, G.O., KIESSLING, R., KLEIN, G. & RODER, J.C. (1980). *In vitro* NK-activity and *in vivo* resistance to leukemia: Studies of beige, beige/nude and wild-type hosts on C57B1 background. Int. J. Cancer. *26*, 789.
10. STUTMAN, O. & CUTTITO, M.J. (1981). Normal levels of natural cytotoxic cells against solid tumours in NK-deficient beige mice. Nature (Lond.) *290*, 254.

**Prostaglandins and Cancer: First
International Conference, pages 783–787
© 1982 Alan R. Liss, Inc., 150 Fifth Avenue, New York, NY 10011**

STIMULATION OF PGI$_2$ BIOSYNTHESIS BY NAFAZATROM (BAY g 6575)

T.E. Eling[1], K.V. Honn[2], W.D. Busse[3], F.
Seuter[3] and L.J. Marnett[2]
[1]National Institute of Enviromental Health
Sciences, [2]Wayne State University, Detroit, MI
[3]Bayer AG, Wuppertal, W. Germany

The experimental drug Nafazatrom (Naf) is a potent
antimetastatic (Honn et al., in press), antithrombotic
(Seuter et al., 1979) agent. Mechanisms for these effects
are not known but they may be mediated by stimulation of
endogenous PGI$_2$ biosynthesis. To test this hypothesis, we
have examined the effect of Naf on several PGI$_2$ biosynthetic systems.

METHODS

Ram seminal vesicles (RSV) were homogenized and the
microsomal fraction (RSVM) prepared as described (Parks and
Eling, 1974). Prostaglandin biosynthesis was determined by
measuring the O$_2$ consumption at 22°C, using a Clark O$_2$ elec-
trode, after addition of 200 µM arachidonic acid (Nu CHEK)
to RSVM. Peroxidatic oxidation of phenylbutazone was determined by measurement of oxygen incorporation into phenylbutazone. PGI$_2$ biosynthesis was estimated by HPLC analysis
of the acid-ethyl acetate extractable products obtained
from an incubation of 1-^{14}C-arachidonic acid (New England
Nuclear) or ^{14}C-PGH$_2$ with RSVM. PGI$_2$ biosynthesis by rat
aortic rings was determined by inhibition of collagen and
ADP-induced platelet aggregation. Rats were pre-treated
with 10-100 mg/kg Naf p.o. before aortic rings were
prepared. Rings of the abdominal aorta were placed in
Tris-buffer (pH 7.4) and incubated for 10 min at 37°C or 30
min at 25°C, respectively. The media was added to the
platelet rich plasma 30 sec prior to addition of the
aggregating agent. Aortas were obtained from 4 groups of

male Wistar rats treated with Naf (10 or 100 mg/kg p.o.) as follows: a) daily for 30 da, b) daily for 10 da, c) two times within 24 hr prior and 90 min prior to sacrifice and d) 90 min prior to sacrifice.

RESULTS

The addition of Naf to RSVM and arachidonic acid (AA) produced a concentration dependent stimulation of prostaglandin biosynthesis as measured by O_2 consumption. 100-200 μM Naf increased the conversion of AA to PGH_2 2 to 3-fold. These data suggest that Naf is functioning as a reducing cofactor for the hydroperoxidase component of prostaglandin endoperoxide synthetase. The hydroperoxidase activity was estimated by measurement of phenylbutazone peroxidatic co-oxidation. As seen in Fig. 1, the addition of Naf to the incubation significantly inhibited phenylbutazone co-oxidation. A concentration dependent inhibition was observed with ID-50 of 20 μM. This is further support that Naf serves as a reducing co-factor for hydroperoxidase activity in RSVM.

The effect of Naf on the biosynthesis of PGI_2 from $1-^{14}C$-AA and $1-^{14}C$-PGH_2 by RSVM was investigated. $1-^{14}C$-PGH_2, at 0.5 and 5 μM, was incubated with RSVM in the presence and absence of 200 μM Naf. At both concentrations of PGH_2 Naf, did not alter the function of PGI_2 from PGH_2. However, 200 μM did alter the biosynthesis of PGI_2 from $1-^{14}C$-AA. The effect of Naf on PGI_2 biosynthesis was dependent on the concentration of AA (Fig. 2). At low concentrations of AA, stimulation of PGI_2 biosynthesis was observed (3 to 6-fold stimulation at 25 μM AA). In the absence of Naf, PGI_2 biosynthesis increased with increasing AA with saturation at 20 μM AA.

Stimulation of PGI_2 synthetase by Naf was also demonstrated using aortic rings. PGI_2 biosynthesis was estimated by inhibition of ADP and collagen-induced platelet aggregation. As seen in Table 1, aortic rings from Naf pretreated rats produced significantly more PGI_2 than rings from untreated rats. These results suggest that Naf stimulates PGI_2 biosynthesis in vivo.

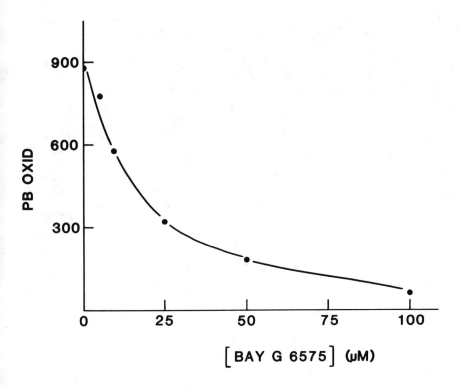

Figure 1. Inhibition of hydrogen peroxide dependent phenylbutazone cooxygenation by Nafazatrom (Bay g 6575). Pheynylbutazone oxidation expressed as µM O$_2$/min/mg.

DISCUSSION

Nafazatrom stimulated the biosynthesis of PGI$_2$ from AA in RSVM preparations. Stimulation was dependent on the concentration of Naf and the concentration of AA used in the incubation systems. At high arachidonic acid concentrations, elevation of PGI$_2$ biosynthesis in the presence of Naf was 3 to 6-fold. At lower AA concentrations, the effect of Naf on PGI$_2$ biosynthesis was less pronounced. Stimulation of PGI$_2$ biosynthesis was also demonstrated using aortic rings from rats pretreated orally with Naf. This effect was measured by the ability of the media from aortic ring incubation mixtures to inhibit platelet aggregation.

These data support the hypothesis that Naf inhibits tumor metastasis by stimulation of PGI2 biosynthesis.

The mechanism for Naf stimulation of PGI2 biosynthesis is not clear. The addition of Naf to incubation mixtures did not alter the conversion of PGH2 to PGI2 suggesting the effect was on the cyclo-oxygenase rather than on PGI2 synthetase. Naf serves as a reducing co-factor for the hydroperoxidase component of fatty acid cyclooxygenase, elevating the conversion of AA to PGH2. Naf is itself co-oxidized by the peroxidase as evidenced by the inhibition of phenylbutazone peroxidatic co-oxidation. PGI2 synthetase is very sensitive to hydro-peroxidase (Salmon, et al., 1978). The stimulation of cyclo-oxygenase and PGI2 synthetase may be mediated by reduction of the steady state level of the hydroperoxide PGG2 by the hydroperoxidase. These results provide additional support for the hypothesis that the anti-metastatic activity of Naf is mediated by stimulation of PGI2 biosynthesis. Further studies are in progress to elucidate the mechanism for stimulation of PGI2 biosynthesis.

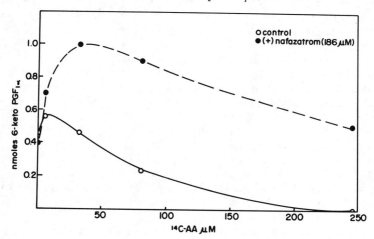

Effect of nafazatrom on biosythesis of PGI2 (6-keto PGF1∝) by RSV microsomes

Figure 2. Effect of Naf on biosynthesis of PGI2 (6-keto PGF1) by RSVM. Open circles = control; closed circles = Naf.

Table 1. Inhibition of Collagen- and ADP-Induced Aggregation by Aortic Rings from Animals Treated with Nafazatrom.

	Collagen-Induced Aggregation				ADP-Induced Aggregation			
	37°C		25°C		37°C		25°C	
Treatment Group	10 [a]	100[a]	10	100	10	100	10	100
A	44[b]	34	34	38	34	38	18	35
B	44	65	66*	56	36	49*	45	47
C	59*	63*	40	61*	15	36*	34	51*
D	36	69	24	25	3	14	1	24

[a]Rats were pretreated with 10 or 100 mg/kg p.o. as described in Methods.
Values expressed as percent inhibition of aggregation.
Astericks indicate value significantly different from control with P ≤ 0.05; n=7.

REFERENCES

Eling T, Warnock R, Dick, Trainer B (1980) Separation of prostaglandins, thromboxanes, hydroxy fatty acids and arachidonic acid by high pressure liquid chromatography. Prost Med 5, 345.

Honn KV, Meyer J, Neagos G, Henderson T, Westley C, Ratanatharathron V. Control of tumor growth and metastasis with prostacyclin and thromboxane synthetase inhibitors: evidence for a new antitumor and antimetastatic agent (Bay g 6575) In Jamieson GA (ed) "Interaction of Platelets and Tumor Cells" New York Alan Liss Inc. (in press).

Parkes D, Eling TE (1974) Characterization of prostaglandin synthetase in guinea pig lung. Isolation of a new prostaglandin derivative from arachidonic acid. Biochemistry 13, 2598.

Salmon JA, Smith DR, Flower RJ, Moncada S, Vane JR (1978) Further studies on the enzymatic conversion of prostaglandin endoperoxide into prostacyclin by porcine aorta microsomes. Biochim. Biophys. Acta. 523, 250.

Seuter F, Busse WD, Meng K, Hoffmeister F, Moeller E, Horstmann H (1979) The antithrombotic activity of Bay g 6575 Arzneim-Forsch/Drug Res 29, 54.

**Prostaglandins and Cancer: First
International Conference, pages 789-792**
© 1982 Alan R. Liss, Inc., 150 Fifth Avenue, New York, NY 10011

LIPOXYGENASE PRODUCTS AS MEDIATORS OF TUMOR CELL LYSOSOMAL ENZYME RELEASE: INHIBITION BY NAFAZATROM

B.F. Sloane, S. Makim, J.R. Dunn, R. Lacoste, M. Theodorou, J. Battista, R. Alex and K.V. Honn
Departments of Pharmacology, Radiation Oncology, Radiology, Chemistry and Biological Sciences
Wayne State University, Detroit, MI 48201

INTRODUCTION

In a recent review Borgeat and Sirois (1981) summarized the relationship between 20:4 metabolites and lysosomal enzyme release thusly: agents which increase cellular levels of cAMP inhibit lysosomal enzyme release, whereas agents which increase cGMP induce release. In contrast to the cyclooxygenase products (PGI_2, PGE_2, etc.) which increase cellular cAMP levels (Hopkins and Gorman, 1981), products of the lipoxygenase pathway have been shown to increase cellular cGMP (Hidaka and Asano, 1977).

In this study we examine the relationship between 20:4 metabolites and lysosomal enzyme release from B16 amelanotic melanoma (B16a) cells grown in tissue culture. We measured activities of three lysosomal enzymes fluorometrically (Sloane et al., 1981): β-N-acetyl glucosaminidase (β-NAG), a marker enzyme for lysosomes; β-glucuronidase (β-GLU), an enzyme whose release from macrophages has been extensively studied, and cathepsin B, a cysteine proteinase whose activity in tumor cells we have shown to correlate positively with metastatic potential (Sloane et al., 1981) and with onset of metastasis. Arachidonic acid metabolism was measured in the microsomal pellet (m.p.) and microsomal supernatant (m.s.) of B16a tumors. Cyclooxygenase activity (indomethacin sensitive) was found in the m.p., whereas lipoxygenase activity was in the m.s. ^{14}C-arachidonic acid conversion into metabolites was determined by TLC.

Release of β-NAG was stimulated 50-60% and of β-GLU 80-100% by a 24 hr exposure to a mixture of lipoxygenase products, 12- and 15-hydroperoxyeicosatetraenoic acid (12- and 15-HPETE) at 0.03 and 3.0 µg/ml. In contrast a 24 hr exposure to 15-HPETE (0.3 and 3.0 µg/ml) did not enhance release of β-NAG, β-GLU or cathepsin B. Release of β-NAG and cathepsin B was significantly decreased (18% and 42%, respectively) after exposure to 15-HPETE at 0.03 µg/ml.

Indomethacin (1 and 10 µM), an inhibitor of the cyclo-oxygenase pathway, did not affect release of β-NAG, β-GLU or cathepsin B. NDGA, an inhibitor of the lipoxygenase pathway, at 0.1 and 1.0 µg/ml decreased the release of β-NAG and β-GLU at 24, 48 and 72 hr (Table 1).

TABLE 1. Effect of NDGA on Lysosomal Enzyme Release From B16a Melanoma Cells in Culture

NDGA	β-NAG			β-GLU		
	24 h	48 h	72 h	24 h	48 h	72 h
0.1 µg/ml	49±1*	48±3*	50±3*	52±2*	67±13*	69±18*
1.0 µg/ml	53±4*	56±6*	52±4*	61±4*	105±14	46±8*

Values are expressed as µM 4-methyl-umbelliferone produced per µg DNA per min as a percentage of the control value; x̄ ± SEM. Asterisks indicate p ≤ 0.05.

We have recently found that Nafazatrom, a potent anti-metastatic and antiproliferative agent (Honn et al., in press), inhibits the formation of an unidentified monohy-droxy fatty acid from the lipoxygenase pathway by B16a cells (Figure 1; ED_{50} = 5 µM). This product was not inhi-bited by indomethacin but was inhibited by ETYA (ED_{50} = 0.9 µM).

Nafazatrom at 1, 5 and 25 µg/ml decreased cathepsin B release from B16a cells after 3 or 7 days of exposure (Figure 2). β-NAG and β-GLU release was inhibited by exposure to 1, 5 or 25 µg/ml of Nafazatrom for 3 days (not illustrated). In vivo administration of Nafazatrom (p.o.) at 0.3 mg/animal/da x 22 da to animals bearing subcutaneous B16a tumors significantly decreased both cathepsin B and β-NAG activity in the tumors and increased the life span of

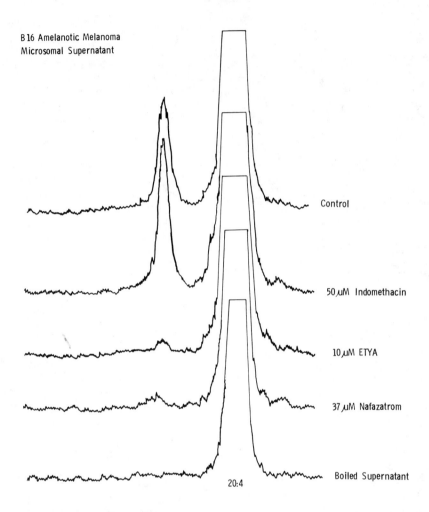

B 16 Amelanotic Melanoma
Microsomal Supernatant

Control

50 µM Indomethacin

10 µM ETYA

37 µM Nafazatrom

Boiled Supernatant

20:4

Figure 1. Radiochromatogram scan of unidentified monohydroxy fatty acid produced by B16a melanoma cells. Product was chromatographed in benzene:ethylether:EtOH: acetic acid (50:40:2:0.2).

these animals (data not shown). These preliminary studies suggest that lysosomal enzyme release by tumor cells may be increased by agents which increase cGMP and decreased by agents which increase cAMP.

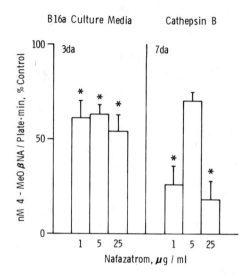

Figure 2. Cathepsin B activity released into the media upon exposure to Nafazatrom (Bay g 6575). Media and drug were changed daily so that the release was measured over a 24 hr period.

REFERENCES

Borgeat P, Sirois P (1981). Leukotrienes: a major step in the understanding of immediate hypersensitivity reactions. J Med Chem 24:121.

Hopkins NK, Gorman RR (1981). Regulation of 3T3-L1 fibroblast differentiation by prostacyclin (prostaglandin I_2). Biochim Biophys Acta 663:457.

Hidaka H, Asano T (1977). Stimulation of human platelet guanylate cyclase by unsaturated fatty acid peroxides. Proc Natl Acad Sci USA 74:3657.

Sloane BF, Dunn JR, Honn KV (1981). Lysosomal cathepsin B: correlation with metastatic potential. Science 212:1151.

Honn KV, Meyer J, Neagos G, Henderson T, Westley C, Ratanatharathron V, Control of tumor growth and metastasis with prostacyclin and thromboxane synthetase inhibitors: Evidence for a new antitumor and antimetastatic agent (Bay g 6575) In Jamieson GA (ed) "Interaction of Platelets and Tumor Cells," New York: Alan R. Liss, in press.

**Prostaglandins and Cancer: First
International Conference, pages 793-797**
© 1982 Alan R. Liss, Inc., 150 Fifth Avenue, New York, NY 10011

PROTECTION AGAINST MISONIDAZOLE-INDUCED TOXICITY IN VITRO
BY FLURBIPROFEN, A NON-STEROIDAL ANTI-INFLAMMATORY AGENT.

Barbara C. Millar[+], Sally Jinks[+] and Trevor J. Powles*

[+]Radiobiology Unit, Physics Department, Institute
of Cancer Research, Sutton, Surrey, U.K.
*Division of Medicine, Royal Marsden Hospital,
Sutton, Surrey, U.K.

INTRODUCTION

Cells which are depleted of oxygen are more resistant to
the lethal effects of ionizing radiation than well-oxygenated
cells and when present in tumours may form foci for regrowth
after radiotherapy. Misonidazole, a 2-nitroimidazole, has
been shown to selectively sensitize hypoxic mammalian cells
to radiation *in vitro* (for review see Adams *et al.*, 1978) and
in vivo (Denekamp and Harris, 1975) and clinical trials are
in progress to determine whether the drug is likely to provide
any therapeutic advantage in radiotherapy regimes (Dische
et al., 1977; Urtason *et al.*, 1977; Jentzch *et al.*, 1977;
Bleehen, 1980).

However, despite the possible advantages of using misonidazole with radiation treatments for cancer, the use of the
drug clinically is limited because of neurotoxicity (Dische
et al., 1977) which may be related to its toxicity to cells
in vitro (Hall and Roizin-Towle, 1975). Nitroaromatic compounds such as misonidazole can be reduced by some enzymes
acting as nitroreductases which could result in the production
of toxic radical anions, superoxide radicals and hydrogen
peroxide (Biaglow *et al.*, 1977; Mason and Holtzman, 1975).

There is some evidence that dexamethasone protects against
misonidazole-induced neurotoxicity in man (Wasserman *et al.*,
1980). Unfortunately, from experiments *in vitro* there is an
indication that the radiation sensitivity of cells is decreased
by this agent (Millar and Jinks, 1981). Thus other agents
are being examined in an attempt to reduce the toxicity of

misonidazole without affecting its radiosensitizing properties. This report concerns the effect of a non-steroidal anti-inflammatory agent (NSAIA), flurbiprofen, on the radiation response and cytotoxic effect of misonidazole in mammalian cells *in vitro*.

MATERIALS AND METHODS

Compounds

Misonidazole and $2\text{-}C^{14}$-misonidazole (53.6 μCi/mg) were kindly supplied by Roche Products (Welwyn Garden City, Herts, England). Flurbiprofen sulphate was a generous gift from the Boots Drug Company (Nottingham, Notts, England).

Cell Culture

Chinese hamster cells V.79-753B were used throughout the work. The routine handling of cells was carried out using methods described previously (Cooke *et al.*, 1976). All experimental procedures have been reported elsewhere (Millar and Jinks, 1981; Millar, Jinks and Powles, 1981). Cultures were routinely treated with 5 x 10^{-5}M flurbiprofen for approximately 20 hr prior to and during experiments.

RESULTS AND DISCUSSION

When cells were pretreated with flurbiprofen they became more resistant to the toxic effects of misonidazole both in air and in hypoxia (Table 1). The protection afforded to flurbiprofen-treated cells was equivalent to a dose reduction factor of two for the amount of misonidazole required to produce a given amount of cell killing (Table 1). This protection could not be explained on the basis of a differential uptake of misonidazole into untreated and flurbiprofen-treated cells since there was no significant difference in the incorporation of $2\text{-}C^{14}$-misonidazole in untreated (24.5%) and treated cultures (29.5%). Furthermore, there was no change in either the radiation sensitivity of flurbiprofen-treated cells in air or in hypoxia or in the degree of hypoxic cell sensitization produced by misonidazole. The lack of change in radiation sensitivity after treatment with flurbiprofen is in contrast to that previously reported for cells treated with dexametha-

Table 1. Toxicity of misonidazole in untreated and flurbiprofen-treated (5×10^{-5}M) Chinese hamster cells, V-79-753B, after a 4 hr exposure time.

Concentration misonidazole (mM)	Hypoxic conditions		Aerobic conditions	
	$Fbf^{(+)}$	$Fbf^{(-)}$ *	$Fbf^{(+)}$	$Fbf^{(-)}$
1.0	100.0	95.0	100.0	100.0
5.0	90.0	24.0	100.0	90.0
10.0	64.0	10.0	100.0	71.0
15.0	23.0	5.5	78.0	48.0
20.0	11.5	2.7	66.0	40.0

*$Fbf^{(+)}$ - flurbiprofen-treated cells.
$Fbf^{(-)}$ - untreated cells.

sone (Millar and Jinks, 1981) which not only protected cells against misonidazole-induced hypoxic cell cytotoxicity but also increased the radiation resistance of the cells by approximately 25%.

Other workers have shown that sulphydryl compounds protect against misonidazole-induced toxicity *in vitro* (Taylor and Rauth, 1981). However, it is unlikely that protection by flurbiprofen is mediated by an increase in endogenous SH since such a change would have increased the radiation resistance of cells (Millar, Fielden and Steele, 1980).

Varghese and Whitmore (1980) have suggested nitro-reduction and the binding of nitro-reduced products to macromolecules as a probable mechanism for the mutagenic and cytotoxic properties of misonidazole. We have recently reported that flurbiprofen does not protect against melphalan toxicity, a compound which does not require metabolic activation. Thus it is arguable that flurbiprofen protection against misonidazole-induced toxicity may be mediated by the inhibition of events leading to the production of toxic products.

Flurbiprofen is a potent inhibitor of prostaglandin biosynthesis and there is evidence that the metabolism of benzidine, a carcinogen, is mediated by enzymes involved in prostaglandin biosynthesis (Zenser, Mattammal and Davis, 1979; Zenser *et al.*, 1980). Further experiments are in progress to determine whether the catabolism of misonidazole is mediated by similar processes.

In conclusion, this report indicates that flurbiprofen, like dexamethasone, reduces the cytotoxicity of misonidazole *in vitro* in air and in hypoxia without affecting the hypoxic cell radiosensitizing properties of the compound. However, unlike dexamethasone it does not increase the radiation resistance of cells. In clinical studies repeated dosage with 50 mg of flurbiprofen given 3 times daily for 10 days produced a mean serum concentration of 2.43 µg/ml (equivalent to 10^{-5}M) (Cardoe *et al.*, 1975). This has important therapeutic implications because of the known toxicity of misonidazole *in vivo*. We are therefore undertaking toxicity studies with flurbiprofen and other similar agents with misonidazole *in vivo*.

ACKNOWLEDGEMENTS

We would like to thank Mr J. Currant for valuable technical assistance and Professor G.E. Adams and Dr E. Martin Fielden for helpful discussions. The work was supported by CRC/MRC funding.

REFERENCES

Adams GE, Fowler JR, Wardman P (1978). Eds. Hypoxic cells in radiobiology and radiotherapy. Br J Cancer 37:Supp. III.
Biaglow JE, Jacobson B, Greenstock CL, Raleigh J (1977). Effect of nitrobenzene derivatives on electron transfer in cellular and chemical models. Molecular Pharmacology 13:269.
Bleehen N (1980). The Cambridge glioma trial of misonidazole and radiation therapy with associated pharmacokinetic studies. Radiation Sensitizers. In Brady LW (ed) "Cancer Management" 5:374.
Cooke BC, Fielden EM, Johnson M, Smithen CE (1976). Polyfunctional Radiosensitizers I. Effect of a nitroxyl biradical on the survival of mammalian cells *in vitro*. Radiat Res 65:152.
Denekamp J, Harris S (1975). Tests of two electron affinic radiosensitizers *in vivo* using regrowth of an experimental carcinoma. Radiat Res 61:191.
Dische S, Saunders MI, Lee ME, Adams GE, Flockhart IR (1977). Clinical testing of the radiosensitizer Ro.07-0582: experiences with multiple dose. Br J Cancer 35:567.

Hall EJ, Roizin-Towle L (1975). Hypoxic sensitizers: radiobiological studies at the cellular level. Radiobiology
117:453.
Jentzch K, Karcher KH, Kogensik HD and 5 other authors (1977).
Initial clinical experience with the radiosensitizing nitro-
imidazole Ro.07-0582. Strahlen Therapie 153:825.
Mason RP, Holtzman JL (1975). The mechanism of microsomal
and mitochondrial nitroreductase. Electron spin resonance
evidence for nitroaromatic free radical intermediates.
Biochemistry 14:1626.
Millar BC, Fielden EM, Steele JJ (1980). Effect of combinations of misonidazole and L-cysteine or DMSO on the survival
of Chinese hamster cells V.79-753B *in vitro*. In Brady LW
(ed) "Cancer Management" 5:450.
Millar BC, Jinks S (1981). The effect of dexamethasone on the
radiation survival response and misonidazole-induced
hypoxic cell cytotoxicity in Chinese hamster cells, V79-753B
in vitro. Br J Radiol (in press).
Millar BC, Jinks S, Powles TJ (1981). Flurbiprofen, a non-
steroidal anti-inflammatory agent, protects against the
cytotoxic effects of hypoxic cell radiosensitizers *in vitro*.
Br J Cancer (in press).
Taylor YC, Rauth AM (1980). Sulphydryls, ascorbate and oxygen
as modifiers of the toxicity of misonidazole *in vitro*.
Br J Cancer 41:892.
Urtason RC, Band PR, Chapman JS, Rabin H, Wilson AF, Fryer GG
(1977). Clinical phase I study of the hypoxic cell radiosensitizer Ro.07-0582, a 2-nitroimidazole derivative.
Radiology 122:801.
Varghese AJ, Whitmore GF (1980). Binding to cellular macro-
molecules as a possible mechanism for the cytotoxicity of
misonidazole. Cancer Res 40:2165.
Wasserman TH, Phillips TL, Van-Raalte G and 6 other authors
(1980). The neurotoxicity of misonidazole: potential
modifying role of phenytoin sodium and dexamethasone. Br
J Cancer 53:172.
Zenser TV, Mattammal MB, Davis BB (1979) . Co-oxidation of
benzidine by renal medullary prostaglandin cyclooxygenase.
J Pharm and Exp Therap 211:460.
Zenser TV, Mattammal MB, Armbrecht HG, David BB (1980)
Benzidine binding to nucleic acids mediated by the peroxi-
dative activity of prostaglandin endoperoxide synthetase.
Cancer Res 40:2839.

**Prostaglandins and Cancer: First
International Conference, pages 799–802
© 1982 Alan R. Liss, Inc., 150 Fifth Avenue, New York, NY 10011**

EFFECTS OF ANTI-INFLAMMATORY AGENTS AND RADIOTHERAPY ON
ESOPHAGEAL MUCOSA AND TUMORS IN ANIMALS

MG Northway, A Bennett, MA Carroll, GL Eastwood,
MS Feldman, HI Libshitz, JJ Mamel and IA Szwarc,
King's College Hospital Medical School, London,
England, University of Texas Systems Cancer Center,
Houston, TX, USA and University of Massachusetts
Medical School, Worcester, MA, USA.

One of the major goals in treatment of neoplastic tumors
with radiotherapy is the radioprotection of normal tissue
without simultaneous protection of tumor. Previous studies
from our laboratory using the opossum (Didelphis virginiana)
have provided evidence that the nonsteroidal anti-inflammatory agent indomethacin significantly decreases experimental
radiation esophagitis whereas treatment with 16,16-dimethyl
prostaglandin E_2 exacerbates the condition (Northway et al,
1980).

The present studies were designed to evaluate the effectiveness of two additional anti-inflammatory drugs, aspirin
and hydrocortisone, as agents to protect normal esophageal
mucosa during irradiation, and to determine whether anti-
inflammatory drugs also protect the mouse WHT-NC transplantable mammary tumor (Bennett et al 1978, 1979) during
radiotherapy.

METHODS

Radiation Esophagitis in Opossums

Eighteen opossums were evaluated by fiberoptic endoscopy
and air contrast barium esophagram prior to irradiation with
2250 rad ^{60}Co in a single exposure to the esophagus as described previously (Northway et al 1979a,b). Six opossums
received 600mg aspirin by suppository, 6 received hydrocortisone 25mg/kg i.m. and 6 controls received 0.5ml saline

i.m., 1 hour prior to irradiation, then twice daily for 10
days.   Each opossum was evaluated 10 days post-irradiation
by repeat endoscopy and barium esophagram, killed, and its
esophagus removed for histology.

Mammary Tumors in Mice

Sixty adult male WHT/HT mice received approximately
1×10^6 cells s.c. in the left flank.   Thirty mice received
flurbiprofen 2.5mg/kg, a newer nonsteroidal anti-inflammatory
agent (The Boots Company Ltd, Nottingham, UK), p.o. in 0.1ml
syrup twice daily throughout the study.   Thirty control mice
received syrup.   Twenty days post-inoculation, 10 mice from
each group received 0, 1000 or 2500 rad x-irradiation (Marconi
TF 1554 250KV therapy unit) to the tumor in a single exposure.
Tumors were measured with calipers on all mice and tumor
volumes were determined before irradiation and immediately
before the mice were killed.   Mice receiving 2500 rad were
killed 6 days post-irradiation; those receiving 0 or 1000
rad were killed 7 days post-irradiation.   All tumors were
removed, weighed, sectioned for histology and extracted and
bioassayed against prostaglandin E_2 (Bennett et al 1973).

RESULTS AND DISCUSSION

Effects of Anti-inflammatory Drugs on Radiation Esophagitis

Histologic, endoscopic and radiologic evaluation of each
esophagus was performed by investigators unaware of the treatment groups.   Each specimen was graded as 0, 1+, 2+ or 3+
for normal mucosa or mild, moderate or severe mucosal changes
respectively.

Table 1.   Evaluation of Irradiated Opossum Esophagus

	Controls	Aspirin	Hydrocortisone
Esophagram	2.6 ± 0.4	1.8 ± 0.3	$1.2 \pm 0.4*$
Endoscopy	2.7 ± 0.3	$0.8 \pm 0.3*$	1.7 ± 0.4
Histology	2.5 ± 0.2	$1.6 \pm 0.2*$	1.8 ± 0.3

Each value is the mean damage score $\pm$ S.E.M. of 6 animals in
each group.
* P<0.05 different from control by Rank Sum Test.

As shown in Table 1, opossums treated with aspirin showed less endoscopic and histologic abnormality of the esophageal mucosa compared to control irradiated animals. Opossums treated with hydrocortisone showed less esophageal abnormality as determined by barium esophagram. These studies confirm our previous findings which showed that indomethacin protected normal opossum esophageal mucosa during radiotherapy. They suggest that nonsteroidal anti-inflammatory drugs should be tried in patients undergoing mediastinal radiotherapy.

Effects of Flurbiprofen on Responses of Mouse Mammary Tumor to Irradiation

Mouse mammary tumor weights decreased in response to each dose of x-irradiation regardless of flurbiprofen or syrup treatment. Tumors from flurbiprofen-treated mice in each irradiation group tended to weigh less. Tumor volumes increased in unirradiated mice from day 20 to day 27. They also increased after 1000 rad in controls but not in flurbi-profen-treated mice. In contrast, tumor volumes decreased in all mice given 2500 rad regardless of flurbiprofen or syrup treatment. Prostaglandin-like material extracted from tumors receiving 0 or 1000 rad was bioassayed on rat gastric fundus as prostaglandin E_2 equivalents. The amount increased after 1000 rad in controls but not in flurbiprofen-treated mice (Table 2).

Treat-ment	Rads	Tumor Wt (mg)	Pre-irrad Volume(ml)	Post-irrad Volume(ml)	PGE_2 Equiv (pg/g)
Syrup	2500	270[b]	0.46	0.18[c]	NA
	1000	400[a]	0.53	0.63[c]	109[a]
	0	610	0.53	0.98[c]	66
Flur	2500	180[b]	0.37	0.18[c]	NA
	1000	340[a]	0.41	0.49	73
	0	520	0.52	0.90[c]	58

Table 2. Effects of flurbiprofen (Flur) treatment on responses of mouse mammary tumor to irradiation (irrad), 8-10 mice/group, mean results shown.
a P<0.05 compared with 0 irradiation
b P<0.05 compared with 1000 rad irradiation
c P<0.01 compared with pre-irradiation volume
NA Not assayed

Our data thus provide evidence that agents such as the non-steroidal anti-inflammatory drugs may have clinical useful-ness in patients undergoing therapeutic thoracic radiotherapy by reducing the untoward effects of radiotherapy on the eso-phagus, without simultaneous radioprotection of malignant tumors.

REFERENCES

Bennett A, Stamford IF, Unger WG (1973). Prostaglandin E_2 and gastric acid secretion in man. J Physiol 229:349.
Bennett A, Houghton J, Leaper DJ, Stamford IF (1978). Tumor growth and response to treatment: beneficial effect of the prostaglandin synthesis inhibitor flurbiprofen. Br J Pharmacol 63:356P.
Bennett A, Houghton J, Leaper DJ, Stamford IF (1979). Cancer growth, response to treatment and survival time in mice: beneficial effects of the prostaglandin synthesis inhibitor flurbiprofen. Prostaglandins 17:179.
Northway MG, Libshitz HI, West JH, Withers HR, Mukhopadhyay AK, Osborne BM, Szwarc IA, Dodd GD (1979). The opossum as an animal model for studying radiation esophagitis. Radiology 131:731.
Northway MG, Libshitz HI, Szwarc IA (1979). A technique for barium esophagram in the opossum. Lab Animal Sci 29:534.
Northway MG, Libshitz HI, Osborne BM, Feldman MS, Mamel JJ, West JH, Szwarc IA (1980). Radiation esophagitis in the opossum: radio-protection with indomethacin. Gastro-enterology 78:833.

**Prostaglandins and Cancer: First
International Conference, pages 803–808
© 1982 Alan R. Liss, Inc., 150 Fifth Avenue, New York, NY 10011**

THE RESULTS OF STUDIES OF FLURBIPROFEN IN CANCER

G. J. Frank

Medical Adviser, Research Department,
The Boots Company Ltd., Nottingham, England.

INTRODUCTION

Flurbiprofen, 2-(2-fluoro-4-biphenylyl) propionic
acid, is a very potent anti-inflammatory agent. Although
it is a most potent inhibitor of the synthesis of prostaglandins by cyclo-oxygenase there is little evidence that
it can antagonise the actions of prostaglandins at therapeutic concentrations. It also inhibits the lipoxygenase
pathway (as suggested by its potent effect at inhibiting
leucocyte migration), and is one of the most potent
inhibitors of platelet aggregation known. Its effects on
tumour growth are summarized in Tables 1 and 2.

THE EFFECT OF FLURBIPROFEN ON THE MURINE MAMMARY NC TUMOUR

Bennett et al in 1978 demonstrated that flurbiprofen
(5 mg/kg orally given from the day of injection of tumour)
significantly reduced primary tumour weight. Another
experiment showed that flurbiprofen could enhance the
effect of radiotherapy and/or chemotherapy.

Leaper et al also demonstrated that the effect of
adjuvant chemotherapy and local radiotherapy on local
metastases and survival time tended to be greater when
flurbiprofen (2.5 mg/kg daily) was given.

TABLE 1

EFFECT OF FLURBIPROFEN ON TUMOUR GROWTH IN VIVO

Assessment of response	In vivo tumour model							
	NC	S180	Lewis lung 1°	Lewis lung 2°	Walker	3LL	TLX5	L1210
Reduces 1° tumour growth	+	+	+				-	-
Enhances survival time	+	+						
" radiotherapy	+	+	+					
" chemotherapy	+	+		-		+	+|	-
Enhances chemotherapy and/or radiotherapy on:								
local recurrence	+							
volume of metastases	+							
survival	+	+						
1° tumour weight	+							
Reduces resistance to chemotherapy					+			
Reduces prostaglandin content of tumour	+	+						

+ = positive effect
- = negative effect

EFFECT OF FLURBIPROFEN ON THE LEWIS LUNG TUMOUR

Professor Hellmann has studied the effect of inhibiting prostaglandin synthesis in various animal tumour systems. Using the Lewis Lung tumour model, he showed that treatment with flurbiprofen alone produced an approximately 30% reduction in primary tumour weight.

When flurbiprofen was given in addition to the cytotoxic compound studied. He also found similar results using the sarcoma S180 tumour model. Flurbiprofen had no effect however on the leukemia L1210 tumour or the lymphoma TLX5 tumour.

EFFECT OF FLURBIPROFEN AS ADJUVANT TO RADIOTHERAPY USING S180 TUMOUR

Hellmann has demonstrated flurbiprofen to be effective at enhancing the effect of radiotherapy on the S180 tumour if given before and after radiotherapy, but it was not effective when only given after radiotherapy. It appears therefore that it is necessary to inhibit prostaglandin synthesis before giving radiotherapy.

EFFECT ON TUMOUR MEDIATED OSTEOLYSIS

Galasko et al (1980) demonstrated that human mammary cancers as well as the rabbit VX2 carcinoma could be cultured against mouse calvarium and that the tumour osteolytic activity could be measured by the amount of calcium released into the culture fluid. It is possible to assess the effect of non-steroidal anti-inflammatory drugs and diphosphonates by adding these compounds in varying concentrations to the culture fluid.

The results for the osteolytically active tumours showed that the most active antiosteolytic agent was the combination of a prostaglandin synthetase inhibitor and a diphosphonate. The most effective sole agent was flurbiprofen $2.4 \times 10^{-6}M$. The results suggest that the osteolysis produced by human mammary cancer can be significantly inhibited by flurbiprofen.

TABLE 2
EFFECT OF FLURBIPROFEN ON TUMOUR GROWTH IN VITRO

Assessment of response	In vitro tumour model		
	Human mammary carcinoma	VX2	B16
Reduces osteolysis	+	+	
Enhances effect of diphosphonates	+	+	
Reduces survival			+

TABLE 3
EFFECT OF FLURBIPROFEN ON TOXICITY OF CHEMOTHERAPY AND RADIOTHERAPY

Toxicity assessment	Toxic agent						
	In vivo				Irradiation	In vitro	
	Anthra-cyclines	Chloram-bucil	ICRF 159	Melphalan		Misoni-dazole	Nitro-furantoin
Median survival time	+		+	+	+		
Gastrointestinal toxicity				+			
Peripheral leukocyte count		+					
Marrow stem cell					+		
Chinese Hamster cells						+	+

PROTECTION OF THE HOST AFTER IRRADIATION OR CYTOTOXIC
THERAPY BY FLURBIPROFEN

Bone marrow removed from animals which have been
heavily irradiated with 900 rads of whole body irradiation
normally develops into very few colonies in the spleens of
donor animals but the results of Powles and Millar (1979)
showed flurbiprofen (14 mg/kg/day for 3 days) to markedly
increase the recovery of the bone marrow from 4.1 to 56.0
stem cells on day 7.

Measurement of the recovery of the peripheral white
cell count 8 days after a single large dose of chlorambucil
(10 mg/kg i.p.) showed adjuvant flurbiprofen (21 mg/kg/day
for 3 days) to increase the peripheral leukocyte recovery
by 66%.

When a high dose of melphalan (20 mg/kg) was given to
mice, over 90% died within 5 days but when this agent was
given with flurbiprofen (12 mg/kg/day for 3 days) the
mortality was markedly reduced, presumably by enhanced
recovery from gut toxicity. (Powles and Millar 1979).
Table 3 summarizes the effects of flurbiprofen on reducing
toxicity.

OUTLINE OF CLINICAL TRIAL PROGRAMME

The above results suggest that flurbiprofen may have a
beneficial adjuvant effect when given with chemotherapy or
radiotherapy, and also reduce the side effects of such
treatment. This reduction of side effects could enable
higher doses to be given. Double-blind clinical trials on
the effect of treatment have been established in patients
suffering from tumours known to normally have a high
prostaglandin content. In addition, clinical trials on the
effect of flurbiprofen at reducing the side effects of
radiotherapy are in progress.

A study of 200 patients with breast cancer will be
completed in 1982.

REFERENCES

Bennett A, Houghton J, Leaper DJ, Stamford IF (1978). Tumour growth and response to treatment: beneficial effect of the prostaglandin synthesis inhibitor flurbiprofen. Brit J Pharmacol 63:356.

Bennett A, Houghton J, Leaper DJ, Stamford IF (1979). Cancer growth, response to treatment and survival time in mice: beneficial effect of the prostaglandin synthesis inhibitor flurbiprofen. Prostaglandins 17:179.

Berstock DA, Houghton J, Bennett A (1980). Improved anti-cancer effect by combining cytotoxic drugs with an inhibitor of prostaglandin synthesis. In "Advances in prostaglandin and thromboxane research", Vol 6, p 567. Ed: Samuelsson B, Ramwell PW, Paoletti R. Raven Press, New York.

Galasko CSB, Rushton S, Lacey E, Samuel AW (1981). Paper presented to the American Orthopaedic Research Society, Las Vegas, February 1981.

Hellmann K (1980). Personal Communication.

Leaper DJ, French BT, Bennett A (1979). Breast cancer and prostaglandins:a new approach to treatment.Br J Surg 66:683.

Powles TJ, Millar JL (1979). Non-steroidal anti-inflammatory drugs and cytotoxics. Cancer treatment reviews 6 (Supplement) 63.

**Prostaglandins and Cancer: First
International Conference, pages 809–813**
© **1982 Alan R. Liss, Inc., 150 Fifth Avenue, New York, NY 10011**

TUMOR CELL INDUCED PLATELET AGGREGATION: INHIBITION BY PROSTACYCLIN, THROMBOXANE A_2 AND PHOSPHODIESTERASE INHIBITORS.

D. Menter, G. Neagos, J. Dunn, R. Palazzo, T.T. Tchen, J.D. Taylor and K.V. Honn
Wayne State University, Detroit, MI 48202

INTRODUCTION

The control of tumor growth and metastasis with prostacyclin (PGI_2) as well as thromboxane A_2 synthetase (TxA_2) inhibitors has been discussed in a recent review (Honn et al., in press). The possible pharmacological management of metastasis via the use of an antimetastatic, tumoricidal agent are also discussed in the aforementioned review. The fact that tumor cells are capable of initiating platelet aggregation in platelet rich plasma (PRP) has been well documented by Gasic and co-workers (Gasic et al., 1973, 1976, 1978).

More recently Hara and co-workers reported that the use of tumor cell membrane fragments also initiated platelet aggregation in PRP as well as washed platelets (Hara, et al., 1980). The actual mechanism by which tumor cells initiate platelet aggregation is yet unknown. In the present studies we have addressed the involvement of TxA_2 in tumor cell induced platelet aggregation. In addition, we discuss aggregatory inhibition by prostacyclin (PGI_2) as well as by TxA_2 synthetase and phosphodiesterase inhibitors.

MATERIALS AND METHODS

B16 amelanotic and Lewis Lung tumor cell lines were maintained via subcutaneous injection into syngeneic C57BL/6J mice. Tumor cells were obtained via dispersion and a high viability fraction was isolated by centrifugal elutriation (Sloane et al., 1981).

Washed platelet preparations were obtained via a modified version of a previously described technique (Hamberg et al., 1974). Platelets were resuspended in Hanks balanced salt solution with Ca^{++} and Mg^{++} divalent cations at various concentrations (optimal concentrations - 1.8 mM Ca^{++} and 4.0 mM Mg^{++}).

Aggregometry cuvettes contained 250 μl of washed platelets in addition to platelet poor plasma (PPP) at 1-10 μl. Tumor cells were added to a final concentration of 1 X 10^4 - 2 X 10^5 cell/ml by volume. Aggregometry studies were carried out on a Sienco DP-247E dual channel aggregometer. Thromboxane A_2 (TxA_2) production was measured via TxB_2 radioimmunoassay (RIA). Aggregometry samples were removed and snap frozen for the RIA at various phases of the aggregation curve. Inhibition of tumor cell induced platelet aggregation was monitored via direct addition of various inhibitors to aggregometry cuvettes.

RESULTS

Washed platelet aggregation was initiated by 1 X 10^4 - 2 X 10^5 tumor cells/ml. The induction of aggregates was shown to be dependent on the presence of divalent cations (1.8mM Ca^{++}, 4.0 mM Mg^{++}) as well as a minimal concentration of platelet poor plasma (0.5%)

Washed platelet aggregation proceeded in two phases. The initial phase appears to be dependent on the production of thromboxane A_2 as indicated by the following lines of evidence: 1) tumor cells stimulate the productions of thromboxane by the platelets (Fig. 2); 2) TxA_2 synthetase inhibitors 9,11-azoprosta-5,13-dienoic acid (4 ng/ml) (Fig. 1,e) and 9,11-imminoepoxyprosta-5,13-dienoic acid (4 ng/ml) (Fig. 1,e) were both shown to eliminate the first phase of aggregation. In addition, PGI_2 (solubilized in benzene/acetone) was shown to delay tumor cell induced washed platelet aggregation at a concentration of 500 pg/ml and completely inhibit the first phase of aggregation at concentrations of 1-5,000 ng/ml (Fig. 1c and d).

The final phase of tumor cell induced washed platelet aggregation appears to be dependent upon the presence of divalent cations and independent of ADP. Washed platelets preincubated with apyrase (0.5 mg/ml), which blocks the action of ADP (Mustard et al., 1972) displayed no loss of the second phase of aggregation. However, the height of the secondary peak was dependent upon the divalent cation concentration. This second phase was totally independent of either PGI$_2$ or TxA$_2$ synthetase inhibitor effects and was observed as a consistent property of all platelet preparations in a 1.8 mM Ca^{++} suspension.

Phosphodiesterase inhibitor M 220 Cl$_2$ on the other hand was more effective at preventing the cation sensitive second phase, whereas isobutyl methylxanthine only increased the lag time. However, when isobutyl methylxanthine was used in conjunction with PGI$_2$ (suspended in .05 M Tris buffer at pH 9.5). There was a signficant decrease in the second phase slope.

DISCUSSION

Previous in vivo studies (Honn et al., 1981) suggested that platelet aggregation is important in metastasis. In order to demonstrate that tumor cells can induce platelets to produce TxA$_2$ and thereby aggregate, we used the in vitro system of tumor cell, Ca^{++} and platelet poor plasma readdition to washed platelets which demonstrated the following: 1) tumor cells induce a biphasic aggregation of platelets; 2) this is accompanied by stimulation of TxA$_2$ synthesis; 3) PGI$_2$ and inhibitors of TxA$_2$ synthetase inhibit platelet aggregation; 4) the PGI$_2$ effects can be synergistically augmented by phosphodiesterase inhibitors. Together, these in vitro and in vivo results establish the important role tumor cell induced TxA$_2$ production plays in metastasis. The mechanism of induction of TxA$_2$ production is yet to be determined.

(Supported in part by NIH grants CA29405, CA29997, AM 13724 and A.C.S. BC-356).

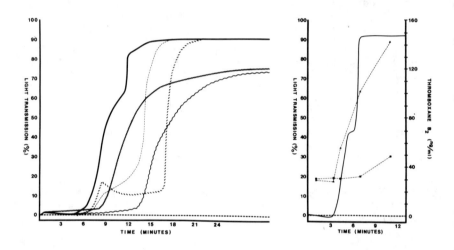

Figure 1. Inhibitor studies: a) ▬▬▬ = standard tumor cell induced platelet aggregation (TCIPA) curve; b) ▬ ▬ ▬ = controls without tumor cells; c) ———— = inhibition of TCIPA by 500 pg/ml of prostacyclin in benzene/acetone $1:10^5$; d)➤➤➤➤= inhibition of TCIPA by 1.0 ng/ml of prostacyclin in benzene/acetone $1:10^5$; e) ◣◣◣◣◣ = inhibition via 4 ng/ml 9,11-azoprosta-5,13-dienoic acid; f) ◣◣◣= inhibition via 4 ng/ml 9,11-iminoepoxyprosta-5,13-dienoic acid; Note: extended lag time.

Figure 2. Standard TCIPA curve as it correlates with radioimmunoassay (RIA) data obtained at various points in the curves. RIA samples at 1) 1 min; 2) bottom of 1st phase; 3) top of 1st phase; 4) top of 2nd phase; 5) 4 min after 2nd phase peak. a) ▬▬▬ = TCIPA curve; ▬ ▬ ▬ = controls without tumor cells; b) ▲——▲ = TCIPA RIA results; ■——■ = control RIA results.

REFERENCES

Gasic GJ, Gasic T, Galanti N, Johnson T, Murphy S (1973) Platelet tumor cell interactions in mice. The role of platelets in the spread of malignant disease. Int J Cancer 11:704.
Gasic GJ, Koch PAG, Hsu B, Gasic TB, Niewiarowski S (1976) Thrombogenic activity of mouse and human tumors: effects on platelets coagulation and fibrinolysis and possible significance for metastasis. Z Krebsforsch 86:283.
Gasic GJ, Boettiger D, Catalfomo JL, Gasic TB, Stewart GJ (1978) Aggregation of platelets and cell membrane vesiculation by rat cells transformed in vitro by rous sarcoma virus. Cancer Res 38:2950.
Hamberg M, Svensson J, Wakabayashi T, Samuelsson B (1974) Isolation and structure of two prostaglandin endoperoxides that cause platelet aggregation. Proc Nat Acad Science 71:345.
Hara H, Steiner M, Baldini MG (1980) Characterization of platelet-aggregating activity of tumor cells. Cancer Res 40:1217.
Honn KV, Cicone B, Skoff A (1981) Prostacyclin: a potent antimetastatic agent. Science 212:1270.
Honn KV, Meyer J, Neagos G, Henderson T, Westley C, Ratanatharatorn V (in press) Control of tumor growth and mestastasis with prostacyclin and thromboxane synthetase inhibitors: evidence for a new antitumor and antimetastatic agent (Bay g 6575). In Jamieson GA (ed): "Interaction of platelets and tumor cells" New York: Alan R Liss.
Mustard JF, Perry DW, Ardlie Ng, Packham MA (1972) Preparation of suspension of washed platelets from humans. Brit J Haematology 22:193.
Sloane BF, Dunn JR, Honn KV (1981) Lysosomal cathepsin B: correlation with metastatic potential. Science 212:1151.

**Prostaglandins and Cancer: First
International Conference, pages 815-817
© 1982 Alan R. Liss, Inc., 150 Fifth Avenue, New York, NY 10011**

FLURBIPROFEN DOES NOT APPEAR TO ENHANCE THE THERAPEUTIC
EFFECT OF CYCLOPHOSPHAMIDE

Susan E. Heckford, Suzanne A. Eccles, T. J.
Powles*, and P. Alexander

The Chester Beatty Research Institute, and
*The Royal Marsden Hospital, Sutton, Surrey,
England

Tumor-bearing animals have received nonsteroidal
anti-inflammatory drugs (NSAIDs) in combination with
cytotoxic agents in a limited number of studies. These
experiments demonstrated that the NSAID, Flurbiprofen,
enhanced the therapeutic effect of alkylating agents and
radiation and prolonged survival of mice with adenocarcinomas (Bennett et al., 1979; Berstock et al., 1980),
and of rats bearing an ascitic tumor (Powles et al., 1978).
The experiments reported here describe the effect of one
such protocol on the growth and dissemination of two
rodent sarcomas.

The animals were supplied by the Chester Beatty
Research Institute Breeding Colony. MC28, a methylcholanthrene-induced fibrosarcoma of Lister Hooded/CBi rats,
and FS6Ml, a benzo(a)pyrene-induced fibrosarcoma of
C57Bl/CBi mice are both poorly immunogenic with high
incidences of spontaneous metastases.

Measurements of subcutaneous (s.c.) sarcoma growth
were made on alternate days following injection of a single
cell suspension (1 x 10^6 cells) prepared with 0.1% trypsin
and 0.05% DNAase. Further small groups of animals received
an intramuscular (i.m.) injection of a mechanically prepared
tumor brei. These sarcomas were excised after 10-14 days
of growth by amputation of the whole limb and the animals
were observed for the development of metastases over a
period of 200 days.

Animals were treated with cyclophosphamide (Cy) (Endox-
ana) alone or in combination with Flurbiprofen (Fp). Flurbiprofen (Froben, The Boots Company, Ltd., England) is a potent
NSAID which inhibits the production of endoperoxides pivotal
in the formation of many prostaglandins. It was administered
s.c. to rats at 7 mg/kg and to mice at 5 mg/kg 3 times daily
during the period of tumor growth as specified in the Figure
Legends. Cy was administered as a single intraperitoneal
(i.p.) injection of 10 or 100 mg/kg to mice and 80 mg/kg to
rats on the second day of Fp treatment. Animal survival data
were analysed using Kaplan-Meier life tables at a 5% level of
significance.

The results of these experiments are illustrated in the
Figures.

FIGURE 1

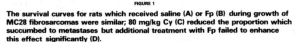

The survival curves for rats which received saline (A) or Fp (B) during growth of
MC28 fibrosarcomas were similar; 80 mg/kg Cy (C) reduced the proportion which
succumbed to metastases but additional treatment with Fp failed to enhance
this effect significantly (D).

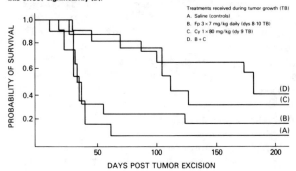

In summary, Flurbiprofen did not affect local growth of
fibrosarcomas (not illustrated here) and the incidence of
distant metastases following resection of the tumors was comparable to that in untreated control groups. Treatment with
high doses of cyclophosphamide retarded growth of the fibrosarcomas and reduced the proportion of animals which succumbed to metastases ($p < 0.05$). There was no statistically
significant effect of additional treatment with Flurbiprofen
($p > 0.05$).

FIGURE 2

Probability of survival following resection of FS6M1. There were no statistically significant differences between the survival curves of control (1) and Fp (2) treated animals, or those which had received 10 mg/kg Cy alone (3) or with Fp (4); 100 mg/kg Cy (5) increased survival but this was not improved significantly by additional treatment with Fp (6).

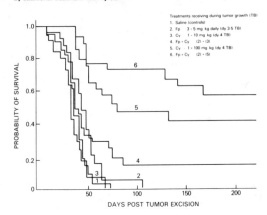

In these studies, we were unable to demonstrate that Flurbiprofen significantly improved the therapeutic effect of cyclophosphamide as determined by measurements of tumor growth and animal survival. However, as only small numbers of animals were used and as these treatment protocols and the histogenic origins of the tumors differ from those used previously, the conflicting results invite further study.

Acknowledgements. This work was supported by grants from the MRC and CRC. We thank The Boots Company, Ltd., England, for the Froben, and Mary Jones of this Institute for statistical analysis of the data.

Bennett A, Houghton J, Leaper DJ, Stamford IF (1979). Cancer growth. Response to treatment and survival time in mice: Beneficial effect of the prostaglandin synthesis inhibitor Flurbiprofen. Prostaglandins 17(2):179.

Berstock DA, Houghton J, Bennett A (1980). Improved anti-cancer effect by combining cytotoxic drugs with an inhibitor of prostaglandin synthesis. Adv in Prostaglandin and Thromboxane Res 6:567.

Powles TJ, Alexander P, Millar JL (1978). Enhancement of anti-cancer activity of cytotoxic chemotherapy with protection of normal tissues by inhibition of P. G. synthesis. Biochem Pharmacol 27:1389.

Prostaglandins and Cancer: First International Conference, pages 819–823
© 1982 Alan R. Liss, Inc., 150 Fifth Avenue, New York, NY 10011

THE EFFECT OF FLURBIPROFEN ON STEM CELL SURVIVAL FOLLOWING X IRRADIATION

R. H. MacDougall, W. Duncan, Barbara M. Clarke

Department of Clinical Oncology, University of Edinburgh, Western General Hospital, Edinburgh, Scotland. EH4 2XU

Salicylate and indomethacin have been shown to protect animals from the effects of X irradiation (Alexander 1955; Northway et al. 1980). Indomethacin has also been shown to protect animals from normally lethal doses of cytotoxic agents and to enhance recovery of bone marrow stem cells following whole body irradiation (Millar et al. 1978; Powles et al. 1979).

These agents are thought to act by inhibition of prostaglandin synthesis. The microcolony survival assay for cells of mouse intestinal mucosa (Withers and Elkind 1970) and the spleen colony assay system for mouse bone marrow cells (Till and McCulloch 1961) were used to investigate the radiobiological basis of this. The non-steroidal anti-inflammatory drug flurbiprofen, which is a more potent inhibitor of prostaglandin synthesis than either salicylate or indomethacin, was used.

MATERIALS AND METHODS

Crypt Microcolony Assay

Groups of four hybrid C57$_{10}$ male mice were given graded doses of 250 kV X rays to the abdomen. Groups were oral dosed 12 hourly with flurbiprofen 2.5 mg/Kg in cellosize or cellosize alone as control:

(i)   7 doses starting 1 hour prior to irradiation
(ii) 3 doses starting 24 hours prior to irradiation

The mice were held in a perspex jig during irradiation
and were not anaesthetised. Segments of jejunum were
removed $3\frac{1}{2}$ days later. Following routine histological
processing, the number of crypts in five transverse sections
were counted for each animal.

Spleen Colony Assay

Hybrid DBA_2 mice were fed either flurbiprofen in cellosize or cellosize alone as above for 3 doses. They were
then given varying doses of 250 kV X rays. Femoral marrow
from these was injected into heavily irradiated recipient
mice. These were sacrificed ten days later. The number of
spleen colonies established and their relationship to the
number of donor cells was noted.

RESULTS

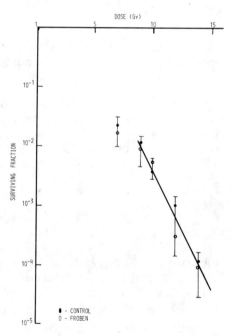

Fig. 1 Jejunal Stem Cell Survival   7 doses

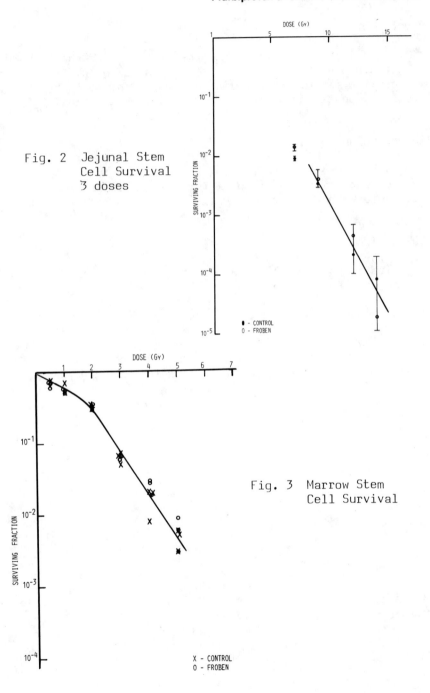

Fig. 2 Jejunal Stem
Cell Survival
3 doses

Fig. 3 Marrow Stem
Cell Survival

Crypt Microcolony Assay

A cell survival curve was constructed after the method
of Withers and Elkind. There is no significant difference
between the flurbiprofen/cellosize and cellosize control
groups. The timing of the drug had no effect. (Figs. 1 & 2)

Spleen Colony Assay

The log surviving fraction of marrow cells is plotted
against radiation dose. No difference is seen between the
flurbiprofen and control groups. (Fig. 3)

CONCLUSION

These experiments do not demonstrate any direct interaction between flurbiprofen and X irradiation in the
response of stem cells in the jejunal crypts or bone marrow
of the mouse. The mechanism of any enhanced repair following X irradiation must be explained by changes in cell
population kinetics. It is suggested that flurbiprofen may
have a "priming effect" on the untreated stem cell population or may stimulate repopulation of irradiated tissues.

ACKNOWLEDGEMENTS

The generous help of F. Donnelly, R. Robertson and
Mrs. Joyce Young is gratefully acknowledged. Flurbiprofen
(Froben) was kindly supplied by The Boots Company Limited,
Nottingham, U.K.

REFERENCES

Alexander P, Bacq ZM, Cousins SF, Fox M, Herve A, Lazav J
(1955). Mode of action of some substances which protect
against the lethal effect of X rays. Radiation Research
2:392.
Millar, JL, Hydspith BN, McElwain TJ, Phelps TA (1978).
Effect of high dose melphalan on marrow and intestinal
epithelium in mice. Br J Cancer 38:137.
Northway MG, Libshitz HI, Osborne BM, Feldman MS, Mamel JJ,
West JH, Szwarc IA (1980). Radiation Oesophagitis in the

Opossum: Radioprotection with Indomethacin. Gastroenterology 78:883.

Powles TJ, Millar JL (1979). Nonsteroidal anti-inflammatory drugs and cytotoxics. Cancer Treatment Reviews 6:63.

Till JE, McCulloch EA (1961). A direct measurement of the radiation sensitivity of normal mouse bone marrow cells. Radiation Research 14:213.

Withers HR, Elkind MM (1970). Microcolony survival assay for cells of mouse intestinal mucosa exposed to radiation. Int J Radiat Biol 17:3:26.

**Prostaglandins and Cancer: First
International Conference, pages 825-830
© 1982 Alan R. Liss, Inc., 150 Fifth Avenue, New York, NY 10011**

PROSTAGLANDIN ADMINISTRATION TO PATIENTS WITH CANCER

T.J. Powles, R.C. Coombes, M. Depledge,
J. Muindi, R. Powles.

Department of Medicine, Royal Marsden Hospital
Downs Road, Sutton, Surrey, U.K.

Some prostaglandins, particularly PGE and PGA, like
cAMP will inhibit cell replication and DNA synthesis in vitro
in many cell systems, including transformed mouse fibroblasts
(Johnson and Pastan, 1971; Honn, Romme and Skoff, 1980).
PGE_2 and its relatively stable analogue 16-16 dimethyl PGE_2
will inhibit cell replication of B_{16} melanoma cells in vitro
(Santoro et al, 1976). Systemic administration of 16-16
dimethyl PGE_2 to mice delayed growth of B_{16} melanoma and
prolonged survival of animals transplanted with the tumour
(Santoro et al, 1976, Santoro et al, 1979). Similar
inhibition of growth of a human colorectal cancer maintained
in mouse xenograft transplantation has been reported by
administration of 16-16 dimethyl PGF_2 associated with
inhibition of cell replication (Tutton and Barkla, 1980).
PGA_1 and PGA_2 the synthetic analogues of PGE_1 and PGE_2
possess similar biological properties to the naturally
occurring PGs. They will inhibit cell replication in vitro
in several cell culture systems, induce differentiation in
erythroleukaemic cells (Santoro et al, 1979) and inhibit
DNA synthesis in Harding Passey melanoma cells (Honn et al
1979, Honn et al, 1979). PGA_1 will also inhibit in vivo
growth of B_{16} melanoma in mice (Faralli et al, 1980).

Short infusions of PGA_1 have been administered to humans
with hypertension and hepato-renal failure. Infusion rates
of 2o ug/kg/min. have been tolerated with only mild nausea,
associated with hypotension (Vincenti et al, 1978; Carr et

al, 1970; Lee et al, 1973; Aruff et al, 1974; Krakoff et al, 1977; Krakoff et al, 1975; Krakoff et al, 1973; Golub et al, 1976).

PGE_2 has been extensively used to induce labour and is available as a pharmaceutical preparation (Prostin, Upjohn) for oral or intravenous administration.

Administration of PGs to patients with cancer has not previously been reported and we have, therefore, tested these agents for anti-tumour activity in a small pilot clinical trial.

Patients and Methods

(a) Six patients were included in the PGE study. Four of the patients had clinically accessible, histologically proven, recurrent soft tissue breast cancer, and two had acute myelogenous leukaemia. All had previously had chemotherapy and/or endocrine therapy and had either relapsed after response, or failed to respond.

PGE (Prostin, Upjohn) was initially administered to four patients by intravenous infusion of approximately 0.05 ug/kg/min. (2.5 Prostin in 500 ml 5% dextrose administered at a rate of 30 mls per hour) for 48 hours. This was followed by oral (sublingual) administration of 1.5 mg Prostin six times per day with dose adjustment according to tolerability. A further two patients had only oral Prostin at the same dose and all patients continued medication until progression of disease or symptoms. At weekly intervals throughout the study, patients were evaluated clinically for toxicity and assessment of response (according to UICC criteria).

(b) Seven patients with clinically assessable, histologically confirmed, metastatic or locally recurrent breast cancer were included in the PGA study. All had previously had chemotherapy and/or endocrine therapy and had previously relapsed after response, or failed to respond.

Pure crystalline PGA_1 and liquid PGA_2 (kindly supplied by Ono Pharmaceuticals, Japan) were dissolved in ethanol and made up into stock solutions containing 10 mg/ml. These were stored in 1 ml ampoules at $-40^{\circ}C$ and the stability checked from time to time by HPLC (Mr. Ed Nice, Ludwig Institute for Cancer Research, London). PGA_1 was given to three patients and PGA_2 to four patients by intravenous injection of appropriate amounts of stock solution diluted in 1 L. of 5% dextrose. Patients were given 1-3 ug/kg/min. of PGA_1 or PGA_2 for six hours once per week. Patients were assessed at weekly intervals for toxicity and response and all continued medication until evidence of progression of disease.

Results.

The patients tolerated Prostin administration for 7-60 days and received a total of 127 - 540 mg. None of the six patients showed evidence of tumour regression and two of the breast cancer patients and both the leukaemic patients showed definite clinical evidence of tumour progression. Intravenous administration of PGE at 0.05 ug/ kg/min. was tolerated satisfactorily with mild diarrhoea occuring in two patients. Oral administration at a dose of 6-9 mg/day was associated with diarrhoea in a further two patients and nausea and vomiting in one patient. These symptoms only occurred when the tablets were swallowed, and not when sucked sublingually. There was no change in pulse rate, blood pressure, respiration rate, renal function, serum calcium or blood count. One patient noticed headache and arthralgia associated with oral administration of the tablets.

All seven patients who received PGA tolerated the medication satisfactorily. They received between 2 and 11 weekly infusions at infusion rates between 1 and 3 ug/kg /min. to a total dose of 40-380 mg. None of the seven patients showed evidence of tumour regression and four showed definite evidence of progression of disease while receiving PGA.

Generally PGA_1 was tolerated better than PGA_2. The main problem which developed during the 18 infusions of PGA_1 were facial flushing (8), pyrexia (8) tachycardia (5) nausea (2), vomiting (2), headache (2) and hypertension (1). During the 19 PGA_2 infusions the main toxicity problems were diarrhoea (13), nausea (8), vomiting (5) headache (9) facial flushing (8) hypertension (6), pyrexia (2) and tachycardia (13). The diarrhoea with PGA_2 infusion was the dose limiting problem usually occurring at between 2-3 ug/kg/min.

Coughing, shortness of breath with some clinical evidence of bronchospasm occurred in two patients with lung metastases during the infusions of PGA_1. In two patients (one of whom developed respiratory symptoms), measurement of peak expiratory flow using the mini-Wright peak flow meter, showed no significant change throughout the infusions. In one asymptomatic patient respiratory function tests revealed no change in dynamic lung volume nor gas transfer pre and post P.G.A. infusion. We could find no cause for the respiratory sumptoms which occurred in the two patients with lung metastases.

No significant changes occurred in haemoglobin, white cell count, platelet count, serum calcium, phosphorous, electrolytes, bicarbonate, liver function tests or blood urea during infusions of PGA_1 or PGA_2.

Discussion

Following the experimental evidence which indicates that PGs might inhibit tumour growth, we have carried out preliminary Phase I studies of PGE_2, PGA_1 and PGA_2 in 11 patients with breast cancer and two patients with leukaemia. Oral administration of PGE_2 up to 9 mg/day was tolerated satisfactorily. The main toxicity problems were gastrointestinal symptoms which were insignificant at this dosage if the tablets were absorbed sublingually. Weekly infusions of PGA_1 and PGA_2 of 20-60 mg. over 6 hours at rates of 1-3 ug/kg/min. were also tolerated satisfactorily the main problems being diarrhoea, vomiting, pyrexia, facial flushing, tachycardia and hypotension.

In these studies we saw no evidence of tumour regression although the numbers of patients studied are not sufficient to exclude anti-tumour activity. Alternatively, intermittent administration of PG's in patients with tumours may not be comparable to the experimental conditions necessary for anti-tumour activity by PGs. With the current interest in development of growth factors and interferon for control of human cancer, further clinical trials of PGs in patients with cancer are indicated.

References

Aruss, AI and Chidsey, CA (1974) Am. J. Med. 56, 695

Carr, AA. (1970) Am; J.∪Med. Sci. 259, 21

Favalli C, Garci E, Santucci L, and Jaffe BM (1980) Prostaglandins 19, 587.

Golub NS, Speckart PF, Zia PK and Horton R (1976) Circ. Res. 39, 574

Honn KV, Davidowicz K, Bienkowski M, Morgan LR, Marnett LJ (1979) Abstracts 4th Int. Prostaglandin Conference p.50.

Honn KV, Romine M, Skoff A, (1980) Proc. Soc. Exptl. Biol. Med. (in press)

Johnson GS and Pastan I. (1971) J.Natl.Cancer Inst. 47, 1357-1360.

Krakoff LR (1977) Prostaglandins 14, 1153

Krakoff LR, Viachakis N, Mendlowitz M and Strickard J. (1975) Clin. Sci. and Mol. Med. 48, 311(s)

Krakoff LR, De Guia D, Viachakis N, Stricker J and Goldstern MH (1973) Circ. Res. 33, 539.

Lee J, McGiff JC, Kennegiesser H et al (1973) Assn. of Int. Med. 74, 703.

Santoro GM, Philpott GW and Jaffe BM (1977) Cancer Research 37, 3774-3779.

Santoro MG, Philpott GW and Jaffe BM (1977) Prostaglandins 14, 645.

Santoro MG, Philpott GW and Jaffe BM (1976) Nature 263, 777-779.

Santoro MG, Benedetto A, and Jaffe BM (1979) Prostaglandins 17, 719.

Tutton PJM and Barkla DH (1980) Br. J. Cancer 41, 47.

Vincenti F and Goldberg L (1978) Prostaglandins 15, 463.

Index

Acetaminophen, 27
Adenylate cyclase, 48, 51, 59, 61, 62, 440, 444
    in bones, 502, 525, 531, 541, 555
    in MDCK line, 493–97
Aging, 163–66, 725–29
Allergic reactions, 8, 29, 775–81; see also asthma
Alveolar-like cells, 465, 467, 472, 476
Amelanotic melanoma, 365–67, 369–72, 378–79; see also B16 melanoma cell; melanoma
Amines, aromatic, 131, 132, 159–61
Aminoazo dyes, 83
Anaphylactic activity, 775–81
Angiogenesis, 685–88
Antibody-dependent cellular cytotoxicity, 713–17
Antibody response, 620, 622, 625–27
Antigens
    fetal, 645–46
    and leukemia myelopoiesis, 399, 402–11
    transplantation-type tumor-specific, 585–88
    tumor, 645, 667–71, 679–83
Anti-inflammatory drugs, 13–14, 613–14
    and bone metastases, 542–51
    and cyclophosphamide, 815–17
    and esophageal mucosa, 799–802
    and prostaglandin synthesis, 25, 33–35

and tumors, 760–64
    see also specific drugs
Antioxidants, 170, 176, 198
Arachidonic acid
    biochemistry of, 14
    and cell proliferation, 754–55
    dependent cooxygenation, 106–8, 114–15, 117–19
    derivatives, 1–14
    and DMSO, 431
    and endothelial cells, 381–82
    and granulopoiesis, 481–84
    inhibition of, 21–37
    and macrophages, 609–15
    metabolism, 22, 37, 260, 262, 281–85
    metabolism, and bone, 501–2, 513–20, 527–31, 534–36
    metabolism, and polymorpho-nuclear leukocytes, 5–7
    metabolites, 281–82, 285; see also specific metabolites
    metabolites, and immunity, 595–604
    metabolites, and tumors, 671
    metabolites, pharmacology of, 47–62
    and murine tumors, 206–9, 212
    and Nafazatrom, 784–85
    and prostaglandin synthesis, 302–3
    release, 223, 225, 256, 242, 281
    source of, 265–70
    and steroids, 35–36
    transformation, 199–200

and uterine cancer, 698–99
and vitamin E/selenium, 149–50
Arginase, 584
Aromatic Amines, 131, 132, 159–61
Arthritis, 612–13
Ascorbate, 167, 170, 447
Aspirin, 172, 174
  and bladder cancer, 136–38
  and bones, 541, 548
  and cyclooxygenase, 5, 14
  and immune system, 603
  and tumors, 198, 776
Aspirin-like drugs, 21–37; see also
  anti-inflammatory drugs
Asthma, 8, 12, 29; see also allergic
  reactions
Atherosclerosis, 32

BALB/c-3T3 cells, 291–94, 298-306
B cells, 598–602, 621–24
Benorylate, 542–44, 551, 764
Benoxaprofen, 543, 548
Benzidine, 126–33
Benzo(a)pyrene, 98–103, 106, 113–20
Benzoyl peroxide, 261–62
Biopsies, 633–47
Bladder cancer, 123, 113–38
Blood cells, 651–54, 679–83
Blood vessels, 4
Bone destruction, 561–65
Bone marrow, 481–84, 610
Bone metastases, 541–51, 567–72
Bone metabolism, 513–20
Bone resorption, 501–7
  lymphokine mediated-, 555–58
  and osteosarcoma, 573–77
  and prostaglandins, 525–36
Breast, 458–59; see also mammary
Breast cancer, 638, 641
  and leukocyte adherence
    inhibition, 668–70
  and osteolysis, 542, 543, 551
  and prostaglandins, 567–72
  see also mammary carcinoma;
    mammary tumor
Bronchoconstriction, 13, 29, 30

B16 melanoma, 789–91
  and flurbiprofen, 771–74
  and prostaglandins, 737–48, 825
Butylated hydroxyanisol (BHA),
  198, 260
Butylated hydroxytoluene (BHT),
  170, 176, 260
Butyric acid, 447, 495

Calcitonin, 525–26
Calcium, 7–8, 50–51, 59–62, 597;
  see also hypercalcemia
cAMP, 48, 60–61, 421
  and bones, 502, 505, 525, 531,
    533, 573
  and cell cycle, 297, 304–6
  and cell growth, 734
  and cytotoxic T cells, 602–3
  in Friend erythroleukemic cells,
    432
  -mediated hormone sensitivity,
    493–95
  and osteolysis, 541
  and platelets, 734–35
  and prostaglandins, 439–40,
    444–45, 448, 597–602
  and T lymphocytes, 620–21
  and tumors, 375–78, 675–76
  see also dibutyryl cAMP
Cancer
  anti-, effect of prostaglandins,
    446–48
  bladder, 123, 133–38
  breast, 657–61, 701–3, 705–8,
    799–803, 805; see also breast
    cancer
  cervical, 697–99
  epithelial, 637–41
  head and neck, 651, 654
  intestinal, 753–76
  lung, 369–71, 691–94, 737–48,
    767–74, 805
  ovarian, 637–41
  pancreatic, 385–88
  and prostaglandins, 415–21,
    825–29

and T cells, 415–21
treatment, 646–47
tumor antigen-induced changes
   in, 679–83
see also carcinogen; malignant; tumor
Carcinogen, 183–88
adherent activity of DES, 143–47
free radical, 167–68
initiation, 81–90
and lung tumor, 155
metabolism, 83–90
promotion, 82, 89
and prostaglandins, 97–103,
   113–20
proximate, 84, 87
structural features of, 82–83
and target organs, 123–38
2-stage carcinogenesis, 189, 205,
   273, 646
ultimate, 87
see also cancer; malignant; tumor
Cell(s)
adherent, 601
alveolar-like, 465, 467, 472, 476
blood, 651–54
bone, 525–36
culture, 382–84, 493–97
differentiation, 427–34, 437–48,
   453–62, 465–78, 487–90, 591
effects of tumor promoters on,
   222–33
endothelial, 381–84
growth, 382–84, 427–34
homologous, 245–61
and interferon, 346
mammary, 167–78
mastocytoma, 8–9
-mediated immunity, 623–25
membranes, protectors of, 149
migration, 612–13
neuroblastoma, 437–38
proliferation, 372, 375–78, 754–
   55
replication, 297–306
squamous differentiation, 453–62

suppressor, 601
transformation, 113–20, 291–95,
   622
tumorigencity, 446–47
see also specific cell lines
Cell cycle, 291–94
disturbance of, 392–95
and prostaglandin receptors,
   430–31
regulation of, 309–28
S phase of, 405–6
Cervical cancer, 697–99
cGMP, 598
and cytotoxic T cells, 602–3
and lipoxygenase products, 789,
   791
and prostaglandins, 444
Chemical carcinogen. *See* carcinogen
Chemokinesis, 614
Chemotaxis, 596, 613
Chemotherapy, 543–44, 548–49, 587,
   589, 803
and anti-inflammatory drugs,
   761–64
and flurbiprofen, 815–17
Choline release, 224–25
Chorio-allantoic membrane, 685–88
Clonogenicity, tumor, 633–47
Coal tars, 81–82
Colcemid, 392–95
Colchicine, 392–95
Collagenase, 541–42
Colony-forming units-
   C, 415
   GM, 399–411
   Tl cells, 416–21
Colony stimulating factor, 481–84
Cooxygenation, 97–108, 113–20
Corticosteroids, 303
and phospholipase inhibition,
   33–35
and prostaglandin inhibition, 5
Cyclic adenine nucleotide, 454, 458,
   462
Cyclic nucleotides. *See* cAMP;
   cGMP; cyclic adenine nucleotide

Cyclooxygenase
    activities, 64
    and arachidonic acid, 22, 37
    and aspirin, 5
    and aspirin-like drugs, 27, 28, 30
    in HeLa cells, 281–82
    inhibition, 23–30, 36–37, 258,
        482–83, 614–15
    and interferon, 351, 356–58, 360
    in MDCK cells, 265–67, 270
    and Nafazatrom, 786
    pathway, 13, 612
    and tumors, 200
Cytochrome P 450, 87, 88, 106,
    116, 124, 152–53
Cytokines, 610–11, 614
Cytotoxicity, 582–84, 602–3, 713–17

Dexamethasone, 33
Dibromoacetophenone, 257, 259
Dibutyryl cAMP, 453–54, 458, 460,
    462
Dibutyryl cGMP, 454, 458–59
Diethylstilbestrol, 143–47
Dimethyl analogues, 370–71
DMBA-induced mammary tumor,
    657–61
DMSO, 425, 427–30, 433
    and myeloid mice tumors, 487–90
    and nude mice tumors, 465, 468,
        470, 473–78
DNA
    and carcinogens, 87, 89–90
    cellular, 297–98
    and DES, 143–47
    strand breaks, 159–61
    synthesis, and growth factors,
        292–93
    synthesis, and Nafazatrom, 747
    synthesis, and prostaglandins,
        309–28, 369–72, 475–76
    synthesis, and tumor promoters,
        244
    synthesis, inhibition of, 445
    synthesis, initiation of, 391–95
    synthesis, thymidine
        incorporation in, 591

Down regulation, receptor, 230–33
D-penicillamine, 613

Eicosatetraenoic acids, 597
    diHETE, 596–97
    HETE, 259–60, 481–84, 596,
        612, 614, 694
    HPETE, 259–62, 738, 790
Eicosatetraynoic acid, 167, 172,
    174, 258, 282–85
Electrophiles, 84–86
Endoperoxide(s)
    analogues, 73
    biological effects of, 4
    metabolism, 31
Endothelial cells, 381–84
Enzyme
    inhibitors, and lipids, 355–56,
        358–59
    inhibitors, mechanisms of, 24–37
    lysosomal, 789–92
    and prostanoids, 149–53
Epidermal growth factor
    and bones, 519, 530–31
    and cell replication, 292–93
    inhibition of binding of, 217,
        222–26
    and prostaglandins, 309, 320,
        325–28
Epidermis
    hyperplasia of, 242–48
    proliferation of, 239–48
    tumors of, 248–49
Epithelial neoplasms, 637–41
Erythropoiesis, 425–34
Esophageal mucosa, 799–802
Esophagitis, 799–801
Estradiol, 176–77
Estrogen, 657, 661

Fetal growth, 644–47
Fibrinolysis, 281
Fibrosarcoma, 514–18, 529, 775–81
5-nitrofuran, 126–31, 138
Flurbiprofen, 543–44, 548–49,
    793–96
    in cancer, 803–7

and cyclophosphamide, 815–17
and lung cancer, 767–74
and mammary tumors, 801–2
and stem cell survival, 819–22
and tumors, 754–56, 761, 763–64
Free radicals, 260, 262
Friend erythroleukemia cells,
 425–34, 477–78

Gamma radiation, 381–84
Glucagon receptors, 494–97
Glucocorticoids, 196, 200
Glutathione, 366–67
Glutathione peroxidase, 176
Glutathione transferase, 151–52
Glycolysis, 446
Gold, 613
Gossypol, 198–99
Granulocyte. See colony-forming
 unit-, GM
Granulopoiesis, 481–84
Growth factors and
 bone metabolism, 513, 519–20
 interferon, 359
 prostaglandins, 191–92, 200, 309,
 320, 325–28; see also specific
 growth factors

Head and neck cancer, 651, 654
HeLa cells, 281–85
Histamine, 620, 775, 778
Histones, 445
HL-60 cell line, 487–90
Hodgkins' disease, 418–20, 601, 651
Hormones
 and breast cancer, 657–61
 as cancer treatment, 646
 and cell cycle, 292–94
 and cell differentiation, 465, 473
 475–76
 and prostaglandins, 441–42
 receptors, 493–97
 and tumors, 581
HSDM₁ fibrosarcoma, 514–18, 529
Humoral growth, 410
Hydrocarbons, 98–103

Hydrocortisone, 33, 433–34, 465,
 473, 475–76
Hypercalcemia, 501–7, 513–20,
 530, 542
Hypersensitivity reactions.
 See allergic reactions

Ibuprofen, 570
Immune system
 cancer patients', 651–54
 impairment by tumor, 590–91
 leukocyte cytotoxicity, 582–84
 tolerance to cancer, 644–46
 trilateral relationships, 333–42
 and tumors, 581–82
Immunity
 and arachidonate metabolites,
 595–604
 cell-mediated, 623–24
 effector mechanisms of, 587–88
 human anti-tumor-, 667–71
 in vivo role of, 585–87
Immunosuppression, 567, 572
 age-related, 725–29
 prostaglandins as mediators of,
 625–27, 663–65
 and tumors, 619, 622–24
Immunotherapy, 628
Indomethacin, 117–19, 172–74
 and bone cancer, 503–5, 543,
 548, 577
 and breast cancer, 570
 and cAMP, 621–22
 and chemotherapeutic drugs, 763
 and cyclooxygenase, 28, 267, 482
 and cytotoxicity, 714
 effect on cancer patients' immune
 system, 651–54
 and growth factors, 519–20
 and humoral response, 600
 and immune system, 603
 and lipoxygenase, 30
 and mouse tumors, 242–48,
 775–81
 and osteolysis, 542
 and osteosarcoma, 577
 and pigment formation, 164

and prostaglandins, 24–26, 33,
196, 306
and T cells, 419, 599
therapy, 601
and TPA, 187, 196–97, 282–83
and tumors, 197–98, 257, 277,
627 , 629, 760–62
Inflammation, 24, 29–30, 32–33,
255, 611–14; see also anti-
inflammatory drugs
Influenza, 600
Injury, 611, 613
Interferon
action in homologous cells,
345–61
and host defense, 333–42
and natural killer cells, 663
Intestinal tumors, 753–56
Intracellular mediators, 596–97

Keratin, 453–62
Kidney, 123, 133–34, 138, 493–97

Lactic acid dehydrogenase, 445–46
Lag phase, 391, 394
Lectin, 601–2
Leukemia, 399–411, 425–34, 487–90
Leukocyte, 5–7, 582–85, 611–13,
667–71, 679–83
Leukotriene
analogues, 69
biochemical pathways, 5–14
and bronchoconstriction, 13
and chemokinesis, 614
formation, 22
and inflammation, 612–13
molecules, 51
naming of, 12
release from monocytes, 667–71
and smooth muscles, 50
structure, 59
and tumors, 679–83
Lewis lung carcinoma, 369–71,
767–74, 805
Lipids(s)
and immunity, 596–97

membranes, 347–61
peroxidation, 149, 155, 158, 163
Lipofuscin, 163–66
Lipoxygenase
activity, 611
and arachidonic acid, 22, 37
and aspirin-like drugs, 27, 30
and bone, 535–36
in HeLa Cells, 281–82, 285
inhibitor, 28–30, 37, 258, 614–15
and interferon, 351
and mammary cells, 171–72, 178
in MDCK cells, 265
in myeloid colony formation,
481–84
pathway, 167, 260, 612
products, 789–92
and tumors, 199–200
Lung cancer, 691–94, 737–48;
see also Lewis lung carcinoma
Lymphocyte, 713–17; see also
B cells; T cells
Lymphoid cells, 595–96
Lymphokine, 555–58, 602, 610
Lysosomal enzymes, 789–92
Lyngbyatoxin A, 221–22

Macrocortin, 35, 36
Macrophage
and arachidonic acid products,
609–15
and cytotoxicity, 716–17
and prostaglandins, 596
role of, in immune system,
725–29
SRS in, 597
and tumors, 583–89, 628, 633–47
see also colony-forming
units-, GM
Macrophage-activating factor,
583–84
Madin-Darby canine kidney cells,
265–70, 493–97
Malignant hypercalcemia, 501–7,
513–20
Malignant melanoma, 713–17
see also melanoma

Malonaldehyde, 163, 166
Mammary cells, 167–78
Mammary carcinoma, 701–3, 705–8,
    see also breast cancer
Mammary glands, human, 458–59
Mammary glands, mouse, 454–57
Mammary glands, rat, 465–78
Mammary tumor, 657–61
    and anti-inflammatory agents,
      799–802
    and flurbiprofen, 803, 805; see
      also breast cancer
Mastocytoma cells, 8–9
Maternal-fetal tolerance, 644–47
Melanoma, 651–52, 653
    malignant, 713–17
    see also amelanotic melanoma;
      B16 melanoma cell
Membranes, cell
    lipid, 347–61
    protectors of, 149
    transmembrane potential, 679–83
Metastasis
    and anti-inflammatory drugs,
      760–61, 763
    and flurbiprofen, 768–71
    prostacyclin/thromboxane ratios
      in, 733–48
    and prostaglandins, 701–3,
      719, 721
Methylcholanthrene, 206
Microtubules, 391–95
Misonidazole, 793–96
Mitogenesis, 601–2
Monocytes, 583–84
    and antibody-dependent cellular
      cytotoxicity, 713–17
    and immune system, 609–10
      612–13
    leukotriene release from, 667–71
    and transmembrane potential,
      679–83
Mononuclear cells, 415–16, 418, 420
Mouse
    fibrosarcoma, 775–81
    neuroblastoma, 367

skin, and prostaglandins, 239–49
skin, and tumors, 256–62
tumor, 465–78, 623–27
Mulitple myeloma, 635–38, 641
Murine. See mouse
Mutagen, 85, 90
Myeloid colony formation, 481–84
Myeloid differentation, 487–90
Myeloma, 505–6, 635–38, 641
Myelopoiesis, 399–411

Nafazatrom, 743–45, 747, 783–92
Naproxen, 26, 28
Natural killer cells, 357–58, 361,
    583, 585, 603
    and cancer, 663–65
    and tumors, 625, 628, 779, 781
Neoplasms, 637–41; see also cancer
Neuroblastoma cells, 437–48
N-hydroxy-2-acetylaminofluorene,
    167–78
Nitroreductase, 124, 126
Nordihydroguaiaretic acid, 198–99,
    282, 284
Nucleic acids, 163–66
Nucleophile, 84, 86

Organs, 454–62
Ornithine decarboxylase, 242–46,
    257, 273–79
Osteoblast, 525–27, 531–35,
    573–74, 577
Osteoclast, 526–27, 532, 541, 562,
    565, 573
Osteoclast activating factor, 504–6
    555, 557–58
Osteocyte, 526, 541
Osteolysis, 541–42, 551, 805
Osteosarcoma cells, 573–77
Ovarian cancer, 637–41

Pancreatic cancer cell line, 385–88
Papaverine, 453, 462
Parathyroid hormone, 502–3,
    525–33, 541–42, 555, 557, 573–74
P-dimethylaminoazobenzene, 155–58

Peripheral blood leukocytes, 679–83
Peripheral blood mononuclear cells,
  651–54
Peroxidase and
  mammary cells, 167–68, 171–78
  xenobiotic cooxygenation, 104–6
Phagocytosis, 356–59, 361, 614
Pharmacology, 47–62
Phenobarbitol, 274–79
Phorboid receptor, 230–33
Phorbol esters
  and cancer, 185, 187–88
  characteristics of binding, 218–22
  and mouse skin, 211–13
  and plasminogen activation,
    281–85
  receptors, 217–33
  and squamous metaplasia,
    460, 462
  stimulation of prostaglandin by,
    189–91
  see also tetradecanoylphorbol
    acetate
Phorbol myristate acetate, 673–77
Phorbol-12, 13-dibutyrate, 220–33
Phosphatidylethanolamine, 266
Phosphodiesterase, 444, 448, 462
  737–38, 811
Phospholipase
  and arachidonic acid, 22
  inhibition, 32–36, 257, 259
  in MDCK cells, 265, 270
  and murine tumors, 207–10, 213
  and phorbol esters, 223, 225
  and virus transformation, 306
Phospholipids, 268–70
Phosphorylation, 445, 602
Pigment formation, 163–66
Plasmalogen, 267
Plasminogen activator, 281–85
Platelet(s) 4, 51
  aggregation, 60
  aggregation, and prostacyclin,
    734–35, 783–85
  aggregation, and thromboxane,
    31, 734–35

  aggregation, tumor cell induced-,
    809–12
Platelet activating factor, 596
Platelet-derived growth factor,
  291–94, 519–20
Plaque-forming cells, 599–600
Polymorphonuclear leukocytes, 5–7
  611–13
Polyoma virus transformation,
  297–306
Polyunsaturated fatty acids
  conversion of, 1–14
  oxygenation of, 1, 3
Prolactin, 657, 661
Promyelocytic leukemia, 487–90
Prostacyclin, 4, 297, 304
  and bones, 533–34
  and cAMP, 597
  effect of gamma radiation on,
    381–84
  formation of, 31, 37
  and inflammation, 613
  instability of, 68, 72, 73
  in macrophages, 596
  metabolism, 22
  metastasis, 737–38
  and platelet aggregation, 809–12
  stimulation of, by Nafazatrom,
    783–87
  and tumor cells, 375–78, 733–48
  See also prostaglandin, I
Prostacyclin synthetase, 32
Prostaglandin
  A, 365–67, 369–72, 432, 434,
    438–40, 442, 448, 477, 598,
    825, 827–28
  administration to cancer patients,
    825–29
  and age-related immuno-
    suppression, 725–29
  and aging pigment, 163–66
  analogues, 47, 61, 67–74
  anti-cancer effects of 446,
    447–48
  B, 366, 453, 459, 708
  binding, 60–61, 705–8

and biochemistry, 1–5, 13–14
442–43
and bone, 513–20, 525–36, 541,
551, 555–58
in breast cancer, 567–72, 657–61
and CFU-GM proliferation,
400–405, 410–11
D, 418, 597
and disease, 21, 24
E, 47–62, 297–306, 367, 376–78,
385–88, 400–411, 415–21,
425–34, 438–42, 448, 453–54,
459, 469, 472–78, 489, 493–97,
501–7, 513–520, 526–535, 541
557–58, 569, 573–77, 598–602,
614, 620, 622, 626–28, 634,
637–41, 645, 651–54, 659–61,
663–65, 673–75, 682, 685–88,
698–99, 707–9, 713–17, 722,
726, 728–29, 747, 767, 775
778–79, 825–27
effect of on cancer patients,
651–54
endogenous production of,
297–306
in endothelial cells, 381–82
F, 47–62, 297–30, 309–28, 391–95,
418, 442, 454, 474–76, 478,
496, 527–28, 534, 598, 620,
634, 659–61, 664, 673–75, 694,
698–703, 707–10, 722, 726,
737, 755, 825
and Friend erythroleukemia cells,
425–34
G, 597, 786
H, 597, 784, 786
and human promyelocytic leukemia, 487–90
I, 297, 304, 674–76, 729, 783–87;
see also prostacyclin
and immune system, 595–611,
620–22
-induced angiogenesis, 685–88
and inflammatory disease, 613–14
inhibition, 5, 187–88
inhibition and tumor growth,

759–64
inhibition of tumor cell
adherence by, 673–77
insensitivity in leukemia patients,
401–2
and intestinal tumors, 753–56
and lung cancer, 691–94
and malignant hypercalcemia,
501–7
in MDCK cells, 493–97
-mediated immunosuppression,
625–27, 663–65
and metastatic beast cancer,
567–72
and microtubules, 391–95
modulation of antibody-
dependent cellular cytotoxicity
by, 713–17
molecules, 51–59
and mouse skin, 239–49
and murine fibrosarcoma, 775,
778–79
and neuroblastoma cells, 437–48
and nude mice tumors, 469–78
and pancreatic cancer, 385–88
and phorbol esters, 223, 225–26
and platelets, 60
and polyoma virus, 297–306
receptor antagonism, 61–62
regulation of DNA replication in,
309–28
response to tumor promoters,
205–13
and retinoic acid, 489
and smooth muscles, 48–50
and squamous carcinoma, 697–99
and squamous metaplasia,
453–54, 459
and stem cells, 472–76
stimulation of, by phorbol esters,
189–91
synthesis, 265–70, 705–8
synthesis, and defense system,
333–42
synthesis, by tumors, 622
synthesis, modulation of, 255–62

and T lymphocyte precursors,
415-21
and TPA, 283, 285
in tumor-associated cells, 701-3
and tumor biopsies, 633-47
and tumor growth, 646-47
and tumors, 274, 278-79, 365-67
369-72, 513-20, 679-83,
767-74
and tumor-host interactions,
581-82, 589-91, 619-29
urinary, 719-22
Prostaglandin dehydrogenase,
150-51
Prostaglandin endoperoxide synthetase, 126-33, 138
Prostaglandin hydroperoxidase, 132
138
Prostaglandin synthetase, 22, 26-27,
167
and carcinogens, 173
-dependent cooxygenation,
97-108, 113-20
and DES, 143-47
DNA strand breaks, 159-61
and interferon, 350-54, 358
and lipofuscin, 165-66
oxygenation of, 4-5
and p-dimethylaminoazobenzene,
155-58
and T cells, 419
and vitamin E/selenium, 150-51
Prostanoid biosynthesis, 149-53
Prostate gland, mouse, 457-58, 460
Proteases, 196
Protein kinase, 532-33
Protein phosphorylation, 602
Protein synthesis, 321
Pulmonary artery endothelium,
381-84
Pyruvate kinase, 445-46

Quiescence, 381

Radiation
and endothelial cells, 381-84

see also gamma radiation; radio-
therapy; X irradiation
Radiotherapy, 589, 761-64, 793-96
799, 802-3, 805, 807
Rama 25 cell line, 465-72, 475-77
Rama 29 cell line, 467, 475
Rama 259, 467-71, 475-77
Rama 521, 468, 471, 475-77
Ram seminal vesicle microsome,
98-106, 114-115, 783-87
Rat liver, 274-79
Renal cell carcinoma, 719-22
Retinoids, 194, 487-90; see also
vitamin A
Retinyl acetate, 273-79
Rheumatoid arthritis, 612-13
Rodent sarcoma, 815-17

Sarcoma 180, 768, 774, 805
Selenium, 149-53, 175-76
Serum factor, human, 225-30
Serum free medium, 437-38,
441-42, 458
Sheep red blood cells, 620-26
Skin, 205-13, 239-49, 273-74,
459-60
Slow reacting substance, 7-9, 597
Slow reacting substance of anaphyl-
axis, 7-8, 10, 12, 22, 29-30
Somatomedins, 292-93
Squamous carcinoma, 561-62,
697-99
Squamous metaplasia, 453-62
Smooth muscle, 48-50, 61-62
Stem cells, 472-76, 819-22
•reoisomerism, 51-59
Steroids, 33-35
Structural activity, 365-67
Sulindoc, 27
Superoxide dismutase, cytoplasmic,
350-54, 357, 360

T cells
cytotoxic, 602-3
precursor, and cancer, 415-21
proliferation, 598-99

and prostaglandins, 600–602,
621–23, 627–28, 645
and tumors, 583, 585–88, 624,
643
Tetradecanoylphorbol acetate (TPA)
and cancer, 185, 187–200
effects of, 217, 255, 273–79
and mouse skin, 205, 208, 209,
212–13, 241–49
and phospholipids, 268–70
and plasminogen activator,
281–85
see also phorbol esters
3T3 L1 mouse fibroblasts, 370
Thromboxanes
biochemical pathways, 1–5, 13–14
and bone resorption, 527–29
chemokinetic movement, 614
and inflammation, 613
inhibition, 258–59
and lung cancer, 694
and macrophages, 596
metabolism, 22
metastasis, 738–42
and platelet aggregation, 809–12
and smooth muscles, 50–51, 62
and tumors, 375–78, 676, 733–48
Thromboxane synthetase, 31–32,
73–74
Thymidine, 591, 598, 601
Thymocytes, 598
Toxicity, 793–96; see also
cytotoxicity
Transmembrane potential, 679–83
Tumor
antigen, 667–71
antigen, and transmembrane,
679–83
and benzo(a)pyrene, 116, 120
biopsies, 633–47
and bone destruction, 561–65
and bone metastases, 502–5, 542
cell adherence, 673–77
cell clonogenicity, 633–47

cell proliferation, 375–78
and chemical carcinogens, 81, 83
155–58
and DES, 143
differentiation, 365–67, 372
growth, 365–367, 661
-host interactions, 581–91, 619–29
inhibitors, 194–200
initiators, 185–86, 205
lysosomal enzyme release, 789–92
-mediated osteolysis, 805
metastases, 542, 673
mouse skin, 239–49
and platelet aggregation, 809–12
promoters, 108, 183–88, 205–13,
217–33, 239–49, 273–79; see
also phorbol esters;
tetradecanoylphorbol acetate
promotion, modulation of,
255–62
prostacyclin/thromboxane ratios
in, 733–48
and prostaglandin inhibition,
759–64
and prostaglandins, 369–72,
437–48, 513–20, 619–29, 701–3
regression, 660
skin, 205–13, 239–49, 273–74

Urinary prostaglandins, 719–22
Uterine cancer, 697–99

Vascular permeability, 611
Viral transformation, 493, 495–96
Virus, 33–42
Vitamin A, 447, 453, 460–62; see
also retinoids; retinyl acetate
Vitamin C, 167, 170, 447
Vitamin D, 531, 573, 574
Vitamin E, 32, 149, 53, 447
VX₂ carcinoma, 514–18, 529–30,
542, 551

X irradiation, 819–22